HEALTH AND CANADIAN SOCIETY:
SOCIOLOGICAL PERSPECTIVES
THIRD EDITION

Health and illness are areas of vital concern both for individuals and for societies. This concern is not surprising given the disruptive consequences of disease and pain, and the relationship of illness to death, religion, and the supernatural. Health is a universal human preoccupation.

The health of the population plays a key role in determining how a society functions. The very survival of a community can be dependent on disease patterns, as the plagues of the Middle Ages and the disappearance of tribal communities from many parts of the world due to epidemics testify. In a more immediate economic sense, the health care system is important simply because of the sheer numbers of people employed and the relative share of a country's economic resources dedicated to it. The study of health and health care in Canada thus presents an analytic and explanatory challenge in integrating historical, personal, interest group, institutional and societal perspectives.

Today in Canada universal state-sponsored health insurance is being challenged and nibbled away at. However, health insurance, health care, and health are not synonymous or equivalent. There is now widespread questioning of the degree to which health care systems actually produce improved health. Arguments about the social determinants of health are now more often heard. However, such arguments can be open to quite different policy and program interpretations. Our ideas and feelings concerning health care are also undergoing change.

Health and Canadian Society provides a comprehensive overview of the relationship between health, health care, and Canadian society. It is a wide-ranging volume that moves from personal and micro concerns to a more macro and institutional focus. It includes chapters of a descriptive nature and others with a more explanatory intent. They have been selected from the major journals or have been expressly written for this book. Ninety-five percent of the contributions are new to this edition. The chapters and the studies reported on are methodologically diverse, ranging from ethnographic studies to statistical analyses of data from large national surveys. Though the chapters are written by anthropologists, economists, historians, political scientists, and physicians, as well as sociologists, they all have a sociological "turn."

Recognized as the standard textbook on the sociology of health in Canada, *Health and Canadian Society* is an essential reference for sociologists, health care providers, health administrators, and policy planners.

DAVID COBURN is a professor in the Department of Public Health Sciences, University of Toronto. His research interests concentrate on the impact of the political economy of health and health care on medical dominance, in which he has published widely. CARL D'ARCY is a professor in the Department of Psychiatry, and Director of Applied Research, at the University of Saskatchewan, Saskatoon. His research interests and numerous publications are in the areas of population health and psychosocial epidemiology. GEORGE TORRANCE is a private consultant in social epidemiology and health services in Ottawa, and adjunct research professor of sociology at Carleton University. His interests are in physical fitness, health promotion, and hospital as institutions and work environments.

David Coburn, Carl D'Arcy,
and George Torrance, editors

Health and Canadian Society: Sociological Perspectives

Third edition

UNIVERSITY OF TORONTO PRESS
Toronto Buffalo London

© University of Toronto Press Incorporated 1998
Toronto Buffalo London
Printed in Canada

ISBN 0-8020-4192-2 (cloth)
ISBN 0-8020-8052-9 (paper)

∞

Printed on acid-free paper

Canadian Cataloguing in Publication Data

Main entry under title:

Health and Canadian society: sociological perspectives

3rd ed., rev. and enl.
ISBN 0-8020-4192-2 (bound)   ISBN 0-8020-8052-9 (pbk.)

1. Social medicine – Canada.   2. Medical care – Canada.   3. Public health –
Canada.   I. Coburn, David, 1938– .   II. D'Arcy, Carl.   III. Torrance, George
Murray, 1941– .

RA418.3.C3H42 1998   362.1'0971   C98-931003-59

University of Toronto Press acknowledges the financial assistance to its publishing
program of the Canada Council for the Arts and the Ontario Arts Council.

Contents

Preface

The third edition of *Health and Canadian Society* is a completely revised book. We started from scratch and looked for articles containing a sociological viewpoint or insights or the application of a sociological perspective to a health issue in Canada. We were more concerned with the content of contributions than with the disciplinary affiliations of the authors. This edition thus includes chapters with a sociological "turn" written by anthropologists, economists, historians, physicians, and political scientists as well as sociologists.

Two chapters have been reprinted from the second edition: one, entitled "Socio-Historical Overview," by George Torrance; and another entitled "Role Strains and Tranquillizer Use," by Ruth Cooperstock and Henry Lennard, which is still timely and illustrative of the role of women and health and health care. Articles were found in the major journals, as well as in the new health journal in Canada (with the same name as this book – no relation), *Health and Canadian Society*. Several chapters were expressly written for this book.

At the time the second edition was written and published (in the mid-1980s) the public debate was about the Canada Health Act and extra-billing by physicians. Today health and health care are even more at issue. This time the emphasis is on cutting costs and attempts to reorganize the health care system to make it more effective and efficient. The "corporate rationalizers," to use Alford's term, are more or less triumphant, at the expense, some would contend, of the power of providers and especially of physicians. There might still be arguments about whether or not medicine is dominant in health care. Newspaper headlines, however, tend to confirm the view that the state, in the context of globalization, the ascendancy of the "New Right," and the hegemony of a business point of view, is now setting the health care agenda. Given the market emphasis of many governments, universal state-sponsored health insurance in Canada is being challenged or is being nibbled away at the edges. Health insurance, health care, and health are not synonymous or equivalent. Today there is widespread questioning of the degree to which health care systems actually produce improved health. Arguments about the social determinants of health are now more popular than they once were, although open to differing policy interpretations.

Now there are more textbooks on the sociology of health in Canada than there were in 1981 when our first edition was the only entry in the field. We present a view of health and health care which is more "structural" than that of some others and one which, we believe, presents a unique view of health and health care in Canada. General readers, academics, students, and others, should find this book useful.

Overview of the Book

This book is divided into five major parts. Part I presents a socio-historical overview of the development of health care in Canada. Part II gives a brief overview of the fiscal dimensions of health care as well as the "bottom-line" insofar as health and health care are concerned, that is, the health status of Canadians.

Part III is the most extensive section, covering the many social factors involved in health and health care, and includes chapters linking social factors and health, Aboriginal health, and the impact of working conditions on health. Indeed, Part III reports research on what are now more fashionably called "the determinants of health." A number of the chapters reflect the influence of feminist theory and theorists in Canada and focus on the impact of social factors on women and health.

The topic of Part IV is health care providers, a subject that embraces one of the largest areas in the sociological literature on health including the often neglected topic of care provided in the home. Part V touches on one of the least studied areas in health care: the hospital. Despite the importance of the hospital as a health care institution and of its role as the new "health factory," few Canadian sociologists have devoted much attention to it. Part VI discusses the Canadian health care system as a whole, with topics ranging from recent provincial health policy changes to a study on community participation in health care in Quebec.

Finally, Part VII delineates factors and forces involved in the relationship between health care and Canadian society as a whole. Here, in a domain where one would expect the role of sociologists to be particularly strong, the field has often been left to economists and to political scientists. Hopefully, this situation is changing. Part VII begins with chapters questioning the "health care = health status" link and ends with a brief and selective overview of the sociology of health in Canada.

The volume moves from micro concerns to a more macro and institutional focus. It includes some chapters of a descriptive nature and others with a more explanatory intent. The chapters are also methodologically diverse and range from ethnographic studies to statistical analysis of data from large national surveys. It is obviously difficult in one volume to do justice to the broad range of writings and insightful studies of those within the sociological tradition in health and health care in this country. We do, however, provide representative writings that cover a wide range of health and health care topics. The overview of the field given in this edition thus provides a comprehensive sampling of the available literature on health and health care in Canada from a broadly sociological perspective. It will introduce the reader to some of the best writers and researchers in the field. We hope you enjoy the book.

A Final Note

Our relationship with our previous publisher, Fitzhenry and Whiteside, was excellent. We are grateful to them for the two previous editions and for permitting us to publish this edition with University of Toronto Press.

We would also like to gratefully acknowledge the hard work and diligence of Freda Elash in the preparation of the manuscript of the book.

David Coburn, Toronto
Carl D'Arcy, Saskatoon
George Torrance, Ottawa

March 1998

HEALTH AND CANADIAN SOCIETY: SOCIOLOGICAL PERSPECTIVES

1

Socio-Historical Overview: The Development of the Canadian Health System[*][1]

George M. Torrance

Studies of the social history of modern health-care systems have burgeoned in the last decade. They include both empirical studies of specific topics and more theoretically oriented accounts of the rise of medicine in relation to the state and other social institutions.[2] This chapter presents a descriptive and interpretive account of the social development of the Canadian health care system, seen against developments elsewhere and using a loose "convergence theory" of development approach.

At a high level of generalization, the health systems of capitalist nations at similar levels of economic development are much alike. In response to similar forces and by diffusion, such nations have adopted fundamentally similar institutions for providing health care: a hierarchy of healing occupations and professions under a dominant medical profession; hospitals as key institutions; public health, industrial health, and environmental legislation; specialized organizations for the training and socialization of health workers, and so on. With some variations, these societies have also developed mechanisms for making increasingly costly health care available to most segments of the population; health insurance schemes have been instituted involving state financing and/or control.

There is also now a fair degree of uniformity in the health values, beliefs, and expectations held by the lay public in different societies. For the most part, there is an acceptance of modern medical science as the basis of valid knowledge in health; a high valuation placed on personal health; a less fatalistic acceptance of disease, illness, and injury; a desire for active intervention in illness episodes; and high expectations for good health care.

A convergence theory view would posit that most advanced industrial societies have followed a broadly similar path in the increased longevity and lowered morbidity of the population and in the evolution of health systems. Infectious and parasitic diseases, which were the scourge of populations throughout history, have been conquered; in their place have come cancer, chronic diseases, and violent injuries. The turning point in health status came in the nineteenth century as changes in agriculture made improved

[*] Reprinted from George M. Torrance, 'Socio-Historical Overview', in *Health and Canadian Society: Sociological Perspectives*, 2nd edition, edited by David Coburn, Carl D'Arcy, George Torrance, and Peter New, pp. 6–32, 1987, with permission from Fitzhenry & Whiteside, Toronto.

food supplies available, the birth rate declined, rising real incomes from an increased economic surplus made improved nutrition and housing possible, and public health measures resulted in improved sanitation. These developments, rather than medical curative techniques, led to improved morbidity and mortality rates (see, for example, McKeown and Record 1962). Immunization made a smaller but significant contribution, more or less coincidentally.

At the same time as disease patterns were changing, a unified medical profession was being forged, attaining professional autonomy and achieving dominance over competing healing occupations. Because of the social origins of physicians, their association with elite educational institutions and their favourable connections with socially and politically dominant groups, physicians with the aid of the state achieved dominance over the healing enterprise. The profession either absorbed competing occupations, drove them into a quasi-illegal status outside the official division of labour, or most common, lent them some legitimacy in exchange for a subordinate status as auxiliaries to medicine (Freidson 1970a). The "strategic accessories" for medical monopoly and dominance, props backed by the coercive power of the state, including such factors as mandatory medical signatures on death certificates, mandatory appointment of physicians as public-health officers, sole access to hospital admitting privileges, exclusive right to prescribe drugs, and so on, were put into place.

Gradually, the scientific discoveries of the late nineteenth century were incorporated, first into public health, then into the curative medical repertoire. Increasingly, the hospital changed from a refuge for the sick poor to a place where medicine and the standardization of medical education created for the first time a situation in which curative medical therapy was visibly effective in limited areas. This, in turn, led a formerly skeptical public to consult doctors more frequently and to give higher prestige to the profession. The support of elite groups, formerly accorded more on social grounds than on grounds of superior effectiveness in healing, was further consolidated. During this period, medicine took the step from a "learned" profession to a "consulting" profession: its nominal legal monopoly became an increasingly real one (Freidson 1970a).

The attainment of professional dominance through the steps sketched above was the first phase of the modernization of health-care systems. The second phase, continuing to the present day, centres on making this newly effective medical care accessible to wider (and lower) social strata in the population. The crucial events here are the emergence of modern systems of state health services or health insurance - the arena of contention is the political system, and the key actors are the organized medical profession, societal elites, working class and labour movements, political parties, bureaucrats, and the state. Although there are substantial national variations in sequences and outcomes, it is again possible to outline a "natural history" that (at a high level of generality) is common to most Western industrialized nations.

A key contingency in health systems was the existence of a cohesive, powerful profession in place before public demand for access to medical care swelled. The first groups to demand access to the new style of care were the middle classes of the industrializing societies. They favoured the insurance principle, the idea of prepaying care through contributions made while they were healthy and working, and demanded no major structural reforms in the organization of care, leaving the poor and the working class to their traditional resorts (Anderson 1972).

The emerging industrial working class in Western Europe was represented by labour unions and socialist political parties. The international labour and social democratic movements aimed for concessions in the package of factory laws, labour legislation, and social insurance similar to those granted the workers by the capitalist elite in Bismarckian Germany. Health insurance was one of the series of social insurance measures advocated, which also included pensions, unemployment insurance, and worker's compensation (Rimlinger 1971).

The extent to which working-class, labour, and socialist movements and parties succeeded in having reforms implemented, and the speed with which they did so, depended on national differences in their strength and political representation, the extent to which they could mobilize other segments, such as farmers and intellectuals, in their support, and the degree of resistance they encountered from organized medicine and from economic elites. Developments in North America diverged from those in Britain, Western Europe, and even Australia and New Zealand. Pressure from working-class groups in Europe led to the gradual extension of health insurance. Industrial workers were the first to be insured. Later, insurance spread to include the families of workers and other groups until virtually universal insurance coverage was attained. Through such developments, health services or health insurance came to be provided through state intervention to most of the population of Western Europe at a relatively early date.

Generally, elites in the European societies acceded to the social insurance and labour measures as a way of preempting more radical political action by an increasingly powerful urban industrial working class. In most countries, however, the medical profession sought to stop or at least to slow changes that threatened its autonomy. In almost all cases, physicians were partly successful; they retained almost total control over the content of their work, and in many cases control as well over the way health care was organized. Although salary and capitation forms of payment were introduced, fee-for-service was still a prevalent form of payment. Medical control over key institutions like hospitals and paramedical occupations went unchallenged. Thus the introduction of state health insurance or health services tended to freeze the patterns of organization that existed at the time of implementation (Anderson 1972: 206).

The outcome of the process gave the health systems of most Western societies the following features: a heavy emphasis on curative medicine as enshrined in private practice and acute-treatment hospitals and little attention to the socio-economic sources of illness, prevention, public health, or rehabilitation; a complex and expensive medical technology; the growth of specialization at the expense of primary care; a rigid division of labour that discouraged the reallocation of roles; the creation of new sources of corporate profits and professional wealth from state-subsidized care; and the intrusion of the medical industry into a range of problems that were formerly considered outside its competence (Illich 1975; Navarro 1976).

A further phase in the evolution of health systems is now occurring in most Western societies. Fed by the growing technological complexity of curative health services and by increases in use (due to such factors as increased lower class accessibility to health-care and to the aging of the population), health-care costs have risen sharply in most countries. Rising costs and direct state involvement brought demands for better control and more efficient organization, chiefly from economic elites who objected to the effects on capital accumulation of increased social spending on "non-productive" services. A desire to control costs also emanated from a new power group that had emerged in health-care systems, in Alford's (1975: 200–209) terms, the "corporate rationalizers." This group of technocratically trained planners and efficiency experts sought to impose organizational controls on the system, frequently through the instrument of state bureaucracies.

The technocrats were initially opposed by the professions whose autonomy they threatened. Later the two groups, technocrats and professionals, tended to come to an accommodation. The result of this uneasy alliance has been that the burden of reducing costs has been pushed onto the least organized, active, and vocal groups in the system, lower level health workers, such as hospital service employees, and the poor and elderly in the patient population (who not infrequently are the first to face direct user charges for their health care).

In many ways, the Canadian experience repeats the main stages undergone by other systems in advanced capitalist societies. There are, however, some distinctive features of the history of health care that provide interesting material for comparative studies. There are two focal points to our discussion, the establishment of medical professional dominance in the Canadian system roughly in the 1800 to 1912 era, and the emergence of nationwide health insurance, which carried through from about 1919 to 1972.

The Emergence of Medical Dominance, 1818–1912

The emergence of medical dominance in preindustrial, nineteenth-century Canadian society illustrates in microcosm the controlled development of Canadian society as contrasted with the more laissez-faire policies and the greater egalitarianism and individualism of American social history in the same period (Lipset 1967; Clark 1976). Medical institutions in Canada developed an elitist character and a close relationship to the state, which has affected developments to the present day.

A social history of the health system in Canada should begin with the native peoples, their health-care systems and then their suppression and decimation by contact with European settlers. Although historical accounts are still sparse, some data are emerging. Ray, for instance, documents how epidemics spread in the wake of the fur trade. In the 1837 smallpox epidemic in the Hudson's Bay Company's Northern Department, "The fur traders estimated that the Indians, chiefly Assiniboine, Blood, Sarsee, Piegan, Blackfoot and Gros Ventre, lost up to three-quarters of their populations" (1981: 66).

Leo Johnson (1974: 14) describes Canadian society as developing through three main stages: a toiler society, a society of independent commodity producers and industrial capitalism. Canadian European society of the early to mid-nineteenth century was chiefly a toiler society of pioneer farmers struggling to scratch out a living from the wilderness and from primary industries, such as lumbering and fishing. There was a small urban colonial and commercial elite.

The health system in Canada in the mid-nineteenth century was shaped by the settler populations and the profile of diseases, beliefs and healing practices, which they brought with them. In the Maritimes and Ontario, and in parts of Quebec, the settlers were chiefly immigrants from the British Isles and Loyalist refugees from the United States. Along the St. Lawrence and inland, the French Canadians still mainly pursued the agrarian way of life into which they were locked by the Conquest and its sequels.

Medicine at this time had little connection with science. In the English-settled areas, physicians and surgeons from Britain, many of them ex-military men who had settled in Canada, were fairly plentiful in the bigger centres. The population in the outlying settlements had limited access to physicians and relied heavily on lay healers and traditional home remedies. The settlers were susceptible to the periodic outbreaks of smallpox, cholera and typhus, as well as to influenza, pneumonia and tuberculosis. The rough conditions in the pioneer era led to many accidents. Often a local farmer could serve as a bone setter, and one or two local women as midwives.

Another feature of pioneer health was self-care through home remedies. As Glazebrook reports of Upper Canada in the 1820s:

In the days when doctors and drug stores were not within hail home remedies and medicine chests were essential. Many of the remedies were herbal and some of these can be traced back for centuries. Roots, bark, leaves, fruit, and seed were the components and often could readily be found in neighbouring woods, as the Indians had long known (1968: 72).

Whisky, brandy, and opium were also used liberally. Patent medicines, often of U.S. manufacture, spread rapidly during the 1830s and 1840s.

By midcentury no cohesive medical profession had emerged. Medical schools were soon established in Upper and Lower Canada and began to graduate doctors. Canada was affected by developments in the United States. After the spread of proprietary medical schools in the U.S. during the Jacksonian era, graduates as well as untrained healers began to trickle into this country. There were many medical occupations at that time. Regular practitioners of various types existed. Added to these were the traditional folk healers who practised part-time. No group enjoyed a monopoly on practice. As in Europe, it is probable that the physicians were the most elite social segment, although surgeons had high status owing to their early military associations with the colonial elite. The rural and urban working classes were somewhat skeptical of medical men of all sorts.

The elitist nature of Canadian social development was shown by the history of Canadian medical licensing laws. In Upper and Lower Canada from 1795 onwards, there were repeated attempts to pass legislation licensing practitioners and suppressing irregular healers. For most of the century, these laws were only partly effective, but still the Canadian experience preceded the U.S. where, after some initial success, attempts at licensing physicians lapsed for a long period. As Stevenson notes:

This Canadian licensing law history is in striking contrast with the situation in the United States where in 1842 a survey revealed that there were eight states which had never had any licensing act; ten where there had been an act which was subsequently repealed; and only four where there had been this unbroken continuity of legal control of licensing (1967: 5).

A crucial stage in the professionalization of an occupation is the exclusion of irregular practitioners and the establishment of a unified, homogeneous occupation (Hughes 1958; Wilensky 1964). Two problems faced Canadian medicine in the nineteenth century in this respect: convincing those who were eligible for membership to become licensed, and devising a solution for others who did not have the desired qualifications but who had enough popular support to resist attempts to make their practice illegal. In the latter case, the marginal segment is usually incorporated within the body of the mainstream profession, as happened in England when the apothecaries were absorbed into the British medical profession.

In Canada in the latter half of the nineteenth century, the major challenge to the hegemony of medicine came from healing sects like the homeopaths and eclectics, which had gained considerable popular following. After much debate in Ontario, they eventually became part of the mainstream medical profession: both homeopaths and eclectics were given representation on the Council of the College of Physicians and Surgeons, the licensing body, where a homeopathic representative continued to sit until 1960 (McNabb 1970: 12–13). Although in Upper and Lower Canada licensing legislation to control entry was in place by 1870, medicine was still a loose conglomeration of conflicting segments until well into the twentieth century.

Establishing schools and upgrading the content and length of training is a key step in professionalization. Although the early history of Canadian medical schools was ridden with crises, the development of medical education in Canada was more orderly than in the U.S., where private diploma mills proliferated (Kett 1967). The Canadian schools became affiliated with universities, which added to their respectability, limited the circle of entrants to those of higher social class origins and ultimately acted to upgrade and standardize the quality of training. In the last decades of the nineteenth century, however, there were continual struggles between the medical schools and the practising professionals to control curriculum and entry to the profession (see Godfrey 1979; Gidney and Millar 1984).

Controlling and narrowing the channels of entry into practice was crucial to solving the problem of "overcrowding," which was perceived as endemic in the late nineteenth century and has persisted in a cyclical fashion to the present. McCaughey (1981) has demonstrated the periodic perceptions of oversupply in the 1851–1911 period in Ontario. Part-time work in other fields was common. MacDermott (1967: 40) notes that, in Montreal in 1875, there were 165 doctors: "Some of them acted as insurance agents, others conducted apothecary shops, etc." When physicians are plentiful, laymen have more choice and control, income remains low and competition for patients inhibits internal unity. Thus, the control of supply, often masked as improvement in standards, is a crucial contingency in forging professional dominance.

The medical profession not only had to suppress quacks and improve training within its own ranks but also had to gain dominance over and restrict the activities of other health occupations on its margins. Willis (1983) distinguishes three main modes of restricting competing occupations: subordination, limitation and exclusion. An occupation subjected to limitation was pharmacy. In keeping with their traditional role of "counter prescribing" drugs for customers who approached them with medical problems, pharmacists functioned as primary care healers, particularly for the poor and for those in areas without doctors. Indeed, there was a considerable overlap in functions between medicine and pharmacy, since most doctors in the nineteenth century (and many well into the twentieth) dispensed their own drugs.

Canadian medicine's drive to professionalize in the nineteenth century involved a struggle to control pharmacy. The medical associations sought to obtain legislation giving them the right to regulate training and practice in pharmacy, but "pharmacists were apparently strong enough to oppose successfully these medical attempts which would have deprived them of any possibility of self-regulation" (Paterson 1967: 851). In 1873 pharmacists in Ontario successfully opposed an amendment to the medical act that would have forbidden counterprescribing. The *Canadian Pharmaceutical Association Journal* disdainfully commented: "It is scarcely worthwhile to discuss the question of counterprescribing. The custom may be abused, but in the main is continued with benefit to all concerned, with the exception of the members of the medical profession, who may not perhaps enjoy that monopoly which they desired" (Canadian Pharmaceutical Association 1967: 108). However, it appears that soon thereafter pharmacy struck a tacit bargain with medicine it gave up counterprescribing in return for an agreement by doctors not to dispense drugs. Bans on counterprescribing were written into the pharmacists' codes of ethics. By the early twentieth century, pharmacy's subordination to medicine was complete.

Occupations that were primarily male in composition were more likely to retain some limited autonomy than those that were female, reflecting gender patterns of domination in the wider society. Aside from pharmacy, the other example of an old occupation that was restricted, this time mainly by subordination rather than limitation, is nursing. Judi Coburn (1974) provides insight into the process whereby the Nightingale reformation of nursing in England, which encouraged middle-class recruitment and emphasized absolute obedience to medicine, spread to Canada and came to dominate nursing in this country. Hospitals became the site for nurse training, and medical control of hospitals by the 1870s ensured that the occupations that grew up there would remain subordinate. As Coburn (1974) and Torrance (this volume) document, a grossly exploitive system emerged of using unpaid nursing students to do most hospital work and casting them out after graduation to make a tenuous living as private duty or home nurses (see Weir 1932 for statistics on the latter).

Community nursing, however, offered some threat to medical markets. Midwifery was a segment of traditional nursing that held such a threat. This role was gradually suppressed in favour of male medical supervision of the birthing process within hospitals (Biggs 1983). Woods (1980: 187) gives a glimpse of how, in 1897, the creation of the Victorian Order of Nurses raised medical apprehension.

Just as the Order appeared to be safely launched, a storm of protest arose from the Canadian medical fraternity. The reason for this sudden outburst was their fear that the nurses would be inadequately trained and would compete with local doctors ... In newspaper advertisements, the Ontario Medical Association trumpeted that the Victorian Order was "a scheme deleterious to the health of the country."

It was only when an American physician was brought in to testify to the value of such an order that the objection was stilled. By then its mandate had been restricted and such duties as midwifery removed from its proposed activities. By the early years of the twentieth century, nursing was subordinated to the organized medical profession, both within hospitals and in community practice. Although nurses functioned as midwives well into the 1930s (and still do to a limited extent in Northern areas), the routine use of either trained nurses or untrained but skilled local women practitioners had largely died out by the Second World War.

Most of the other "paramedical" occupations now within the official medical division of labour are relatively new, that is, born in the hospital under medical control. This holds for such occupations as physiotherapy, occupational therapy, medical laboratory and X-ray technology. Larkin (1983) has demonstrated how, in the U.K., whether a health occupation had a history of independent practice outside the hospitals and whether it was primarily male or female affected its fate in the health division of labour. In Canada, such emerging occupations as X-ray technology, physiotherapy, and occupational therapy tended to be largely female, hospital based, and created under medical tutelage, a recipe for subordination. Most remained under direct control in education and association affairs until very recently. For instance, Maxwell and Maxwell (1983: 347) note that it was not until 1966 that occupational therapy in Canada had an occupational therapist as president of the national association.

Although medicine was to have its internal problems and its border skirmishes with competing occupations, such as osteopathy and chiropractic, until well into the twentieth century, institutions for professional dominance were in place before the beginning of the First World War. The year 1912 marks a convenient if arbitrary turning point in

this process. This was the year in which Dr. Thomas Roddick, one of Canada's most celebrated medical men turned politician, succeeded in effecting the passage of the Canada
Medical Act, standardizing medical licensing procedures across Canada. One of Roddick's motives was to limit the number of practitioners in Canada (Stevenson 1967:
6–7), a step that, as noted above, has the effect of raising incomes through creating an
artificial scarcity. High incomes and high education enhance social prestige, which further consolidates a profession's position.

The years around 1912 were also the years in which the Flexner report on medical
education in the United States and Canada appeared and resulted in both upgrading and
"scientizing" the medical education process. Its impact was not as dramatic in reducing
medical graduates in Canada as in the U.S., because by this time, the Canadian profession had already got supply under control (see Coburn, Torrance, and Kaufert 1983:
414–415). Benefactions for laboratories to Canadian universities by American foundations in the wake of Flexner, however, did enhance the public perception that medicine
was now scientific and capable of producing tangible results in curing (see Shortt 1983,
for a skeptical account of the latter). The hegemony of this new scientific medicine practised by a closed, elite circle of men was consolidated.

Canadian society at the turn of the century was becoming increasingly industrialized
and urbanized. Montreal, Toronto, Hamilton, and Vancouver were on the way to becoming big cities. Winnipeg was booming as the gateway to Prairie settlement. Canada's
population was becoming more heterogeneous. Large numbers of immigrants had been
brought in to do the country's dirty work during the early canal- and railway-building
era. The Irish, fleeing famine in their home country and subjected to horrible cholera
epidemics, worked on the canals and railways. Large numbers of Chinese were imported
to work on the construction of the Canadian Pacific Railways. The risks to which they
were exposed and the primitive health care available to them are documented in Pierre
Berton's books (1970, 1971). Slavic immigrants, many of whom came to settle the Prairies, gravitated to railway construction in Northern Ontario. The abysmal living and
health conditions, especially in the subzero winters, are described in Bradman's *The
Bunkhouse Man* (1928), an early sociological classic.

Many of the immigrants gravitated to the growing cities. Large numbers of Irish
immigrants moved into the slums of Montreal, where they were joined by impoverished
French-Canadian migrants from the farm and by Eastern Europeans, including the Jews
who moved into the sweatshops of the needle trades. Ames's *The City Below the Hill*
(1897) and Copp's *The Anatomy of Poverty* (1974) document their misery. Housing and
public health measures in the new industrial cities were primitive, and diseases such as
smallpox, typhoid, influenza, and tuberculosis took a fearful toll. Montreal, Toronto,
Winnipeg, and Vancouver came to vie among the worst cities in the world in health conditions, infant mortality and death rates (Copp 1974: 25–26, 100; Arbitise 1977: 104;
Piva 1979: 123).

The development of the Francophone health system up to this time deserves consideration. French-Canadian society was moving from a rural to an urban basis. Largely
because of the accommodation that developed between the Anglophone industrial elite
and the traditional Francophone elite, social welfare, education, health, and other service institutions remained under the Church, with the state acting to retard rather than to
promote modernization. Squeezed by pressure on the land and consequent colonization
of marginal farmland as well as large-scale migration to the bottom rung of the urban
labour force, French-Canadian society developed particular health problems. There was
much rural and urban poverty. Death rates and infant and maternal mortality rates

remained higher than the national average until well into this century, partly due to the high birth rates and large families and partly to the pervasive poverty.

Copp (1974: 96) concludes that, in urban Montreal, the French-Canadian working class had higher rates of infant and maternal mortality than did migrants from Europe. Ironically, McGill University Medical School was emerging at this time as a world leader, but its expertise failed to filter down to the Francophone and immigrant population. The wealth and progress of the Anglophone elite who controlled the largest part of the Quebec economy stood in contrast to the situation of the French Canadians.

The Development of Government Health Insurance, 1919–1972

Although Canadians like to think of themselves as progressive, Canada actually lagged behind other countries in the development of social-welfare legislation (Wilensky 1975: 30–31). Government health insurance has been debated at least since 1919 in Canada, but it was only in 1968 that the legislation for a relatively complete system was in place. Thus, Canada trailed most Western European countries, Britain, and New Zealand in making health care economically accessible to most of the population.

Health insurance must be seen as a social movement and its enactment as part of an international diffusion of ideas. It is essentially a reformist rather than revolutionary notion, involving changes in the way people pay for health services rather than reorganization of the way services are provided. The alternative to health insurance, a system of state-provided services as exemplified by the Soviet health system, did have its followers in North America, particularly in socialist circles. Norman Bethune, for one, became an exponent of these ideas in his Montreal days (Park 1978: 102–112). However, state-provided services were much less popular and influential than the social insurance ideas as weakly espoused by Mackenzie King and, more forcibly, by the League for Social Reconstruction and the Co-operative Commonwealth Federation (CCF).

In the advocacy of health insurance, Canada was initially behind even the United States. There was a move towards health insurance in the United States in the 1910–1920 era when a number of states developed, but never implemented, legislation. Again in the early 1930s, U.S. policy proposals derived from the Committee on the Costs of Medical Care were in advance of thinking in Canada (Anderson 1972: 65–68). The United States, however, fell behind Canada in following up state-sponsored health insurance, and today Canadian experience is frequently held up as a model for the U.S.

We have mentioned that, on the international scene, health insurance was part of the package of social insurance and labour legislation that emerged in Germany in the late 1880s and spread to other European countries in the early years of this century. Canada and the United States were affected by this current as their industrialization progressed. Unlike Europe, however, social forces here prevented a rapid adoption of the European models.

Although industrialization proceeded rapidly in early twentieth-century Canada, the spread of industry was uneven. Manufacturing was concentrated largely in southern Ontario and Quebec. Large segments of the population were still employed in the resource industries or on family farms in the Prairies, the Maritimes, and rural areas of the central provinces. The lack of an effective political alliance between farmers and urban industrial workers was one reason why social welfare legislation, including health insurance, was slow to develop in Canada. (See Brady 1947, for a discussion "of differences" in this respect among white Commonwealth countries.)

The health-care system that had developed by the 1920s in this country was vastly different from its pioneer origins. Public health, fed by discoveries in bacteriology and immunology, was beginning to tackle successfully the problems of epidemics and health in the cities. Antiseptic surgery and other advances modestly improved the effectiveness of curative medical therapy. New medical specialities were created. Technology was increasingly concentrated in the institution of the hospital, which was changing to a place where the skills of surgery and obstetrics were practised and diagnostic techniques such as X-rays and laboratory tests were used. Hospitals were gradually replacing the doctor's office and the patient's home as the locus of serious treatment for middle- and upper-class patients as well as for the indigent. Hospitals were becoming "doctors' workshops" not only, as in Europe, for a special breed of hospital consultants but for all doctors in the community. Medicine, having earlier consolidated its authority over competing healers, was building an establishment of subordinate workers to assist with auxiliary tasks within the hospital.

More people were coming to accept the claims of medicine to effective treatment. Although pockets of resistance remained, the problem was becoming more that of obtaining access to medical care than of staying out of the clutches of the doctor. Barriers to health care were of two kinds: the shortage of practitioners and facilities in some regions and the problems of paying for the increasingly costly services. Paying for physician and hospital services was difficult not only for the poor but also for members of the prosperous working and middle classes. Since free care had traditionally been provided to the indigent in the public wards of hospitals, the problem was particularly acute for the latter groups. It was to them that the idea of health insurance had a strong appeal. A limited conception of health insurance, as a risk-sharing device for prosperous working- and middle-class people, leaving the poor to state-subsidized charity care and the rich to self-payment, became a dominant idea behind later discussions of health insurance. Although the doctors felt that lower income groups should have mandatory coverage in order to pay fees, most aspects of this model, especially its nonintervention in private practice and fee setting, proved attractive to the medical profession when alteration in the traditional system of paying for medical services became inevitable.

Early medical reaction to health insurance was conditioned by fears of lay control. Peterson (1978) shows in the U.K. how difficult was the struggle to exclude laymen from judgment in professional matters and keep professional ranks closed to lay interference, especially from organized third parties. In Europe, contract practice, sick funds, and industrial plans were common. Although such plans were rarer in Canada, they were seen as posing a menace. In the 1890s, the Ontario Medical Association warned against "lodge practice" (Godfrey 1979: 240). That this dependency could lead to miserable conditions is suggested in a discipline case before the Ontario College of Physicians and Surgeons in which a doctor who worked for two mines near Kenora for a stipend of 50 cents per month per miner was prosecuted for turning to market "Kamama Hindoo Remedies" to make a living (Godfrey 1979: 229). Such were the dangers, along with that of political interference, that the profession feared.

Although the Canadian Medical Association (CMA) had existed since 1867, it remained weak and divided until the reforms implemented by Dr. T.C. Routley in the late 1920s. Thenceforth, it became a forum for interpreting emergent developments like the health insurance movement and formulating a coherent response from the profession. CMA concern with the health insurance issue was initially muted. The development of national health insurance in Britain after 1912 raised questions, but the main response was that "it couldn't happen here." The idea of large-scale lay intervention in the medical field, in the form of government health insurance or worse, state medicine, seemed remote.

Perhaps allaying the fears of organized medicine were the close connections the Canadian medical profession had developed with government and bureaucratic elites. From colonial days, the regular medical profession had received a sympathetic ear from Canadian governments. Canadian doctors were well represented in elective political office, and career doctors became dominant in local, provincial, and federal departments of health where they acted as liaisons between governments and the organized profession. In essence, as Malcolm Taylor (1960) has pointed out, public government had ceded to the organized profession many of the powers of a "private government" within the health sphere. The doctors had reasons to feel proud of their discharge of these powers: in the years from 1900 to 1930 they had succeeded in upgrading medical education, creating an advanced system of practitioners and hospitals and had co-operated in developing public health measures. In wartime, their effort to organize a medical service within the armed services was a striking model of the coalescence of public and private efforts. To the medical men, it seemed unlikely that this symbiotic relationship would be disturbed.

On the part of most Canadian governments of the day, intervention was equally unthinkable. As Bryden (1974) suggests, most were captives of the "market ethos," under which large-scale state intervention in social welfare was considered beyond the limited functions and resources of government. The state was, in part, a creature of the economic elite and was preoccupied with creating the conditions for economic growth by parcelling out resource concessions and tariff protection to private interests and building an infrastructure of transportation, communications, and services to facilitate industrial development. Although a modest income tax had been introduced in the First World War, the resistance of individuals and corporations to taxation made it inconceivable to many government leaders that state resources could also be found to finance social welfare schemes.

Governments could also fall back on the constitutional dilemma as an excuse for inaction. Under the British North American Act, responsibility for health rested with the provinces. When a province wanted federal aid to implement measures, or later when the federal government wanted to introduce national programs, constitutional disputes delayed implementation.

As elsewhere, the history of the enactment of state health insurance in Canada is largely a history of increasing popular pressure for change. Channelled through interest groups and political parties of the left, public pressure forced reluctant governments and a mostly resisting medical profession to implement limited reforms. In Canada's case, a decisive role was played by the province of Saskatchewan, which elected the first social democratic provincial government in Canada and went on to pioneer health insurance legislation. Although universal hospital insurance in Saskatchewan was not enacted until 1947, its political history went back much further. Periods of agitation in the health field tended to follow periods of social and economic turbulence in Canadian social development.

The period immediately following the First World War saw the first stirrings. In 1919, social insurance, including health insurance, became a plank in the platform of the federal Liberal party. Under pressure from the labour movement and from returning soldiers, the B.C. government appointed the first legislative committee to investigate health insurance (Matters 1974). These initiatives faded in the 1920s as prosperity returned to the country and political radicalism diminished (although a second legislative commit-tee on health insurance was appointed in British Columbia in the late 1920s).

The 1920s and 1930s were the time of farmers' parties and governments in Alberta, Saskatchewan and Ontario, and of Progressive party representation in the federal gov-ernment. Building on their experience of municipal doctor and hospital schemes in the Prairies, the farmers' movement in Alberta and British Columbia favoured state-spon-sored health insurance.

Whittaker (1977: 54) makes the point that the political trend in Canada in the 1920s was more reformist than revolutionary because the urban working class, too weak and fragmented to act independently, was co-opted into supporting the petit bourgeois, mainly farmers, in their struggle with the capitalist class. As Whittaker notes:

"The petit bourgeois influence ... militated against the adoption of social welfare legislation which was a concern for working-class people but only of marginal importance to farmers who were more self-sufficient by the nature of their occupation. Thus, the only social legislation passed by the Liberals during the decade of the 1920s was the old age pension program, virtually forced down King's throat by J.S. Woodsworth at a crucial time for the minority Liberal government" (1977: 56).

The agrarian movements that developed in Alberta and Saskatchewan in the 1920s did foster state intervention. These movements inherited some of the populist, anti-elite, antimonopoly sentiment that had emerged in the United States and was also manifest in the antimedical activities of the Patrons of Industry in Ontario in the 1890s (McNabb 1970: 15). Saskatchewan was a seedbed of innovation in health care. Lipset (1968) has discussed the social conditions that facilitated cooperation and social innovations in the province. Saskatchewan's municipal doctor plan, union hospital plan, and municipal hospital care plans, begun during the First World War to enable thinly populated com-munities to tax their populations in order to build hospitals, hire doctors, and prepay hospital care, were important precursors of later state involvement.

The 1930s was another period of social turbulence, which created a demand for social change. The Great Depression had a devastating effect on Canada, particularly on the single-crop economy of the Prairies. A series of droughts in the Western provinces wors-ened the effects of the collapsed wheat market. Much of the western farm population and many industrial workers in the large cities across the country were on relief. Politi-cal radicalism was rife and was manifest in events such as the On-to-Ottawa Trek initi-ated by unemployed men from work camps in the west. The political climate was polarized to a high degree. In Ottawa, R.B. Bennett's Conservatives replaced Mackenzie King's Liberals in power. Bennett raised the bogey of a Bolshevist revolution.

The Canadian health care system came under a serious strain as the Depression wore on. Many people could not pay for medical and hospital care. Indigent patients flooded the hospitals. On the Prairies, many of the municipalities were bankrupt, and the local authorities across the country were hard pressed to pay for the indigent patients and to meet hospital deficits. Doctors' incomes declined as patients failed to pay their bills. Medical relief plans were introduced to pay a portion of the medical bills and provide the doctors with some income. Poverty, poor nutrition, and inability to afford health care exacerbated the health problems of the population. Communicable diseases like pneu-monia, influenza, and tuberculosis, the spread of which is fostered by poor living condi-tions, flourished.

Among some minorities like the native Indians, the inequalities in health status stood out starkly. In the late 1930s in Manitoba, it was noted that "the tuberculosis rate among

Treaty Indians is fourteen times the rate for the province as a whole and 24 times the rate for the white races" (Mitchell 1940: 92). In 1937 Treaty Indians made up less than 2 percent of the population of Manitoba but accounted for 40 percent of the tuberculosis deaths.

The 1930s saw the first significant political initiatives for government health insurance at the national level. In 1932, the League for Social Reconstruction, an alliance of socialist intellectuals, was formed. The League made state health insurance one of the proposals in *Social Planning for Canada* (1935), their blueprint for a planned society. The following year, League intellectuals, along with farm and labour groups, helped form the new CCF party. State medicine and health insurance was a key plank in the Regina Manifesto of the new party. The first actual legislation was passed in Alberta by the United Farmers of Alberta (UFA) government in 1934. However, Social Credit came to power the next year, and the act was never implemented.

British Columbia, whose polarized politics and strong labour movement had produced earlier agitation for health insurance, became the next province to take legislative initiatives. In 1935, the Patullo Liberal government passed a health insurance act, later holding a plebiscite on the issue. The Patullo government was under pressure from the CCF, which for the first time was running candidates in the provincial elections. The B.C. legislation was designed by George Weir, who had earlier conducted a study of the nursing profession, and was supported by Ian MacKenzie, then a B.C. government minister. Despite public support expressed in the plebiscite, the B.C. legislation was never implemented, partly because of the opposition from the medical profession and its conservative allies, partly because of the failure of the federal government to provide financial support (see Ormsby 1962; Robin 1973).

In the late 1920s and 1930s the CMA paid increasing attention to the issue of health insurance. The Committee on Medical Economics began to investigate the issue and in 1934 produced a report setting out the principles they believed should guide the development of health insurance. The principles included administration by a nonpolitical commission with a majority professional representation, free choice by physicians of payment method, medical control over fee schedules and compulsory coverage up to certain income levels (Taylor 1978: 25). Although the report accepted the principle of state involvement in financing health insurance, it reflected the profession's strong insistence on protecting its autonomy in fee setting and control of work. The profession's opposition to any government plan that violated these principles was demonstrated by its vigorous resistance to the B.C. plan.

At the federal level, Bennett's Conservative government of 1930 to 1935 grappled with the problem of relief. In a desperate departure from his previous laissez-faire policies, Bennett introduced a "New Deal" package of legislation that included a health insurance scheme. After Bennett's defeat in 1935 by MacKenzie King, this legislation was declared unconstitutional. King appointed a Royal Commission on Federal-Provincial Relations to seek solutions to the constitutional impasse. The Commission's work, however, was hampered by opposition from Ontario and Quebec, which resented any extension of federal power in their domains.

As the Dirty Thirties drew to a close, Canadian society and Canadian politics were in a demoralized state. The economic crisis and the constitutional conflict had frozen social development. Disparities between provinces, regions and social classes had become glaringly apparent. Some important movements of political reform were gaining support, but they were still relatively weak. Fostered by the CCF, a tentative class politics was emerging, but the division between agrarian interests and industrial workers, reinforced by factors such as the doctrinal opposition to socialism by Canadian Roman Catholics, hindered the effectiveness of the new movement. For its part, the Canadian labour movement was only beginning to regain some reformist momentum from the aggressive new industrial unions that were organizing in the automobile and steel industries after the breakup of earlier political action in the First World War and postwar era (Robin 1968: 293).

The coming of the Second World War marked a turning point in the stalemate. Even though the cautious Mackenzie King Liberals were in power in Ottawa, the mobilization of Canadian resources by the war effort and the fears of Canadian elites of increased radicalism after the war created a climate of government activism that was unique in Canadian history. To avert economic depression and social unrest after the war and spurred by the threat of CCF gains, the government put a great deal of effort into planning for postwar reconstruction. It was anticipated that the federal government, strengthened by the new powers advocated by the Rowell-Sirois Commission, would assume a leading role.

Health insurance, along with other social security measures, received attention. Dr. J.J. Heagerty, director of federal Public Health Services, was appointed to head a committee to investigate health insurance. The CMA, influenced by the experience of the Depression and the spirit of wartime unity, gave full cooperation to the committee. The result of the Heagerty Committee's deliberations, later to be adopted in large part as government policy, was a recommendation for a universal, comprehensive, government-administered system of health insurance to be financed jointly by federal and provincial governments. As the war came to an end, national health insurance at last seemed imminent.

There is little need to recount in detail the protracted implementation of this program in the postwar years, since this story has been admirably told in several sources (see especially Taylor 1978; Leclair 1975; Swartz 1977; and on the Saskatchewan Medicare crisis, Badgley and Wolfe 1967). A chronicle of the major legislative events includes the breakdown of the Federal-Provincial Conference on Reconstruction in 1945 and the failure of immediate reform, Saskatchewan's implementation of universal hospital insurance in 1947, introduction of the Federal Health Grants in 1948 and the enactment of a nationwide hospital insurance program in 1957. Saskatchewan pioneered again with medical care insurance in 1962, and in 1964, the federal Royal Commission on Health Services (Hall Commission) recommended a comprehensive universal health insurance program, similar to Saskatchewan's, for the country as a whole. This was followed by the bitter struggle to implement medical care insurance. Federal legislation was passed in 1966, delayed until 1968, but in 1972, with the entry of the Yukon and Northwest Territories, Canada had finally fulfilled the design for universal health insurance covering hospitalization, physician care and some ancillary services.

As Clark (1976) has stated, post-Second World War Canadian society had greatly changed from prewar days. Prosperity had returned, population had dramatically increased through immigration and the baby boom, and the new suburbs had spread outward as urbanization grew. Major shifts took place in the labour force out of agriculture and the primary industries towards secondary manufacturing and especially towards services of all kinds. Women entered the labour force in increasing numbers. A new middle class of white collar and professional workers in the expanding education, health, government, and business sectors arose alongside the old middle class of merchants, professionals, and entrepreneurs. The Canadian economic elite was joined by members of the "Comprador" elite (see Clement 1975) as the American takeover of Canadian industry accelerated. Although the economic elite extended its power over Canadian industry, in some ways Canadian society was becoming less elitist. This was particularly true in the educational sphere where, for the first time, the proportion of the school-age population going on to postsecondary education almost equalled that of the United States (even while the lower classes were still substantially underrepresented).

Rapid change also took place in the health system. The postwar era witnessed the blooming of the medical industrial complex. Research, mainly at centres and corporations outside Canada, generated new technologies, which were imported into the system. Federal Health Grants poured money into hospital building and renovation, which had been neglected during the war and Depression. Medical specialization grew rapidly. The paramedical occupations, especially those dealing with technology and centred in the hospital, expanded. Profit-making industries, such as the private insurance, pharmaceutical, and hospital supply industries, most under foreign control, prospered.

With the development of the sulfa and antibiotic drugs, which were effective against diseases such as pneumonia and bacterial infections, and with the emergence of new diagnostic tools, the ordinary medical practitioner gained prestige and confidence from his clients. The influence of the mass media and mass education contributed to lay acceptance of medical knowledge and to the decline of alternative belief systems and practitioners. While as late as the 1930s a substantial proportion of the population remained skeptical about doctors and their craft, by the postwar period such groups were a small fringe of society. Quasi-medical healers like chiropractors still held on, but their theories of disease, if not the actual services they offered, could hardly withstand the onslaught of the sciences identified with the regular medical profession.

In the Depression and war years, organized medicine in Canada had displayed a co-operative if highly qualified attitude towards government health insurance. After the war, it changed its stand, particularly on medical insurance. Postwar prosperity meant that clients were better able to pay for services. Medical incomes rose. The spectre of the Depression receded. More important, the success of the hospital- and profession-sponsored voluntary health insurance seemed to offer an alternative to government-administered schemes. These plans, which began in the late thirties, grew by the 1950s to provide partial coverage to large sections of the population. When in 1949 the CMA adopted a new policy opposing a strong government role in health insurance and advocating expansion of the voluntary plans, the private health insurance industry had also developed a strong vested interest in a nongovernmental system. And, in the postwar era, such traditional opponents of the welfare state as the Canadian Manufacturers Association had regrouped their forces.

Although it had no strong objections to federal-provincial hospital insurance in 1957, organized medicine as represented by the CMA and the provincial associations opposed government medical care insurance. The most direct confrontation took place in Saskatchewan. The government plan there came into effect only after a bitter doctors' strike had forced many compromises (Badgley and Wolfe 1967). But the withdrawal of services by a group supposedly dedicated to the client helped erode the profession's mystique. In conservative provinces such as Alberta and Ontario, medicine had cooperated with the provincial governments' limited Medicare plans in an attempt to pre-empt federal intentions. That the profession itself was not a monolithic entity in its response to change is indicated by the case of Quebec, where the general practitioners cooperated with the government, but the specialists went on strike before finally acceding (Taylor 1978: 379–413). Across the country, however, organized medicine generally fought a strong rearguard campaign before succumbing to government medical care insurance.

The national health insurance program, which was enacted by 1970, largely followed the blueprint drawn by the Hall Commission Report of 1964. It opted for compulsory universal coverage and public administration, rejecting the role of voluntary plans as intermediaries. But, in most ways, it did little to challenge the medical establishment. Private practice and fee-for-service were left in place. No major structural changes in the organization or content of medical work were made.

Why should the medical profession have resisted as strongly as they did what were, after all, a rather limited set of changes in how they were paid? Blishen (1969) has ana-lyzed the social roots of the profession's ideology on the health-insurance issue. In essence, Blishen sees the defensiveness largely as a reaction to strains arising from the changing conditions of medical work, the growing dependence of the ordinary practi-tioner on specialist colleagues and paramedical workers, new controls from peers and administrators in the hospital, and from the self-regulating colleges. These strains were then projected upon the external bogey of government intervention. While Blishen's analysis usefully draws attention to the role of underlying strains and ideological motives, especially the theme of autonomy, it seems plain that less complex motives were paramount. The profession had a clear conception of its material self-interest, and the spectre of interference in this area was a strong concern.

Bothwell and English (1981) claim that relative to the U.S. and Britain, Canadian medicine in the 1930s and early 1940s was receptive to health insurance. But, as they conclude: "It was always a qualified support and enthusiasm varied inversely with the economic condition of the profession" (1981: 492).

On a wider front, Walters (1982) argues with Swartz (1977) that Canadian medical insurance was not primarily a response to high levels of class conflict but was rather a response by the state "acting in the long-term interests of the capitalist class by seeking to increase the productive capacity of labour and reduce the economic costs of illness" (1982: 157). Her argument, however, hinges on a very narrow definition of class conflict and mainly concentrates on the period of the 1950s and 1960s, minimizing the impor-tance of activity in the First World War era and the later decisive part played by the CCF-NDP, either acting directly when in power or as a spur to other parties facing an electoral threat or a minority government situation.

While they appear to understate the degree of conflict involved, both the Bothwell and English (1981) and Walters (1982) arguments capture important elements in the process. The Canadian medical profession was more receptive to state action than the American, and, although late, the Canadian state did come to implement a measure that, as both Swartz and Walters agree, was perceived to be in the long-term interests of the capitalist class. These themes indicate the continuity of Canadian patterns of elite accommodation between the early era of consolidating medical dominance and the later era of health insurance. They also illustrate Canadian society's historically greater penchant than the U.S. for public over private institutions, institutions that nevertheless buttress the ruling elite and perpetuate inequality of power and wealth among their participants.

The health insurance program that was in operation in Canadian society by the early 1970s, a program that had taken half a century to realize, had a range of effects on the broader health system. Some were relatively superficial, others more significant.

Undoubtedly, in the area of equalizing access to curative health care, health insurance had positive effects. The size of the disparities between geographic regions and income groups in access to physician's services had been reduced. Although disparities in access between regions and by social class remain, the situation that existed as recently as the early 1950s whereby higher income groups were more than twice as likely to visit physicians as the lower groups (Department of National Health and Welfare 1960: 50) had changed. Class differences in utilization had lessened. The crippling financial burden of serious illness had receded.

However, in other ways, the main impact of the Canadian health insurance program was to institutionalize the status quo and hence increase the difficulty of structural changes needed to make health care more responsive to society. Despite their resistance to the programs, some of the main beneficiaries, at least initially, were the provider groups themselves. But the problems of conceiving health in a broader sense than crisis intervention in acute-illness episodes or of providing appropriate care to those for whom no cure is possible remained problems to be tackled.

Notes

1   Much of the section on the rise of health insurance in the original was inspired by work done from 1970 to 1974 on a project directed by Robin Badgley with the assistance of Catherine Charles and myself on "The Canadian Experience with Universal Health Insurance" (Badgley, Charles, and Torrance 1975). Odin Anderson was a collaborator on that project. Although never formalized, my theoretical thinking in the project, and especially in the paper, was influenced by Freidson (1970a, 1970b) and by structural-comparative-historical works such as Anderson (1972) and Glazer (1970a, 1970b) on health systems, Rimlinger (1971) and Wilensky (1975) on social welfare systems, and Moore (1966) and Bendix (1956) on the social transformation of modern societies in general. The "convergence theory" model, presented as a simplifying device to place Canadian developments in context, owes more to the above sources than to the functionalist perspective on modernization and the professions identified with Parsons's (1966) or Lipset's (1967) emphasis on value orientations. An attempt to incorporate a Marxist explanation into the analysis and to look at recent developments in medical dominance is contained in Coburn, Torrance, and Kaufert (1983). Such Marxist insights as are included in the original of the present chapter and the current revision owe much to Robin Badgley's work on the original project, to David Coburn's influence, and to Swartz's (1977) article.

2   Two collections of articles on medical history are Shortt (1981) and Roland (1984). Major theoretically oriented books dealing with the rise of medicine in other countries include Larson (1977), Peterson (1978), Starr (1982) and Willis (1983). Much of the sociological interest in this topic can be traced to the contributions of Freidson (1970a; 1970b), and subsequent works that have attempted to extend or correct Freidson's focus on the medical profession within the health division of labour to include a more complete account of relations between capitalist institutions, the state and the health system; see especially Navarro (1976) and McKinlay (1977). Canadian articles dealing with this include Swartz (1977), Walters (1982) and Coburn, Torrance, and Kaufert (1983).

References

Alford, RR. 1975. *Health Care Politics: Ideological and Interest Group Barriers to Reform.* Chicago: University of Chicago Press.

Ames, RB. 1897. *The City below the Hill.* Montreal: Bishop.

Anderson, OW. 1972. *Health Care: Can There Be Equity?* New York: Wiley.

Arbitise, AFJ. 1977. *Winnipeg: An Illustrated History.* Toronto: Lorimer.

Badgley, RF, and S Wolfe. 1967. *Doctors' Strike - Medical Care and Conflict in Saskatchewan.* Toronto: MacMillan.

Badgley, RF, C Charles, and GM Torrance. 1975. *National Health Insurance in Canada.* Department of Behavioural Science, University of Toronto. Mimeograph.

Bendix, R. 1956. *Work and Authority in Industry.* New York: Wiley.

Berton, P. 1970. *The National Dream.* Toronto: McClelland and Stewart.

Berton, P. 1971. *The Last Spike.* Toronto: McClelland and Stewart.

Biggs, LC. 1983. The Case of the Missing Midwives: A History of Midwifery in Ontario from 1795–1900. *Ontario History* 75(1): 21–35.

Blishen, B. 1969. *Doctors and Doctrines: The Ideology of Medical Care in Canada.* Toronto: University of Toronto Press.

Bothwell, RS, and JR English. 1981. Pragmatic Physicians: Canadian Medicine and Health Care Insurance, 1910–1945. In SED Shortt ed. *Medicine in Canadian Society: Historical Perspectives.* Montreal: McGill-Queen's University Press.

Bradman, E. 1928. *The Bunkhouse Man.* Reprinted with a new introduction. Toronto: University of Toronto Press, 1972.

Brady, A. 1947. *Democracy in the Dominions.* Toronto: University of Toronto Press.

Bryden, K. 1974. *Old Age Pensions and Policy Making in Canada.* Montreal: McGill-Queen's University Press.

Canada. 1940. *Report of the Royal Commission on Dominion-Provincial Relations.* Ottawa: King's Printer.

Canada. 1964. *Report of the Royal Commission on Health Services.* Ottawa: Queen's Printer.

Canadian Pharmaceutical Association. 1967. *A Brief History of Pharmacy in Canada.* Toronto.

Clark, SD. 1976. *Canadian Society in Historical Perspective.* Toronto: McGraw-Hill-Ryerson.

Clement, W. 1975. *The Canadian Corporate Elite.* Toronto: McClelland and Stewart.

Coburn, D, GM Torrance, and JM Kaufert. 1983. Medical Dominance in Canada in Historical Perspective: The Rise and Fall of Medicine? *International Journal of Health Services* 13: 407–432.

Coburn, J. 1974. I See and Am Silent: A Short History of Nursing in Ontario. In J Acton, P Goldsmith, and B Shepard eds. *Women at Work, Ontario 1850–1930.* Toronto: Canadian Women's Educational Press.

Committee on the Costs of Medical Care. 1932. *Medical Care for the American People.* Chicago: University of Chicago Press.

Copp, T. 1974. *The Anatomy of Poverty: The Condition of the Working Class in Montreal, 1897–1929,* Toronto: McClelland and Stewart.

Department of National Health and Welfare. 1960. *Illness and Health Care in Canada: Canadian Sickness Survey 1950–51.* Ottawa: Dominion Bureau of Statistics (Catalogue no. 82–518).

Freidson, E. 1970a. *Profession of Medicine.* New York: Dodd Mead and Company.

Freidson, E. 1970b. *Professional Dominance: The Social Structure of Medical Care.* New York: Atherton.

Gidney, RD, and WPJ Millar. 1984. The Origins of Organized Medicine in Ontario, 1850–1869. In CG Roland ed. *Health, Disease and Medicine.* Hannah Institute for the History of Medicine. Toronto: Clarke Irwin.

Glazebrook, GP. 1968. *Life in Ontario: A Social History.* Toronto: University of Toronto Press.

Glazer, WA. 1970a. *Paying the Doctor.* Baltimore: Johns Hopkins.

Glazer, WA. 1970b. *Social Settings and Medical Organization.* New York: Atherton.

Godfrey, CM. 1979. *Medicine for Ontario: A History.* Belleville: Mika Publishing.

Hughes, EC. 1958. *Men and Their Work.* Chicago: University of Chicago Press.

Illich, I. 1975. *Medical Nemesis: The Expropriation of Health.* London: Calder and Boyars.

Johnson, LA. 1974. The Political Economy of Ontario Women in the Nineteenth Century. In J Acton, P Goldsmith and B Shepard eds. *Women at Work, Ontario 1850–1930.* Toronto: Canadian Women's Educational Press.

Kett, JF. 1967. American and Canadian Medical Institutions 1800–1870. *Journal of the History of Medicine* 22: 343–356.

Larkin, G. 1983. *Occupational Monopoly and Modern Medicine.* London: Tavistock.

Larson, MS. 1977. *The Rise of Professionalism: A Sociological Analysis.* Berkeley: University of California Press.

League for Social Reconstruction. Research Committee. 1935. *Social Planning for Canada.* Reprinted with a new introduction. Toronto: University of Toronto Press, 1975.

Leclair, M. 1975. The Canadian Health Care System. In S Andreopoulos ed. *National Health Insurance: Can We Learn From Canada?,* 11-93. New York: Wiley.

Lipset, SM. 1967. *The First New Nation: The United States in Historical and Comparative Perspective.* New York: Doubleday.

Lipset, SM. 1968. *Agrarian Socialism.* (Rev. ed.) Garden City, N.Y.: Doubleday and Company.

MacDermott, HD. 1967. *One Hundred Years of Medicine in Canada.* Toronto: McClelland and Stewart.

Matters, DL. 1974. A Report on Health Insurance: 1919. *B.C. Studies* 21: 28–32.

Maxwell, ID, and MP Maxwell. 1983. Inner Fraternity and Outer Sorority: Social Structure and the Professionalization of Occupational Therapy. In A Wipper ed. *The Sociology of Work: Papers in Honour of Oswald Hall.* Carleton Library series number 129. Ottawa: Carleton University Press.

McCaughey, D. 1981. The Overcrowding of the Medical Profession in Ontario: 1851–1911. Paper presented to the annual meeting of the American Association for the History of Medicine, Toronto.

McKeown, T, and C Record. 1962. Reasons for the Decline in Mortality in England and Wales in the Nineteenth Century. *Population Studies* 29: 391–422.

McKinlay, JB. 1977. The Business of Good Doctoring or Doctoring as Good Business: Reflections on Freidson's View of the Medical Game. *International Journal of Health Services* 7: 459–483.

McNabb, E. 1970. *A Legal History of the Health Professions in Ontario.* Committee on the Healing Arts. Toronto: Queen's Printer.

Mitchell, R. 1940. Public Health in Manitoba. In Canadian Public Health Association. *The Development of Public Health in Canada.* Toronto: University of Toronto Press.

Moore, B. 1966. *Social Origins of Dictatorship and Democracy.* Boston: Beacon Press.

Navarro, V. 1976. *Medicine Under Capitalism.* New York: Prodist.

Ormsby, M. 1962. T. Dufferin Patullo and the Little New Deal. *Canadian Historical Review* 43: 277–297.

Park, L. 1978. Norman Bethune as I knew him. In W MacLeod, L Park, and S Ryerson eds. *Bethune: The Montreal Years.* Toronto: Lorimer.

Parsons, T. 1966. *Societies: Evolutionary and Comparative Perspectives.* Englewood Cliffs: Prentice-Hall.

Paterson, GR. 1967. Canadian Pharmacy in Pre-Confederation Medical Legislation. *Journal of the American Medical Association* 200: 849–852.

Peterson, MJ. 1978. *The Medical Profession in Mid-Victorian London.* Berkeley: University of California Press.

Piva, MJ. 1979. *The Condition of the Working Class in Toronto - 1900–1921.* Ottawa: University of Ottawa Press.

Ray, AJ. 1981. Diffusion of Diseases in the Western Interior of Canada. In SED Shortt ed. *Medicine in Canadian Society: Historical Perspectives.* Montreal: McGill-Queen's University Press.

Rimlinger, GV. 1971. *Welfare Policy and Industrialization in Europe, America and Russia.* New York: Wiley.

Robin, M. 1968. *Radical Politics and Canadian Labour.* Kingston: Industrial Relations Centre, Queen's University.

Robin, M. 1973. *Pillars of Profit: The Company Province 1934–72.* Toronto: McClelland and Stewart.

Roland, CG. ed. 1984. *Health, Disease and Medicine.* Hannah Institute for the History of Medicine. Toronto: Clark Irwin.

Shortt, SED. ed. 1981. *Medicine in Canadian Society.* Montreal: McGill-Queen's University Press.

Shortt, SED. 1983. Physicians, Science and Status: Issues in the Professionalization of Anglo-American Medicine in the Nineteenth Century. *Medical History* 27: 51–68.

Starr, P. 1982. *The Social Transformation of American Medicine.* New York: Basic Books.

Stevenson, A. 1967. *Physicians' Panel on Canadian Medical History.* Toronto: Schering Corporation.

Swartz, D. 1977. The Politics of Reform: Conflict and Accommodation in Canadian Health Policy. In L Panich ed. *The Canadian State: Political Economy and Political Power.* Toronto: University of Toronto Press.

Taylor, MG. 1960. The Role of the Medical Profession in the Formulation and Execution of Public Policy. *Canadian Journal of Economics and Political Science* 26: 108–127.

Taylor, MG. 1978. *Health Insurance and Canadian Public Policy.* Montreal: McGill-Queen's University Press.

Walters, V. 1982. State, Capital and Labour: The Introduction of Federal-Provincial Insurance for Physician Care in Canada. *Canadian Review of Sociology and Anthropology* 19: 157–172.

Weir, GM. 1932. *Survey of Nursing Education in Canada.* Toronto: University of Toronto Press.

Whittaker, R. 1977. Images of the state in Canada. In L Panich ed. *The Canadian State: Political Economy and Political Power.* Toronto: University of Toronto Press.

Wilensky, HL. 1964. The Professionalization of Everyone. *American Journal of Sociology* 70: 137–158.

Wilensky, HL. 1975. *The Welfare State and Equality.* Berkeley: University of California Press.

Willis, E. 1983. *Medical Dominance: The Division of Labour in Australian Health Care.* Sydney: Allen and Unwin.

Woods, SE. 1980. *Ottawa: The Capital of Canada.* Toronto: Doubleday.

2

Health Care Costs: Canada in Perspective*

Douglas E. Angus

Health services researchers have been busy during the past decade particularly since each province has completed major examinations of its health care system (Angus 1991). They have never been so occupied as they are at present, while costs in the health care system have always been of some concern in Canada (Angus 1987), during the latter part of the 1980s and early 1990s the pressures on costs and budgets have increased significantly.

The situation has been exacerbated further by two recent (and severe) recessions, and by federal Conservative and Liberal governments downloading the federal deficit problems to the provincial governments. Everyone, including governments, providers, and the public at large, is concerned about such issues as our capacity to fund health care services at the present level, the efficiency and effectiveness in the system, the impact of new technologies, the quality of care being provided, the way in which the system is organized and managed; and the overall impact of health care on population health status.

Certainly the cost of providing health care services in Canada is high. At present we spend more than $68 billion, or 10 percent of our Gross Domestic Product - GDP, on health care services (Health and Welfare Canada 1994). Of all countries in the Organization for Economic Cooperation and Development (OECD) group that maintain predominantly publicly funded systems of health insurance, Canada spends the highest amount per person on its health care services. Indeed, only one country, the United States, spends more per capita and a higher proportion of its GDP on health care than does Canada (Schieber 1987; U.S. GAO 1991; Health and Welfare Canada 1990).

The challenge for Canada with respect to health care costs is multidimensional. First, and foremost, it is clear that we must reverse the continual internal expansion of the health care system which, by and large, has been the norm for the past couple of decades. Then, we must improve the way in which health care resources are allocated and managed. The World Bank in a recent (and excellent) report has argued that governments around the world must redirect their spending on health to more cost-effective programs and towards improving health outcomes while, at the same time, containing costs (World Bank 1993). Given the popularity of Canada's health care system, the trick is to achieve greater efficiency. At the same time the system is being

* Material used for this Chapter is based on work done for the Project on Cost-Effectiveness of the Canadian Health Care System and for the Canadian Nurses Association. The author is grateful to Queens-University of Ottawa Economic projects and the Canadian Nurses' Association for allowing aspects of their material to be incorporated into this paper.

called upon to improve performance, it is also being asked to increase accountability, responsibility, and responsiveness (Angus 1991).

In the rest of this chapter, the Canadian trends in health expenditures will be examined. Then, to put Canada into perspective, Canada's experiences will be compared and contrasted with countries in the OECD. Finally, there will be a discussion of the implication of actions that governments in Canada are taking to address the costs and effectiveness of the Canadian health care system.

Trends in Size and Composition of Canadian Health Care Expenditures

During the past three decades (from 1960–1990) health care expenditures went through three distinct phases. In the first, 1960–1970, while Canada was expanding public coverage of hospital and medical services, health care costs as a percentage of GDP went from 5.5 percent in 1960 to 7.1 percent in 1970. During the 1970s, the second distinct phase, health care costs as a proportion of GDP remained relatively stable due primarily to two notable factors: (externally) the oil price increases of the early 1970s, which forced attention to national budgets; and, (internally), national price and wage controls. Both factors helped keep the lid on the growth in costs. During the third phase, however, health care costs have climbed even more significantly than during the 1960s, going from 7.7 percent in 1981 to 9.9 percent in 1991 (Table 1). As will be seen later, Canada was one of the few OECD countries to experience such rapid escalation during the 1980s and early 1990s.[1] In fact, "even when expressed in constant dollars, the increases from 1975 to 1987 are dramatic (in total, an increase of 83.3 percent) far exceeding the 12.3 percent increase in population over the same period" (Taylor 1990: 188).

TABLE 1
Total health care expenditures as a percentage of gross domestic product (GDP), 1960 - 1993

Year	Percentage of GDP	Year	Percentage of GDP
1960	5.5	1977	7.3
1961	5.9	1978	7.3
1962	5.9	1979	7.2
1963	6.0	1980	7.3
1964	6.0	1981	7.7
1965	6.0	1982	8.6
1966	6.1	1983	8.8
1967	6.4	1984	8.7
1968	6.6	1985	8.5
1969	6.7	1986	8.5
1970	7.1	1987	8.8
1971	7.4	1988	8.7
1972	7.3	1989	8.9
1973	6.9	1990	9.3
1974	6.8	1991	9.9
1975	7.2	1992	10.1
1976	7.3	1993	10.1

Note: Data for 1987–1993 are "preliminary estimates".

Source: Health and Welfare Canada 1990; 1994, and Angus 1987

The composition of health care expenditures changed also. Spending on institutional care increased significantly throughout the 1960s and 1970s, going from about 45 percent of total health care costs in 1960 to 54 percent in 1980 (Table 2). During the 1980s, however, the proportion of health care spending on institutions decreased to 49 percent in 1990. Acute care hospitals (at 39 percent of health care expenditures in 1990) still represent the largest single category of costs. The direct cost of physicians' services has remained at about 15 percent of total health care costs in the 1980s. Still, while this proportion may be constant and relatively small, decisions made by physicians have a significant impact on the use of the other sub-sectors in the system (hospitals, pharmaceuticals, personnel, other technology) which are paid for by the third-party payers in the system (Angus 1993).

In examining issues related to cost containment other researchers have observed that "although the share of the total expended on hospitals declined from 44.4 percent to 39.2 percent, nevertheless total absolute expenditures by hospitals increased 62.2 percent and for all other institutions (mainly due to the increase in long-term care facilities), 93.6 percent. Expenditures on physicians' services in constant dollars increased 87.3 percent, owing in part to an increase of 21.6 percent in physician supply. Some other increases were even more extraordinary: home care, 373 percent over the twelve years; ambulance services, 247 percent; and drugs and appliances, 138 percent. This latter increase is due, in part, to the fact that all provinces have drug programs for various groups and also subsidize the purchase of prostheses and wheelchairs" (Taylor 1990: 188).

TABLE 2
Percentage distribution of total health expenditures by major category, Canada, selected years,1960 - 1990

	Percentage Distribution			
	1960	1970	1980	1990
Institutions	45.1	52.2	54.1	49.0
General & Applied Special Hospitals	30.3	36.6	41.0	39.0
Homes for Special Care	5.1	7.2	13.1	10.0
Others	9.7	8.4		
Professional Services	24.6	22.5	22.0	22.0
Physicians	16.8	16.6	15.1	15.0
Others	7.8	5.9	6.9	7.0
Drugs and Appliances	14.8	12.5	10.8	13.0
Other Health Costs	15.6	12.8	13.1	16.0
Total	100.0	100.0	100.0	100.0

Source: See Table 1

International Comparisons

While there are data and conceptual problems at the international level, comparison of experiences among the industrialized countries of the OECD can provide valuable insights into cross-country differences with respect to the important determinants of health expenditures. These comparisons highlight common problems, common solutions, and a point of reference for Canada on the international scene.

Health care systems in the OECD can be characterized in one of three ways. First, there are the "National Health Service" or Beveridge-type care systems where one can find universal coverage for the country's residents, financing derived by national general taxes, and some form of national ownership/control of the factors of production. Countries in this category are Australia, Canada, Denmark, Finland, Greece, Ireland, Italy, New Zealand, Norway, Portugal, Spain, Sweden, and the United Kingdom.

In the second category of health care systems is the "Social Insurance" or Bismarck-type which is characterized by compulsory universal coverage within a social security framework, financing by employer and individual contributions through non-profit insurance funds, and a combination of public/private ownership of the factors of production. Countries here include Austria, Belgium, France, Germany, Japan, Luxembourg, the Netherlands, and Switzerland.

The final category of health care system is the "private insurance" or consumer-sovereignty model where one finds individual or employer-based purchase of private health insurance coverage, financing through individual and/or employer contributions and (generally) private sector ownership of the factors of production. The United States is the best example of countries in this category, with Turkey being another.

While these categories generally hold for the countries identified, none are mutually exclusive. For instance, in the Beveridge countries of Canada and the United Kingdom, we do find some private insurance and ownership of the factors of production. In Canada, hospitals are non-profit corporations governed by independent boards of trustees, and the vast majority of physicians are self-employed on a fee-for-service basis. As well, at the other extreme, more than 40 percent of total health care expenditures in the United States are funded publicly for such programs as Medicare and Medicaid. Although the OECD countries have diverse health care systems, they (by and large) are remarkably similar in their objectives and incentives.

Generally, the proportion of overall health care expenditures which are sourced in the public sector is about 77 percent (Table 3). The OECD pointed out that "at least 95 percent of the population is eligible for public coverage against the risk of hospitalization ... in 20 of 23 OECD countries (excluding Turkey) in 1983" (OECD 1987: 25). At about 40 percent, the United States is the clear outlier.

The benefits covered under the various health care systems vary from country to country. One usually finds total coverage for hospital inpatient physician and diagnostic services under each of the three major categories of systems. For other services such as pharmaceuticals, eyeglasses, appliances, and nursing homes, coverage differs according to various criteria, for example, income levels, employment status, region of responsibility, age restrictions, cost and sharing. Cost sharing for pharmaceuticals is quite common throughout much of the OECD. Still, in many of the Beveridge and Bismarck systems, "significant cost sharing on *basic services* (emphasis added) is generally perceived as inconsistent with the underlying social welfare aims of the public health programs ... interestingly, virtually all countries waive cost-sharing for the poor, and impose limits on cumulative cost-sharing payment" (OECD 1987: 25).

TABLE 3
Health care expenditures in OECD countries, as percent of GDP, and percent in the public sector, 1991

Model Type and Country	Health Expenditures as percent of GDP	Public Health Care Expenditures as percent of Total
A. Beveridge Model		
Australia	8.6	72
Canada	9.9	76
Denmark	7.0	87
Finland	8.9	78
Greece	4.8	75
Ireland	8.0	86
Italy	8.3	78
New Zealand	7.7	83
Norway	8.4	99
Portugal	6.2	61
Spain	6.5	72
Sweden	8.8	91
United Kingdom	6.6	87
B. Bismarck Model		
Austria	8.5	68
Belgium	8.1	76
France	9.1	78
Germany	9.1	77
Japan	6.8	74
Luxembourg	6.6	92
Netherlands	8.7	78
Switzerland	8.0	68
C. Private Insurance		
Turkey	4.1	40
United States	13.3	41
OECD Average	8.1	77

Source: OECD 1993, OECD Health Systems: Facts and Trends 1960-1991, Health Policy Studies No. 3, Paris

Hospital and physician reimbursement mechanisms vary significantly among OECD countries. Since hospital expenditures are the largest single item of total health care expenditures, it is this sector where much of the effort to control costs has occurred. Most countries use some form of global budgeting, and a few others use such mechanisms as payments per day, payments per case (e.g., diagnostic related groupings - DRGs), or payments per service. In some countries, for example, the United Kingdom and Germany, and public hospitals in France, payments to hospitals usually include the reimbursement to physicians. However, in other countries such as Canada, the United States and Japan, and private hospitals in France, payments to hospitals and physicians (usually fee-for-service) are kept separate. It has been observed that "... prospective total budget approaches inclusive of inpatient physician services ... results in lower expenditures than ... a retrospective per diem cost or charge-based system with physicians being paid on a fee-for-service basis. In fact, most OECD countries have implemented, or are moving towards, either total budget approaches (the United Kingdom, Canada, France) or prospective per diem (Germany) or per case (the United States) systems" (OECD 1987: 27).

Another major item of health care expenditures is that for physicians services. In virtually all systems, decisions made by physicians have a significant impact on the other resources in the system, that is hospitals, technology, pharmaceuticals, and other health personnel, which are paid for (in most cases) by the same funders in the system. "Thus, the incentives inherent in physician payment systems are critical in determining overall systems costs" (OECD 1987: 27). The general reimbursement mechanisms used are fee-for-service, capitation, salary or variants of these methods. Most countries reimburse hospital-based physicians differently than physicians in ambulatory care settings, with Canada clearly being different than all of the other Beveridge health care systems. In some countries, the United Kingdom for example, general practitioners (GPs) are used as "gatekeepers" for patient access to inpatient hospital services, diagnostic tests and so on. In addition, unlike those in Canada and the United States, consumers in most OECD countries do not have unfettered freedom of choice regarding physicians; rather, they are required to choose a physician for given periods of time (OECD 1987).

In the Bismarck-type and private insurance countries (e.g., Belgium, France, Germany, Japan, and the United States) the basic way of reimbursing ambulatory care physicians is the fee-for-service mechanism. In many of the Beveridge-type health care systems, for example, the United Kingdom, Denmark (in Copenhagen), and Spain, physicians are reimbursed through a capitation method after patients have selected their GPs and have become members of their practice groups. "In Germany, medical services are allotted an overall budget, which is divided among physicians. Other countries maintain a relatively low fee schedule and authorize fee supplements to be paid by patients (Australia, France, Denmark [outside Copenhagen], New Zealand)" (Contandriopoulos et al. 1993: 36).

Patient or household contributions to cover costs of medical services have increased substantially in many OECD countries. "Patient participation" has been established or expanded (usually in the form of user fees) to include all or parts of the population in Belgium, France, Luxembourg, Norway, Portugal and Sweden; in countries such as Denmark and Ireland, user fees are being applied to only certain population groups.

In addition to hospitals and physicians, the other significant component of health care expenditures in the OECD countries is that for pharmaceuticals. Generally, pharmaceuticals are reimbursed on a fee-for-service basis, with fees being established on such criteria as retail prices, wholesale prices, acquisition costs and the lowest cost generic equivalent drug. Either the patient or pharmacist is reimbursed directly. When patients are in institutions for care, pharmaceuticals are supplied free of charge, that is, they are considered part of the overall service and, hence, are part of the hospital's overall budget (OECD 1987).

The ways in which health care systems are organized, managed, and regulated can have an impact on health care expenditures as well. We note that, throughout most of the industrialized countries, the two major areas of emphasis are control over supply and influences on demand, usually through the application of some form of "patient participation." In fact, "some types have been widely utilized, such as spending ceilings (especially in the hospital environment), control over service fees, control over practice activities, use of less costly alternatives to institutional services (especially in hospitals), and the increase or introduction of user contributions to financing" (Contandriopoulos et al. 1993: 63–64). Furthermore, market mechanisms for financing and/or delivery of health care have been implemented in a few OECD countries. For example, competition between public and private insurance exists in the Netherlands and the U.S. (especially with respect to Health Maintenance Organizations (HMOs)). In the United Kingdom and one part of the health care system in France, competition between public and private producers or between care purchasers and providers is in place (Contandri-opoulos et al. 1993).

When the previous characteristics of the various OECD countries health care systems are considered in relation to their health care system spending performance, one can generally observe an association between the two (Contandriopoulos et al. 1993). On average in OECD countries since 1980, health care expenditures as a percentage of GDP have ranged between 7 and 8 percent. Notable exceptions are Canada, Finland, Sweden, France, Germany, the Netherlands, the United States (at the outer range), and the United Kingdom (at the lower range) (Table 4). Not only is it important to compare countries on the basis of their allocations to health care from GDP, but if we are interested in learning which countries are most successful at controlling the growth of health care expenditures, it is essential to examine the elasticities of total health care expenditures to GDP (see Table 4).

Since most OECD countries expanded their public health programs during the 1960s, health care expenditures relative to GDP grew fastest during that period, that is, about 40 percent faster than GDP. Two countries which stand out with the most significant growth in health care expenditures during that period were Switzerland (70 percent) and Sweden (63 percent). In the 1970s, its early years marked by the oil shock, the growth of health care expenditures decreased on average, to 24 percent. Notable exceptions (with higher than average growth) were Switzerland (63 percent), Belgium (46 percent), Germany (44 percent) and Luxembourg (44 percent). At the other end of the scale were Canada (1 percent), Denmark (5 percent), Finland (12 percent) and the United Kingdom (15 percent), all of which are Beveridge health care type countries. It is worth recalling that in Canada, provincial constraints and country-wide wage and price controls (in the early 1970s) were also significant factors working to control the growth of health care costs during that period.

As a result of recessions experienced by most OECD countries throughout the 1980s, growth of health care expenditures was even less than the previous decade, i.e., 9 percent (on average). The only Beveridge-type country where health care expenditures growth far exceeded the growth in GDP, as well as the OECD average, was Canada (21 percent). In some of the Beveridge countries, health care expenditures growth actually decreased (Sweden, Denmark, Ireland, and the United Kingdom). Of the Bismarck-type health care systems, only the Netherlands experienced a decrease in the growth in health care expenditures, which is in direct contrast to Belgium and France, where health care costs grew 27 percent and 19 percent respectively, faster than GDP. Of all OECD countries during the 1980-90 period, the most significant outlier was the United States (with 30 percent growth in health care expenditures). Factors that contribute to effective cost control in successful OECD countries are discussed later in this chapter.

TABLE 4
Health care expenditures in OECD countries, 1960-1991 by type of model

Model Type and Country	Health Care Expenditures as % of GDP					Elasticity Ratios		
	1960	1970	1980	1990	1991	1960-1970	1970-1980	1980-1990
A. Beveridge								
Australia	4.8	5.6	7.1	8.3	8.6	1.08	1.21	1.11
Canada	5.3	7.2	7.5	9.5	9.9	1.28	1.01	1.21
Denmark	3.6	5.9	6.7	6.7	7.0	1.47	1.05	0.93
Finland	3.8	5.7	6.4	7.8	8.9	1.46	1.12	1.16
Greece	2.6	3.7	4.0	4.9	4.8	1.31	1.05	1.12
Ireland	3.8	5.1	8.1	7.6	8.0	1.37	1.17	0.96
Italy	3.6	5.2	6.6	8.1	8.3	1.48	1.07	1.16
New Zealand	4.2	5.1	7.2	7.3	7.7	1.16	1.26	1.07
Norway	3.2	4.9	7.1	8.0	8.4	1.47	1.27	1.09
Portugal	–	3.0	5.1	6.1	6.2	–	1.20	1.13
Spain	1.6	3.6	5.4	6.4	6.5	1.63	1.21	1.08
Sweden	4.7	7.1	9.2	8.6	8.8	1.54	1.22	0.87
U.K.	3.9	4.6	5.9	6.0	6.6	1.23	1.15	0.96
B. Bismarck								
Belgium	3.4	4.2	6.5	7.9	8.1	1.31	1.46	1.27
France	4.3	5.9	7.5	8.8	9.1	1.31	1.20	1.19
Germany	4.9	6.0	8.4	8.8	9.1	1.32	1.44	1.11
Japan	3.0	4.6	6.5	6.7	6.8	1.30	1.27	1.03
Luxembourg	–	4.7	6.8	7.0	6.6	–	1.44	1.05
Netherlands	4.0	5.9	8.0	8.4	8.7	1.35	1.24	0.96
Switzerland	3.3	5.1	7.0	7.9	8.0	1.70	1.63	1.13
C. Private Insurance								
Turkey	–	–	3.7	3.8	4.1	–	–	1.01
U.S.	5.3	7.4	9.2	12.2	13.3	1.41	1.21	1.30
OECD Total	3.9	5.1	7.0	7.8	8.1	1.41	1.24	1.09

Note: Elasticity ratios - elasticity of total health expenditure growth to total domestic expenditure growth.

Source: OECD 1993, OECD Health Systems: Facts and Trends, Table 1

Changes in rates of medical-specific inflation and health benefits per capita during 1960-1990 reflect changes in economic conditions and changes in government and provider approaches to incomes during that period. In the 1960s, governments were increasing the scope and coverage of health care services to their populations, which also contributed to an "inflationary pull" on medical prices. The range of insured health care benefits expanded more in the 1960s and 1970s than in the 1980s. As a result of severe inflation in most countries in the 1970s, "professional incomes were often frozen and real wages of public employees sometimes cut; the price of many health services declined in relative terms" (OECD 1993: 23). As the data in Table 5 suggest, while professionals were able to recoup some of their earlier losses, they were able to do so less successfully in the 1980s than in the 1960s, primarily because purchasers had introduced a number of relatively effective cost-containment mechanisms (which are elaborated upon later in this chapter). Still, while health care inflation in Canada was about twice that for the OECD average, real health spending/benefits per capita were consistent with that throughout the OECD in general.

Throughout most of the OECD countries, particularly in Europe, the rate of growth of health-care-specific prices has slowed considerably. Notable exceptions are Canada, Finland, and the United States where, it appears, "expenditure on health still grows faster, on average, than total private consumption" (OECD 1993: 26). It is suggested that the changing age structure of the population and decisions related to the use of new technology could exacerbate this situation, all of which points to the necessity to better allocate and manage health care resources.

TABLE 5

Annual rates of increase (%) in health care inflation and benefits, OECD countries, 1960-1990

Model Type and Country	Health Care Inflation			Real Health Benefits/ Spending per Capita		
	1960-1970	1970-1980	1980-1990	1960-1970	1970-1980	1980-1990
A. Beveridge						
Australia	3.2	1.0	0.3	2.6	3.3	2.3
Canada	1.4	0.3	1.8	4.7	3.8	2.5
Denmark	0.8	-1.3	0.2	8.5	3.8	1.0
Finland	-1.8	-0.9	1.7	10.9	5.0	3.1
Greece	-0.6	0.1	-1.2	10.5	4.0	4.4
Ireland	-0.6	-1.5	2.2	8.3	9.2	-1.6
Italy	1.0	-0.5	0.6	7.8	6.1	3.5
New Zealand	-0.1	2.8	1.6	3.7	1.3	0.2
Norway	3.2	0.7	-0.1	5.0	6.3	2.4
Portugal	–	0.9	0.4	–	8.0	1.3
Spain	1.1	-0.1	0.4	14.9	6.7	1.2
Sweden	-0.6	0.8	-0.6	8.9	3.1	1.4
U.K.	-0.8	-0.6	1.3	4.6	4.9	1.9
B. Bismarck						
Belgium	1.5	0.0	0.6	4.6	7.8	2.7
France	0.1	-1.5	-0.9	7.6	6.6	4.5
Germany	0.9	1.0	0.7	4.4	5.7	1.2
Japan	1.1	-1.1	0.9	12.5	7.7	3.0
Luxembourg	–	-0.7	0.4	–	6.8	2.8
Netherlands	1.3	3.2	0.5	7.0	1.4	1.3
Switzerland	1.6	2.5	0.9	6.5	2.0	1.9
C. Private Insurance						
Turkey	–	–	2.0	–	–	0.2
U.S.	0.8	0.0	2.7	5.2	3.8	2.3
OECD Total	0.9	0.4	0.7	7.0	5.1	2.4

Note: Health Care inflation is the excess of health care price increases over those on all goods and services. OECD averages are arithmetic and exclude Turkey; in 1960-70, Luxembourg and Portugal are excluded.

Source: OECD 1993, OECD Health Systems: Facts and Trends, Table 3

It is important to examine the composition of health care expenditures, for the way in which health care is provided across OECD countries can impact expenditures and, hence, can provide some potentially useful organizational possibilities for Canada to consider. Table 6 shows the composition of health care expenditures by major sub-sector: hospitals, ambulatory care, and pharmaceuticals. A few significant trends emerge. For instance, "pervasive incentives steer patients towards hospitals in the Nordic countries; the same patients are driven to consult office-based physicians in Germany (whose offices are often well equipped with sophisticated diagnostic machinery) and in the United States where a large share of light surgery takes place" (OECD 1993: 26). Inpatient hospital care usually is more costly than ambulatory care. In countries where the shares of health care expenditures are more balanced between hospital and ambulatory care (e.g., Japan and Germany), overall cost control is more evident than in countries where hospital care accounts for the largest share of expenditures. In Canada hospital care accounts for more than twice the ambulatory care expenditures. Canada, Sweden, and Germany are the only countries to see the share of pharmaceutical expenditures rise noticeably during the past decade.

In the same way that most OECD countries were able to slow the rate of growth of medical-specific prices, similar success was achieved in controlling hospital-specific and pharmaceutical inflation (Table 7). The only industrialized countries still experiencing greater-than-OECD average hospital-specific inflation are Switzerland, United States, Germany, Belgium, and Canada. As well, Canada, the United States, and Germany have also experienced higher than average pharmaceutical-specific inflation during the 1980-90 period.

During the past decade, many countries in Europe (and elsewhere in the OECD) have been restricting and reforming their health care systems to try to deliver effective services more efficiently. An integral aspect of these reforms is the cost control mechanisms which are in place in various countries and which have been highlighted earlier in this chapter. After all is considered at the international level, what seems to work reasonably well, both in terms of cost control and health outcomes performance?

Recently, Contandriopoulos and his colleagues (1993) undertook to examine patterns and characteristics of regulation in OECD countries and to assess their impact on health care expenditures and on health status of the population in their respective countries. Table 8 summarizes the rankings of countries on the basis of their success in controlling costs and in improving health status. The results are interesting. Perhaps not surprisingly the United States is the outlier (in the negative sense) when it comes to both cost-control and health system performance variables. Canada, however, does not fare much better. It ranks in the second to last group in both categories, being 18th of 21 on cost control and 17th of 21 on health system performance. The latter variable is a composite measure that encompasses both health status (as measured by life expectancy and infant mortality) and the level of expenditures on health care services. At the other end, "Denmark has the best cost-control indicator: Japan, the best health outcomes" (Contandriopoulos et al. 1993: 20). Whether the health care system is Beveridge or Bismarck-type does not appear to determine the level of performance. Countries from both types of systems appear as the high performers as well as low performers.

TABLE 6
Composition (%) of health care expenditures, OECD countries by major sub-sector, 1960-1990

Model Type and Countries	Hospitals				Ambulatory Care				Pharmaceuticals			
	1960	1970	1980	1990	1960	1970	1980	1990	1960	1970	1980	1990
A. Beveridge												
Australia	–	29.1	52.9	48.1	–	–	22.3	25.5	–	–	7.9	8.8
Canada	43.6	52.2	52.6	49.1	23.9	22.4	22.1	21.9	12.9	11.2	8.9	13.3
Denmark	50.3	55.8	65.1	62.2	–	38.4	30.1	31.3	–	9.1	9.1	9.2
Finland	41.2	50.4	49.2	44.7	21.7	21.5	27.2	33.9	16.2	12.6	10.7	9.4
Greece	63.0	46.4	48.9	57.5	–	–	–	–	35.2	43.3	34.8	24.4
Ireland	–	–	46.1	51.1	–	–	–	–	–	22.2	14.7	18.3
Italy	43.2	47.6	54.0	46.7	35.8	36.2	29.5	27.3	19.8	15.5	13.9	18.4
New Zealand	52.4	55.7	55.3	49.5	–	–	–	–	–	–	–	9.6
Norway	38.1	68.2	73.8	70.4	–	–	21.3	23.8	9.7	7.8	10.0	10.4
Portugal	–	27.5	29.9	25.5	–	–	16.3	–	–	15.6	22.4	17.6
Spain	–	52.5	54.1	47.2	–	–	12.6	–	–	23.5	21.0	18.0
Sweden	69.0	59.7	68.5	51.3	–	–	–	–	3.5	4.2	6.5	8.2
U.K.	44.5	49.0	56.1	44.0	–	–	–	–	–	–	11.2	10.7
B. Bismarck												
Belgium	38.4	25.7	32.9	32.8	41.3	42.5	38.9	40.0	24.3	28.1	17.3	15.5
France	34.7	38.0	48.1	44.2	27.6	26.6	24.8	28.4	22.1	23.2	15.9	16.8
Germany	–	35.7	36.1	36.6	–	29.0	26.6	28.0	–	19.5	18.7	21.3
Japan	34.1	26.4	30.7	30.2	–	48.4	44.3	40.5	–	–	22.1	17.3
Luxembourg	–	–	31.3	27.7	–	22.4	49.5	52.1	–	19.7	14.5	15.0
Netherlands	–	55.1	57.3	51.8	–	–	27.7	26.9	9.5	7.5	7.9	9.9
Switzerland	44.6	41.7	42.6	42.8	30.9	–	45.5	–	–	19.1	15.2	12.3
C. Private Insurance												
Turkey	–	–	11.5	19.1	–	–	–	–	–	–	–	–
U.S.	37.8	44.1	48.9	46.2	29.1	26.8	26.5	29.4	15.7	11.8	8.6	8.1

Notes: Hospitals includes all in-patient care, ambulatory care includes all out-patient medical and paramedical services. Pharmaceuticals includes purchase of medicines (as well as over-the-counter). OECD averages are arithmetic and exclude Turkey; in 1970 they exclude Luxembourg and Portugal.

Source: OECD 1993, OECD Health Systems: Facts and Trends, Table 4

TABLE 7
Annual rates of increase (%) in hospital inflation and pharmaceutical inflation, OECD countries, 1960-1990

Model Type and Country	Hospital-Specific Inflation			Pharmaceutical-Specific Inflation		
	1960-1970	1970-1980	1980-1990	1960-1970	1970-1980	1980-1990
A. Beveridge						
Australia	1.1	0.8	0.0	-0.5	-4.7	-0.6
Canada	3.2	2.8	1.7	-3.4	-3.2	4.4
Denmark	7.4	0.8	0.3	–	-3.5	1.2
Finland	1.5	-0.3	1.1	-2.8	-2.3	1.4
Greece	0.5	4.0	2.6	-2.8	-2.5	-4.3
Ireland	9.0	-1.0	1.1	–	-3.1	1.1
Italy	5.8	0.7	2.2	-3.7	-9.4	-3.9
New Zealand	2.1	2.4	0.1	–	-2.7	0.1
Norway	3.7	0.4	0.0	0.4	-0.6	0.9
Portugal	–	0.8	-0.8	–	-5.4	-0.2
Spain	1.1	-0.6	1.8	–	-8.5	0.2
Sweden	-0.6	2.1	-1.3	–	-1.4	-2.2
U.K.	2.9	3.2	0.7	-4.4	-1.7	-0.8
B. Bismarck						
Belgium	5.8	1.5	2.1	-1.5	-4.8	0.1
France	1.6	0.3	0.1	-3.0	-5.4	-3.4
Germany	5.6	7.2	2.2	-0.8	-0.8	2.2
Japan	-1.8	-2.4	0.7	-4.3	-3.0	1.4
Luxembourg	–	-0.7	0.5	–	-5.1	1.1
Netherlands	1.6	6.5	1.1	–	-3.7	-0.2
Switzerland	1.6	4.9	3.1	–	-1.3	-1.1
C. Private Insurance						
Turkey	–	–	–	–	-2.5	–
U.S.	3.5	0.6	2.2	-3.1	–	3.8
OECD Total	3.1	1.9	1.1	3.8	-3.3	0.0

Note: Specific inflation is the excess of in-patient care or pharmaceutical price increases over those on all goods and services. OECD averages are arithmetic and exclude Turkey; in 1960-70 they exclude Luxembourg and Portugal.

Source: OECD 1993, OECD Health Systems: Facts and Trends, Table 5

In trying to "explain" the factors that account for the high level of success enjoyed by some countries in controlling expenditures, Contandriopoulos et al. (1993) found:
- Centralized health care systems are better able to control expenditures and perform better than decentralized systems. "Performance" encompasses composite measures of health status and level of health expenditures.
- The greater the number of financing sources that exist, the greater are health care expenditures, the greater is the increase in these health care expenditures, and the lower is system performance.

TABLE 8
International rankings of cost control and health system performance in the 1980s

		Value of the group score[1]
Cost-control variables[2]		
Group 1	Denmark	1.37
Group 2	Ireland, Sweden	0.58
Group 3	Japan, Luxembourg, Switzerland, Spain, United Kingdom	0.46
Group 4	Austria, Netherlands, Germany, Australia, New Zealand	-0.46
Group 5	Belgium, Finland, Italy, Norway, Canada, France, Greece	-0.07
Group 6	United States	-0.37
Cronbach's alpha=0.75		-2.22
Performance variables[3]		
Group 1	Japan	1.40
Group 2	Ireland, Italy, Germany, Austria, Sweden	0.70
Group 3	Netherlands, United Kingdom, Switzerland, Greece	0.39
Group 4	Australia, France	-0.07
Group 5	Denmark, Finland, Spain, New Zealand	-0.28
Group 6	Canada, Norway, Luxembourg, Belgium	-0.85
Group 7	United States	-2.11
Cronbach's alpha=0.50		

Notes:
1   Variation from the mean index, set at zero. Measures have been standardized to account for relative wealth and size of country.
2   The difference between projected and actual expenditures per capita on health care. Projections are based on GDP.
3   A composite of overall health expenditure indexes standardized for GDP and population and of the state of public health (life expectancy and infant mortality).

Source: André-Pierre Contandriopolous et al. 1993, "Cost-control measures in the health care systems of Canada and other countries: Description and assessment," Health Care Working Paper No. 93-01, University of Ottawa

* The greater is the share of private sector financing, the less is the ability to control expenditures.
* The greater the control on physician compensation, the lower are total health expenditures, the greater is system performance, and the lower is the health sector's share of GDP (and the less it tends to increase).
* Whichever health care system is examined, there is the inevitable balance to strike among equity, freedom of choice, and efficiency. Different regulatory mechanisms will impact this balance in different ways, for example:

–   "Technocratic regulation" (also known as the "command and control plan-
    ning model"), by legislative and regulatory constraints, forces the health
    care system to adopt specific goals. Agents in the system learn to circum-
    vent bureaucratic controls and to manipulate information so as to project a
    favourable image to the technocratic authority. This, then, gives rise to a
    gradual increase in technocratic controls in order to compensate for these
    dysfunctions.
–   "Professional self-regulation" is a responsibility delegated by the public,
    through government, to members of the professions in exchange for the
    right to practice their skills. The laws creating and governing professional
    associations refer explicitly to this delegation process. As with the techno-
    cratic model, professional self-regulation occupies a dominant position
    within the regulatory structure of a health care system. From a pragmatic
    viewpoint it seems difficult to undertake reforms in a health care system
    without attempting to co-opt professionals in these changes, i.e., perhaps
    the use of managerial and professional incentives would be relevant.
–   "Laissez-faire" regulation (also known as market-based regulation) is
    based on the existence of a market economy where all goods and services
    are traded in competitive markets. In contrast with the other two models,
    laissez-faire has not received serious consideration as a primary mecha-
    nism for regulating health care costs, mainly because of the characteristics
    of the health care services market. Consequently, only certain mechanisms
    in the competitive model have been marginally considered in the organiza-
    tion of mixed markets, e.g., the reforms of the UK National Health Service.

Since these three models are "pure paradigms ... no health care system is likely to be
governed exclusively by any one of them. Four other regulatory approaches arise in the
interface between the three poles of authority, public competition, the mixed market,
regulation by professional incentives, and regulation by management incentives"
(Contandriopoulos et al. 1993: 122). That many processes are followed in various
countries reflects the "multidisciplinary nature of health care regulation ... and the combination of technocratic and professional regulation of activities within the system in
the context of public competition seems to offer the possibility of achieving the goals
of efficiency and effectiveness while respecting the principles of equity, individual freedom, and cost control in health care. These multiple regulatory tools do not, however,
guarantee cooperative behaviour and innovation among health care managers. A management incentives system must also be implemented in order to promote the active
participation of organizations in such an environment" (Contandriopoulos et al. 1993:
40).[2]

As a result of their analysis, Contandriopoulos et al. concluded that, on the one hand,
countries that have managed market systems tempered by technocratic management
techniques have been the most successful at controlling health care costs: these are
Denmark, Ireland and Sweden. On the other hand, countries that rely primarily on the
professional or management incentives models are notably less successful at controlling health care expenditures: countries in this group are the Netherlands, Germany,
Australia, New Zealand, Finland, Norway, and Canada. With respect to this latter
group,

"even though these regulatory systems may have promoted a certain level of equity and professional freedom through sharing the responsibility for resource allocation, the quest for equity was offset by the failure to reach a satisfactory level of cost control. It can also be seen that where trade-offs between efficiency, equity, and freedom are difficult - as in the United States - the compromise that underlies such tensions involves a fragmentation (emphasis added) of the health care system which ... hinders its capacity to control expenditures" (Contandriopoulos et al. 1993: 141).

Canadian Initiatives to Control Health Care Costs

It is obvious that major reforms to health care systems have been under way in many OECD countries and many are beginning to realize some important gains in overall health systems performance. In view of the fact that we are spending some 10 percent of our GDP on health care services – second only to the United States – it is legitimate to ask what Canada has been doing to reform and/or restructure its health care system and to control health care costs. The short answer is that Canada has been studying, reviewing and examining health care delivery very extensively since the early 1980s, and, only recently, have various initiatives been implemented in some jurisdictions in the country.

Each province and territory in Canada has completed major reviews of its health care system. When one examines the terms of reference of each review "concerns for rising health care costs, dissatisfaction with the existing organizational structure of health care delivery, human resources requirements, technology and quality and accessibility of care were common themes throughout the country. Although the order or emphasis of these issues varied from one commission to the next, there was no doubt that fiscal concerns represented a major underlying thread" (Angus 1991: 3).

The fiscal concerns that brought about the provincial royal commissions and task forces (beginning in 1983 with Newfoundland) have become more intense and the need to reverse the trend of continual internal expansion of the health care system has become more pronounced. Spending on health care has to be redirected to more cost-effective programs and the system has to be managed in ways that will not only contain costs but also improve health outcomes. Provinces are moving in directions to reform their health care systems in three basic ways, i.e., "toward greater emphasis on disease prevention and health promotion, toward community-based care alternatives, and toward greater accountability" (Angus 1991: 75).

These initiatives, directions and reform activities have been reviewed by a number of health care analysts (Angus 1991, 1993, 1995; Mhatre and Deber 1992, and elsewhere in this volume; Canadian Hospital Association 1993; Canadian College of Health Service Executives 1994). In this section, the principal implications of such reforms are summarized under four major categories: finance/funding; health human resources; organization/structure; management.

Finance/Funding

Generally, governments across Canada will maintain tight control of health care costs and likely will begin to reduce the proportion of public health care resources earmarked for the health care system. This implies significant reductions in the acute-care sector, shifts of some of the savings from such cuts to less costly community-based services, continued capping of payments for physicians' services, and shifting from the fee-for-service reimbursement system to other forms of payment, for example salary and capitation, and lower cost pharmaceutical solutions (including greater use of co-payments).

During the past couple of years, governments – principally by containing the growth of costs for hospital care and physicians' services – have been bringing health care costs under control. Still there is much more that could be done to bring about more appropriate and more cost-effective and cost-efficient use of the health care system. By making more appropriate use of facilities and services, and by provinces moving to adopt the "better practice" aspects of each other's health care delivery systems, significant savings are possible, without undermining the existing health status of the population (Angus et al. 1995). Methods to incorporate incentive structures that could bring about such efficiencies need to be developed – provinces still "have not found mechanisms that will lead to effective cost control at the micro level, which is where health care providers are making decisions every day about which services to use in given situations" (Angus et al. 1995: 127).

Health Human Resources

Most of the emphasis on developing more efficient use of health human resources is on physicians and nurses. Government concern over the growth in physician supply, the resulting increase in expenditures for medical services and the lack of incentives for physicians to control use of medical services, has led to specific actions to control both the growth in their supply and compensation. While certain initiatives are under way with respect to nursing and midwifery, there has been much less effort at developing an integrated approach to overall health human resources in Canada. As was recently observed, "Canada's experience in health human resource planning highlights the need for a more coordinated and integrated approach to personnel planning that acknowledges the multiple disciplines involved in health care and seeks a mix of practitioners that uses the lowest-cost provider, appropriate for the services to be delivered. Efficiencies as a result of substituting health human resources and incentives for using appropriate services and settings have yet to be realized" (Angus et al. 1995: 105).

Organization/Structure

The major reforms to health care systems in Canada are taking place in the organization and management of the delivery of services. Restructuring, rationalization, regionalization, and decentralization of health care are happening in one form or another in the provinces. Structural changes in the health care sector are putting new emphasis on cross-functional and multidisciplinary team approaches to health care delivery.

Traditional hierarchical organizations are shifting to more decentralized structures where resources will be allocated on the basis of the health needs of the population. Hospital boards are being replaced by regional boards, resulting in increased pressure on new board members to become more accountable, both politically and administratively. The increasing reduction in acute care facilities and the emphasis on alternative approaches to delivering services are placing greater pressures on organizations and management to create new and innovative linkages among and between different service areas. Overall, governments are strategically redirecting the systems towards ways which will effectively address the maldistribution services and inefficient use of health care resources.

Management

In order to strengthen management of the health care sector, better information is required. Much can be done to improve the efficiency and effectiveness of the system, a major element of which is more effective management. If planning and management of the health system are to be improved, a necessary step is to begin to relate health services to the health needs of the community's population and, very important, to their impact on health outcomes.

Much has to be done to close the many significant gaps that exist in the data. One of the most important needs is for "reliable and relevant health outcome measures against which health care resource use can be evaluated [and] there is still insufficient information on the outcomes of pharmaceuticals and on out-of-hospital services. [Furthermore] national data on community-based services – the other major component of continuing care – are required to complement those on residential care facilities. [As well] data on the effectiveness of medical, surgical, pharmaceutical, and technology-based interventions and their substitutability are needed, [and finally] more up-to-date data are needed" (Angus et al. 1995: 124).

Conclusions and Implications

Canadians are proud of their past achievements in providing universal and comprehensive medical and hospital services to all residents. Yet, as has been shown in this chapter, evidence has been accumulating that shows that our health care system does have flaws and is in need of restructuring and reform. In addition to the fiscal situation facing all levels of government in Canada, several other trends are challenging Canada's health care sector. Issues related to changing demographics; the use of new (and existing) technology; the supply, mix and distribution of health human resources; changing needs and expectations (both from the consumer and provider); and the organization and funding/reimbursement mechanisms affect the management of human and financial resources and the choice of direction for facilities and services. Adding to the complexity of the situation, the system at the same time is being called upon to improve performance and to increase accountability, responsibility and responsiveness.

What, then, are some of the major conclusions we can draw from the international evidence and from some provincial initiatives to control costs, and what are the implications? First, and foremost, by constantly comparing our health care system with that of the United States, we tend to affirm the belief that our system is better. However, by doing only this, we breed complacency. As has been shown earlier, health care systems in most other parts of the OECD (especially in Europe) are more like our system. Importantly, the evidence suggests that many of their systems perform much better than ours. Hence, we should be paying much more serious attention to experiences in those high-performing countries so that we may adopt some of their approaches to delivering effective and efficient health care services. We should focus on countries such as Denmark, Sweden, the United Kingdom, Switzerland, and Japan. As part of that broad-based evidence, the various activities under way in various parts of Canada suggest that provinces can (and should) learn much from each other with respect to effective management of their health care systems. This means that we must look far beyond evidence in the United States for lessons and directions: how much can be learned from a country that is the worst performer both in terms of cost control and of health status success?

Another important observation is that countries that have the following key characteristics are consistently better at controlling health care costs while at the same time
remaining capable of providing a more comprehensive range of services than does
Canada: (Contandriopoulos et al. 1993)

- The hospital and ambulatory care sectors account for similar shares of health care
  expenditures. In Canada, hospital care accounts for more than twice the ambulatory care expenditures.
- Health care systems are centralized. It is important to ascertain what should (and
  what should not) be centralized and decentralized, especially in view of the fact
  that some provinces are decentralizing parts of their health care systems.
- Health care systems are financed by single (or few) funders. The corollary is that
  the greater is the share of private sector financing (the United States being a good
  example), the less is the ability to control expenditures.
- Control over physician compensation is relatively high. As well, according physicians greater financial accountability for their clinical decisions helps to control
  overall health care expenditures.
- Managed market systems that are tempered by technocratic management techniques, for example, Denmark and Sweden.

Finally, while Canada appears to be embarking on the road to health care reform, it
still is only a beginning. Given the foreseeable fiscal situation in Canada, major reform
or restructuring likely will have to occur. Canada can maintain its primarily egalitarian
system of health insurance and still deliver a wide range of effective health care services for a smaller proportion of its GDP than at present. Examples to which we can
refer are Denmark, Japan, the United Kingdom (at about 7 percent of GDP), Norway,
New Zealand (at 8 percent), and Sweden, Germany, and France (at about 9 percent). In
fact, during the past few years Sweden has actually decreased the share of its GDP
going to health care. Alternative delivery mechanisms and reimbursement approaches
should be seriously examined and implemented. Important aspects of this are the development of feasible incentive programs and adaption of certain private sector techniques
(e.g., competition for funds, purchaser-provider splits) as means to improve efficiency
in the system. Given the significance of physicians and their decisions affecting
resource use in the system, it is not surprising that issues around physician resource
management and planning have absorbed the provinces during the past few years.
However, because of real issues related to health human resource substitution, it is
essential that *integrated* health human resource planning be addressed as vigorously as
are issues related to physicians. With respect to organization and management changes
in Canada's health care system, careful consideration should be given to all issues surrounding decentralization of health care delivery and management, to best ascertain
what should (and should not) be decentralized. Europe's experiences here would be
most relevant for Canada.

Overall, then, health care systems around the world have been under reform. Canada
is no exception. Spending on health care has to be redirected to more cost-effective
programs, and the system has to be managed in ways that will not only contain costs
but also improve health outcomes. Since Canadians generally accept the egalitarian
nature of their health care system, the equity criteria inherent in this system are
accepted as a "given." Within that equity framework, however, there is significant
capacity to increase efficiency. In the future, one might hope to see a health care system
where consumers are wiser and better users of appropriate services, and where health
care professionals work more closely together to deliver only effective and appropriate

services in the most efficient way possible and that other factors such as employment, education, and so on, which contribute as much (if not more) to health status, *are* beneficiaries of some of the resources "freed up" from the health care system.

Notes

1   Some "explanations" for this cost escalation are the recessions of the early 1980s and early 1990s (CMA 1993). While they may have had some impact on the rise in the proportion of GDP going towards health care, most of the increase is due to health care inflation in Canada, which was about twice that for all OECD countries (OECD 1993).
2   The reader is referred to Pazderka (1993) for a comprehensive review of issues related to the manager-funder interface in the health care system.

References

Angus, DE. 1987. Health Care Costs: A Review of Past Experience and Potential Impact of the Aging Phenomenon. In D Coburn, P New, C D'Arcy and G Torrance eds. *Health and Canadian Society: Sociological Perspectives*, 57-82. Markham: Fitzhenry and Whiteside.

Angus, DE. 1991. *Review of Significant Health Care Commissions and Task Forces in Canada Since 1983-84.* Ottawa: Canadian Hospital Association, Canadian Medical Association, Canadian Nurses Association.

Angus, DE. 1993. *Health Care Reform: Revisiting the Review of Significant Health Care Commissions and Task Forces.* Ottawa: Canadian Nurses Association.

Angus, D, L Auer, JE Cloutier, and T Albert. 1995. *Sustainable Health Care for Canada.* Ottawa: Queen's–University of Ottawa Economic Projects, University of Ottawa.

Angus, DE, and E Turbayne. 1995. *Path to the Future: A Synopsis of Health and Health Care Issues, National Nursing Competency Project.* Ottawa: Canadian Nurses Association.

Auer, L, DE Angus, JE Cloutier, and J Comis. 1995. *Cost–Effectiveness of Canadian Health Care.* Ottawa: Queen's–University of Ottawa Economic Projects, University of Ottawa.

Barer, ML, and GL Stoddart. 1991. *Toward Integrated Medical Resource Policies for Canada.* Report prepared for the federal/provincial/territorial Conference of Deputy Ministers of Health. Winnipeg: Manitoba Health.

Canadian College of Health Service Executives. 1994. *External Environmental Analysis and Health Reform Update: Special Report.* Ottawa: CCHSE.

Canadian Hospital Association. 1993. *Briefing Report for the National Health Policy Reform Project.* Ottawa: CHA Press.

Canadian Medical Association. 1993. *Toward a New Consensus on Health Care Financing in Canada.* Ottawa: Working Group on Health Care Financing in Canada, Canadian Medical Association.

Contandriopoulos, AP, et al. 1993. *Regulatory Mechanisms in the Health Care Systems in Canada and Other Industrialized Countries: Description and Assessment.* Ottawa: Queen's–University of Ottawa Economic Projects, University of Ottawa.

Health and Welfare Canada. 1990. *National Health Expenditures in Canada 1975-1987.* Ottawa: Supply and Services Canada.

Health and Welfare Canada. 1994. *National Health Expenditures in Canada 1975-1993.* Ottawa: Supply and Services Canada.

MacKenzie, T, B Tholl, and G Brimacombe. 1992. *Physician Compensation in Canada: The Economics of Balancing Patient, Provider and Payer Interests.* Ottawa: Canada Medical Association. Mimeograph.

Manga, P. 1993. *Avoiding Fundamental Reforms: Current Cost Containment Strategies in Canada*. Ottawa: Queen's–University of Ottawa Economic Projects, University of Ottawa.

Mhatre, S, and RB Deber. 1992. From Equal Access to Health Care to Equitable Access to Health: A Review of Canadian Provincial Health Commissions and Reports. *The International Journal of Health Services,* 22(4): 645–668.

OECD. 1987. *Financing and Delivering Health Care: A Comparative Analysis of OECD Countries*. Paris: OECD.

OECD. 1993. *OECD Health Systems: Facts and Trends 1960-1991, Health Policy Studies No. 3*. Paris: OECD.

Pazderka, B. 1993. *Managing the Funder-Provider Interface in the Health Care System*. Ottawa: Queen's–University of Ottawa Economic Projects, University of Ottawa.

Taylor, MG. 1990. *Insuring National Health Care: The Canadian Experience*. Chapel Hill: University of North Carolina Press.

U.S.G.A.O. 1991. Canadian Health Insurance: Lessons for the United States. Report to the Chairman. Washington: Committee on Government Operations, House of Representatives.

World Bank. 1993. *World Development Report 1993: Investing in Health*. Oxford: Oxford University Press.

3

Health Status of Canadians

Carl D'Arcy

What is the current health status of Canadians? What has been the general trend in health status? Using a variety of institutional and national survey data we attempt to provide some answers to the questions.

There is no single indicator of health status of a population. Life expectancy, morbidity, disability, hospital use and alternate health care are among the variety of measures that can be used. Each measure contributes an item of information to the overall assessment of the health of a population. However, practical limitations indictate that we must focus on a limited set of indicators. Choices have to be made. In making those choices of indicators to review we have focussed on major issues. For those interested in more details and other indicators our references provide a good starting point. We review data on mortality, life-expectancy, prevalence of health problems (morbidity), mental health, disability/functional limitation, hazards at work, health protective behaviors, utilization of health services including alternate therapies and well-being. Each set of data reviewed provides us with a particular view of that multifaceted entity – the health status of Canadians.

Mortality

Mortality (death) rates in Canada have shown a general and substantial decline. The crude death rate per 1,000 population per year has declined from 11.6 in 1921 to 7.2 in 1991. The standardized death rate, which takes into account changing age and gender composition of Canada's population, shows an even greater change from 12.9 per 1,000 population in 1921 to 5.3 deaths per 1,000 population in 1991 (Peron and Strohmenger 1985; Statistics Canada *Mortality*). These changes in rates are shown in Figure 1.

These declines in death rates have not been uniformly distributed throughout the population. Between 1951 and 1990 the age-standardized all-cause mortality rates for Canadian women fell by 49.5% from 1,025 to 518 deaths per 100,000; while for Canadian men the drop was 32.8% from 1,322 to 888 deaths per 100,000 population (Nair 1993).

Death rates from specific diseases also show a diverse pattern. While most diseases have generally declined, some specific diseases have shown increases in death rates. Cardiovascular diseases are the most frequent cause of death in Canada. Age standardized (to the 1986 Canadian population) mortality rates for all cardiovascular diseases for women in Canada fell 64% from 522 deaths per 100,000 population in 1951 to 187 deaths per 100,000 population in 1992. For men the mortality rates for cardiovascular disease fell 52% from an estimated 660 deaths to 314 deaths per 100,000 population over the four decade period from 1951 to 1992 (Heart and Stroke Foundation 1995). See Figure 2.

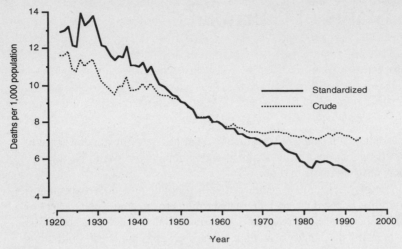

Figure 1
Crude and standardized mortality rates, Canada, 1921-1991

Note: Standardized Rate - standardized to 1971 Census population.

Source: Peron and Strohmenger 1985 and Statistics Canada, *Mortality - Summary List of Causes*, relevant years

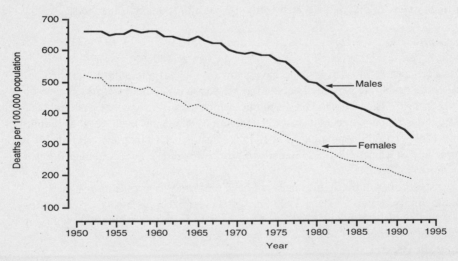

Figure 2
All cardiovascular diseases: Age-standardized mortality rates by gender, Canada 1951-1992

Note: Rates standardized to the 1986 Census population.

Source: Based on data in Heart and Stroke Foundation of Canada 1995

In contrast, age standardized rates for cancer, the second leading cause of death in Canada, have generally continued to increase during the last several decades although there is significant gender differences and variable patterns for specific cancers.

For men the age standardized mortality rates for *all* cancers increased 8.5% over the years 1969 to 1991, from 222.4 deaths per 100,000 population in 1969 to an estimated 241.3 deaths per 100,000 in 1996 (rate standardized to the age distribution for the 1991 census of Canada). In men the death rate from *all* cancers appears to have peaked at 253 deaths per 100,000 population in 1988 and has shown a slight decline and general levelling off to date during the 1990s. By comparison the age standardized mortality rate from *all* cancers for women has remained essentially flat being 152.5 deaths per 100,000 population in 1969 and an estimated 153.3 deaths per 100,000 population in 1996 (National Cancer Institute of Canada 1996). These trends in *all* cancers deaths are shown in Figure 3a.

The age standardized mortality rates from lung cancer for both sexes has shown a more striking upward trend. For males, deaths from lung cancer has increased 48.3% rising from 52.4 deaths per 100,000 population per year in 1969 to 77.7 deaths per 100,000 per year in 1996 (National Cancer Institute of Canada 1996). For women the increased deaths from lung cancers have been much more dramatic rising from 7.8 deaths per 100,000 population per year in 1969 to 34.0 deaths per 100,000 population per year in 1996 – a 335.9% increase! See Figure 3b. While the trend in deaths from lung cancer for males has essentially flattened out in the 1980s and the 90s, lung cancer deaths for females continued steadily increasing into the 1990s. Deaths from lung cancer for women now exceed deaths from breast cancer; the mortality rate for breast cancer was 29.4 deaths per 100,000 population per year in 1996 (National Cancer Institute of Canada 1996).

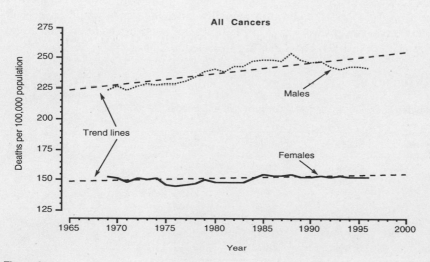

Figure 3a

Age standardized mortality rates (ages 25-74) all cancers, by gender, Canada, 1969-1996

Note: Rates standardized to 1991 census population.

Source: Based on data in National Cancer Institute of Canada 1996

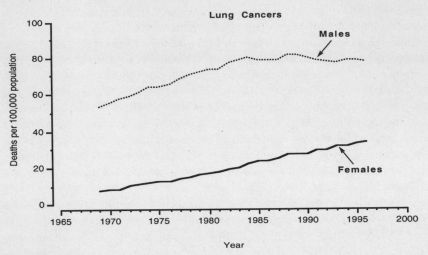

Figure 3b
Age standardized mortality rates (ages 25-74) lung cancers, by gender, Canada, 1969-1996

Note: Rates standardized to 1991 census population.

Source: Based on data in National Cancer Institute of Canada 1996

Another way to look at the impact of trends in mortality rates in the Canadian population is to look at deaths avoided as a result in changes in mortality rates over time. We estimate, using Ng's (1992) figures on mortality rates, that there would have been almost 53,000 more deaths in Canada in 1989 if the risk of death had remained at the same level as it was in 1971. These data are presented in Table 1.

TABLE 1
Deaths avoided due to declining risk of death by age and gender, Canada 1989

Age	Males	Females	Total
<1	2,336	1,680	4,016
1-14	896	599	1,495
15-34	1,373	822	2,195
35-54	5,547	2,597	8,144
55-74	12,265	7,238	19,503
75+	5,707	12,037	17,744
Totals	**28,124**	**24,973**	**53,097**

Note: The extra number of deaths that would have occurred in 1989 if the risk of death by gender and age had remained at the 1971 levels.

Source: Derived from data on age/gender specific mortality rate reduction in Ng 1992 and national estimates for the population of Canada for 1989

About 30% of "avoided deaths" involved individuals less than 55 years of age; 70% of "avoided" deaths involved individuals over 55. There were more avoided deaths among men than among women (53% versus 47%). While the above comments apply to absolute declines in mortality it is also important to look at proportional changes, since younger individuals generally have much lower absolute levels of mortality than senior adults. The same amount of absolute decline in child and youth mortality would result in a much greater proportional change for the younger age ranges than for the older age ranges. The same type of argument would apply to proportional changes for men and women. Both the absolute and proportional perspectives on "avoided deaths" is required to fully appreciate the nature of the decline in mortality that has occurred in Canada in the last decades of this century. Figure 4 shows information on the proportionate reduction in age specific mortality rates by age and gender between 1971 and 1989 per capita. A large decline in mortality is evident in younger age groups; a lesser decline in deaths among young adults; a greater decline in mortality among the middle aged groups; and a subsequent lesser decline in mortality in the older age groups.

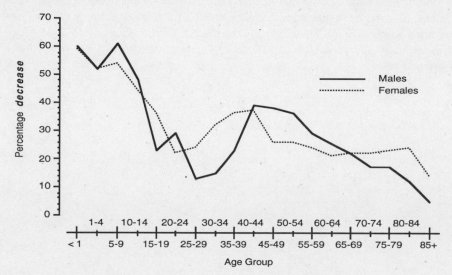

Figure 4
Proportional reduction in age specific mortality rates by gender, Canada 1971-1989

Source: Based on data in Ng 1992

Life Expectancy

In contrast to most of the measures of health status, data on estimated life expectancy has been available for Canada and for the provinces for the last seven decades. Life expectancy covering shorter periods have been calculated for various reasons and social groupings in Canada. Life expectancy is a derived measure of the mean length of life of a population cohort assuming that the mortality pattern is stabilized at the level observed during a given period. It is seen as a good indicator of the overall health of the population. Not surprisingly, given the decline in death rates, there has been a steady increase in life expectancy over the last several decades. For men life expectancy at birth has gone from 58.4 years in 1921 to 75.1 years in 1994. For women life expectancy has risen from 60.6 years in 1921 to 81.1 years in 1994. See Figure 5. The gains in life expectancy over the last seven decades has been 16.7 years for men and 20.5 years for women. Throughout the century women have reported greater gains in life expectancy than men (Statistics Canada *Deaths*).

While improvements in the health of children and reduction in child mortality have been most significant in increasing the life expectancy of Canadians, there has however been improvement in life expectancy throughout the age span, and women have benefited more than men from this improvement in life expectancy. For example, the expectancy for further life, of men 65 years of age and over, has increased 2.76 years from 13.04 more years in 1921 to 15.80 more years in 1991. For women 65 years of age and older, the increase in longevity has been greater at 6.43 years; from 13.55 further years of life in 1921 to 19.98 further years of life in 1991.

In International comparisons of life expectancy for 1993 Canada is surpassed by Japan, Sweden and Hong Kong. However Canada's life expectancy is better than that reported for the United States, Norway, France, the United Kingdom, Germany and Ireland. In the Netherlands, Spain and Australia life expectancy for males is greater than in Canada, however life expectancy in those countries for females is lower than in Canada (United Nations 1996). These data are reported in Table 2. Generally Canada fares well in terms of International comparisons of life expectancy but there is room for improvement.

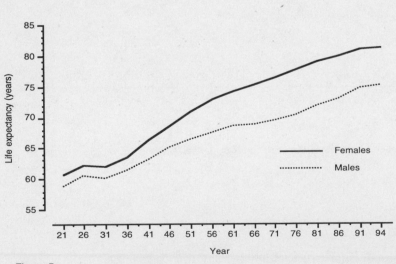

Figure 5
Life expectancy at birth by gender, Canada 1921-1994

Source: Based on data in Nagnur 1986 and Statistics Canada *Deaths*, relevant years

TABLE 2
Average life expectancy at birth, selected countries, 1993

Country	Females	Males
Japan	82.6	76.5
Hong Kong	81.9	75.7
Sweden	81.2	75.5
Canada	**80.8**	**74.3**
Netherlands	80.5	74.5
Norway	80.4	73.7
France	80.9	73.1
Spain	80.6	74.7
Australia	80.7	74.9
United Kingdom	78.8	73.7
Germany	79.1	72.8
Ireland	78.2	72.7
Italy	80.7	74.3
Brazil	68.9	64.1
Iraq	67.6	64.5
Guatemala	67.6	62.7
India	60.7	60.6
Kenya	57.1	54.1

Source: Based on data in United Nations Development Programme, *Human Development Report* 1996

Health Problems

Physical Health Problems

The General Social Survey of 1991, a large recurrent national survey of the Canadian adult population (n = 11,924), reports that almost two-thirds of Canadian adults (63%) report at least one chronic health problem. Of the 13 health conditions presented to the survey respondents the most commonly reported conditions were skin and other allergies, arthritis and rheumatism, and hypertension: the proportion of the population reporting these conditions were 21%, 21%, and 16% respectively. The likelihood of having a health condition increased with age. However, hay fever and allergies were the exception to this trend and decreased with age. More women than men reported chronic health conditions and women had higher prevalances of arthritis and rheumatism, hay fever and allergies, migraines and emotional disorders. High cholesterol, heart trouble and diabetes are the exception to this differential, being more frequently reported as health problems by men. Figure 6 shows the data on the prevalence of these selected health conditions by gender among Canadians.

The most frequent complaints that the general population report are much more prosaic continuing problems and they stand in stark comparison to the health problems discussed and shown in the media and portrayed in popular entertainment. Also worthy of note is that while women have greater longevity, they report more health problems.

Chronic health problems

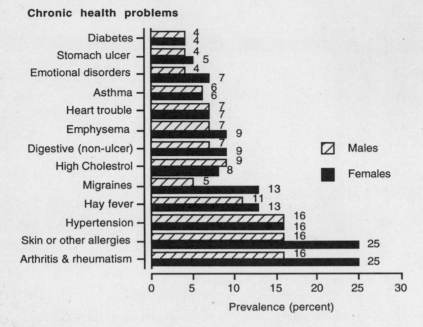

Figure 6
Prevalence of chronic health problems among Canadians aged 15+, by gender, 1991

Source: Based on data in Statistics Canada 1994

Mental Health

The previous section dealt with largely self-reported physical health problems, however some 5% of Canadian adults in that survey (4% of males and 7% of females) reported that they suffer from "emotional disorders" (Figure 6 above). Using a more rigorous and detailed interview and using more refined diagnostic criteria for a major psychiatric disorder called *Major Depressive Disorder* (MDE), the National Population Health Survey estimated that 5.6% of Canadians aged 18 and over had recently experienced depression. MDE was much more frequent among females in comparison to males, 7.3% in contrast to 3.7%. Depression also has a distinct age gradient, being more prevalent in younger adults than in older adults. Depression is three times more prevalent among those aged 18 to 24 in comparison to those 65+ (Figure 7).

Extrapolating the survey data, 5.6% of Canadians reporting MDE means some 1.1 million adult Canadians report symptoms of significant depression. While depression is a frequently occurring psychiatric disorder, generally community epidemiology surveys using standardized diagnostic interview schedules find that anxiety (panic) and phobic disorders are more frequent (Bland et al. 1988). These data suggest that mental health disorders are frequently experienced by Canadians as continuing chronic conditions.

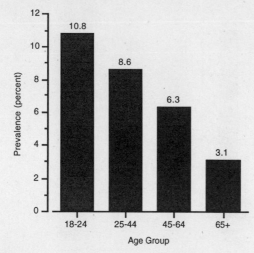

Figure 7
Prevalence of major depressive episode among Canadians by age group, 1994-95

Source: Based on data in Beaudet 1996

*the definition of
"disability" is somewhat
a value judgement*

Disability/Activity Functional Limitation

Another indicator of health status is the extent to which Canadians are disabled or feel restricted in performing their usual social roles.

The 1991 Health and Activity Limitations Survey (HALS 1991) is a very large post-censal survey of approximately 150,000 individuals living in the community and an additional 10,000 individuals living in health related institutions. The HALS 1991 survey defined three groups of individuals as having a disability: 1) those individuals who are limited in activities at home, school, work or leisure because of physical or physiological conditions; 2) those individuals who have been told by a health professional that they had a learning disability or a mental health handicap, or that they were developmentally delayed or mentally retarded; and 3) those individuals who have difficulties with learning or remembering. Using that definition of disability the survey estimated that, in 1991, 4.2 million or 16% of the Canadian population had some disability. Forty-seven percent of all those defined as being disabled had mild disability; 32% had moderate disability and a further 22% were severe disability – that is 3.7% of the adult Canadian population were considered to have severe disabilities (Statistics Canada 1995). Disabilities were more prevalent among seniors and the *severity* of disability was greatest in seniors. Major sources of disability were in the areas of mobility, agility and hearing. Approximately two-thirds of the population *with* disabilities under 55 years of age were employed in some capacity. Figure 8 shows the HALS 1986 and HALS 1991 data on disability by age in Canada for 1986 and 1991. These data indicate increasing disability throughout the life span and a slight increase in overall disability in the Canadian population between 1985 and 1991.

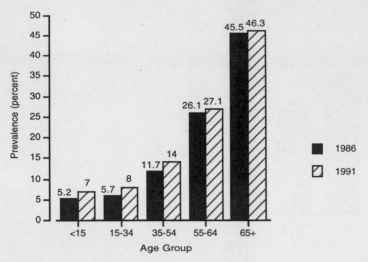

Figure 8
Percent of population with disabilities by age group, Canada, 1986 and 1991

Source: Statistics Canada 1995

Another measure of activity limitation is that of the activity restrictions that occurs in the general population called "disability days." Two-week disability-days are a combination of days spent in bed because of sickness or reduced activity days due to sickness occurring in a two week period prior to a survey interview. The General Social Survey of 1991 found the mean disability days for the general population was 0.64 days in the previous two-week period. The prevalence of disability days increases with age and are more frequent in women than in men, however, there is a decline in disability days for women during child-bearing years. Figure 9 shows the data on the average number of disability days in 1991 for Canada by age and gender.

Still another measure of functional health status is a global self-assessment of health which emphasizes abilities required to perform daily tasks. The Comprehensive Health Status Measurement System (CHSMS) is composed of a series of questions about vision, hearing, speech, mobility, use of hands and fingers, memory and thinking, feelings and pain and discomforts. The 1994-95 National Population Health Survey (NPHS) used this measure to assess the "functional" health of Canadians. The CHSMS score is from 0 (death) to 1 (perfect health). On this measure the Canadian average is 0.9 out of 1.0, nearly perfect health. Eighty-eight percent of men and 83% of women are reported to have a high level of health on this scale, a score of 0.80 or greater. Twenty-seven percent of men and 24% of women reported that they had perfect health (Federal, Provincial and Territorial Advisory Committee on Population Health 1996b). Of those who reported less than perfect health most ailments were of a minor nature that could be corrected such as farsightedness or hearing loss. Figure 10 shows the percent of Canadians with excellent and very good health by age group. It is clearly evident that with increasing age a declining portion of Canadians have excellent or very good health. A sharp decline in the proportion of Canadians in excellent health occurs among those 45-65. On the positive side however, 60% of Canadians 75+ had very good or excellent health.

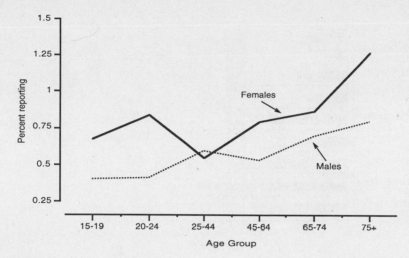

Figure 9
Mean disability days in last two weeks by age group and gender, population aged 15+, Canada, 1991

Source: Statistics Canada 1994

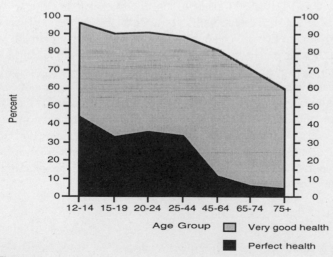

Figure 10
Proportion of Canadians aged 12+ in "perfect" or "very good" functional health, 1994-95

Source: Based on data in Federal, Provincial and Territorial Advisory Committee on Population Health 1996b

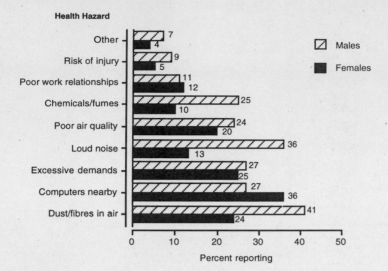

Health Hazard

Figure 11
Perceived exposure to health hazards at work by Canadians aged 15+ working at a job or business, by gender, 1991

Source: Statistics Canada 1994

Health Risks

Exposures to Health Hazards

The General Social Survey of 1991 asked Canadians a series of questions about work and health. One set of those questions dealt with exposures to largely physical work place health hazards. Two-thirds of Canadian adults who were working at a paid job or in a business believe that they were exposed to some sort of health hazard in the physical work place environment in the preceeding year. Figure 11 graphically displays exposure by type of physical hazard. Most commonly perceived exposures are due to dust fibres in the air, proximity to computer screen or video display terminals. "Excessive demands," loud noise, poor air quality and exposure to chemicals and toxic fumes were the next most frequently reported exposures. Two-thirds of individuals reporting exposures believe that these exposures had negatively affected their health. Generally more men than women reported hazard exposures at work and women were somewhat less likely to report health effects resulting from that work exposure.

Risk Factors (for disease)

High blood pressure, high cholesterol and being overweight are core risk factors for heart disease, stroke, and adult onset diabetes. Data from the National Population Health Survey and the Provincial Heart Health Surveys report that 22% of the adult population between 18 and 74 years of age have high blood pressure; 15% have high cholesterol (6.2 +mmol/L); and 32% are overweight as measured by the body mass index (BMI of 27 or more) (see Figure 12). Indeed trend data show that there has been a significant increase in obesity in the Canadian population since the mid 1980's, espe-

cially among women (Federal, Provincial and Territorial Advisory Committee on Population Health 1996b).

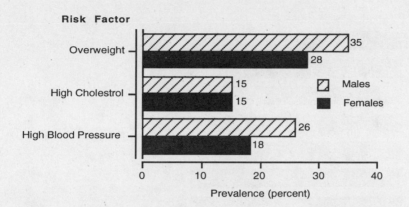

Risk Factor

Figure 12
Prevalence of selected risk factors, high blood pressure,[1] high cholesterol,[2] being overweight,[3]
among Canadians aged 18 to 74, 1994-95

Notes: [1] High blood pressure = 140/90 mm or greater and/or treatment for hypertension.
         [2] High Cholesterol = 6.2+ mmol/L.
         [3] Overweight = BMI of 27.0 or more.

Source: Federal, Provincial and Territorial Advisory Committee on Population Health 1996a

Preventive Health Practices

Some diseases are largely avoidable by practicing appropriate personal health behaviours. We recognize of course that the practice of preventive health behaviors depend
not only on individual action but also on social and institutional support, facilitation,
and dissemination of information. Data on four health practices that have been strongly
related to health outcomes are reviewed.

Immunization

Immunization, particularly of children, is essential to protect against various disabling
and even fatal diseases such as polio, measles and diptheria. Public health authorities
also recommend that senior citizens receive vaccinations against influenza which can
sometimes prove fatal in the frail elderly. Foreign travellers are also recommended to
be immunized against diseases that are endemic in the areas that they may travel to.
Figure 13 shows data on immunization coverage of children at two years of age in Canada during 1993-94. This data is taken from nationwide mail surveys of children who
had turned two but not three years of age. The greatest level of immunization in children was found to be for the diseases of measles, mumps and rubella at 97% coverage;
followed by the immunization for diptheria, pertussis (whooping cough), and tetanus
at 85 to 87%. The immunization level for polio was 90% and influenza B was 70%.
Immunization against any mengiococal disease was much more limited and is largely
confined to the provinces of Quebec and Saskatchewan. While these data indicate a rea-

sonably good level of coverage, there are still in the order of 5 to 15% of Canada's children that aren't receiving adequate immunization for potentially fatal diseases.

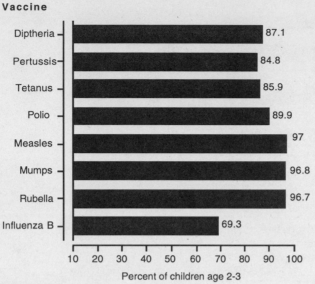

Vaccine

Figure 13
Immunization coverage of children at 2 years of age, Canada 1993-94 (95% CI)

Source: Health Canada 1997

Pap Test

Cervical cancer is a treatable disease if caught early, otherwise it is fatal. Regular Pap tests for cervical cancer have been shown to substantially reduce the mortality from cervical cancer in women. The National Population Health Survey of 1994-95 shows that some 82% of women 15 years of age and over report having a Pap test in the last three years before the survey; 55% of women report having a Pap test in the last 12 months; 15% report never having had a Pap test (Federal, Provincial and Territorial Advisory Committee on Population Health 1996b). Figure 14 shows trend data in Pap smear testing for Canada from 1985 to 1994-95. Data from three national surveys, the *1985 Health Promotional Survey*, the *1990 Health Promotional Survey* and the *1994-95 National Population Health Survey* are used. These data show a moderate increase in the proportion of women having a Pap test in the last three years and a corresponding decline in the proportion of women reporting "never" having had a Pap test.

Smoking

Smoking is a behaviour with major consequences. Makomashi-Illing and Kaiserman (1995) estimate that smoking caused the death of 41,000 Canadians in 1991. For males smoking attributable deaths comprised 26% of all male deaths: for women 15% of all deaths were attributable to smoking.

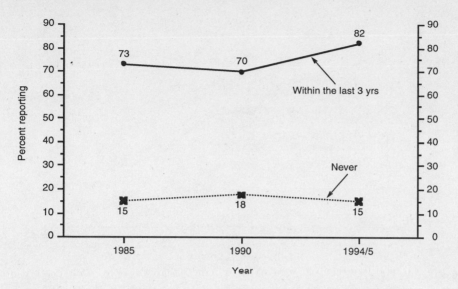

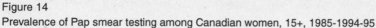

Figure 14
Prevalence of Pap smear testing among Canadian women, 15+, 1985-1994-95

Source: O'Connor 1993 and Federal, Provincial and Territorial Advisory Committee on Population
Health 1996b

The NPHS of 1994-95 found that 29% of Canadians 12 years of age and older smoked either on a daily (24%) or non-daily (5%) basis, 41% report they never smoked and 30% reported they were ex-smokers. The seven million Canadians who smoked consumed an average of 19 cigarettes a day. It should be noted that these data underestimate tobacco usage, as data on those who smoke pipes or cigars or chew tobacco are not reported here. Men are more likely to smoke than women. Cigarette smoking increases until middle years and then declines in older age groups. This age profile for smoking may be the result of both aging and birth cohort effects. Smoking as a social habit really gained prominence during the 1940's and 50's and early 1960's. From 1970 to 1990 the prevalence of cigarette smoking declined substantially from 47% to 30% of Canadians.

Figure 15 shows data from a variety of national surveys on trends in "current smoking" by gender in Canada since 1965; the decline in smoking from 1965 to 1990 is clearly evident. Since 1990 the decline in smoking appears to have levelled off. Additional data from several smaller surveys suggest that the decline in cigarette smoking has stopped and there may have been a slight increase in cigarette smoking since 1993 (Stephens 1995). Particularly disturbing is the increasing rate of smoking among young women. Canada compares favorably with other industrial countries in having a lower than average rate of smoking in its population.

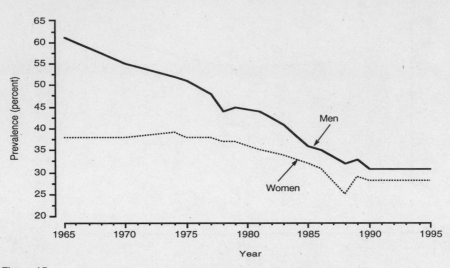

Figure 15
Trends in current cigarette smoking, Canadian population, by gender, 1965 to 1994-95

Note: Current cigarette smokers = regular daily smokers + occasional smokers. Data from 1965 to 1990 based on population 15+; data for 1994-95 includes those 12+.

Source: Based on data in Pederson 1993 and Federal, Provincial and Territorial Advisory Committee on Population Health 1996b

Exercise

A fourth preventive health measure is that of exercise. Physical activity is connected to cardiovascular health and mental health and is positively related to well-being throughout the age span. The 1991 General Social Survey found that 32% of Canadians were physically active, that is 39% of males and 26% of females. These figures are up from the similar data from the 1985 General Social Survey where 31% of males and 23% of females, 27% of the overall population, reported themselves to be active (Statistics Canada 1994). Activity as reported here is based on an index of energy expenditure. Survey respondents were classified as *sedentary* (less than 500 Kcal/wk), *moderately active* (500 to 2000 Kcal/wk), or *active* (a minimum of 2000 Kcal/wk). Survey respondents were asked a series of questions about their usual total time per week spent on various activities. The level of exertion on these activities was described as light, moderate or vigorous. Energy expenditure estimates were assigned according to the demands of the type and intensity of the physical activity engaged in. A summary measure of energy expenditure per week was then calculated for each survey respondent. While approximately one third of Canadians reported themselves active, one fifth of Canadians (22%) reported that they had a sedentary lifestyle. Women reported themselves to be more sedentary than men, 25% versus 19%. Figure 16 shows data on the percent of the population who report themselves to be active by age and gender.

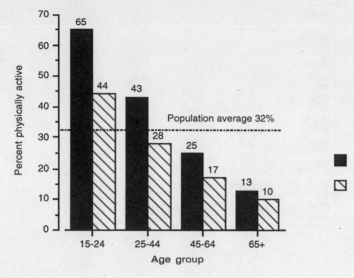

Figure 16
Percent of Canadians aged 15+, physically active, 1991

Source: Based on data in Statistics Canada 1994

Utilization of Health Services

Practitioners

Data from the NPHS of 1994-95 shows that 80% of Canadians, 73% of men and 86% of women, report that they visited a doctor during the previous 12 months. That figure increases to 92% if the same question is asked about visiting any health professional (Federal, Provincial and Territorial Advisory Committee on Population Health 1996b). Figure 17, using slightly different data from the 1991 GSS, shows data on the use of a variety of health care practitioners. General practitioners were the most frequently contacted followed by dentists, optometrists and medical specialists. Auxiliary health professionals such as psychologists or physiotherapists were contacted at a much lower rate (Statistics Canada 1994). These data clearly reaffirm that the general practitioner plays the role of gatekeeper for the Canadian health care system.

In contrast to the data reported above, during 1994-95 a much smaller 5% of Canadians aged 12+ report having used some sort of alternative therapist during the previous 12 months. Of those using alternative therapists, massage therapy was the most commonly used (46%), followed by homeopath and naturopath (31%), and acupuncturists (4.8%). Women were more likely than men to use alternate therapists, 7% versus 3%. Alternate therapist use is highest in our younger adults aged 25-44 (7% of that age group use alternative therapists). Figure 18 presents data on the percent of Canadians using various alternate therapists (Federal, Provincial and Territorial Advisory Committee on Population Health 1996b). It is usual for individuals to use regular biomedical practitioners and alternative therapists during the same time period.

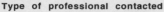

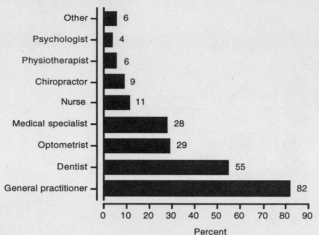

Type of professional contacted

Figure 17
Contact with selected health professionals in the past 12 months by Canadians, aged 15+, 1991

Source: Statistics Canada 1994

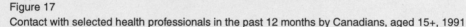

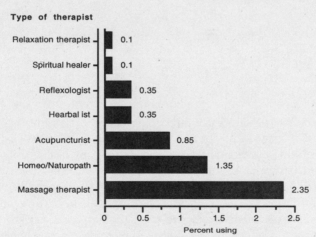

Type of therapist

Figure 18
Use of alternative health therapists in the past 12 months by Canadians, aged 12+, 1994-95

Source: Federal, Provincial and Territorial Advisory Committee on Population Health 1996b

Hospital Use

In 1992-93 Canadians spent almost 40 million days in general and special hospitals, excluding long-term psychiatric hospitals. There were 3.5 million separations (patient stays) and an average stay of 11 days in hospitals. Diseases of the circulatory system account for most of the hospital days, 19%, followed by mental disorders and cancers (Federal, Provincial and Territorial Advisory Committee on Population Health 1996b).

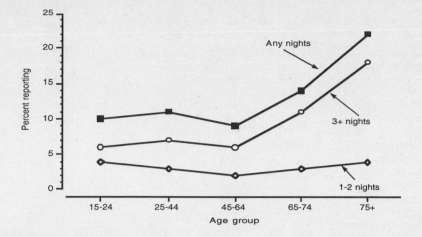

Figure 19
Percent of Canadians aged 15+ spending nights in health institutions by age group, 1991
Source: Statistics Canada, 1994

The GSS of 1991 reports that 11% of Canadians living in the community (as opposed to those living full time in institutions) spent at least one night as a patient in a hospital, nursing home or convalescent home during the past 12 months. Three percent of Canadians spent one or two nights in institutions; 8 percent spent three or more nights in such institutions. Nights in institutions are more frequent among the younger adults, decrease in middle age and rise substantially in the older age groups. Not only does the frequency of institutional nights increase in the older age groups but the proportion staying three or more nights increases (Statistics Canada 1994). Women generally report a higher number of institutional nights throughout the life span. Figure 19 shows these age related changes in hospital, nursing and convalescent home use.

Though the data reviewed here generally indicate a high level of use of health services, and some might say a higher than necessary level of use, the National Population Health Survey found that some 4% of the Canadians reported that during the last 12 months they had required some health care or advice on at least one occasion and that they *did not* receive it (Federal, Provincial and Territorial Advisory Committee on Population Health 1996a).

Medication Use

Table 3 provides national data on the use of selected medications by Canadians. The self report data are from the National Population Health Survey (NPHS) of 1994-95.

The NPHS surveyed Canadians concerning the use of prescription and non-prescription (over-the-counter, OTC) medications during the month preceding their interview. Almost 77% of Canadians reported some medication use during the *past* month. Pain relievers were by far the most often used type of medication with 61% of Canadians reporting use during the month proceeding their interview. Not surprisingly, cough and cold remedies were the next most often used type of drug, at 16%. Allergy medicines were the third most often type of medication used – 10%. Penicillin and other antibiotics were used during the past month by 9.4% of Canadians; stomach medicines were used by 8.2% of Canadians.

TABLE 3
Medications most frequently used by Canadians aged 12+ during the past month, including both prescription and over-the-counter medications, percent using, 1994-95

Medication Type	Percent of Population Using
Pain relievers	61.0
Cough/Cold remedies	16.0
Allergy medicines	9.8
Penicillin and other antibiotics	9.4
Stomach remedies	8.2
Blood Pressure medications (excluding diuretics)	7.6
Birth Control pills	5.1
Asthma medications	4.8
Heart medicine	4.2
Codeine/morphine/demerol	4.2
Menopause/aging hormones	3.4
Laxatives	2.9
Diuretics	2.8
Anti-depressants	2.8
Sleeping Pills	2.7
Tranquilizers	2.6

Source: Original analysis of the National Population Health Survey of 1994-95 public use micro dataset

Medication use appears to be generally concerned with relatively minor but frequent aches and pains, cold and flu symptoms and allergy relief. However, it is true that size-able numbers of Canadians also reported medication use for infections, blood pressure and heart disease.

A different view of medication use is provided by data on prescription drug use in the province of Saskatchewan for 1989. As Saskatchewan had a universal prescription drug plan at the time, it provides a unique opportunity to look at medication use in the general population. Quinn et al. 1992 report that during the twelve months of 1989, 66% of the provincial population received at least one prescription for a medication, and the mean number of prescriptions *per user* during the year was 8.2. Females received substantially more prescriptions than males; the most noticeable gender differences are for cardiovascular drugs, antidepressants, and benzodiazapenes. In general drug use increased with age. Among seniors (those 65+) 80.8% had received at least one prescription during the year in contrast to 63.4% of those under 65; the mean numbers of prescriptions during the year for seniors was 18.4. Seniors represented 14.6% of the study population but accounted for 40.1% of all prescriptions filled in the province and 40.2% of drug costs. Table 4 provides data on the use of select types of drugs by the Saskatchewan population. Anti-infective agents including antibiotics were the most frequently prescribed drug, painkillers including anti-inflammatory medications are the next most frequently prescribed drugs, followed by skin preparations, and hormones and hormone substitutes (including oral contraceptives, estrogen and insulin). Among the psychotherapeutic agents, anti-anxiety drugs (anxioltics, sedatives and hypnotics) were the most frequently prescribed followed by antidepressants and tranquilizers (Quinn et al. 1992).

TABLE 4
Use of selected types of prescription medications by the Saskatchewan population (%) during the year 1988

Medication	Population receiving a prescription
Antibiotics	26.2
Cardiovascular	7.5
Analgesics (pain relief)[1]	11.4
Antidepressant	2.2
Tranquilizer	0.9
Anxiolytic, sedative or hypnotic[2]	4.4
Eye, ear, nose and throat drugs	6.5
Gastrointenstinal	6.7
Hormones and substitutes[3]	8.3
Skin and mucous membrane preparations	9.4

Notes: (1) includes NSAIDs; (2) includes benzodiazepines;
(3) includes oral contraceptives, estrogen, insulin.

Source: Quinn et al. 1992

While there are regional differences in medication use in Canada and some provinces such as Quebec consume more prescription drugs than others, the Saskatchewan data provides a good picture of the extent and type of prescription medication in use in Canada.

Well-Being

In this section of the chapter we shall look at several more subjective measures of health, personal well-being, the presence or absence of stress, positive psychological health and self-reported health.

Chronic Stress

Although stress has not been implicated as a *direct* risk factor for many conditions, both chronic stress and negative life events are repeatedly reported to have a strong impact on physical and mental health. Stress in its various manifestations can affect the physiology and morphology of the circulatory system, and by psychoneuroimmunilogical mechanism, stress affects the response of organisms to external stimuli and toxic agents.

The NPHS of 1994-95 asked Canadians up to18 questions on stress in everyday life. Responses to the questions were used to assess the *relative* amount of stress in people's lives. Scores on the scale were arbitrarily divided into three intuitive categories – high, moderate, and low. The NPHS reports 26% of Canadians were rated as experiencing high chronic stress with almost equal numbers of Canadians reporting moderate (38%) and low (36%) chronic stress levels. Women report more chronic stress than men, and chronic stress, in contrast to other health conditions, is more prevalent in the younger age groups. Figure 20 provides data on the age and gender distribution of chronic stress in the Canadian population (Federal, Provincial and Territorial Advisory Committee on Population Health 1996b).

64   Health Status of Canadians

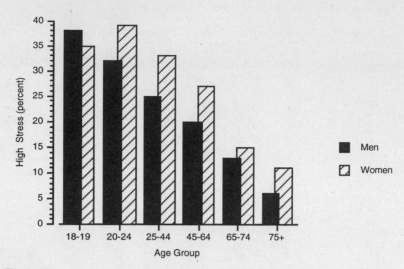

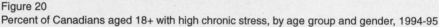

Figure 20
Percent of Canadians aged 18+ with high chronic stress, by age group and gender, 1994-95

Source: Based on data in Federal, Provincial and Territorial Advisory Committee on Population
Health 1996b

Psychological Well-Being

One problem with most health status measures is that they are largely "negative" in that
they measure illness or the absence of illness rather than health as a positive. One definition of personal well-being is that of having the mental and social attributes that permit an individual to successfully deal with the challenges one faces in life.
Antonowsky's *Sense of Coherence* scale is designed to measure that generalized resistance in individuals which facilitates "making sense out of the countless stresses with
which we are constantly bombarded" (Antonowsky 1987). The SOC scale measures the
extent to which a person views life events and challenges as comprehensible, manageable and meaningful. The concept of a *sense of coherence* is similar to notions of psychological hardiness (Kobasa, Maddi and Courington 1981) and control and mastery
(Pearlin et al. 1981; Pearlin and Schooler 1978). The SOC is a salutogenic, positive,
measure of health. The NPHS used the short 13 item version of the SOC scale to measure the psychological well-being of Canadians.

Canadians on average scored 59 out of 78, which is three-quarters of the way up the
SOC scale. On average men scored slightly higher than women on this measure of psychological well-being, however age differentials were much larger that gender differentials – sense of coherence increases significantly with age (Federal, Provincial and
Territorial Advisory Committee on Population Health 1996b). Figure 21 shows the
level of psychological well-being among adult Canadians by age group and gender.

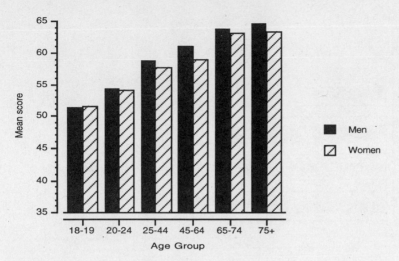

Figure 21
Psychological well-being among Canadians aged 18+, by age groups and gender, 1994-95

Source: Based on data in Federal, Provincial and Territorial Advisory Committee on Population Health 1996b

Self-rated Health

Self-rated health is the final measure we shall consider. It is considered a good predictor of health care utilization, longevity and health problems. Self-rated health provides us with the individual's summary of their current mental and physical health. Twenty-six percent of Canadians aged 12+ rate their health as *excellent*; 38% rate their health as *very good*; 10% rate their health as *poor*. When compared over time Canadians' rating of their health has remained virtually unchanged since 1985; see Figure 22. Men are more likely than women to rate their health as excellent or good but these gender differences are small. Self-reported health status deteriorates markedly with age: 4% of 15 to 19 year olds rate their health as fair or poor, this compares with 31% of Canadians aged 75 and older (Federal, Provincial and Territorial Advisory Committee on Population Health 1996b).

Conclusion

This chapter has reported on the health status of the Canadian population using a variety of measures – mortality, life expectancy, diseases, chronic problems, disability/functional limitations, risk factors, preventive health practices, utilization of health services, and general well-being. These data indicate that the health status of the Canadian population has substantially improved during this century. There have been decreases in the risk of mortality, particularly early death, increased life expectancy, increased access to health care and considerable individual satisfaction with health. However, there are some troublesome areas such as lung cancer mortality, especially in women, and obesity, which do not conform to the general trend of improving health.

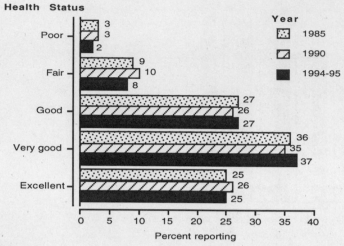

Figure 22
Self-rated health status among Canadians, aged 15+, 1985 to 1994-95

Source: Adams 1993 and original analysis of the *National Population Health Survey, 1994-95* public use dataset

Equally clear is the fact that in comparison to some other countries, Canada could still improve the health of its population, for example, in terms of overall life expectancy, perinatal mortality, and levels of immunization.

The recent Federal, Provincial and Territorial Advisory Committee on Population Health's report on *The Health Status of Canadians* notes a number of current trends: high and persistently high unemployment; high child poverty rates; growing inequalities in income; increasing obesity; smoking among teenagers and young women; and teen pregnancy rates; that, if unchanged, could have a significantly negative impact on the future health of the Canadian population (Federal, Provincial and Territorial Advisory Committee on Population Health 1996a).

Finally, not everyone in Canada shares equally in the general good health of the country. On most measures of health a sizeable proportion of Canadians fare poorly. Those suffering from *one* health problem are likely to be also afflicted by another *additional* health problem. There are also significant variations by age, gender, geographic region and socio-economic status. Aboriginal Canadians' health status is substantially lower than that of other Canadians. The average life expectancy of Status Indians, both men and women, is a full *seven years less* than that of Canadian men and women (Health Canada 1991; Statistics Canada 1993).

References

Adams, O. 1993. Health Status. In Health and Welfare Canada, T Stephens and GD Fowler, eds. *Canada's Health Promotion Survey 1990: Technical Report,* 23-31. Ottawa: Minister of Supply and Services Canada (Catalogue no. H39-263/2-1990E).

Antonovsky, A. 1987. *Unraveling the Mystery of Health: How People Manage Stress and Stay Well.* San Francisco: Jossey-Bass Publishers.

Beaudet, MP. 1996. Depression. *Health Reports* 7: 11-24.

Bland, RC, SC Newman and H Orn eds. 1988. Epidemiology of Psychiatric Disorders in Edmonton. *Acta Psychiatrica Scandinavica* 77 (Suppl. 338).

Federal, Provincial and Territorial Advisory Committee on Population Health. 1996a. *Report on the Health of Canadians.* Ottawa: Health Canada (Catalogue no. H39-385/1996-1E).

Federal, Provincial and Territorial Advisory Committee on Population Health. 1996b. *Report on the Health of Canadians: Technical Appendix.* Ottawa: Health Canada (Catalogue no. H39-385/1-1996E).

Health and Welfare Canada. T Stephens, GD Fowler, eds. 1993. *Canada's Health Promotion Survey 1990: Technical Report.* Ottawa: Minister of Supply and Services Canada (Catalogue no. H39-263/2-1990E).

Health Canada. 1997. *Canadian National Report on Immunization, 1996.* Canada Communicable Disease Report - Suppl. Vol 24S4 May, 1997. Ottawa: Health Protection Branch, Laboratory Centre for Disease Control.

Health Canada. 1991. *Health Status of Canadian Indians and Inuit - 1990.* Ottawa.

Heart and Stroke Foundation of Canada. 1995. *Heart Disease and Stroke in Canada.* Ottawa.

Kobasa, SC, SR Maddi, and S Courington. 1981. Personality and Constitution as Mediators in the Stress-Illness Relationship. *Journal of Health and Social Behaviour* 22: 268-378.

Makomaski-Illing, EM and MJ Kaiserman. 1995. Mortality Attributable to Tobacco Use in Canada and its Regions, 1991. *Canadian Journal of Public Health* 86(4): 257-265.

Nagnur, D. 1986. *Longevity and Historical Life Tables - 1921-1981 (Abridged): Canada and the Provinces.* Ottawa: Statistics Canada.

National Cancer Institute of Canada. 1996. *Canadian Cancer Statistics, 1996.* Toronto: National Cancer Institute of Canada.

Ng, E. 1992. Reductions in Age-Specific Mortality Among Children and Seniors in Canada and the United States, 1971-1989. *Health Reports* 4(4): 367-378.

O'Connor, A. 1993. Women's Cancer Prevention Practices. In Health and Welfare Canada, T Stephens and GD Fowler eds. *Canada's Health Promotion Survey 1990: Technical Report,* 169-180. Ottawa: Minister of Supply and Services Canada (Catalogue no. H39-263/2-1990E).

Pearlin, LI, MA Lieberman, EG Menaghan, and JT Mullan. 1981. The Stress Process. *Journal of Health and Social Behavior* 22: 337-356.

Pearlin, LI, and C. Schooler. 1978. The Structure of Coping. *Journal of Health and Social Behavior* 19: 2-21.

Pederson, L. 1993. Smoking. In Health and Welfare Canada, T. Stephens and Graham D. Fowler, eds. *Canada's Health Promotion Survey 1990: Technical Report,* 91-101. Ottawa: Minister of Supply and Services Canada (Catalogue no. H39-263/2-1990E).

Peron, Y. and C. Strohmenger. 1985. *Demographic and Health Indicators: Presentation and Interpretation.* Ottawa: Statistics Canada (Catalogue no. 82-543E).

Quinn, K, MJ Baker, and B Evan. 1992. A Population-Wide Profile of Prescription Drug Use in Saskatchewan, 1989. *Canadian Medical Association Journal* 146(12): 2177-2186.

Statistics Canada. *Mortality - Summary List of Causes.* Relevant Years. Ottawa: Minister of Industry, Science and Technology.

Statistics Canada. *Deaths.* Relevant Years. Ottawa: Minister of Industry, Science and Technonology (Catalogue no. 84-21.1).

Statistics Canada. 1994. *Health Status of Canadians: Report of the 1991 General Social Survey.* Ottawa: Minister of Industry, Science and Technology.

Statistics Canada. 1995. *A Portrait of Persons with Disabilities.* Ottawa: Minister of Industry, Science and Technology (Catalogue no. 89-542E).

Stephens, T. 1995. Trends in the Prevalence of Smoking, 1991-94. (Workshop Report) *Chronic Diseases in Canada*, 16:27-32.

United Nations Development Programme. 1996. *Human Development Report.* New York: Oxford University Press.

Part III
Social Factors in Health and Illness

That a variety of social factors such as education, income, gender, ethnicity, culture, work environment, social roles, and aging strongly influence the etiology, course, and outcome of disease has long been recognized and written about in the literature on the sociology of health and illness. Today some of these relationships have been "redis-covered" by some economists and epidemiologists and relabeled "determinants of health" (see *Daedalus* Fall 1994; Evans et al. 1994). Determinants of health are a major factor in the current debate about the role of health care in our society and indeed whether or not health care is really responsible for the health of the Canadian population.

Health and illness is not uniformably distributed in Canada. There are regional, gender, education, income, and ethnic differences in its distribution. These social differences in the distribution of health are evident whether one looks at mortality, specific diseases, utilization of services, or health preventive practices. But the precise nature of these relationships and the mechanisms of action underlying them are not always clearly understood. More importantly the policy implications of the connections between the social environment and health are rarely drawn out and more infrequently acted on.

Leonard Syme, the noted epidemiologist, wrote recently that "we have known for hundreds of years the people in the lowest level of the social class hierarchy have the highest rates of virtually every disease condition. Despite universal recognition, epidemiologists have not studied the reason for this phenomena" (Syme 1994). The list of possible explanations is long, but we know little of the various subcomponents that are associated with social class. Syme goes on to comment that perhaps the reluctance to examine in more detail the relationships between the social environment and health is the fact

... we do not feel that anything can be done about it. Social class is a product of vast historical, economic and cultural forces, and, short of revolution, it is not something one targets for intervention. So we give up and instead urge people to lower their fat intake. But this view is not based on fact. For example, if research were to show that people in the lower social classes had higher rates of disease because they were poor, it might be true that interventions would be difficult. In reality we have no evidence that lack of money is the major culprit. It seems premature to conclude that social class is too difficult to consider or deal with. (Syme 1994)

The chapters in this section of the book show no reluctance to examine the role of the social environment in affecting the cause, course, and outcome of illness. They deal with a variety of social factors or contingencies that influence health, illness and the use of health services. There are chapters on socioeconomic status and health, health among aboriginal Canadians, ethnicity and health, cultural constructions and health, women and health, mental health, work and health, and aging and health. Some chapters deal with several of these issues at the same time. Uniformly, the chapters explore the issue of how various social factors influence and determine health. They explore the mechanisms by which social statuses (broadly defined) and social roles shape the occurrence and the experience of health and illness.

In this Part

Carl D'Arcy's chapter, specifically written for this book, deals with the broad issues of inequalities and health. He reviews data from a variety of sources on mortality, health problems, disability, risk factors, preventive health practices, utilization of services, and well-being. Evident in these data are significant socioeconomic differentials in which those at the lowest end of the social scale suffer significantly more health problems and have higher rates of mortality. Several possible mechanisms of action whereby we can understand how socioeconomic status affects health status are delineated. The implication of these inequalities for health policy and social policy are discussed.

Wilkins and Sherman's short chapter summarizes what is known statistically about the relationship between low income, premature birth, low birth weight and other indicators of child health in Canada. The authors findings are placed in the larger context of child health. While the data indicate a narrowing of the gap of excess mortality between those at the lowest income and those at the highest income since 1971, differentials still exist and excess deaths among low income children should be reduced.

The focus of Kue Young's article is an historical review of health and demographic data for sub-arctic aboriginal Canadians. These data are examined in light of the theoretical construct of "the demographic transition." While the data reviewed showed a significant improvement in the health of sub-arctic aboriginal Canadians during the last century, they also clearly demonstrate that the health of Canada's aboriginal population lags significantly behind that of the Canadian population as a whole. Kue Young concludes his article by noting,

The health experience of sub-arctic Indians does not fit well with either the First or Third World. Increasingly, scholars have used the term 'Fourth World' to describe the 'internal colonial' situation of indigenous people in industrialized countries such as Canada. There is some justification for such a category on epidemiological grounds also. The health care debate, however, need not center on the medical care versus socioeconomic development dichotomy. It would appear that concurrent action in both areas are necessary, with neither one being the 'prerequisite' of the other. For indigenous people, medical care will perhaps ensure that the 'floor' does not sink any lower, while broad social measures will push the 'ceiling' upwards.

Kaufert and O'Neil's chapter on aboriginal health interpreters deals with the issue of consent for treatment as a pivotal event in the treatment of aboriginal Canadians from remote areas of Northern Canada. For aboriginal clients, agreements reflect the emergence of trust relationships brought about through an extended, incremental process of exchange rather than a formal final contract. Interpreters act as intermediaries in the cross cultural negotiation between doctor and patients and strongly influence that process.

Migliore focuses on punctuality, pain, and time-orientation among Sicilian Canadians. In his article, Migliore provides a cultural (meaning) interpretation for why Sicilian Canadians may arrive late for medical appointments, seek immediate relief from pain, and why their illness behaviour is often characterized by a high degree of emotion and expression.

Anderson, Blue, and Lau's article on women's perspective on chronic illness inquires into the lives of women living with a chronic illness and draws attention to the complex processes that frame the meaning of chronic illness for those that have to live with one.

Data from immigrant Chinese and Anglo-Canadian women with diabetes show that illness as a socially real entity is constructed in a complex social, political, and economic context. Styles of managing illness that could be attributed to the ethnicity are in contrast seen as pragmatic ways of dealing with the harsh realities of material existence. The authors note that individualizing social problems and shifting responsibilities for caregiving from the state to the individual obscures the social context of illness and excludes the socially disadvantaged from adequate health care.

Cultural differences in the experience and reality of menopause by women in Japan and Canada is the focus of the chapter by Kaufert and Lock. The authors central concern is to "... compare the ways in which Canadian and Japanese women, and their physicians, select, organize, and interpret the bundle of physiologic changes that occur in women as they age." The authors see in menopause a unique opportunity to explore how differences in class and culture and in economic and political power find expression to the bodies of women. Implicit and explicit in this discussion is the issue of the "medicalization" of "normal" life events and changes.

Cooperstock and Lennard deal with the issue of antianxiety drugs as solutions to "problems of living." Their study of a (mainly female) group of Toronto residents examines the social and behavioural consequences and the meaning of tranquilizer use for maintaining given social roles. Analysis of the data responds to three major questions: What are the consequences that ensue from the use of these drugs? What functions do they serve for the individual? What functions do they serve for the families and intimates of users? Although the authors caution that the nature of their sampling prohibits generalizing to the larger population, they emphasize that "... in order to understand the functions served by those drugs, it is necessary to look beyond the medical model of disease to the structural factors creating the stresses that bring many people to the attention of the health care system."

Continuing the theme of psychotherapeutic drug use Rawson and D'Arcy's article on the use of sedatives (minor tranquillizers) and hypnotics (sleeping pills) examines data on the self reported use of these drugs in national surveys of Canadians over the last two decades. The results of the analyses suggest that the use of these drugs in Canada is about average for an industrialized society. The use of sedative hypnotics was higher among women, the elderly, separated, divorced, or widowed individuals, those who had a secondary school education or less, individuals with low family income, the retired and the unemployed. Among women, higher rates of use were reported by those whose main activity was keeping house, as compared with those who were employed outside the home, and by those who lived alone. Higher rates of use were also found for individuals who had consulted a physician or had been hospitalized recently, individuals taking multiple drugs, those who scored highly on an anxiety scale, persons in whom negative feelings predominate, and those who experience the high frequency of psycho-physiological symptoms of anxiety and depression. From a regional point of view the highest rates of use for women were consistently reported from Quebec, while the lowest rates were consistently found in the Prairies. No consistent regional pattern was found for men.

It has been suggested that higher levels of distress among women may be partially a function of their nurturant roles. Role related differences in exposure and/or responsiveness to events occurring to network members are hypothesized to represent a "cost of caring" for women that translates into elevated levels of depressive symptoms. Turner and Avison examine the significance for depressive symptoms of gender differences in exposure and vulnerability to eventful stress among a sample of physically disabled subjects. They find that indeed the well established relationship between gender and depression (women report more depressive symptoms) can at least be partially understood as arising from systematic sex differences in exposure and/or vulnerability to stressful life events. Women were found in this study to report more negative events than men. This difference did not primarily involve events occurring to the respondent but rather resulted from differences in the number of events reported as happening to important "others" in their network.

Pursuing the issue of gender differences in health and illness, particularly mental health, Lowe and Northcott explore how job conditions influence overall physical and psychological well-being among unionized postal workers employed by Canada Post in Edmonton. The results of the study emphasize the dominant, direct, and pervasive influence of job characteristics on the psychological well being of both men and women.

While it is clear that lay persons do indeed routinely self-evaluate and self-treat many of their health problems as part of daily living, the nature and extent of the self-care practices are not well understood. Segall and Goldstein examine the issue of self-care in a random sample of Winnipeg residents. The results of their study suggest that select social characteristics and skeptical attitudes towards physicians are important correlates of self-care. Women, younger people, and those with a university education were more likely to engage in self-care practices.

In the final chapter of this section of the book, Roos and Havens use data from the Manitoba Longitudinal Study on Aging to examine predictors of successful aging. Three questions are addressed: 1) what proportion of a seniors cohort will age successfully?; 2) what are the health care expenditure patterns associated with successful aging?; and, 3) which characteristics of individuals predict successful aging? For this study successful aging was defined in terms of an individual retaining the ability to function independently. Twenty percent of the cohort were judged to have aged successfully. Those who aged successfully reported greater satisfaction with life, made fewer demands on the health care system and were less likely to have their spouses die or enter a nursing home.

References

Evan, RG, ML Barer and TR Marmor. 1994. *Why are Some People Healthy and Others Not?*: *The Determinants of Health of Populations.* New York: Aldine DeGruyter.

Daedulus. Special Issue. Health and Wealth. 1994; 123(4) (Fall).

Syme, SL. 1994. The Social Environment and Health. *Daedulus* 123(4): 79–86.

4

Social Distribution of Health Among Canadians[*]

Carl D'Arcy

Introduction

Social and socio-economic differences in health status have been a persistent character-istic of Canadian society. Currently, and traditionally, there have been and are substan-tial age, gender, regional, educational, occupational, income, and ethnic differences in mortality, morbidity, and well-being.

Cross-sectional data on morbidity, the utilization of services, mortality, disability, health information and knowledge, health related behaviors, and general well being show that significant inequalities in health currently exist in Canada (e.g., Billette and Hill 1978; Cadman et al. 1986; D'Arcy 1986, 1987, 1989; Canada 1980; Evers and Rand 1982, 1983; Evers et al. 1987; Federal, Provincial and Territorial Advisory Com-mittee on Population Health 1996; Hay 1988; Jarvis and Boldt 1982; Kue Young 1988a; Health and Welfare Canada 1986, 1987; Miller and Wigle 1986; Morrison et al. 1986; Rootman 1986; Wigle and Mao 1980; Wilkins and Adams 1983).

For example, physical and mental health problems and disability vary by age and sex. Women report more episodes of illness and use more medical services than males but live longer. Males report higher levels of more severe illnesses such as heart dis-ease, cancers, and accidents etc. than females. These gender differences are obviously a function of the complex interplay of physiological and social factors.

There are regional and educational differences in self-protective behaviors such as immunization, Pap smear testing, breast self-examination, exercise, cigarette smoking, etc. Health protective behaviors are generally practiced more frequently by those with higher education and by those with higher income levels. There are socio-economic differences in disability with those reporting higher levels of disability having signifi-cantly lower income (Statistics Canada 1995).

There are occupational and income differences in overall mortality and in mortality from specific disorders. In the lowest income category, accidents, neoplasms and dis-eases of the respiratory system in males, and congenital abnormalities in females, are relatively more frequent for those aged 1-14 years. Diseases of the circulatory system are the major source of income-related mortality differentials in the 35-64 age group.

* This is a much revised and updated version of a paper entitled "Reducing Inequalities in Health in Canada? Trends and Implications" presented at the session on "Social Dimensions of Health and Ill-ness" at the 25th Annual Conference of the Canadian Sociology and Anthropology Association at the Learned Societies Conferences, University of Victoria, May 26-30, 1990.

Circulatory diseases are relatively more frequent causes of death in lower income groups (Wigle and Mao 1980).

The unemployed are found to report significantly higher levels of psychological distress, short-term disability, major activity limitation, health problems, hospitalizations, and health service utilization. Though health effects of unemployment persisted across various socio-economic and demographic statuses, they were more pronounced for some groups. Females and older unemployed individuals reported more health problems and physician visits whereas the "low-income" unemployed who were also the principal family earners, reported much more psychological distress (D'Arcy 1986).

Native Indian and Inuit populations have significantly poorer health and much shorter life expectancy than the rest of Canadians. The greatest risk to life among the status Indian population occurs in the time from birth to one year and in adolescence and young adulthood. The stillbirth rate for the Indian population is one-third higher than the national average. Indian death rates from violence, either self- or other-inflicted, or accidents, are substantially higher than national rates. These discrepancies in health are no doubt a reflection of the substantially poorer economic conditions and living standards that confront Canada's native populations (Canada 1980; Jarvis & Boldt 1982; Kue Young 1988b, and Waldram et al. 1995).

Socio-economic status variables, in addition to the demographic variables of age and gender, emerge as dominant defining social characteristics that affect health status. Socio-economic status also substantially modifies the effect of demographic variables on health.

Evidence of regional and socio-economic differences in health were central to the movement for the development of public comprehensive health programs in Canada during the early and middle decades of this century (Canada Sickness Survey 1960).

During the last several decades significant improvements have occurred in basic measures of the health status of Canadians.

Mortality rates in Canada have shown a general and substantial decrease, while mortality from specific categories of diseases show a more diverse pattern with decreases in the age-standardized mortality rates for cardiovascular disease (the leading cause of death in Canada) while the age-standardized rates for cancer, the second leading cause of death in Canada, continues to increase, although there are variable patterns for specific cancers, e.g., there has been a large increase in lung cancer deaths in women (see Chapter 3).

This Chapter

This chapter reviews current data on the social distribution of health in Canada, and by implication data on social inequalities in health in Canada. Data is presented on the distribution of life expectancy, mortality, health problems, disability and activity limitation, risk factors, preventative health practices and well-being. The dominant role of socio-economic status (SES) in determining health is evident in those data.

The question of whether or not there have been decreases or increases in social inequalities in health in Canada during the last several decades is also addressed. We also discuss the possible mechanisms of action underlying this SES-health connection and point to some of the policy implications that emanate from these data.

Life Expectancy

In contrast to most other measures of health status, data on estimated life expectancies has been available for Canada and the provinces for the last seven decades. Life expectancies covering shorter periods have been calculated for various social groupings in Canada. Life expectancy is a measure of the mean length of life of a cohort assuming that the mortality pattern is stabilized at the level observed during a given period. It is seen as a good indicator of the overall health of a population. It is considered the best summary indicator of general trends in inequalities in health in Canada.

Age and Gender Trends

For men, life expectancy at birth has gone from 58.4 years in 1921 to 75.1 years in 1994. For women, life expectancy has risen from 60.6 years in 1921 to 81.1 in 1994. The gains for men over the seven decades have been 16.7 years; for women the gains have been 20.5 years. Generally, throughout these decades women have reported greater gains in life expectancy than men (See Figure 5 in Chapter 3).

While improvements in the reduction in child mortality and improvements in the health of children have been the most significant factor in increasing the life expectancy of Canadians, there has been improvements in life expectancy throughout all age groups. Women have benefited more than men in the improvements of life expectancy of middle and older age groups. For example, the expectancy for further life of men aged 65 has increased 2.76 years from 13.04 more years in 1921 to 15.80 years in 1991. For women aged 65 the increase in longevity has been greater at 6.43; from 13.55 further years of life in 1921 to 19.98 further years of life in 1991.

These increases in life expectancy for those aged 65 are shown in Figure 1.

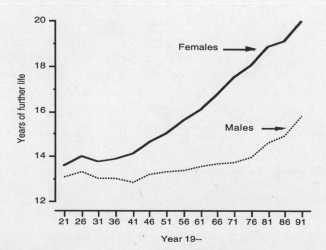

Figure 1
Life expectancy at age 65 by gender, Canada, 1921 to 1991

Source: Nagnur 1986 and Statistics Canada *Deaths,* relevant years

Regional Trends

During the earlier part of the century life expectancy at birth and other ages differed significantly from province to province; however, with few exceptions, there has been a strong trend towards the convergence of life expectancies and survival probabilities not only at birth but also for other age groups since 1931. The provincial difference in life expectancy at birth was greatest in 1931, being approximately 8 years for both males and females. In 1931, Quebec had the lowest life expectancy for males and females at 56.2 and 57.7 years respectively; the highest life expectancies for males and females was in Saskatchewan at 64.2 and 65.9 years respectively. In 1991, the provincial difference in life expectancy had declined to 2.1 years for both men and women. Saskatchewan had the longest life expectancy for males and females at 72.8 and 80.5 years respectively. Prince Edward Island had the lowest life expectancy for men at 73.2 years and Newfoundland had the lowest life expectancy for women at 79.5 year (Nagnur 1986; Statistics Canada, *Deaths*).

Figure 2 shows differences between highest and lowest life expectancies among the provinces at age 15 and at age 65. The trend toward convergence – reducing provincial inequalities – is most evident for the younger age groups.

Intra-regional variations also exist. Substantial variations in life expectancy have been noted for various community sizes with larger metropolitan areas registering longer life expectancies (Wilkins and Adams 1983). Similar substantial variations have also been found within a single metropolitan area (Wilkens 1986).

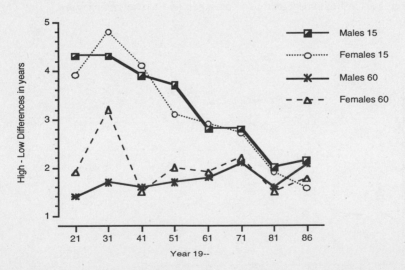

Figure 2
Difference between highest and lowest life expectancies among Canadian provinces at age 15 and 60 by gender, 1921-1986

Source: Nagnur 1986 and Statistics Canada 1990

Income Trends

Data on life expectancy for various socio-economic groupings shows some encouraging and some discouraging patterns. Life expectancy by income for metropolitan Canada in 1971 was reported to be 72.47 years for males in the highest income quintile and 66.33 years for those in the lowest income category. The comparable 1971 figures for females were 77.45 years and 74.62 years (Wigle and Mao 1980). The same life expectancy estimates for 1986 are 76.0 years in the highest income quintile years and 70.5 years in the lowest income quintile for males. For females the 1986 figures are 81.1 years and 78.9 years (Adams 1990: 13). Thus, during the 1970s and the early 1980s there was a reduction in the life expectancy differentials between the highest and lowest income quintiles for both men and women while at the same time there has been an overall increase in life expectancy. The life expectancy income differential for men decreased from 6.2 years in 1971 to 5.5 years in 1986. For women, the differential decreased from 3.2 years to 2.2 years. Gender differences in life expectancy are greatest in the lowest income quintile. For men the greater gains in life expectancy have been registered by the lowest income quintile, 4.2 years, in contrast to gains of 3.5 years in the highest income quintile. For women there were similar greater gains in the lowest income quintile, 4.3 years in contrast to gains of 3.3 years in the highest income quintile; see Figure 3.

But, if we look at gains in life expectancy at age 60, greater gains are recorded by the highest income quintiles than the lowest income quintiles.

Aborignal Life Expectancy

Comparisons of life expectancy between Indian and non-Indian are not very encouraging in terms of reducing inequalities in health. Although average life expectancy at birth for both Indians and the national population has improved, the discrepancy in life expectancy between Indians and the national population has largely remained unchanged or increased. In 1961, 1971, 1981, and 1986 the life expectancy at birth for male Canadian aboriginals were 59.7, 60.2, 62.4 and 63.8 years - some 8.8, 9.1, 9.5, and 9.2 fewer years of life expectancy than the national population. For women aborginals life expectancies were 63.4, 66.2, 68.9, and 71.0 years of life respectively. Thus, female Indians had 10.8, 10.1, 10.0, and 8.7 fewer years of life expectancy in 1961, 1971, 1981, and 1986 (Health and Welfare Canada 1986, 1991); see Figure 4.

However, other data on the health status of native Indians is a bit more encouraging. These data show declines in Aboriginal mortality from infections, parasitic and respiratory diseases, as well as from perinatal conditions (see Kue Young, Chapter 6). However, the crude mortality rates for accidents and circulatory diseases show sharp rises during the 1940s, 1950s, 1960s, and early 1970s with a peak appearing in the late 1970s and some slight decline since then. Mortality from neoplasms for Indians, like that of the rest of the Canadian population, shows a gradual upward trend since 1950.

Immigrants Life Expectancy

Chen et al. (1996a) in reviewing the health of Canada's immigrants based on an analysis of data from the large-scale National Population Health Survey (NPHS) of 1994-5 notes that when they arrive in Canada immigrants are a relatively healthy group. This is not surprising given that individuals in good health are more inclined to emigrate –

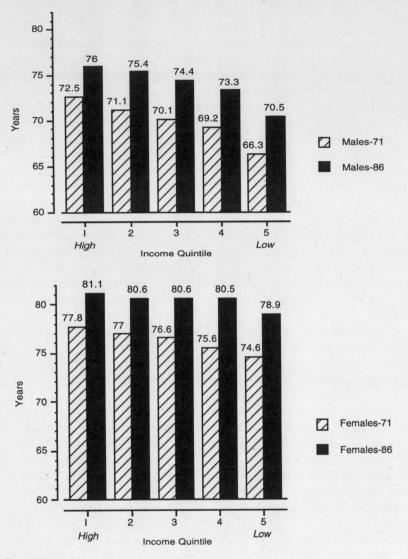

Figure 3
Life expectancy at birth by income quintile and gender, Canada 1971 and 1986

Source: Wigle and Mao 1980 and Adams 1990

the healthy emigrant effect. Second, potential immigrants to Canada are subject to screening to ensure that they do not suffer from serious medical conditions and that they are fit enough to seek employment in Canada. Recent immigrants (less then 10 years since time of arrival), regardless of their country of birth, were found to be healthier than the Canadian-born; this was particularly true of immigrants from non-European countries. But among immigrants who have lived in Canada for more than 10 years the prevalence of chronic conditions and long term disability approaches the levels found in the Canadian-born population. As time in Canada lengthens, immigrants lifestyles and health related behaviours come to resemble those of the Canadian-born.

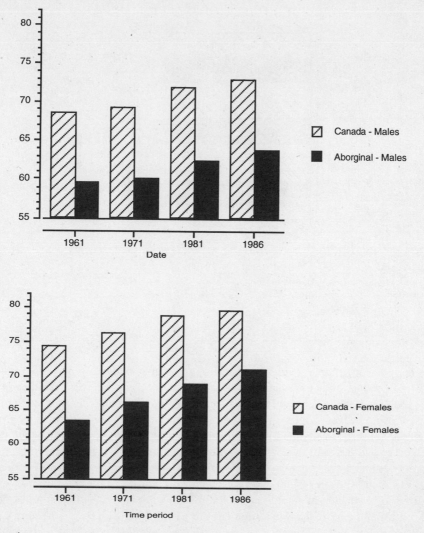

Figure 4
Aboriginal Life Expectancy, Canada 1961-1986

Source: Health and Welfare Canada 1986 and 1991

In a separate article Chen et al. (1996b) found that immigrants, especially those from non-Europoean countries, had longer life expectancy and more years of life free of disability and dependency than did the Canadian-born. However, while immigrants were less likely than the Canadian-born to be disabled, they were only slightly less likely to be dependent on others for help with activities of daily living. The data on life expectancy for Canadian-born, European immigrants and non-European immigrants are presented in Figure 5.

Chen et al. (1996b) conclude that the most likely reason for immigrants longevity and relative good health is the healthy immigrant effect.

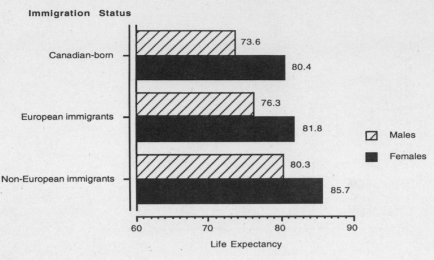

Figure 5
Immigrants Life Expectancy, Canada, 1991

Source:　Chen et al. 1996b

Career Earnings and Survival

There is good longitudinal evidence of a strong positive association between mid-to-late career earnings and subsequent survival after 65 for Canadian men. Wolfson et al. (1993) used the Canada Pension Plan as a source of data on income in order to examine the relationship between income and mortality. The Canada Pension Plan is a compulsory public earnings-related pension plan which (along with the identical Quebec Pension Plan) covers 100% of the Canadian paid labour force. Employment earnings, both of employees and the self-employed, are subject to a payroll tax administered annually as part of the income tax system. Everyone who has contributed for at least three years is eligible for a pension at age 65, and a lump sum death benefit. (Provision has been made recently for a more flexible retirement age.) Thus those who have worked in Canada outside the province of Quebec and have attained the age of 65 are (or will become) beneficiaries of the Canada Pension Plan. The year and month of death is recorded on the file of the CPP for the purposes of terminating the pension and disbursing the lump sum death benefit. The CPP was started in 1966; the beneficiary file contains over 5 million records. Wolfson et al. focused their analysis on the records of males who had attained the age of 65 on or after September 1, 1979. The analysis covers the records of 545,769 individuals. The sample was restricted to males because their pre-retirement earnings history was considered more indicative of family SES than that of females.

The authors conclude that their analysis of these data clearly show a significant income-related mortality gradient. Higher earnings decades prior to age 65 are associated with lower mortality during the following nine years. Being married, not retiring early, not being disabled and experiencing improvements in earnings (above inflation) during the latter decades of one's career, are all significantly associated with higher survival probabilities. Figure 6 shows data from this study on survival by income quintile to age 74.

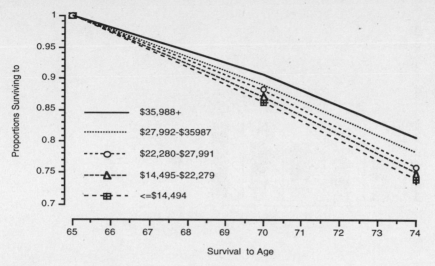

Figure 6
Proportion of CPP retiree's surviving to age 74 by income quintile

Source: Wolfson et al. 1993, Table 2

Wolfson et al. note that if all of the CPP cohort they studied had experienced the mortality rates of the highest income quintile (the top 20 percent of average earners) then survival probabilities would have been increased by 8 percentage points. That increase is equivalent to increase in survival that would occur if cancer as a cause of death among males was eliminated (Nagnur and Nagrodski 1987).

Comment

Though there has been a reduction in income inequalities in life expectancy in Canada during the last two decades it is still evident that irrespective of age, significant differentials in life expectancy by income and aboriginal/non-aboriginal status still exist. If we look internationally there is certainly room for improvement in the overall life expectancy of Canadians.

Mortality

Infant Mortality

Infant mortality in urban Canada has generally shown considerable improvement during the last several decades. In 1971 infant mortality in the lowest income quintile was 20 per 1,000 live births, twice as high as the 10 per 1,000 live births in the highest income quintile. By 1986 infant mortality had been cut almost in half with the mortality rate being 11 per 1,000 live births in the lowest income quintile and 6 per 1,000 live births in the highest income group. Though there has been a substantial improvement in the overall reduction of infant mortality in Canada and some lessening in the income gradient in infant mortality, there nevertheless remains a substantial income gradient in infant mortality rates in Canada. Infants in the lowest income quintile are 83 percent more likely to die than those in the highest income quintile. These data on income and infant mortality are shown in Figure 7.

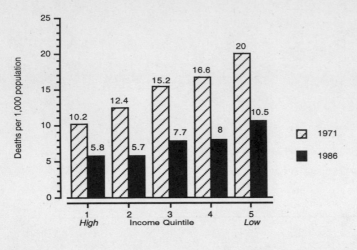

Figure 7
Infant mortality by income quintile, by sex, urban Canada, 1971 and 1986

Source: Wilkins, Adams, and Brancker 1989, Table 4

Selected Causes of Deaths by Income

We noted in the introduction that Wigle and Mao (1980) in their study of socio-economic differences in mortality found that there were, in 1971, significant differences in frequency and cause of death by income categories and that there were age/income interactions in these patterns. Large mortality differences by income category were observed for a variety of diseases. Among adult men and women the income differential was greatest for circulatory diseases. Wilkins, Adams, and Brancher (1990) updated the Wigle and Mao study looking at data on 88,129 deaths occurring in Canada's census metropolitan areas during 1986. These deaths were categorized as to cause of death, and the residence location of the deceased were categorized in terms of detailed census track economic characteristics of the area classifying them into five income quintiles.

Wilkins et al. found that the major causes of death in 1986 which contributed most to income inequalities in mortality were circulatory diseases, accidents, poisonings and violence, and neoplasms. Using the measure of potential years of life lost (PYLL) prior to age 75, circulatory diseases were found to account for twenty-five percent of excess PYLL related to income differentials in mortality; accidents, poisonings and violent causes of death account for 17 percent of excess PYLL; and neoplasms (cancers) account 15 percent. Respiratory diseases, ill-defined conditions, metabolic diseases and perinatal conditions were each found to contribute six or seven percent of excess PYLL related to income differentials (Wilkin et al. 1989).

In order to highlight "success" and "failures" with respect to reducing income inequalities in mortality, Wilkins et al. categorized causes of death in three categories: "successes," were diseases where overall mortality had declined during the 1971-86 period and the income gradient in mortality had diminished; "little change" were diseases for which there was little change in the mortality associated with income gradients or in which there was somewhat less inequality but in the context of higher mortality; and "failures," diseases in which mortality was higher and there was also increased inequality in mortality associated income gradient.

Improvement ("success") was registered in the overall mortality and income gradients of perinatal conditions, infectious diseases, cervical cancer, stomach cancer, diabetes mellitus, respiratory diseases, digestive system diseases, cirrhosis of the liver, motor vehicle traffic accidents, pedestrian accidents, accidental poisonings, drownings, and fires over the 1971-84 period.

"Little change" was evident in the mortality characteristics of breast cancer, colon and rectal cancer, circulatory diseases except ischemic heart disease and cerebrovascular disease, alcoholism, and nervous system diseases.

"Failures" include lung cancer, suicide, mental conditions, metabolic diseases other than diabetes, and undefined conditions. These "failures" are most evident in males.

Figure 8 provides data on trends in age standardized mortality rates by income quintiles for infectious diseases (a success), breast cancer (little change), and lung cancer for males and suicide (both failures), in urban Canada, for the years 1971 and 1986.

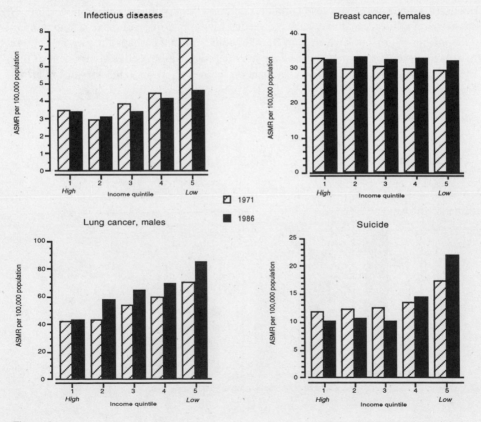

Figure 8
Age standardized mortality rates (ASMR) for selected causes of death, by income quintile, urban Canada, 1971 and 1986

Source: Wilkens, Adams, and Brancher 1989, Chart 6

Health Problems and Socio-Economic Status

Heart Disease

The National Population Health Survey of 1994-95 (NPHS) asked respondents whether or not those surveyed had a long-term condition diagnosed by a health professional. Heart disease was among the many conditions the survey inquired about. Extrapolating survey results to the national population, Figure 9 shows the effects of income on the prevalence of heart disease in those aged 45+. NPHS respondents were classified into five income adequacy categories depending on household income and size of household. For example, the dollar cutoff for the lowest income is less than $10,000 for household sizes of 1 to 4 persons, and less than $15,000 for household sizes of 5 or more persons. The highest income category includes those with $60,000 income for households of 1 or 2 persons, and $80,000 for households of 3 or more persons (NPHS 1996).

The data show that for both men and women the lowest rates of heart disease occur among those with the highest income. For men the highest rates of heart disease occurred among men with lower middle incomes. Men with lowest income category appear anomalous in that they have the second lowest rate of heart disease among men. The reasons for this is unclear. One could hypothesize that perhaps the physical nature of work that lowest income men engage in may provide a protective component or that there is an age interaction effect. The data on women show a straightforward relationship increased between income and the declining prevalence of heart disease.

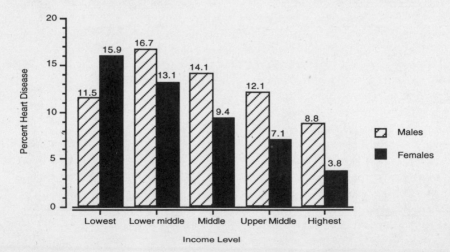

Figure 9
Prevalence of Heart Disease among Canadians, 45 years of age and older, by gender and income level, 1994-95

Source: Original analysis of the National Population Health Survey public access micro dataset

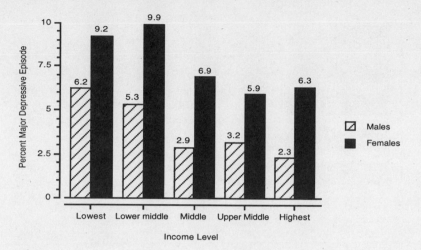

Figure 10
Prevalence of Major Depressive Episode among Canadians, 18+, by gender and income level, 1994-95

Source: Original analysis of the National Population Health Survey public access micro dataset

Major Depressive Episode

The NPHS of 1994-95 also asked a detailed set of questions on an individual's mood in order to assess the prevalence of a major psychiatric disorder called Major Depressive Episode (MDE). Some 5.6% of Canadians 18 and over had recently experienced depression. Evident in that data is a clear cut inverse relationship between income adequacy and risk of depression. Those with the lowest incomes have the highest risk of MDE; those in the high income category have the lowest risk of depression. That finding holds true for both men and women. These data also show higher rates of depression being consistently reported by females in all income categories.

Dental Health

A population's dental health is an indirect measure of the dental hygiene, access to dental care, and nutrition in that population. Canada's Health Promotion Survey of 1990 asked a variety of questions on dental health. Although there is a strong relationship between age and dentate status, a very basic measure of the dental health of a population is that of the percent of the population who have at least one natural tooth.

Only fifty percent of Canadians 65 years of age and older have one or more natural teeth. Figure 11 shows the strong direct relationship between income and having one or more natural teeth. Evidence in these data is a strong positive relationship between having natural teeth and income. In 1990, 36% of Canadians aged 15+ in the lowest income category had no natural teeth. In contrast only 3% of those in the highest income category did not have any natural teeth.

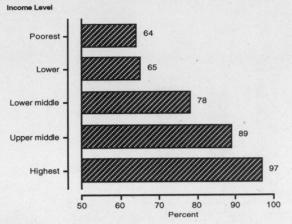

Figure 11
Persons with 1+ natural teeth among Canadians aged 15+, by income level, 1990

Source: Charette 1993

Disability/Activity Limitation

The General Social Survey of 1991 asked Canadians a series of questions about whether or not they were limited in the activities they could carry out at home and at work. Figure 12 shows data on Activity Limitation by income among Canadians 15 years of age and older. The income categories reported here are similar to those used in the NPHS analysis but of course reflect income levels in 1991 (Statistics Canada 1994). These data again show an inverse relationship between income and activity limitation. Those in the lowest income category were three times more likely to report some activity limitation.

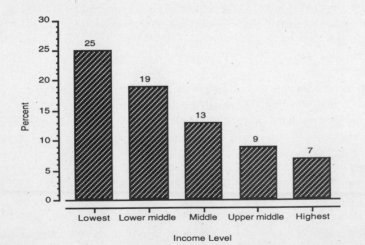

Figure 12
Prevalence of activity limitation among Canadians, aged 15+, by income level, 1991

Source: Statistics Canada 1994

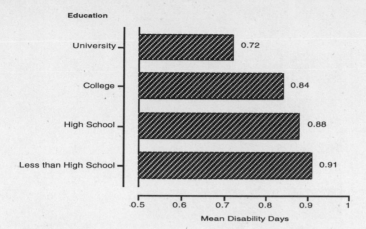

Figure 13
Frequency of disability days in the two previous weeks among Canadians, by educational level (age-standardized), 1994-95

Source: Federal, Provincial and Territorial Advisory Committee on Population Health 1996b

Disability Days

Another measure of activity limitation is that of "disability days." Two-week disability days are a combination of days spent in bed because of sickness, or reduced activity days due to sickness occurring in a two-week period prior to a survey interview. The National Population Health Survey of 1994-5 asked several questions on days sick and reduced activity days. Figure 13 show data on the occurrence of "two-week disability days" by education level among Canadians. These data show the lowest number of disability days occurs among those who have completed university training.

Disability

The 1991 Health and Activity Limitation Survey (HALS), a very large postcensal survey of Canadians shows very clearly that persons with disability have much lower incomes than those without disability. This income disparity is evident at all ages. Table 1 shows the data on the average income of persons 15+ by disability status.

TABLE 1
Average income of persons aged 15 and over living in households, Canada, 1990

Age Group	Average Income - Dollars	
	With disabilities	Without disabilities
15-34	15,650	19,015
35-54	24,160	33,330
55-64	20,320	31,040
65 and over	16,940	19,605

Note: Excludes persons with no income in 1990.

Source: Statistics Canada 1995

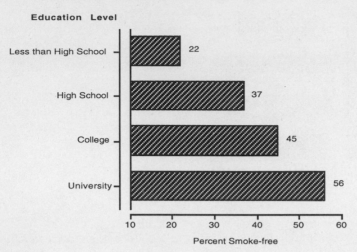

Figure 14
Prevalence of smoke-free workplaces among working Canadians, aged 15+, by education, 1994

Source: Health Canada 1994

Risks

Smoke-Free Workplace

One measure of exposure to health risks in the workplace is that of working in a "smoke-free" environment. The NPHS of 1994-95 asked survey respondents about smoking at work and restrictions in smoking at work. Thirty-nine percent of Canadians aged 15+ reported that smoking was not allowed at their workplace. Smoking was allowed in some places in 31 percent of worksites. Twenty-nine percent of workplaces allowed smoking in most places at the worksite. Figure 14 shows the percent of Canadians 15+ who reported that smoking was not allowed at their workplace by education level obtained. Those with less than a high school education were most likely to be exposed to smoke at the workplace, whereas those with a university degree were the least likely to be exposed to smoke at the workplace. These data hint at a class-based relationship in smoking behaviour.

Risk Factors for Disease

High blood pressure, high cholesterol and being overweight are core risk factors for heart disease, stroke and adult onset diabetes. The Provincial Heart Health Surveys of 1986 to 1992 which undertook physical examination of Canadians report that 22% of Canadians age 18 to 84 have high blood pressure; 15% have high cholesterol levels, and 32% have a body mass index (BMI) equal to or greater than 27. The data in Figure 15 show the relationship between the prevalence of those risk factors and education. For all three risk factors there is a clear inverted SES gradient. Higher rates of high blood pressure, high cholesterol, and a BMI ≥ 27 are found in those with 12 or fewer years of education; in contrast those with 16+ years of education had the lowest prevalence of these three risk factors.

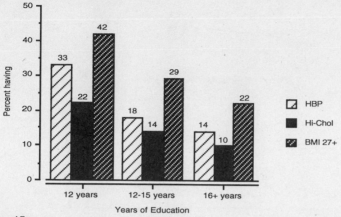

Figure 15
Prevalence of high blood pressure, high plasma cholesterol, and obesity, Canada 1986-92, population aged 18-74

Note: High blood pressure = 140/90 mm
       High cholesterol = 6.2 + mmol/L
       Overweight = BMI of 27.0 or greater

Source: Federal, Provincial and Territorial Advisory Committee on Population Health 1996

Preventive Health Practices

It is strongly suggested in the research literature that some diseases, such as cervical cancer, lung cancer, heart diseases, adult onset diabetes, etc. are largely avoidable through the practice of appropriate personal health behaviours.

Pap Test

Cervical cancer is a treatable disease if caught early. Regular Pap tests have been shown to substantially reduce the mortality from cervical cancer in women. The NPHS of 1994-95 report 85 percent of women 16+ report that they had a Pap smear at some point in their lives. Fifteen percent reported they never had a Pap smear. However this health practice of having a Pap smear is not uniformly distributed in the population. As Figure 16 shows, women with less than a high school education were more likely *never to have had* a pap smear test (20%) and less likely *to have had* a Pap test in the last 3 years (recommended practice).

Smoking

Smoking is a behaviour with major health consequences. Smoking is attributed with causing 26 percent of all male deaths and 15 percent of all female deaths (Makomashi-Illing and Kaiserman 1995).

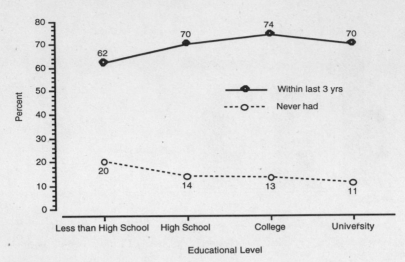

Figure 16
Percent *never had Pap smear* and *having Pap smear within last 3 years*, among women aged 16+, by education (age-standardized), Canada, 1994-95

Source: Federal, Provincial and Territorial Advisory Committee on Population Health 1996b

The data from the NPHS 1994-95 show a strong inverse relationship between smoking and education; see Figure 17. Fourteen percent of those with a University education report that they are current smokers; those that smoke report smoking an average of 15 cigarettes per day. In stark contrast 41% of those with less than high school education report that they are current smokers; those that smoke consume on average 19 cigarettes per day. These and other data strongly indicate that smoking is concentrated in the lower socio-economic strata of Canada. Smoking appears to be emerging as a class based health behaviour.

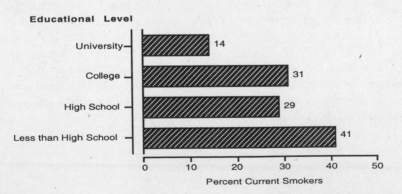

Figure 17
Percent current smokers by education (age standardized), Canada, population 12+, 1994

Source: Federal, Provincial and Territorial Advisory Committee on Population Health 1996b

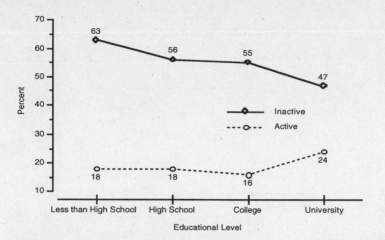

Figure 18
Percent reporting active and inactive leisure time activity, by education (age standardized), Canada, population 12+, 1994-95

Source: Federal, Provincial and Territorial Advisory Committee on Population Health 1996b

Exercise

A third preventive health practice we shall look at is that of exercise. Physical activity is connected to cardiovascular health. The NPHS also asked questions about leisure time physical activity. Again these data on leisure time physical activity show a strong positive relationship between more education and moderately active and active leisure time activities; see Figure 18. Those with a university education were more active than those with less than a high school education. Those with less than a high school education were most likely to be sedentary in their leisure time.

Utilization of Health Services

The NPHS of 1994-95 like most other national health surveys before it, asked Canadians about their use of health and medical services during the previous 12 months.

Non-use Physician Services

Figure 19 shows data from the NPHS on the percent of Canadians not using a physician during the past 12 months by level of education. The NPHS showed that 20 percent of Canadians aged 12+ had not seen a physician during the past 12 months. However those with less than high school education were more likely *not* to have seen a physician (23%) in comparison to those with a university education (16%). There is no direct financial impediment to using physician services in Canada because they are covered by various provincial and federal compulsory public health insurance programs.

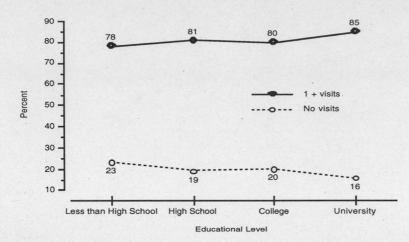

Figure 19
Percent of Canadians reporting *no visits* and *1+ visits* to a physician during the past 12 months, 1994-95, population age 12+

Source: Federal, Provincial and Territorial Advisory Committee on Population Health 1996a

Dental Services

The NPHS data reveals a much stronger socio-economic gradient in "visits to a dentist" in the past 12 months. This is not surprising given that dental services are not a publicly insured service and are variably available as a benefit of employment. Data in Figure 20 shows the relationship between not having visited a dentist in the past 12 months and income. While only 25% of those in the highest income category had not seen a dentist in the past 12 months, 62% of those in the lower middle income category and 59% of those in the lowest income category report not having visited a dentist in the past 12 months.

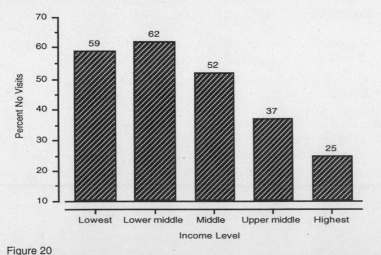

Figure 20
Percent of Canadians reporting *no visits* to a dentist/orthodontist in the past 12 months, 1994-95

Source: Original analysis of the National Population Health Survey public access micro dataset

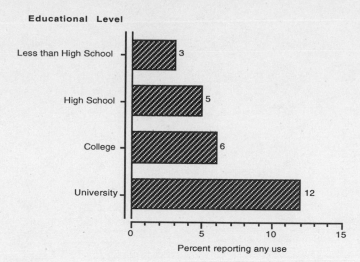

Figure 21
Percent of Canadians aged 12+ reporting use of an alternative health care therapist by education (age standardized), 1994-95

Source: Federal, Provincial and Territorial Advisory Committee on Population Health 1996b

Alternative Care

During 1994-95, five percent of Canadians aged 12+ reported having used the services of an alternative therapist. Massage therapists were the most commonly used therapists followed by homeopaths and naturopaths. When we look at the distribution of the use of alternative services among Canadians, we find that those with a university education are *most likely* to use the services of an alternative therapist whereas those with less than high school education were the least likely to use such a therapist. This is perhaps not all that surprising given that alternative therapists are not usually available as a part of public health services or as part of any health insurance program.

Well-Being

In terms of well-being we shall briefly look at the social distribution of three more subjective measures of health – chronic stress or the absence of it, psychological well-being and self-reported health.

Chronic Stress

Stress has been repeatedly implicated as a causative factor in physical and mental disorder. The NPHS asked Canadians a series of questions on stresses in everyday life. Responses to these questions were used to construct indices of the relative amount of stress in Canadian's lives. The level of chronic stress in individuals' lives was categorized as *high*, *moderate*, and *low*. Twenty-six percent of Canadians reported themselves experiencing a high level of chronic stress, 38% a moderate level of stress; 36% report low stress levels.

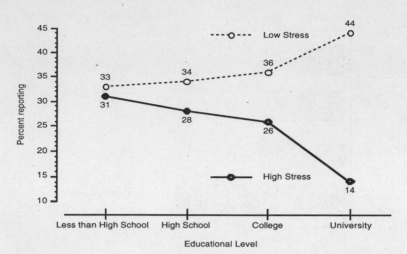

Figure 22
Percent of Canadians 18+ reporting 'high' and 'low' chronic stress levels by education (age standardized), 1994-95

Source: Federal, Provincial and Territorial Advisory Committee on Population Health 1996b

When we look at the distribution of stress in terms of socio-economic status the NPHS data show that high stress levels are more prevalent among those with less than a high school education and least prevalent among those with a university education. Conversely low chronic stress levels were most prevalent among those with a university education and *least* prevalent among those with less than a high school education; see Figure 22.

It may be suggested that the differences in stress exposures between socio-economic strata is largely responsible for the SES gradient in studies of psychological distress (Turner et al. 1995).

Psychological Well-Being

The NPHS used a measure called the Sense of Coherence (SOC) scale to assess the psychological well-being of Canadians. The SOC is designed to measure the extent to which a person views life and its events as comprehensible, meaningful and manageable (Antonowsky 1987). The SOC is seen as a measure of positive well-being.

Canadians on average scored an average of 59 out of 78 on this scale. Little gender difference in this scale is evident but scores on the scale increase with age, with those in the 65+ age categories reporting the highest levels of psychological well-being. When we look at scores on this SOC scale by education there is an education gradient – those with the lowest level of education report the lowest level of psychological well-being; see Figure 23.

However while the differences reported between education levels is statistically significant (largely because of the survey's large sample size), it is difficult to understand a 2.2 (out of 78) point spread as being socially significant. Variation *within* an educational level no doubt far exceeds the differences *between* educational levels.

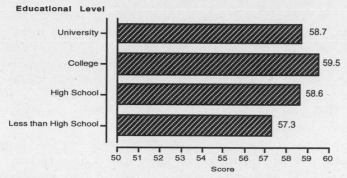

Figure 23
Mean psychological well-being score by education (age standardized), Canada, population 18+, 1994-95

Source: Federal, Provincial and Territorial Advisory Committee on Population Health 1996b

Self-rated Health

Self-rated health is considered a very good predictor of future health care utilization, health problems, and longevity. Self-rated health is the individual's summarization of how they see their health. Data from the 1994-95 NPHS show that 26% of Canadians rated their health as excellent; 38% rated their health as very good; 27% as good; 8% as fair; and 2% rated their health as poor. Figure 24 shows the distribution of self-rated health status among Canadians by education (age-standardized to remove age-education interactions). Again evident in these data is a clear educational gradient with excellent and very good self-rated health being much more prevalent among those with higher levels of education.

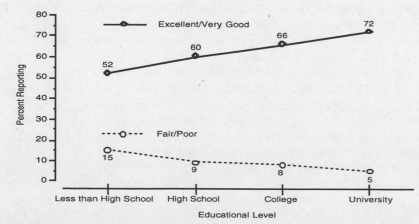

Figure 24
Percent of Canadians reporting their health to be "excellent/very good" and "fair/poor" by education (age standardized), population 12+, 1994-95

Source: Federal, Provincial and Territorial Advisory Committee on Population Health 1996b

Summary

The data reviewed here strongly suggests that we as Canadians are obviously doing better in terms of longevity – greater life expectancy and lower mortality – but perhaps feeling worse, physically – more chronic health problems, more disability days, and use of physicians services. But, we seem to feel happy about ourselves. Regional inequalities in health evident in the early and middle parts of this century appear to be diminishing. However, while life expectancy for Aboriginal Canadians shows a general increase, they still have a life expectancy substantially shorter than the non-Aboriginal population. That gap has not decreased in the last quarter century.

With regard to socio-economic differences in health, all income groups are doing better in terms of mortality and life expectancy. And differences between upper and lower income quintiles have narrowed overtime. However, mortality data for some diseases which have a significant lifestyle component show a widening of the income gradient.

Data presented on specific chronic diseases such as heart disease and depression show a significant socio-economic gradient in the prevalence of these diseases. That socio-economic gradient is also evident in the data on activity limitation and disability, in risk factors for diseases, the practice of preventive health behaviours, the utilization of health services (though less so) and in terms of personal well-being.

It is unfortunate that there does not appear to be any narrowing of the income gradient in preventive health behaviours. The implication of health preventive practices for future mortality may be debatable, however the continued and widening gradient with respect to smoking is particularly troublesome. Social differentials in smoking contribute to the increasing income differentials in lung cancer (Wilkens et al. 1990).

Inequalities and/or Inequities?

Not surprising, there is some ambiguity in the literature as to whether the social differences in health documented here are inequalities, that is uneven but implying no judgement as to "rightness" (if anything there is a hint of individual responsibility), or inequities, that is unevenness that is unjust, the result of bias and unfairness. Inequalities may be noted. Inequities demand action.

There are three criteria that can and should be used in judging whether social differences in health are inequities or inequalities.

First, can the health outcome be modified? To a large extent this is a function of our existing knowledge; however, the very fact that the health outcome is differentially distributed socially implies that it is in most cases amenable to modification.

Second, it can be argued that social inequalities which start early in the individuals life span are not merely inequalities but are, in fact, inequities – a result of the unfairness or bias in the social stratification system. Inequalities that start early in life are circumstances or events over which the developing human individual has little or no control. Furthermore, health differentials early in life not only affect one's immediate health but also may affect the developmental process and the acquisition of other relevant skills essential or useful to "success" in later life (e.g., schooling). The data for Canada do indeed show significant social inequities in terms of peri- and neo-natal mortality and morbidity. These social inequities also persist through childhood. Currently available evidence would suggest that with respect to life expectancy at birth significant inequities exist; however, there has been some reduction in the magnitude of these inequities during the last decades.

Third, inequalities in health can be perceived as inequities insofar as they result from factors that are outside the *reasonable control* of the individual. For example, consider mortality-associated "risk factors." These risk factors are differentially distributed socially with higher prevalence among the lower socio-economic groups. It is argued here that these risk factors are themselves inequities if:

1) relevant information and comprehension concerning potential risk factors is similarly differentially distributed;
2) there is a differential cost attached to the avoidance of the risk factor(s);
3) the risk factors and associated behaviours provide positive reinforcement and no alternative positive reinforcements are readily accessible.

These later points really refer to the role of the social environment in health. Though "environment" issues in promoting health and preventing disease were prominently featured in the Lalonde Report of 1975, they have been neglected and overlooked (Buck 1985). There is sufficient evidence to suggest that health information is differentially distributed socially, and that there are some significant increased economic and social costs associated with pursuing healthy lifestyles. In the sense that these risk factors, the precursors to health, are unevenly distributed, then the resulting health inequalities observed are indeed inequities.

Mechanisms of Action

It is easy to understand how material deprivation such as nutrition, crowding and shelter can affect health. It is also understandable how social deprivation can affect self-esteem, impulse control and coping skills. It is also plausible that different social strata are exposed to more physical stress (hazards) and more psychological stress (unemployment, death, etc.).

There are animal studies that show how enriching the social environment can affect brain structure. Stress has been shown to affect the human immune system.

In these senses social facts can become biological factors. Miller (1995) points to the importance of the 3Rs of social science: *resource position* – material resources both direct and indirect; *relational position* – respect, coping and social support; and *relative position* – power and powerlessness, all affecting all human life including health.

Implications

When confronted with the fact that there are inequalities in health the average Canadian is perplexed. Canada has medical care and hospital insurance programs. Everybody, more or less, has access to good quality medical care. So why should there be social differences in health? Isn't that what comprehensive public medical and hospital programs are all about; ensuring access to care and thus decreasing inequities in health?

Of course medical and hospital care are in reality part of the "sick" (as opposed to "health") care system. By and large they do relatively little to promote the health and general well-being of the population. They generally deal with people who have become "unhealthy."

Health does not solely or even largely come from the "sickness" care delivery system. It has a genetic and environmental (physical, nutritional, and psycho-social) base. Health also does not just occur at one point in life, it occurs through time as various experiences throughout the life span are connected. However, the human individual is perhaps more vulnerable to physical and psycho-social damage during specific points of personal development during the life span.

We have in this paper shown data on the existence and persistence of social differences in health in Canada. The socially descriptive categories used such as age, gender, socio-economic status, etc. are in fact shorthand for a constellation of factors that involve:

Experiences – physical, social and psychological

Attitudes and values – perception of choices, willingness to take action, etc.

Resources – material, psychological and social.

In essence, in describing social groups, we are referring to individuals and groups of individuals that have had different experiences both physical, social and psychological, have differential access to resources both physical and social, and develop different attitudes and values, which in turn lead to different experiences ...

Various constellations of experiences, values and resources may be more or less favorable to positive health outcomes.

Also important is the cumulative nature of life experiences, the notion of a life span in which experiences in earlier stages of life affect the development of, and reactions and responses to, symptoms in later life (see Richman and Flaherty 1985).

Theories that seek to explain social inequalities in health have to take into account these differentials in experiences, resources, attitudes and values and their effects through the life span.

A variety of theoretical approaches have been put forward to explain these inequalities in health. These approaches can be grouped under the headings of artifact, natural and social selection, and cultural and behavioural factors (Townsend and Davidson 1982; Blane 1985). Of these explanations, those that emphasize the material and non-material (cultural and behavioural) aspects of social structure appear to be the most plausible; Verbrugge (1985) provides a good example of this approach in explaining gender differences in health.

The fact that publicly accessible comprehensive health care (both medical and hospital) programs have not eradicated inequalities in health suggests that 'health' is broadly based.

Others have more eloquently documented the importance of traditional sanitation and public health measures in reducing mortality and improving health during the late nineteenth and early twentieth century (McKeown 1976). It is suggested that our major illness problems today are of a chronic illness and disability nature rather than the result of acute infectious diseases (Fries 1983). New strategies have to be developed to meet these changed circumstances. More access to the traditional health care delivery system will not necessarily reduce social inequalities in health. We need to look beyond traditional service delivery and access to service solutions in order to improve the health status of the population at large and its constituent parts.

There are significant social differences in the practice of health protective behaviors. These behaviors can have a significant impact on health status. More effort needs to be placed on health promotion and disease prevention. However, in pursuing such a strategy the emphasis must be away from a 'blaming the victim' approach and towards an approach that attempts to understand the context in which negative health-related behavior occurs. There needs to be an understanding of the incentives and positive reinforcing elements of the "risk" behaviors in order to get the leverage necessary to effect change in those behaviors.

In terms of illness prevention, we need to earmark for action those areas in which substantial improvements can be made. Examples include the provision of adequate sewer and water systems in native communities, vaccination levels, adherence to diabetic diet treatment regimens, Pap smear register and reminder systems, anti-smoking campaigns, etc.

These health promotion and prevention activities should be broadly conceived to include nutrition, good housing, interpersonal skills and other aspects of the physical and social environment conducive to well-being.

Real health reform would focus on native health issues, occupational health and safety measures, healthy pregnancy programs, early childhood programs, school based health education programs.

Finally there is a need to focus upstream, to use Millers phrase, on the underlying economic industrial and social policies that shape our society and our health as a population. Economically we have to promote better paying jobs and reduce differentials in payment between jobs. Better basic packages of benefits (dental care, prescription medications, pensions) need to be attached to all employment – including part-time employment. We need to supplement low wages, promote employee ownership. More emphasis is needed on social housing and early childhood education programs.

Effort is needed on social and economic fronts as well as on the health fronts if we are going to reduce further the social inequities in health present in Canada. Good health should be as basic to citizenship as the right to vote.

References

Amick, BC, S Levine, AR Tarlov, and DC Walsh eds. 1995. *Society and Health*. New York: Oxford University Press.

Antonovsky, A. 1987. *Unraveling the Mystery of Health: How People Manage Stress and Stay Well*. San Francisco: Jossey-Bass.

Billette, A, and CB Hill. 1978. Risque relatif de mortale masculine et les clases sociales au Canada 1974. *L'Union Medicin du Canada* 107: 583-590.

Blane, D. 1985. An Assessment of the Black Report's Explanations of Health Inequalities. *Sociology of Health & Illness* 7(3 Nov): 423-445.

Beck, RG, and JM Horne. 1976. Economic Class and Risk Avoidance: Experience under Public Medical Care Insurance. *Journal of Risk and Insurance* 43(1): 73-86.

Buck, C. 1985. Beyond Lalonde - Creating Health. *Canadian Journal of Public Health* 76 (Suppl. 1, May/June): 19-24.

Burke, MA. 1986. Changing Health Risks. *Canadian Social Trends* (Summer): 22-26.

Cadman, D, MH Boyle, DR Offord, P Szatmari, NI Rae-Grant, J Crawford and J Byles. 1986. Chronic Illness and Functional Limitation in Ontario Children: Findings of the Ontario Child Health Study. *Canadian Medical Association Journal* 135: 761-767.

Canada. Department of Indian and Northern Affairs. 1980. Indian and Inuit Affairs Program. *Indian Conditions: A Survey*. Ottawa: Minister of Indian Affairs and Northern Development.

Canada. Department of National Health and Welfare. 1960. Illness and Health Care in Canada - Canadian Sickness Survey 1950-51. Ottawa: The Queen's Printer.

Canada Health Survey. 1981. The Health of Canadians. Report of the Canada Health Survey. Ottawa: Minister of Supply and Services (Catalogue no. 82-538E).

Charette A. 1993. Dental Health. In Health and Welfare Canada, T Stephens and GD Fowler eds. *Canada's Health Promotion Survey 1990: Technical Report*. Ottawa: Minister of Supply and Services Canada (Catalogue no. H39-263/2-1990E).

Chen, J, E Ng, and R Wilkins. 1996. The Health of Canada's Immigrants in 1994-95. *Health Reports* 7: 4.

D'Arcy, C. 1986. Unemployment and Health: Data and Implications. *Canadian Journal of Public Health* 77(Suppl 1): 124-131.

D'Arcy, C. 1987. Social Inequalities in Health: Implications for Priority Setting. A paper presented at the Second Biennial Conference on Health Care in Canada: Setting Priorities, Wilfrid Laurier University, Waterloo, Ont., April/May, 1987.

D'Arcy, C. 1989. Reducing Inequalities in Health: A Review of Literature. In Knowledge Development for Health Promotion: A Call for Action. Ottawa: Health Services and Promotion Branch of Health and Welfare, Canada (Catalogue no. H39-147/1989E).

Evers, SE, and CG Rand. 1982. Morbidity in Canadian Indian and Non-Indian Children in the First Year of Life. *Canadian Medical Association Journal* 126: 249-252.

Evers, SE, and CG Rand. 1983. Morbidity in Canadian Indian and Non-Indian Children in the Second Year. *Canadian Journal of Public Health* 74(3): 191-194.

Federal, Provincial and Territorial Advisory Committee on Population Health. 1996a. *Report on the Health of Canadians.* Ottawa: Health Canada (Catalogue no. H39-385/1996-1E).

Federal, Provincial and Territorial Advisory Committee on Population Health. 1996b. *Report on the Health of Canadians: Technical Appendix.* Ottawa: Health Canada (Catalogue no. H39-385/1-1996E).

Fries, JF. 1983. The Compression of Morbidity. *Milbank Memorial Fund Quarterly/Health and Society* 61(3): 397A19.

Hay, D. 1988. Socio-Economic Status and Health Status: A Study of Males in the Canada Health Survey. *Social Science and Medicine* 27(12): 1317-1325

Health and Welfare Canada. 1986. *Issues of Health Promotion in Family and Child Health - A Source Book.* Ottawa: Indian and Inuit Services, Medical Services Branch, Health and Welfare, Canada

Health and Welfare Canada. 1987. *The Active Health Report - Perspectives on Canada's Health Promotion Survey.* Ottawa: Health and Welfare Canada.

Health and Welfare Canada. 1991. *Health States of Canadian Indians and Inuit 1990.* Medical Services Branch. Ottawa: Ministry of Supply and Services (Catalogue no. H 34-48/1991E).

Health Canada. 1994. *Survey of Smoking in Canada, Cycle 2.* Fact Sheet #7, Ottawa.

Kue Young, T. 1988a. Are Subarctic Indians Undergoing the Epidemiologic Transition? *Social Science and Medicine* 26(6): 659-671.

Kue Young, T. 1988b. *Health Care and Cultural Change: The Indian Experience in the Central Subarctic.* Toronto: University of Toronto Press

Jarvis, GK, and M Boldt. 1982. Death Styles Among Canada's Indians. *Social Science & Medicine* 16(14): 1346-1352.

Makomaski-Illing, EM, and MJ Kaiserman. 1995. Mortality Attributable to Tobacco Use in Canada and Its Regions, 1991. *Canadian Journal of Public Health* 86(4): 257-265.

Marmot, MG, AM Adelstein, and L Bulusu. 1983. Immigrant Mortality in England and Wales 1970-78. *Population Trends* 33: 14-17

McKeown, T. 1976. *The Role of Medicine: Dream. Mirage or Nemesis?* London, Nuffield Provincial Hospitals Trust.

Miller, SM. 1995. Thinking Strategically About Society and Health. In BC Amick III, S Levine, AR Tarlov and DC Walsh eds. *Society and Health,* 342-358. New York: Oxford University Press.

Miller, WJ, and DT Wigle. 1986. Socio-Economic Disparities in Risk Factors for Cardiovascular Disease. *Canadian Medical Association Journal* 134: 127-132.

Morrison, HL, RM Semenciw, Y Mao, and DT Wigle. 1986. Infant Mortality on Canadian Indian Reserves, 1976-1983. *Canadian Journal of Public Health* 77(4): 269-273.

Nagnur, D. 1986 *Longevity and Historical Life Tables 1921-1881 (Abridged). Canada and the Provinces.* Ottawa: Statistics Canada (Ministry of Supply and Services) (Catalogue no. 89-506).

Nagnur, DN, and M Nagrodski. 1987. *Cause-Deleted Life Tables for Canada (1921 to 1981): An Approach Towards Analysing Epidemiologic Transition.* Analytical Studies Branch Research Paper Series No. 13. Ottawa: Statistics Canada.

Nicholls, E, C Nair, L MacWilliam, J Moen and Y Moa. 1986. *Cardio-Vascular Disease in Canada.* Ottawa: Statistics Canada and Health and Welfare, Canada (Ministry of Supply and Services) (Catalogue no. 82-544).

Peron, Y, and C Strohmenger. 1985. *Demographic and Health Indicators.* Ottawa: Statistics Canada, (Ministry of Supply and Services) (Catalogue no. 82-543E).

Richman, JA, and JA Haherty. 1985. Stress, Coping Resources and Psychiatric Disorders: Alternative Paradigms from a Life Cycle Perspective. *Comprehensive Psychiatry* 26(5): 456-465.

Rootman, I. 1986. Socio-Economic Status and Self-Perceived Health in Canada: Some Findings From Canada's Health Promotion Survey. A paper presented at the Ontario Sociological Association, Waterloo, Ont., Oct 24.

Statistics Canada. 1987. *Cancer in Canada 1982.* Ottawa: Minister of Supply & Services (Catalogue no. 82-207).

Statistics Canada. 1987. *Health and Social Support.* 1985 - General Social Survey Analyses Series. Ottawa: Minister of Supply & Services (Catalogue no. 11-612, No.1).

Statistics Canada. Relevant years. *Mortality - Summary List of Causes.* Ottawa: Minister of Industry, Science, and Technology.

Statistics Canada. Relevant years. *Deaths.* Ottawa: Minister of Industry, Science, and Technology (Catalogue no. 84-21.1).

Statistics Canada. 1994. *Health Status of Canadians: Report of the 1991 General Social Survey.* Ottawa: Minister of Industry, Science, and Technology.

Statistics Canada. 1995. *A Portrait of Persons with Disabilities.* Ottawa: Minister of Industry, Science, and Technology (Catalogue no. 89-542E).

Townsend, P, and N Davidson. 1982. *Inequalities in Health: The Black Report.* Harmondsworth: Penguin Books.

Turner, RJ, B Wheaton, and DA Lloyd. 1995. The Epidemiology of Social Stress. *American Sociological Review* 60(1): 104-125.

Ugnat, AM, and E Mark. 1987. Life Expectancy by Sex, Age and Income Level. *Chronic Diseases in Canada* 8(1): 12-13.

Verbrugge, LM. 1985. Gender and Health, an Update on Hypotheses and Evidence. *Journal of Health and Social Behavior* 26(Sept): 156-182.

Whitehead, M. 1987. *The Health Divide: Inequalities in Health in the 1980's.* London: The Health Education Authority.

Wigle, DT, and Y Mao. 1980. *Mortality by Income Level in Urban Canada.* Ottawa: Dept of National Health and Welfare, Non-communicable Disease Division, Health Promotion Branch.

Wilkins, R, and O Adams. 1983. Health Expectancy in Canada, Late 1970s: Demographic, Regional and Social Dimensions. *American Journal of Public Health* 73(9): 1073-80.

Wilkens, R, O Adams, and A Brancher. 1990. Changes in Mortality by Income in Urban Canada from 1971 to 1986. *Health Reports* 1(2): 137-174.

Wolfson, M, G Rowe, JF Gentleman and M Tomiak. 1993. Career Earnings and Death: A Longitudinal Analysis of Older Canadian Men. *Journal of Gerontology* 48:(4): S167-S179.

5

Low Income and Child Health in Canada[*]

Russell Wilkins and Gregory J. Sherman

Introduction

This presentation summarizes what we know statistically about the relationship between low income, prematurity and low birth weight, as well as other indicators of child health. It is based on the most recent population-based data available for Canada. Much of this research was co-sponsored by Health Canada and Statistics Canada. An earlier version of this work was presented in testimony to the House of Commons Sub-Committee on Poverty (Wilkins and Sherman 1990).

In order to place our findings with regard to low birth weight and prematurity into the larger context of child health, we start with a brief review of some population-based findings concerning the relationship of low income to several indicators of child health, based on mortality and morbidity data from vital statistics and health surveys.

Life Expectancy

Based on the best data currently available for Canada, it appears that the health problems of poor children begin before birth, and continue to place these children at greater risk of death, disability and other health problems throughout infancy, childhood and adolescence.

At birth, children from the poorest neighbourhoods (Quintile 5) in urban Canada have a life expectancy which is 5 1/2 years shorter than that of children from the richest neighborhoods (Quintile 1) in the case of boys, and 2 years shorter for girls. Moreover, a higher proportion of those fewer years of life can be expected to be lived with disability and other health problems.

These mortality differences are based on an analysis of 104,000 deaths (including 1,650 infant deaths) which occurred in 1986 in Canada's 25 Census Metropolitan Areas. The results were published in Statistics Canada's *Health Reports* (Wilkins et al. 1990).

Infant Mortality

In urban Canada in 1986 infant mortality in Quintile 5 (the poorest neighborhoods) was 11 per thousand live births compared with 6 per thousand in Quintile 1 (the richest).

---

* Revised version of a presentation to the Symposium on Prematurity and Low Birth Weight organized by the Canadian Council on Children and Youth and the Canadian Institute of Child Health, Ottawa, 28-29 October 1990.

That is to say, infant mortality was nearly twice as high (1.8 times) among the poor as it was among the rich. Moreover, the relative difference was nearly as great in 1986 as it had been in 1971.

However, another way to look at the differences between the quintiles is to estimate the number of "excess" deaths related to income differences. To do this, we simply assume that the rates observed in the richest quintile had applied to all quintiles of urban Canada, and that the same relative differences by income also affected rural areas and small towns. Had that been the case in 1986, there would have been approximately 700 fewer infant deaths. That represented 23% of the 3,000 infant deaths which actually occurred.

In 1971 there were 6,400 infant deaths in Canada, including an estimated 2,000 "excess" deaths related to low income, which represented 32% of the total. In other words, although the relative disparity in infant death rates between rich and poor decreased only slightly, the absolute number of excess deaths related to low income fell by 1,300 – a decrease of 65%.

Deaths of Children Aged 1-14

Approximately 1,500 children aged 1-14 died in Canada in 1986. In urban Canada, the death rate in the poorest quintile was 1.5 times higher than the rate in the richest quintile. Assuming that the relative differences between quintiles also applied to rural areas and small towns, we estimate that 150 (10%) of the total deaths of children aged 1-14 were "excess," compared with what might have been the case had all children experienced the same low risks as the children of the richest quintile.

In 1971 there were 3,200 deaths of children aged 1-14 in Canada, including an estimated 730 "excess" deaths related to low income (23% of the total).

In 1986, the major causes of death for children aged 1-14 in urban Canada were accidents, poisoning and violence, which accounted for approximately 40% of deaths. Tumors accounted for an additional 20%, congenital anomalies for 14%, nervous system diseases for 7%, and respiratory diseases for 5% of all deaths of children of those ages.

It should be emphasized, however, that in absolute terms, death rates among children in Canada are very low, as are rates of institutionalization.

Institutionalization of Children Aged 0-14

In 1986 only 2,500 children aged 0-14 were residents of long-term health care-related institutions in Canada (Statistics Canada 1988). Unfortunately, we have no data on the socioeconomic backgrounds of the families of these children.

However, we know considerably more about the situation of disabled children living at home, of whom there were 275,000 aged 0-14 in 1986.

Disability in Children Aged 0-14

According to special tabulations from Statistics Canada's Health and Activity Limitation Survey (HALS) of 1986, the rate of childhood disability was over twice as high among children from poor families compared to rich families. Note that these data apply to all Canada, and are based on family rather than neighborhood income. Seven percent (7%) of children from the poorest quintile had some degree of disability, compared to 3.5% of children from the richest quintile.

Had the same low rate of childhood disability observed for the rich applied to all Canadian children, then there would have been 89,000 fewer disabled children in Canada.

The differences between income quintiles were even more pronounced when only severe disability was considered, in which case the rate was 2.7 times higher among the poor compared to the rich – and we estimate that there were 9,400 "excess" cases of severe childhood disability related to income differences.

Injuries to Child Pedestrians and Bicyclists

We saw earlier that accidents are by far the largest cause of death among children aged 1-14, and we know that is also the case for young adults. However, for every death of a child due to accidents, there are over 70 admissions to hospital, and for every admission to hospital, at least 25 injuries treated by outpatient services.

According to a study of neighborhood differences in rates of injury from traffic accidents to child pedestrians and bicyclists in the Montreal area (Dougherty et al. 1990), the rate of serious injury in the poorest quintile was approximately 4 times higher than that of the richest quintile. We do not have the data needed to determine if such marked differences by income apply to other parts of Canada or to other kinds of injuries and diseases.

The Impacts of Low Birth Weight and Prematurity

Various short-, medium- and long-term consequences can arise as a sequel to low birth weight and prematurity. These include increased risk of mortality, morbidity, developmental delay and disability.

Data from the Quebec Health Survey of 1987 (Wilkins 1988) showed that 45% of children with long-term disability had been disabled since birth or before age one. In other words, their disability was probably related to congenital or perinatal causes.

In this regard, we know that low birth weight and prematurity are the most important risk factors for infant mortality and disability of congenital and perinatal origins.

For example, a British Columbia study which linked infant death and birth records for 1977 found that over half of all infants who died in that province before age one weighed 2500 g (5 1/2 lbs) or less at birth (Dunn 1984). The prevalence of health and developmental problems of various sorts was also far higher in low birth weight compared with normal weight babies.

About 20,000 of the 370,000 babies born each year in Canada weigh less than 2500 g, and 22,000 are born prior to 37 weeks gestation (Statistics Canada 1971-1986). Thus, the full impact of any disadvantage related to low birth weight and prematurity is potentially very large.

A rough but objective indicator of the effect of low birth weight on infant morbidity in the early neonatal period, and of direct costs for hospital care, can be obtained from Quebec data on the average number of initial hospital days for infants according to their birth weight (Colin and Desrosiers 1989; Charbonneau et al. 1989). These figures show that in each successively lower 500 g interval below 2500 g, the number of days of stay approximately doubled: from about 4 at 2500 g or over to approximately 7 or 8 at 2000-2500 g, to 17 or 18 at 1750-2000 g, to about 32 at less than 1500 g.

Low Birth Weight and Prematurity by Income

In our current study of 220,000 births by neighborhood income in urban Canada in 1986 (Wilkins et al. 1991), we found that the average rate of low birth weight – using the World Health Organization standard of <2,500 g as the upper limit – was 6% in Canada in 1986, but that the rate of low birth weight varied according to income. The rate of low birth weight was 7% in the poorest quintile, compared to 5% in the richest quintile. The ratio of Quintile 5 to Quintile 1 was thus 1.4, and using the rate in Quintile 1 (the richest quintile, and lowest rate) as a standard, we estimate that an additional 2,900 babies were born with low birth weight compared with what would have been the case had the rate in the richest quintile applied to all quintiles.

Low birth weight is frequently caused by simple prematurity, which with modern neonatal intensive care need not necessarily be too dangerous. However, when an infant is born at full term and is still low birth weight, or is born prematurely and weighing much less than most other babies born at that gestational age, then that infant is said to be "small for gestational age" (SGA), and intrauterine *growth retardation* is indicated. The criteria used to determine SGA status take into consideration the sex of the child, whether there was a single or multiple birth, as well as the gestational age and birth weight of the baby (Arbuckle and Sherman 1991).

In urban Canada in 1986, we found that the poorer the neighborhood, the higher was the proportion of infants which were SGA. While 10% of all babies were SGA, the rate was only 8% in Quintile 1 compared with 12% in Quintile 5. The ratio of rates in Quintile 5 compared to Quintile 1 was thus 1.5, and we calculate that there would have been 6,700 (or 18%) fewer SGA babies in the absence of the "excess" related to income differences in the rates.

Births to Teenage Mothers

While healthy teenagers with adequate resources, support, a healthy environment, early prenatal care and good nutrition usually produce healthy, normal birth weight babies, far too many teenage mothers are lacking in one or several of these desirable attributes. On average in Canada, 15% of births to teenage mothers, regardless of the neighborhood income quintile, are small for gestational age – which is a much higher rate than that of even the lowest income quintile for women aged 20-34.

Compared to women in their twenties and thirties, teenage mothers are far more likely to be poor, unmarried, and having their first baby. Statistically speaking, at least, our results show that those factors seem to account for virtually all of the additional risk of low birth weight and prematurity which is so consistently associated with teenage mothers. That was also the conclusion of a recent meta-analysis for the World Health Organization (Kramer 1987).

In urban Canada in 1986, there were four or five times as many births to teenage mothers in the poorest neighborhood income quintile as in the richest. Since there were approximately the same number of young women in each quintile, the trend was the same in terms of fertility rates as well.

In all parts of Canada in 1986, there were 22,000 births to teenage mothers, which represented 6% of total births to mothers of all ages. Had the teenage birth rate been as low in all quintiles as it was in Quintile 1, there would have been only half as many births to teenage mothers in 1986. Let us remember, however, that as recently as 1971, there were 40,000 births to teenage mothers, which represented 12% of all births.

Our results also show that while women in poor neighborhoods tended to begin childbearing earlier, by age 25, their fertility was well below that of their counterparts in wealthier neighborhoods.

Trends in Infant Mortality and Low Birth Weight

While enormous progress has been made in lowering the infant mortality rate in recent years, much less progress has been made in reducing the rate of low birth weight.

The infant mortality rate has been lowered in large part by increasingly effective and sophisticated treatment of high risk infants – and anyone who has had any personal experience with a low birth weight baby can attest to how extremely important that capability is. But at the same time, comparatively little progress has been made in terms of preventing low birth weight – which as we have seen is one of the major causes of infant mortality and childhood disability.

Low Income and Very Low Income by Age Group

Special tabulations of census data indicate that the nature of low income may not be the same by age group. Low income is usually defined as below the Statistics Canada low income cut-off, regardless of how far below the line that income may be. However, the income of the families of low income children tends to be substantially farther below the cut-off than the income of low income seniors, for example.

In the case of Montreal at the time of the 1986 census, 32% of seniors were poor compared to 28% of children. However, 16% of children were very poor (living in families whose income was less than 60% of the low-income cut-off), compared to 3% of seniors. These figures are based on unpublished special tabulations prepared by Statistics Canada for the *Regroupement des Départements de Santé Communautaire du Montréal-Métropolitain*, and are similar to earlier results obtained from the 1981 census (Wilkins 1985).

Trends in Life Expectancy and Infant Mortality Disparities

All of the member states of the World Health Organization, including Canada, have endorsed the goal of "Health for All by the Year 2000." It is increasingly recognized that in order to make progress towards this goal, a substantial reduction of socio-economic inequities in health will be necessary (Epp 1986). Some historical comparisons may help place the possibility of attaining this goal into perspective.

In Canada today, the disparity in life expectancy at birth between rich and poor (of all ages) is over twice as great as the disparity in life expectancy between the highest and lowest of Canada's five regions (the Atlantic provinces, Quebec, Ontario, the Prairie provinces, and British Columbia) (Wilkins et al. 1990). However, the current rich-poor disparity in life expectancy at birth is about as large as regional disparities were in the early 1950s.

Similarly with infant mortality, the rich-poor disparity (5 per thousand) is currently over twice as great as the regional disparity (2 per thousand). However, the rich-poor disparity in infant mortality is no greater now than was the regional disparity in the late 1960s, and it is far smaller than were the regional disparities in infant mortality which prevailed during the 1940s and 1950s.

Summary and Conclusion

Poor children in Canada have substantially poorer health than do the children of other Canadians. Compared to children from rich neighborhoods, poor children are 40-50% more likely to be born too small, too soon, or with growth retardation; they are almost twice as likely to die before their first birthday; and they are over twice as likely to suffer long term disability and other health problems. These differences are summarized in Table 1.

TABLE 1

Child health and low income: Indicators and estimates for Canada, 1971 and 1986[1]

Indicator	Year	Total (#)	Rich-poor[2] disparity (Q5/Q1)	Excess related to low income[3] (#)	(%)
Infant deaths (< 1 year)	1986	3,000	1.8	700	(23)
	1971	6,400	2.0	2,000	(32)
Deaths of children 1 - 14 years	1986	1,500	1.5	150	(10)
	1971	3,200	1.7	730	(23)
Institutionalization among children <15 years	1986	2,400	?	?	?
Children <15 years					
-with any degree of disability	1986	275,000	2.1	89,000	(32)
-with severe disability	1986	24,000	2.7	9,400	(40)
Newborn infants with					
-growth retardation (SGA: <10p)	1986	37,000	1.5	6,700	(18)
-low birth weight (LBW: <2500g)	1986	20,000	1.4	2,900	(14)
-low birth weight (LBW: <2500g)	1971	26,000[4]	?	?	?
Births to teenage mothers <20 yrs	1986	22,000	4.0	11,000	(50)
	1971	40,000	?	?	?

Notes:

(1) Rich-poor disparity and excess related to low income are based on data for urban Canada (25 Census Metropolitan Areas), except for disability estimates, which are based on data for all Canada.

(2) Rich-poor disparity: Ratio of rate in Quintile 5 (poorest) compared to rate in Quintile 1 (least poor).

(3) Excess related to low income: Assuming rates observed in Quintile 1 (least poor) applied to all quintiles. Except for disability estimates, the percentage excess calculated for urban areas was applied to events in all of Canada.

(4) Newfoundland excluded from 1971 data (because weight not reported on birth registration), but included for 1986 (from provincial Health Department data).

Source: Birth, death and disability data from Statistics Canada, compiled in the course of joint studies with Health and Welfare Canada, and presented in testimony to the House of Commons Subcommittee on Poverty (Wilkins and Sherman 1990)

In terms of the population-based indicators of child health outcomes presented here, it is apparent that the gap between rich and poor is still wide in Canada. Nevertheless, the differences in terms of excess mortality related to low income have been narrowing since 1971.

Unfortunately, we do not yet have the data needed to examine trends regarding disability or risk factors such as low birth weight and prematurity. There is also a great need for individually-based data on various measures of socioeconomic status to complement the mostly ecologically-based data which we have examined.

In conclusion, we can say that a large part of Canadian society has already obtained low rates of infant and child mortality and disability. Tracking Canada's future progress in terms of the objective of reducing socio-economic inequities in child health implies, however, that we continue to monitor the extent to which the rates already obtained by many Canadians are attained by all, regardless of income.

Notes

The views of the authors are their own and not necessarily those of Statistics Canada or Health Canada.

References

Arbuckle, TE, and GJ Sherman. 1989. An Analysis of Birth Weight by Gestational Age in Canada. *Canadian Medical Association Journal* 140: 157–165.

Charbonneau, L, G Forget, JY Frappier, A Gaudreault, E Guilbert, and N Marquis. 1989. *Adolescence et Fertilité: Une Responsabilité Personnelle et Sociale.* La Périnatalité au Québec 2. Quebec: Ministère de la Santé et des Services Sociaux en Collaboration avec l'Association des Hôpitaux du Québec.

Colin, C, and H Desrosiers. 1989. *Naître Égaux et en Santé: Avis sur la Grossesse en Milieu Défavorisé.* La Périnatalité au Québec 3. Quebec: Ministère de la Santé et des Services Sociaux en Collaboration avec l'Association des Hôpitaux du Québec.

Dougherty, G, IB Pless, and R Wilkins. 1990. Social Class and the Occurrence of Traffic Injuries and Deaths in Urban Children. *Canadian Journal of Public Health* 81: 204–209.

Dunn, HG. 1984. Social Aspects of Low Birth Weight. *Canadian Medical Association Journal* 130: 1131–1140.

Epp, J. 1986. *Achieving Health for All: A Framework for Health Promotion.* Health and Welfare Canada. Ottawa: Minister of Supply and Services Canada (Catalogue no. H39-102/1986E).

Kramer, M. 1987. Determinants of Low Birth Weight: Methodological Assessment and Meta-analysis. *Bulletin of the World Health Organization* 65(5): 663–737.

Statistics Canada. 1988. *The Health and Activity Limitation Survey. Selected data for Canada, Provinces and Territories.* Ottawa: Disability Data-base Program, Statistics Canada.

Statistics Canada. 1971-1986. *Vital Statistics: Births and Deaths, 1971-1986.* Various years. Ottawa: Information Canada and Minister of Industry, Trade and Commerce (Catalogue no. 84–204).

Wilkins, R. 1985. *Données sur la Pauvreté Dans la Région Métropolitaine de Montréal.* Montreal: Départment de Santé Vommunautaire, Hôpital Général de Montréal.

Wilkins, R. 1988. L'incapacité. Chapter 8 in A Émond ed. *Et la Santé, ca va? Rapport de l'Enquête Santé Québec.* Quebec: Les Publications du Québec.

Wilkins, R, and GJ Sherman. 1990. *Child Health and Low Income: Data for Canada.* Testimony presented to the House of Commons Sub-Committee on Poverty (Nicole Roy-Arcelin, Chairman) Standing Committee on Health and Welfare, Social Affairs, Seniors and the Status of Women, in relation to its study of child poverty. Ottawa, Ontario: House of Commons, February 21.

Wilkins, R, A Brancker, and OB Adams. 1990. Changes in Mortality by Income in Urban Canada from 1971 to 1986. *Health Reports* 1(2): 137–174.

Wilkins, R, GJ Sherman, and PAF Best. 1991. Birth Outcomes and Infant Mortality by Income in Urban Canada, 1986. *Health Reports* 3(1): 7–31.

6

Are Subarctic Indians Undergoing the Epidemiologic Transition?[*][1]

T. Kue Young[2]

Introduction

The long term temporal changes in the pattern of health and sickness in a population has been described as its 'epidemiologic transition.' First formulated by A.R. Omran in 1971, the theory was modelled after that of the better known 'demographic transition' (Omran 1971). Most populations supposedly undergo three 'ages'–the age of pestilence and famines, the age of receding pandemics, and the age of degenerative and man-made diseases. The pace of transition differs between populations, and Omran distinguished between the classical or western model (exemplified by England and the United States), the accelerated transition model (Japan and Eastern Europe), and the contemporary delayed model where most so-called Third World countries today would belong. Other propositions in this theory include the preeminence of mortality in population dynamics, the important role played by children and young women in mortality decline, and the interplay of demographic, socioeconomic and ecological determinants of health and disease (Omran 1971, 1977a).

Omran's theory has not been tested in many historical populations, probably because of the difficulty in reconstructing past disease rates in the absence of adequate records. Subsequent to his original formulation, Omran attempted to validate the 'classical' model based on U.S. data (Omran 1977a; 1977b). Despite the lack of other confirmatory analyses, the concept has found its way into the medical literature (Anonymous 1977) and its broad outlines, if not its detailed propositions, are more or less accepted as useful descriptive tools in historical epidemiology.

No mention was made in Omran's papers regarding the aboriginal populations in North America. Presumably they would fall under the 'contemporary delayed' model, among countries in the Third World, where massive modern medical technology heralded the relatively recent mortality declines. Kunitz, in his monograph on the health status and health care among Navajo Indians in southwestern U.S.A., made specific reference to the epidemiologic transition (Kunitz 1983). The validity of this theory, however, needs to be demonstrated in other Amerindian groups with different cultural histories, social organizations and ecological adaptations. Such an

* Reprinted from *Social Science and Medicine*, Vol 26, T. Kue Young, 'Are Subarctic Indians Undergoing the Epidemiologic Transition?', pp. 659–71, 1988, with permission from Elsevier Science Ltd., Oxford, England.

examination has policy implications in that Omran's theory (and Kunitz's validation) made implicit judgement as to the relative roles of health services and socioeconomic development in effecting changes in health status. If the model can be shown to fit the past, it might conceivably be predictive of the future. In the debate over the role of health care – two extreme positions can be discerned. On the one hand, the 'left' perspective views the redistribution of health services to the poor and underscored as an important social goal, even if such services have not been proven to be effective. This is contrasted with the 'right' view which embraces the charge of ineffectiveness to justify service cutbacks and rationing.

This paper reviews the health and demographic data of Canadian Indians, primarily Algonkians in the central subarctic boreal forest. It investigates if the epidemiologic transition theory is applicable in general to subarctic Indians, and if yet a fourth 'model' should be established to account for their experience in North America.

Ethnohistorians have divided the post-contact history of Indians in the Canadian subarctic into various periods (Bishop and Ray 1976). I have adhered to this scheme in Table 1, but have also included changes in health status and medical care. This paper will concentrate on health status. The historical development of health services for Canadian Indians has been detailed in a previous paper in this journal (Young 1984a).

Health Consequences of Contact

There is little paleopathological data from the Canadian subarctic to shed light on the prevalence of diseases among the Indians prior to the arrival of Europeans and recorded history (Jarcho 1984; Buikstra and Cook 1980). One could, of course, apply studies of contemporary hunter-gatherers (Dunn 1968; Wadsworth 1984; Eaton and Konner 1985) and extrapolate them to prehistoric Algonkians, with due allowance made for ecological differences. Thus one could perhaps assume that in pre-contact times, the Indians consumed a high protein diet based on meat and fish and rarely suffered from chronic malnutrition, although acute starvation occurred occasionally. Some infections existed, primarily zoonotic parasitic infestations, but these were probably of low virulence. Particular genotypes in both man and pathogen had evolved over long periods of time to allow both to coexist. Chronic and degenerative diseases – those now termed 'diseases of westernization' (Trowell 1981) – were probably rare. In a bibliographic review of the North American Indian demographic change, Johansson concluded that pre-contact Indians were unlikely to have been disease-free or enjoyed low death rates (with violence and accidents playing a major role in mortality). He estimated that life expectancy at birth was probably in the 20s range, comparable to the 'average' of modern hunter-gatherers and primitive agriculturalists (Johansson 1982).

By the early and mid-18th century, various accounts of the Indian's health began to appear in the journals of fur traders and explorers in the hinterland of Hudson Bay. I have provided a more detailed description of these sources elsewhere (Young 1979). The near unanimity of these utterances regarding the Indian's excellent health could have been the result of the observers' idealized notion of the 'noble savage', the poor health of contemporary Europeans from the lower classes, and the 'healthy survivor' bias to which cross-sectional observations are always susceptible. Nevertheless, while life was no doubt short, harsh and at times violent, early and pre-contact Indians probably did enjoy a relatively healthy and vigorous existence, at least in comparison to what was to follow.

TABLE 1
Historical periods of Indians in the eastern subarctic

Period	Years	Socio-cultural changes	Health and disease pattern	Health care delivery
Pre-historic	Before 17th century	Hunter-gatherers in small bands.	Scanty paleopathological data; well adapted to ecosystem? Healthy, blissful existence?	Traditional medicine: concepts, beliefs, worldview, practitioners, therapies.
Early fur trade era	Late 17th to mid 18th centuries	Earliest visits of European explorers and traders to Indian territories.	Excellent health reported by contemporary European observers.	
Competitive trade era	1763-1821	Numerous competing trading centers and unbridled slaughter of game.	Famines and epidemics: Smallpox, Measles, Influenza, Pertusis, Tuberculosis.	Famine relief and lay dispensing by traders and missionaries.
Trading post dependency	1821-1890	Trapping as a basic subsistence pattern necessary to survival.		
Early government influence	1890-1945	A transitional era when government agents, missionaries, and a more modern technology had modest impact. Trapping continued.	Struggle for survival.	MD with annual Treaty Party.
Modern era	1945-present	Establishment of permanent villages with schools, medical facilities, etc. while trapping, hunting, and fishing continues; government subsidies provide an increasing proportion of income.	Infectious diseases brought under control; rise of new epidemics - accidents and violence, chronic diseases.	Organized health services.

Source: Modified from Bishop and Ray 1976

Infectious diseases such as measles, smallpox and influenza, which spread rapidly and immunize a large proportion of the people, were not favored by natural selection and were probably absent among the small, widely scattered bands of Indians in pre-contact times (Black 1975; Cockburn 1971). It has been estimated that, due to the absence of alternative animal hosts and the short period of infectivity, the number of new cases per year required to sustain the infection would have greatly exceeded the average population size of hunter-gatherer bands (Fenner 1971). When outsiders introduced these new diseases into the 'virgin soil', the impact on the indigenous population was often devastating. The shift from what geneticist J.V. Neel called 'small band' to 'large herd' epidemiology (Neel 1968) has been repeatedly demonstrated around the world, and Indians in the subarctic were no exception.

One of the earliest recorded epidemics in the subarctic was the smallpox epidemic of 1781, which spread through the boreal forest west of Hudson Bay and across the Plains to the Rocky Mountains. It was graphically described by contemporary observers such as Edward Umfreville and David Thompson (Young 1979). The virulence of the disease and the Indians' response (e.g., plunging into cold water in a febrile state, abandoning the sick, and giving up the will to survive) combined to produce a high case-fatality rate.

It is possible that subarctic Indians could have experienced the disease earlier through contact with other tribes further to the east and south. In the first half of the 17th century, the *Jesuit Relations* recorded various epidemics among the Montagnais and other woodlands Algonkians along the St. Lawrence Valley (Heagerty 1926, Bailey 1969). Smallpox was believed to have been introduced by ships from France or indirectly from settlers in New England. Through Indian travellers and European missionaries and traders, the disease spread to the Iroquoians in southern Ontario. In a 7-year period during the 1630s, reportedly half of the Huron population succumbed (Trigger 1985).

Among historical demographers there is some dispute over the role of disease in population decline among Amerindians. The estimation of prehistoric Indian populations is fraught with difficulties and uncertainties, and the results show wide ranging variation (Dobyns 1966). Yet it is important to know the pre-contact population, the approximate time the population began to decline, and when it reached its nadir, if one were to assess accurately the impact of disease as a result of European contact.

According to Dobyns, based on archival research dealing primarily with Mesoamerica and Florida, indirect contact between tribes could have resulted in long-distance transmission of diseases. Many tribes could have been affected by 'European diseases' long before they ever came face to face with a European (Dobyns 1983). There may in fact have been massive epidemics in eastern Canada preceding the historically recorded epidemics in the 17th century (Martin 1978). Thus, according to Trigger, "the extraordinary levels of mortality and other misfortunes that followed European contact must have caused [many Indian informants] to idealize earlier times as a halcyon age of physical health, economic prosperity, and social harmony" (Trigger 1985: 244).

Regardless of the onset, duration, frequency and severity of introduced epidemics, their impact on Indian societies extended beyond the merely demographic. Virgin-soil epidemics characteristically kill off or debilitate a high proportion of adults in their prime years, people who are responsible for food procurement, defense and procreation (Crosby 1976). The social disruption which followed involved changes in kinship pattern, band membership and clan organization (Krech 1978). The impotence of indigenous belief and healing systems to deal with the new catastrophes prepared the way for inroads by European missionaries. Martin even proposed a spiritual origin of the fur trade: the Indians interpreted their misfortunes as the animals declaring war on them, and they retaliated by embracing fur trade technologies such as guns and traps (Martin 1978). Such a novel theory, however, has been seriously challenged by other fur trade scholars (Krech 1981).

For the subarctic, one could only speculate if there were large-scale epidemics earlier than the mid-18th century. What is beyond dispute is the many more documented epidemics which came in the 19th century, when diseases such as measles, influenza, whooping cough, and scarlet fever – in addition to smallpox – took regular toll of the Indians (Young 1979; Hurlich 1983; Graham-Cumming 1967). Many of these epidemics can be traced from their origins in the new settler colony on the Red River and Norway House, a major trading post on Lake Winnipeg. From these they spread along fur trading routes into the forests of northern Ontario, Manitoba and Saskatchewan (Ray 1976). Similar epidemics were also documented among the northern Athaspaskans in the MacKenzie Valley with equally devastating effects (Krech 1978; 1983). The impact of introduced diseases in depopulation, however, has been disputed by some scholars. The same historical records led Helm to conclude that there were no severe epidemics among Athapaskans living in the MacKenzie/Laird drainage basins before 1820. Instead, it was intermittent starvation and female infanticide which had kept population at low levels (Helm 1980).

At any rate, according to one tally, there was hardly a 50-year period without a major outbreak in the subarctic. The frequency of epidemics occurring in 'overlapping clusters' with very short intervals of respite allowed little chance for population recovery (Hurlich 1983).

Compounding the problem of epidemics were periodic famines resulting from the depletion of game due to both natural cycles and overtrapping and hunting (Hurlich 1983; Steegman 1983). To counter the environmental threats the Indians adopted various strategies such as limitation of population, diversification of food sources, innovation in food gathering and preservation, and just plain endurance. Those living near trading posts also came to rely on relief rations or borrowed against future fur harvests. (Here again, one should also be cautious in examining historical materials, particularly fur traders' journals. While starvation undoubtedly occurred, its magnitude and extent may have been exaggerated. Scholars in semantics have pointed out the biased view of Indian culture in such sources, and the use of such terms as 'starving' and its variants carried metaphysical and ritual messages in addition to their literal and technical meanings (Black-Rogers 1986).)

The Struggle for Survival

By the beginning of the 20th century, the Indians in the subarctic had been involved in the fur trade for over 200 years. While greatly debilitated by ever present famines and epidemics, they had probably recovered from the depopulation of the initial 'contact shock.' Still, from the descriptions of contemporary physicians, a generally bleak picture emerges. Thus Dr. Meindl, a physician who accompanied the Treaty No. 9 Commissioner to Indian settlements in northern Ontario, observed that the Indians were "far below the average size and weight of the white man, their muscles and bones underdeveloped, their stature stooping, with long narrow, thin chest" (Young 1979).

Tuberculosis was already rife in many communities, as were scabies, pediculosis, impetigo, and intestinal infections, reflecting the poor personal hygiene, housing conditions, and environmental sanitation in the permanent settlements, where the Indians were by then increasingly congregated.

Venereal diseases were prevalent in areas closer to the towns but were relatively rare in the more remote settlements. The ethnologist Alanson Skinner who travelled down the Albany River, reported that "pneumonia, consumption and la grippe were the best known and most fatal diseases", while "in spite of their great immorality [sic], syphilis and gonorrhea were almost unknown" (Skinner 1912).

During the first decade of this century, statistics on notifiable diseases began to be collected, and these were appended to the Annual Reports of the Chief Medical Officer of the Department of Indian Affairs. Among the infectious diseases reported, in descending order of frequency, were: tuberculosis and scrofula, diarrhea, dysentery, enteritis, syphilis, malarial fever, erysipelas, septicemia, influenza, measles, whooping cough, diphtheria, croup, smallpox, scarlet fever, and typhoid fever.

During the inter-war years the overwhelming problem among Indians in the subarctic, indeed Indians anywhere in Canada, was tuberculosis. Doubts were often entertained by physicians and administrators as to the very survival of the Indian 'race'. In the 1920s a study in the Norway House Agency in northern Manitoba showed that the tuberculosis mortality rate was 20/1000, while the average mortality rate from all causes was about 25/1000, if one excluded the flu year of 1919 when mortality reached 140/1000 (Stone 1925).

With the institution of vaccination by the Hudson's Bay Company since the early-19th century and later by the Canadian government (particularly at annual Treaty visits), the threat of smallpox was substantially reduced, although there were still sporadic outbreaks during the first three decades of this century. It was in 1946 that the last two indigenous cases in Canada occurred (Graham-Cumming 1967). The importance of smallpox in subarctic settlements a century or two ago caused some concern recently. In York Factory on the Hudson Bay coast, the erosion of gravesites led to the disinterment of bodies of victims who might have died of smallpox, raising the spectre of dormant viruses re-emerging in a smallpox-eradicated world (Ewart 1983).

In the 1940s among the Cree and Ojibwa Indians in northern Manitoba and the James Bay coast two health and nutrition surveys were conducted (Moore et al. 1946; Vivian et al. 1948). The Indians surveyed showed deficient intakes of calories and most types of nutrients, far below the recommended allowances of the time. They also suffered from an excessive disease burden, particularly turberculosis and childhood diseases. The findings of these two teams, composed of leading public health and nutrition experts of the day, underscored the plight of the Indians, and gave impetus to the massive government intervention in the post-War years.

Rapid changes occurred in subarctic Canada in the 4 decades since the end of World War II. Government involvement in the areas of health care, social assistance, education, and economic development increased substantially. While these efforts resulted in increasing dependence of Indian communities on external Euro-Canadian institutions and personnel, they nevertheless assured a basic level of living that was superior to that of the 1940s and before.

The recent changes in the health pattern of subarctic Indians will be discussed in terms of population trends, causes of mortality, incidence of selected diseases, and nutritional status. Attempts will be made to reconstruct trends from the 1920s onwards but I will caution that historical statistical data for Indians prior to the 1960s should be viewed with a healthy dose of skepticism.

Trends in Fertility and Mortality

Romaniuc has constructed a time series of fertility rates for Canadian Indians from 1900 to 1973 and the James Bay Cree from 1927 to 1972. He showed that the crude birth rate increased from about 40/1000 in the pre-World War II years to just under 50/ 1000 in the early 1960s (Romaniuk 1981). The increase in fertility during the early stages of the 'modernization' period was believed to occur as a result of the weakening or removal of biocultural inhibitions of childbearing in traditional societies. Some of the contributing factors include a decline in birth intervals, breast-feeding, pregnancy wastage and spousal separation (Romaniuk 1974). From the mid 1960s, the birth rate began to decline (Figure 1). Similar fertility trends have also been observed among Alaska Natives (Blackwood 1981). The relatively high fertility rate has resulted in an age-sex pyramid which is more typical of developing countries today or that of Canada half a century or more ago (Figure 2).

In terms of mortality an impressive decline in the infant mortality rate has occurred over the past several decades, although the gap between Indians and Canadians nationally has still not been closed (Figure 3). It is important to note that the Indian/non-Indian disparity in infant mortality is primarily due to the high Indian postneonatal (28 days to 1 year) mortality rate. The neonatal mortality rate among Canadian Indians is in fact quite close to that of the Canadian population nationally.

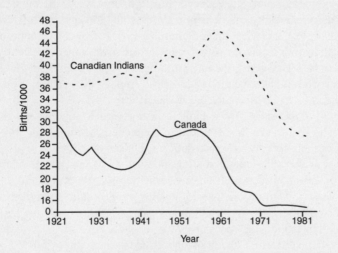

Figure 1
Change in birth rate in Canadian Indian and Canadian national population, 1921-1984

Source: 1921-1974 Canadian data from Leacy F. H. (Ed.) *Historical Statistics of Canada*, 2nd edn. Statistics Canada, Ottawa 1983. 1975-1984 Canadian data from Statistics Canada, *Vital Statistics*, Vol. I. *Births and Deaths* for relevant years. 1921-1973 Canadian Indian data from Romaniuc (Ref. (Romaniuk 1981)). 1974-1981 Canadian Indian rates computed from estimated number of births in Ram B. and Romaniuc A. Fertility Projections of Registered Indians 1982-1996. Indian and Northern Affairs Canada, Ottawa, 1985, Table 5, p. 11, and estimated Indian population data from Perreault J., Paquette L. and George M. V. Population Projections of Registered Indian Population 1982-1996. Indian and Northern Affairs Canada, Ottawa, 1985, Table 6.1, p. 58.

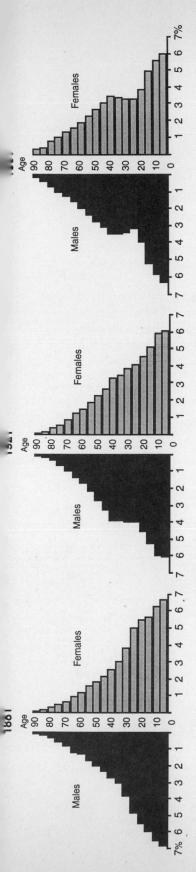
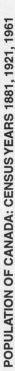

POPULATION OF CANADA: CENSUS YEARS 1881, 1921, 1961

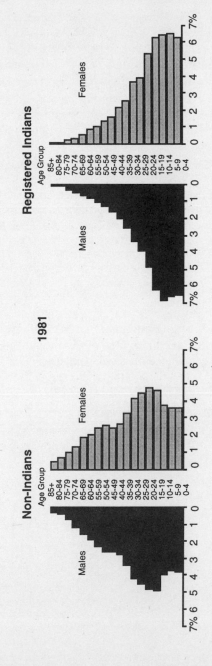
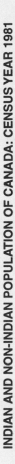

INDIAN AND NON-INDIAN POPULATION OF CANADA: CENSUS YEAR 1981

Figure 2
Population structure of Canadian Indians 1981 compared with Canada 1881, 1921, 1961 and 1981

Source: Canadian data for 1881-1961 from Peron Y. and Strohmenger C. Demographic and Health Indicators. Statistics Canada. Ottawa, 1985, Fig. 4, p. 7. Indian and non-Indian data for 1981 from Statistics Canada 1981 Census of Canada: Canada's Native People, 1984, chart 4

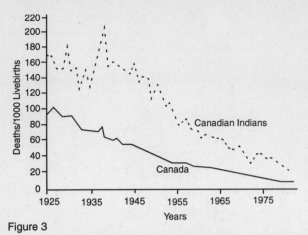

Figure 3
Change in infant mortality rate: Canadian Indians and Canada, 1925-1984

Source: 1925-1974 Canadian data from Leacy F. H. (Ed.) *Historical Statistics of Canada*. 2nd edn.
Statistics Canada, Ottawa, 1983. 1925-1963 Canadian Indian data from Latulippe-Sakamoto C.
Estimation de la mortalité des indiens du Canada. 1900-1968. MA dissertation, Université de
Ottawa, 1971. 1964-76 Canadian Indian data from Siggnir A. *J. An Overview of Demographic,
Social and Economic Conditions Among Canada's Registered Indian Population*. Ottawa: Indian
and Northern Affairs Canada, 1979. 1977-83 Canadian Indian data from Medical Services Branch,
Health and Welfare Canada, Annual Reviews, for relevant years.

A review of the causes of death of the Cree-Ojibwa in northwestern Ontario during
1972-1981 indicated that tuberculosis and other infectious diseases were, by then, no
longer important causes, their places having been taken over by accidents and violence,
which constituted over a third of the deaths (Figure 4) (Young 1983a).

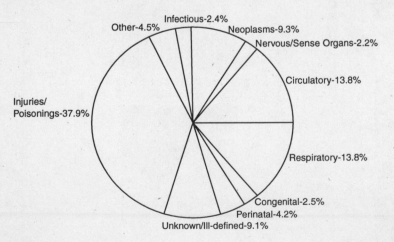

Figure 4
Distribution of deaths by cause for Indians in northwestern Ontario, 1972-1981

Source: Based on data in Young 1983

By computing standardized mortality ratios one can determine the risk of death from particular diseases in the Indian population relative to the Canadian population, taking the different age structures into consideration. In most categories of causes, there were excessive risks of death among Indians (Figure 5). Exceptions included circulatory diseases where the risks were lower, and neoplasms, where the risks were not significantly different.

Similar mortality patterns have been demonstrated in other regional studies of Indians, e.g. in Alberta (Millar 1982), among the James Bay Cree in northern Quebec (Robinson 1985), and Natives in Labrador (Wotton 1985).

Nationally, data on Indian mortality in seven provinces for the years 1977-1982 have been compiled (Mao et al. 1986). Of note is that no infectious diseases were within the 10 highest ranking causes of death. For coronary heart disease and stroke, Indians were either close to or have already exceeded Canadian national rates (Figure 6). For the more isolated (and presumably less 'acculturated') Indians in the subarctic, this may be a portent of things to come.

It is difficult to construct time trends for cause-specific mortality rates for Canadian Indians, whether national or for regional groups, due to incomplete reporting and inconsistent coding practices in official sources. Figure 7 shows the changes in the crude mortality rate for major groups of causes from the 1940s to 1980. It is evident that a shift from infectious diseases to the chronic diseases and accidents and violence has indeed occurred.

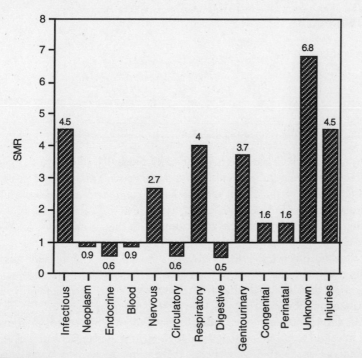

Figure 5
Standardized mortality ratios for selected causes among Indians in northwestern Ontario, 1972-1981

Source: Based on data in Young 1983

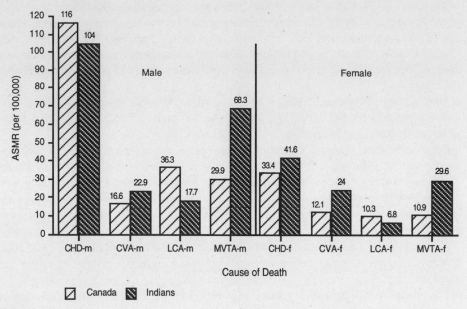

Figure 6
Age-standardized mortality rates for selected causes: Canada and Canadian Indians, 1977-1982

Notes: CHD–coronary heart disease, CVA–cerebrovascular disease, LCA–lung cancer, MVTA–motor vehicle traffic accidents.

Source: Based on data in Mao et al. 1986

The Decline and Persistence of Infectious Diseases

The rapid decline in tuberculosis incidence is graphically presented in Figure 8, narrowing somewhat the gap between Indians and Canadians in general. TB is one disease where medical care factors in the short term seem to have been remarkably successful in reducing the disease burden (Enarson and Grzybowski 1986). The problem, however, is far from being eradicated and outbreaks continue to occur sporadically in different parts of the country.

The dramatic decline in infectious diseases notwithstanding, the risk of such diseases among Indians relative to the whole of Canada is still substantial. Table 2 provides hospital separation data from Manitoba. It can be seen that the standardized morbidity ratio are quite high for most diseases with an infectious etiology.

Clinical studies on respiratory infections indicate that Indian children suffer from more severe illness, multiple recurrent episodes and long term sequalae (Houston et al. 1979). While death and severe morbidity rarely result from infections with organisms such as diphtheria, their presence in the Indian population is still regularly demonstrated (Young 1984b). Epidemics of viral and bacterial gastroenteritis still occur in Indian communities periodically, particularly in areas with deficient water and sanitation facilities (Robinson and Moffatt 1985).

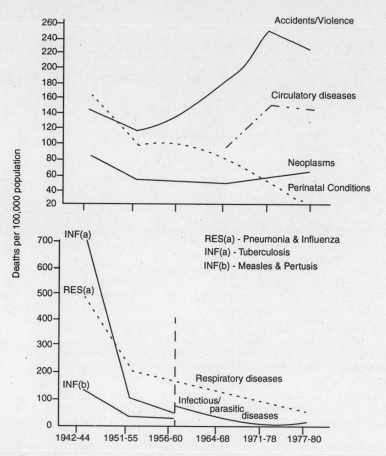

Figure 7

Changes in Canadian Indian crude mortality rates for selected causes

Note: All mortality rates expressed as deaths per 100,000.

Source: 1944 data from the submission to the Senate-House of Commons Committee on the Indian Act by the Minister of National Health and Welfare, in Minutes, Appendix B, p. 91, 1947. 1964-68 data from Latulippe-Sakamoto C. Estimation de la mortalité des indiens du Canada, 1900-1968. MA dissertation, Université de Ottawa. 1971. 1951-60, 1971-76, 1977-80 data from Medical Services Branch, Health and Welfare Canada, Annual Reviews, relevant years

The Emergence of New Diseases

Of increasing interest is the emergence of chronic diseases such as cancer, heart disease, stroke and diabetes among Indians. In terms of mortality, previously discussed national data suggest that some Indians may have 'caught up' with the rest of the Canadian population. The hospital morbidity data from Manitoba (Table 2) also show slight excess in circulatory diseases and four-fold excess of endocrine diseases, mainly due to diabetes.

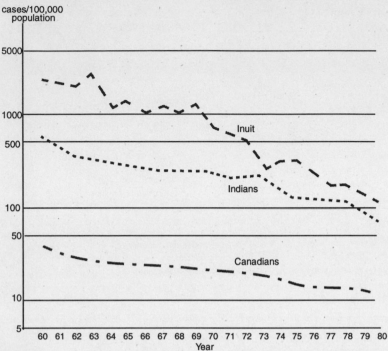

Figure 8
Decline in incidence of new and reactivated cases of tuberculosis among Indians, Inuit and
Canadians, 1960-1980

Source: Unpublished data from Medical Services Branch, Health and Welfare Canada

TABLE 2
Standardized morbidity ratios for selected causes among Manitoba Indians, 1981-82

	ICD-9 code	Diagnosis	SMR
I	001-139	Infectious/parasitic	4.3
	001-009	intestinal infections	5.0
	010-018	tuberculosis	23.8
II	140-239	Neoplasms	0.7
III	240-279	Endocrine/nutritional/metabolic	3.9
VI	320-389	Nervous system/sense organs	2.7
	320-322	meningitis	3.3
VII	390-459	Circulatory system	1.8
VIII	460-519	Respiratory system	3.0
	480-487	pneumonia/influenza	6.7
XV	760-779	Perinatal conditions	1.9
XVII	E800-E999	Injury/poisoning	3.3

Note: The SMR compares the rate of hospitalization for Indians with that of the total Manitoba
provincial population adjusting for age.

Source: Computed from unpublished data provided by the Manitoba Health Services Commission

Baseline epidemiologic studies have only begun to be conducted in the past several years, on cancer (Young and Frank 1983; Young and Choi 1985), diabetes (Young et al. 1985; Szathmary and Holt 1983) and hypertension (McIntyre and Shah 1986). Continuing surveillance is required to determine if an upward trend in these diseases is present.

While Indians are at lower risk for cancer compared with Canadians nationally, large excesses have been found for several sites, namely gallbladder and kidney, while deficits are observed for sites such as lung and breast (Young and Frank 1983; Young and Choi 1985). A variety of environmental and genetic factors are likely to be responsible for such a pattern. It is, however, reasonable to project that the gap between Indians and Canadians in the so-called cancers of 'westernization' would be narrowed in the future.

The prevalence of physician-diagnosed diabetes among the Cree-Ojibwa in north-western Ontario and northeastern Manitoba was higher than Canadians nationally, with a female:male ratio of 2.5:1. Almost half of the known cases were diagnosed within the past five years of a 25-year period, suggesting an increase in incidence as well (Young et al. 1985). In southwestern Ontario the age-adjusted prevalence rate of diabetes among one group of Indians was seven times that of whites living in surrounding rural areas (Evers et al. 1987). Among the Athapaskan-speaking Dogribs, where clinical diabetes is reputedly rare, a glucose tolerance survey revealed abnormal curves for 10% of the subjects tested (Szathmary and Holt, 1983).

There is still a large gap in our understanding and knowledge of circulatory diseases such as ischemic heart disease, stroke and hypertension. Research is currently underway among the Cree and Ojibwa of northern Ontario and Manitoba to establish the prevalence of various risk factors and their associations with the development of various chronic diseases.

Dietary Change and Nutritional Status

Health and nutritional status are intimately related. Indeed, the poor health status of Indians is often attributed to their poor nutrition. Although protein-calorie malnutrition is generally absent, other nutritionally associated health problems include obesity, iron-deficiency anemia, vitamin inadequacy, and dental caries.

According to the Nutrition Canada Indian Survey conducted during the 1970s (Canada Department of National Health and Welfare 1974), the intakes of calories, proteins, and B vitamins among Indians were comparable to Canadians nationally. The intake of vitamin C and A, however, was lower than the national group. Among Indians, those living in remote, isolated areas such as the James Bay coast in northern Quebec had even lower intakes of these vitamins (Hoffer et al. 1981). The low dietary intake of vitamin D and the short daylight during the winter months put many Indian children in the subarctic at risk for rickets. This disease is still being diagnosed in northern Ontario and Manitoba during the 1980s (Haworth and Dilling 1984).

The Nutrition Canada survey also indicated that Indian men had lower mean weight-for-age than Canadians up to age 40-49, but showed substantial gain beyond 50. Among women, Indians were heavier at all age groups (Canada Department of National Health and Welfare 1980) (Figure 9). Current research among the Athapaskans and Algonkians in the subarctic will provide more data on the problem of obesity, overweight, fat patterning and their role in chronic diseases such as diabetes and ischemic heart disease.

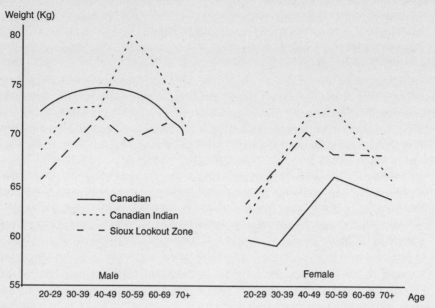

Weight (Kg)

Figure 9
Mean body weight by age: Canadian, Canadian Indian, and Indians in the Sioux lookout zone (northwestern Ontario), early 1970s

Source: Canadian and Canadian Indian data from nutrition Canada survey (Canada Department of National Health and Welfare 1974). Sioux Lookout Zone data from author's unpublished survey data

The change from a state of inadequate calories in the pre-War years to one of excessive obesity among Indians is due to the profound changes in their food habits. With the establishment of trading posts, European foods such as flour, oatmeal, sugar, lard and tea were introduced. After World War II and the trend towards permanent settlements and abandoning of hunting and fishing, dependence on store bought foods became more important, a fact documented by ethnographers working in many subarctic communities (Rogers 1962; Bishop 1974). Dietary changes can also occur relatively rapidly as a result of modern resource development projects, as was demonstrated in a northern Manitoba band affected by a hydroelectric power project (Waldram 1985). Despite their nutritional superiority (Berkes and Farkas 1978) and the lower costs, 'country foods' are decreasing in importance in the diet of many Indian groups. At particular risk are children, with their predilection for sweetened carbonated drinks and sugary snacks. The immediate consequences could be seen in the deplorable dental health status (Titley and Mayhall 1976) – the long term effects have yet to be assessed.

The Social Pathologies

Kunitz (1983) coined the term 'social pathologies' to include accidents, violence (self-inflicted and interpersonal) and the health effects of alcohol abuse. Among Canadian Indians, these causes contribute to about a third or more of all deaths (Young 1983a; Mao et al. 1986). Historically the rising trend can be seen to begin steadily from the end of the Second World War (Figure 7). Detailed sociological inquiries have provided further information on the circumstances surrounding 'accidental' deaths, many of which were in fact associated with alcohol intoxication (Jarvis and Boldt 1982). In many Indian communities across Canada, suicide 'epidemics', especially among the young, are periodically reported (Ward and Fox 1977).

An indication of the severity of alcohol related health problems among Indians can be obtained indirectly from a geographical study of Ontario counties. The District of Kenora, which has one of the highest proportion of Indians in the population among all Ontario counties (about 30%), ranked highest in terms of alcohol consumption, alcohol-related offences, and hospital admissions (under the diagnostic rubrics of 'alcoholism', 'alcoholic psychoses', and 'liver cirrhosis'). Interestingly, the District of Kenora ranked quite low in terms of mortality from liver cirrhosis (Adrian 1983). This finding supports the observation that drinking among northern Indians is mainly of the 'binge' type, which results in deaths from accidents and violence rather than from cirrhosis.

The Indian experience with alcohol has been studied extensively (e.g., Hamer and Steinbring 1980). While initially alcohol may have served some beneficial communal integrating function (Dailey 1968), in recent times excessive drinking has become a widespread social and health problem. Research on the one hand has attempted to seek a 'biological' explanation, i.e. genetically determined enzyme deficiency (Fenna et al. 1971), and on the other, attributed causes to social, economic and political factors (Price 1975; Robbins 1973). The devastation of social pathologies mediated by alcohol – a 'poison stronger than love' – in one northwestern Ontario Ojibwa community, has been meticulously documented (Shkilnyk 1985).

Whatever their causes, the impact of accidents and violence on population change and the epidemiologic transition lies in their exceedingly high rates among young adults. This is reminiscent of the 'virgin soil' epidemics of infectious diseases during early contact. These conditions now serve as 'competing causes' for the chronic diseases by removing a large number of potentially at risk individuals earlier on in life.

The Epidemiological Transition

To the extent that disease patterns have changed during the past 3 centuries, one can say that subarctic Indians and indeed Canadian Indians nationally, have undergone an epidemiologic transition. While the three 'ages' of Omran can be broadly discerned, there are several notable features which distinguish sub-arctic Indians from any of the 3 basic models proposed (western accelerated, and delayed modern).

The 'age of pestilence and famines' for subarctic Indians probably did not begin until contact with Europeans (during the late 17th century in the Hudson Bay hinterland), or perhaps up to a century before actual contact if one accepts the possibility of long-distance transmission of diseases via other Indians with an earlier contact date. There should be a pre-contact 'age' not characterized by pestilence and famines, though not necessarily of low mortality. There was no allowance for this in Omran's original theory, which appeared not to have considered widely scattered nonagricultural, pre-industrial, 'primitive' hunter-gatherer societies.

After contact, the health history of subarctic Indians followed roughly the 'rise-and-fall' course of infectious diseases. Smallpox was one of the earliest to be recorded, and appeared to have been largely controlled by the late 19th and early 20th centuries. Tuberculosis did not show a dramatic decline until the 1960s.

In the post World War II decades, by virtue of their being incorporated into the larger Euro-Canadian society, Canadian Indians have been subjected to massive interventions in social welfare, medical care and economic development. While these measures are sometimes arguably of dubious benefits, one must concede that they have resulted in overall reduction in the incidence and mortality of many infectious diseases and in infant mortality rate (largely the result also of infectious diseases). Canadian Indians therefore cannot be considered to be comparable to the developing countries, particularly the 'least developed' ones, which are still suffering from an exceedingly high infant mortality rate and infectious disease burden. Yet, these countries can only muster perhaps less than 1% of the resources in health and social services per capita currently enjoyed by Canadian Indians (Young 1983b).

While collectively subarctic Indians do not share the epidemiologic pattern of countries in the 'contemporary delayed model', they have also not followed exactly the patterns set by either the 'western' or 'accelerated' models. There is disturbing evidence that the decline in infectious diseases among Indians has stabilized and persisted at a level still higher than that experienced by other Canadians, and the risk of recrudescence still remains.

Against such a background, other 'new' diseases – the chronic, degenerative diseases – have slowly but unmistakably been rising in importance. However, even among this group of diseases, genetic factors peculiar to the Amerindians may favor some diseases, such as diabetes and gallbladder diseases, over others such as ischemic heart disease. The 'New World Syndrome' hypothesis (Weiss et al. 1984) maintains that underlying metabolic defects mediating through obesity have resulted in the emergence of extremely high rates of diabetes and gallbladder disease, over and above that which could have been attributed to lifestyle change alone.

Another major deviation from the 'age of degenerative and man-made diseases' of Omran is the high mortality rate from accidents and violence – a rate that is perhaps unparalleled in the world – which 'compete' with the chronic diseases. Unfortunately there is no purely medical strategy which can reduce these largely socially determined conditions.

At present, it would appear that the health of Canadian Indians has reached a sort of limbo. They seem to occupy an unenviable position of having more of just about every category of disease than their co-nationals. This situation has been depicted by Kunitz, writing about the Navajos:

[The] stagnant reservation economy coupled with an increasing sophisticated social service and health care system had placed a floor under the [Indians] below which immiseration was unlikely to fall and a ceiling above which development was unlikely to rise (Kunitz 1983: 179).

A clear understanding of past, current and likely future epidemiological situation of a population is fundamental to establishing public health policies. Which one of Omran's models of epidemiological transition fits a particular region or country best has important policy implications. Under the western model the steepest decline in mortality occurred primarily as a result of improvement on living standards, while in the contemporary delayed model changes in health status has often been attributed to medical-technological interventions. There is indeed widespread perception among many health policy makers in developing countries that they cannot 'wait' for socio-economic development to occur.

The health experience of subarctic Indians does not fit well with either the First or Third World. Increasingly, scholars have used the term 'Fourth World' to describe the 'internal colonial' situation of indigenous peoples in industrialized countries such as Canada (O'Neil 1986). There is some justification for such a category on epidemiological grounds also. The health care debate, however, need not center on the medical care versus socioeconomic development dichotomy.   It would appear that concurrent action in both areas are necessary, with neither one being the 'prerequisite' of the other. For indigenous peoples, medical care will perhaps ensure that the 'floor' does not sink any lower, while broad social measures will push the 'ceiling' upwards.

Notes

1 This paper is based on a lecture delivered at the course on "Anthropology and Health: Native Populations of the Arctic and Subarctic", held at the Inter-University Centre for Postgraduate Studies, Dubrovnik, Yugoslavia. 17-23 August, 1986.
2 Dr. Young is recipient of a National Health Research Scholar career award from Health and Welfare Canada (6607-1377-48).

References

Adrian, M. 1983. Mapping the Severity of Alcohol and Drug Problem in Ontario. *Canadian Journal of Public Health* 74: 335.

Anonymous. 1977. The Epidemiological Transition. *Lancet* 2: 670.

Bailey, AG. 1969. *The Conflict of European and Eastern Algonkian Cultures, 1504-1700: A Study in Canadian Civilisation,* 2nd ed. Toronto: University of Toronto Press.

Berkes, F, and CS Farkas. 1978. Eastern James Bay Cree Indians: Changing Patterns of Wild Food Use and Nutrition. *Ecology of Food and Nutrition* 7: 155.

Bishop, CA, and AJ Ray. 1976. Ethnohistorical Research in the Central Subarctic: Some Conceptual and Methodological Problems. *Western Canadian Journal of Anthropology* 6: 116.

Bishop, CA. 1974. *The Northern Ojibwa and the Fur Trade: An Historical and Ecological Study.* Toronto: Holt, Rinehart and Winston.

Black, F. 1975. Infectious Diseases in Primitive Societies. *Science* 187: 515.

Black-Rogers, M. 1986. Varieties of "Starving": Semantics and Survival in the Subarctic Fur Trade, 1750-1850. *Ethnohistory* 33: 353.

Blackwood, L. 1981. Alaska Native Fertility Trends, 1950-1978. *Demography* 18: 173.

Buikstra, JE, and DC Cook. 1980. Paleopathology: An American Account. *American Review of Anthropology* 9: 433.

Canada Department of National Health and Welfare. 1980. *Nutrition Canada: Anthropometry Report.* Ottawa.

Canada Department of National Health and Welfare. 1974. *Nutrition Canada: Indian Survey.* Ottawa: Information Canada.

Cockburn, TA. 1971. Infectious Diseases in Ancient Populations. *Current Anthropology* 12: 45.

Crosby, AW. 1976. Virgin Soil Epidemics as a Factor in the Aboriginal Depopulation in America. *William and Mary Quarterly* 33: 289.

Dailey, RC. 1968. The Role of Alcohol Among North American Indian Tribes as Reported in the Jesuit Relations. *Anthropologica* 10: 45.

Dobyns, HF. 1983. *Their Number Become Thinned.* Knoxville, Tenn: University of Tennessee Press.

Dobyns, HF. 1966. Estimating Aboriginal American Population: An Appraisal of Techniques with a New Hemispheric Estimate. *Current Anthropology* 7: 395.

Dunn, FL. 1968. Epidemiological Factors: Health and Disease in Hunter–Gatherers. In RB Lee and I DeVore eds. *Man the Hunter,* 221. Chicago, Ill: Aldine.

Eaton, SB, and M Konner. 1985. Paleolithic Nutrition: A Consideration of its Nature and Current Implications. *New England Journal of Medicine* 312: 283.

Enarson, DA, and S Grzybowski. 1986. Incidence of Active Tuberculosis in the Native Population of Canada. *Canadian Medical Association Journal* 134: 1149.

Evers, S, E McCracken, I Antone, and G Deagle. 1987. Prevalence of Diabetes in Indians and Caucasians Living in Southwestern Ontario. *Canadian Journal of Public Health* 78: 240.

Ewart, WB. 1983. Causes of Mortality in a Subarctic Settlement (York Factory, Manitoba) 1714-1946. *Canadian Medical Association Journal* 129: 571.

Fenna, DL, O Mix, O Schaefer, and J Gilbert. 1971. Ethanol Metabolism in Various Racial Groups. *Canadian Medical Association Journal* 105: 472.

Fenner, F. 1971. Infectious Disease and Social Change. *Medical Journal of Australia* 1: 1043.

Graham-Cumming, G. 1967. The Health of the Original Canadians, 1867-1967. *Medical Services Journal,* Canada 23: 115.

Hamer, J, and J Steinbring eds. 1980. *Alcohol and Native Peoples of the North.* Lanham, Md: University Press of America.

Haworth, JC, and LA Dilling. 1984. Vitamin-D-Deficient Rickets in Manitoba, 1972-84. *Canadian Medical Association Journal* 134: 237.

Heagerty, JJ. 1926. The Story of Smallpox Among the Indians of Canada. *Public Health Journal* 17: 51.

Helm, J. 1980. Female Infanticide. European Diseases, and Population Levels Among the MacKenzie Dene. *American Ethnologist* 7: 259.

Hoffer, J, J Ruedy, and P Verdier. 1981. Nutritional Status of Quebec Indians. *American Journal of Clinical Nutrition* 34: 2784.

Houston, CS, RL Weiler, and BF Habbick. 1979. Severity of Lung Diseases in Indian Children. *Canadian Medical Association Journal* 120: 116.

Hurlich, MG. 1983. Historical and Recent Demography of the Algonkians of Northern Ontario. In AT Steegman ed. *Boreal Forest Adaptations: The Northern Algonkians,* 143. New York: Plenum Press.

Jarcho, S. 1964. Some Observations on Disease in Prehistoric North America. *Bulletin of the History of Medicine* 38: 1.

Jarvis, GK, and M Boldt. 1982. Death Styles Among Canada's Indians. *Social Science and Medicine* 16: 2345.

Johansson, SR. 1982. The Demographic History of the Native Peoples of North America: A Selective Bibliography. *Yearbook of Physical Anthropology* 25: 133.

Krech, S. 1983. The Influence of Disease and the Fur Trade on Arctic Drainage Lowlands Dene, 1800-1850. *Journal of Anthropological Research* 39: 123.

Krech, S. 1981. *Indians, Animals, and the Fur Trade: A Critique of Keepers of the Game.* Athens, Ga: University of Georgia Press, .

Krech, S. 1978. Disease, Starvation and Northern Athapaskan Social Organization. *American Ethnologist* 5: 710.

Kunitz, SJ. 1983. *Disease Change and the Role of Medicine: The Navajo Experience.* Berkeley, Calif: University of California Press.

Mao, Y, H Morrison, R Semenciw, and D Wigle. 1986. Mortality on Canadian Indian Reserves. *Canadian Journal of Public Health* 77: 263.

Martin, C. 1978. *Keepers of the Game: Indian–Animal Relationships and the Fur Trade.* Berkeley, Calif: University of California Press.

McIntyre, L, and CP Shah. 1986. Prevalence of Hypertension, Obesity and Smoking in Three Indian Communities in Northwestern Ontario. *Canadian Medical Association Journal* 134: 345.

Millar, WJ. 1982. Mortality Patterns in a Canadian Indian Population. *Canadian Studies in Population* 9: 17.

Moore, PE, HD Druse, FF Tiskall, and RSC Corrigan. 1946. Medical Survey of Nutrition Among the Northern Manitoba Indians. *Canadian Medical Association Journal* 54: 223.

Neel, JV. 1968. Opening Statement. In *Biomedical Challenges Presented by the American Indians.* Washington, DC: Pan American Health Organization.

Omran, AR. 1977a. Epidemiologic Transition in the United States: The Health Factor in Population Change. *Population Bulletin* 32: 3.

Omran, AR. 1977b. A Century of Epidemiologic Transition in the United States. *Preventive Medicine* 6: 30.

Omran, AR. 1971. The Epidemiologic Transition: A Theory of the Epidemiology of Population Change. *Milbank Memorial Fund Quarterly* 49: 509.

O'Neil, JD. 1986. The Politics of Health in the Fourth World: A Northern Canadian Example. *Human Organization* 45: 119.

Price, JA. 1975. An Applied Analysis of North American Indian Drinking Patterns. *Human Organization* 34: 17.

Ray, AJ. 1976. Diffusion of Diseases in the Western Interior of Canada, 1830-1850. *The Geographical Review* 66: 139.

Robbins, RH. 1973. Alcohol and the Identity Struggle: Some Effects of Economic Change on Interpersonal Relations. *American Anthropologist* 75: 49.

Robinson, E. 1985. Mortality Among the James Bay Cree, 1975-1982. In R Fortuine ed. *Circumpolar Health 84: Proceedings of the Sixth International Symposium on Circumpolar Health,* 116. Seattle, Wash: University of Washington Press.

Robinson, EJ, and MEK Moffatt. 1985. Outbreak of Rotavirus Gastroenteritis in a James Bay Cree Community. *Canadian Journal of Public Health* 75: 21.

Rogers, ES. 1962. *The Round Lake Ojibwa.* Occasional Paper 5, Art Archeology Division. Toronto: Royal Ontario Museum.

Romaniuk, A. 1981. Increase in Natural Fertility During the Early Stages of Modernization: Canadian Indian Case Study. *Demography* 18: 157.

Romaniuk, A. 1974. Modernization and Fertility: The Case of the James Bay Indian. *Canadian Review of Sociology and Anthropology* 11: 344.

Shkilnyk, AM. 1985. *A Poison Stronger Than Love.* New Haven, Conn: Yale University Press.

Skinner, A. 1912. Notes on the Eastern Cree and Northern Saulteaux. *American Museum of National History in Anthropology Papers* 9(1): 7.

Steegman, AT. 1983. Boreal Forest Hazards and Adaptations: The Past. In AT Steegman ed. *Boreal Forest Adaptations: The Northern Algonkians,* 243. New York: Plenum Press.

Stone, EL. 1925. Tuberculosis Among the Indians of the Norway House Agency. *Public Health Journal* 16(2): 76.

Szathmary, EJE, and N Holt. 1983. Hyperglycemia in Dogrib Indians of the Northwest Territories of Canada: Association with Age and a Centripetal Distribution of Body Fat. *Human Biology* 55: 493.

Titley, KC, and JT Mayhall. 1976. The Dental Disease Status of Indian Residents in the Sioux Lookout Zone of Northern Ontario. In *Circumpolar Health: Proceedings of the Third International Symposium.* Toronto: University of Toronto Press.

Trigger, BG. 1985. *Natives and New Comers: Canada's "Heroic Age" Reconsidered.* Montreal: McGill-Queen's University Press.

Trowell, HC, and DP Burkitt eds. 1981. *Western Diseases: Their Emergence and Prevention.* Cambridge, Mass: Harvard University Press.

Vivian, RP, C McMillan, PE Moore, EC Robertson, WH Sebrell, FF Tisdall, and WG McIntosh. 1948. The Nutrition and Health of the James Bay Indian. *Canadian Medical Association Journal* 59: 505.

Wadsworth, G. 1984. *The Diet and Health of Isolated Populations.* Boca Raton, Fla: CRC Press.

Waldram, JB. 1985. Hydroelectric Development and Dietary Delocalization in Northern Manitoba, Canada. *Human Organization* 44: 41.

Ward, JA, and JA Fox. 1977. A Suicide Epidemic in an Indian Reserve. *Canadian Psychiatric Association Journal* 22: 423.

Weiss, KM, RE Ferrell, and CL Hanis. 1984. A New World Syndrome of Metabolic Diseases with a Genetic and Evolutionary Basis. *Yearbook of Physical Anthropology* 27: 153.

Wotton, KA. 1985. Mortality of Labrador Innu and Inuit, 1971–1982. In R Fortuine ed. *Circumpolar Health 84: Proceedings of the Sixth International Symposium on Circumpolar Health,* 139. Seattle, Wash: University of Washington Press.

Young, TK. 1984a. Indian Health Services in Canada: A Sociohistorical Perspective. *Social Science and Medicine* 18: 257.

Young, TK. 1984b. Endemicity of Diphtheria in an Indian Population in Northwestern Ontario. *Canadian Journal of Public Health* 75: 310.

Young, TK. 1983a. Mortality Pattern of Isolated Indians in Northwestern Ontario. *Public Health Reports* 98: 467.

Young, TK. 1983b. The Canadian North and the Third World: Is the Analogy Appropriate? *Canadian Journal of Public Health* 74: 239.

Young, TK. 1979. Changing Patterns of Health and Sickness Among the Cree-Ojibwa of Northwestern Ontario. *Medical Anthropology* 3: 191.

Young, TK, and NW Choi. 1985. Cancer Risks Among Residents of Manitoba Indian Reserves, 1970-79. *Canadian Medical Association Journal* 132: 1269.

Young, TK, and JW Frank. 1983. Cancer Surveillance in a Remote Indian Population in Northwestern Ontario. *American Journal of Public Health* 73: 515.

Young, TK, LL McIntyre, J Dooley, and J Rodriguez. 1985. Epidemiologic Features of Diabetes Mellitus Among Indians in Northeastern Manitoba and Northwestern Ontario. *Canadian Medical Association Journal* 132: 793.

7

Culture, Power and Informed Consent: The Impact of Aboriginal Health Interpreters on Decision-Making*

Joseph M. Kaufert and John D. O'Neil

Introduction

The signing of a consent agreement prior to surgery or invasive diagnostic or treatment procedures is a pivotal event in the negotiation of trust in the doctor-patient relationship. Most analysts have focused on the legal, ethical or procedural aspects of consent. However, there is growing recognition of the importance of considering political and cultural factors which lie outside the immediate context of the medical encounter and beyond the control of either physician or patient. This chapter will examine the processes through which consent is negotiated when the patient is a Native from one of the remote areas of northern Canada. It will explore the application of ethnomedical approaches emphasizing explanatory models and an interactionist framework to understanding the impact of intermediaries in cross-cultural negotiation of consent.

In our research on cross-cultural health communication in urban hospitals, it was apparent that negotiations around the signing of a consent form provided the clearest illustration of the unequal knowledge and power of the clinician and the patient. The clinician's approach to obtaining consent was based primarily on a biomedical understanding of a particular disease and associated treatment procedures; the approach of the Native patient to giving consent was based on experiential and cultural knowledge of past and present illnesses, interpretations of the social meaning of hospital regulations and health professional behaviour, and general attitudes defining intergroup relations in the wider society.

Legal approaches to informed consent and those rooted in biomedical ethics have not dealt adequately with situations in which clients and clinicians speak different languages and have different understandings of illness states and treatment options. This paper suggests an alternative approach which is rooted in the social sciences and uses both ethnomedical and socio-interactionist frameworks, rather than ethical or legal models. Ethnomedical approaches focusing on explanatory models allow both the biomedical perspectives of the clinician and the lay or tradi-

* This manuscript contains sections of a previously published manuscript, 'Biomedical Rituals and Informed Consent' originally printed in Weisz, G. (ed.) *Social Science Perspectives on Medical Ethics*, University of Pennsylvania Press, 1991.

tional perspectives of the client to be incorporated into the analysis. Similarly, where the consent-giving process is seen as the negotiation of shared meanings embedded in broader cultural contexts, we emphasize that analysis must also incorporate the perspective of social interactionism to understand the power relationships in clinical communication.

A single case study recorded during our research focusing on the work of Native language interpreters will be used to describe more general problems of achieving meaningful informed consent. The case study will illustrate differences in the culturally based explanatory models held by clinician and client. These alternative models or interpretive frameworks influence both power relationships and adequacy of communication between all participants in the clinical encounter.

A central focus of this chapter is on the pivotal impact of intermediaries. Specifically, our examination of the process of negotiating consent emphasizes an understanding of the cultural, linguistic and socio-political impact of the intermediary in cross-cultural communication. Language interpreters, patient advocates, family members, and bilingual health workers function as culture brokers as well as language translators. In negotiating consent agreements we observed that some of the interpreters functioned as a negotiator for the clinician who wants the trust of the client. In other interactions, interpreters functioned as advocate for the client who wants some understanding and control over what is planned by the clinician. The case study suggests that cross-cultural consent negotiation continues to be influenced by historical relations of inequality. We conclude that interpreters and other culture brokers function as agents empowering the patient to assert rights that might otherwise be ignored or denied.

Ethical and Legal Perspectives on Informed Consent

Medical ethicists, legal scholars and philosophers discuss informed consent in terms of idealized standards, using landmark legal decisions as examples and emphasizing the medical and legal mechanisms for effective management (White 1983). In common law, consent to medical treatment is a legal requirement with origins in rules governing surgical practice which held a physician liable for battery if they "touched" a patient without prior permission. The process of consenting to treatment emphasizes the principals of autonomy and self-determination protecting the client's right to exercise control over their own body (Faulder 1985).

Prior to 1950, consent was primarily an agreement by the patient to proposed treatment in which the client freely conceded personal autonomy to the legitimate authority of the physician (Barber 1978).

However, during the past three decades the changes in the law of informed consent in the United States and Canada have modified the standards for determining whether a client is appropriately informed from more clinician-oriented to more consumer-oriented criteria. Recent decisions in Canada and the United States have shifted physician-oriented standards to criteria which emphasize the need for "full disclosure" from the objective standard of the "reasonable patient." The standard which had previously applied focused on what a "reasonable physician" should reveal (Somerville 1981). Recent decisions have even evaluated the impact of the constraints on patients in situations where they were not provided with adequate information or were directly coerced (Lautt 1987). In both Canada and the United States the concept of the "reasonable patient," emphasizing what a competent client would need to know to make an informed decision, has emerged as the dominant criteria. The reasonable patient standard serves as a guide to physicians and courts in deciding which treatment alternatives and risks or benefits are salient to the patient; and therefore must be disclosed (Hopp v Lepp and Reibl v Hughes).

Despite this trend in the evolution of legal precedents to reinforce the patient's right to self-determination and support for more consumer-oriented standards of disclosure, consent agreements continue to raise a wide range of ethical and legal questions which social scientists may address using methodological and theoretical approaches different from those of lawyer or ethicist. Unfortunately in much of the legal and biomedical ethics literature the actual decision-making process is ignored or described in formal, ritualistic terms. Key decisions are described in formal legal briefs which retrospectively reconstruct events to support legal or ethical decision criteria (Sharp 1979). Although precedent cases are also framed within the context of adversarial relations, most do not convey a sense of the sequence of social interaction or a feeling for the problems of communication between participants who do not share the same sociocultural framework or socioeconomic status. Case studies therefore seldom provide information for assessing the power relationships between participants and the impact of wider contextual factors which influence consent proceedings. For these reasons much of the legal and clinical literature on consent does not adequately engage the issue of mediating between cultural frameworks and balancing the unequal power of participants.

Consent in Cross-Cultural Communication

As we have emphasized, legal and ethical analysis of consent decisions has not adequately considered situations in which clients and clinicians speak different languages and apply alternative culturally-based explanatory frameworks. Individual and shared group language and culture influence the interpretation of illness and treatment options. With minimal reference to the influence of language and culture, the legal and ethical literature emphasizes that for valid consent decisions to be achieved: (1) full information about risks, benefits, and alternative treatments must be provided; (2) patient competency must be established; (3) patients must be able to understand the information presented; and (4) patients must be placed in situations in which they can act voluntarily (Meisel et al. 1977).

Despite the clarity of these criteria for assessing the validity of generalized consent agreements, situations involving cross-cultural exchanges of information about risks and benefits of treatment depend on accurate and culturally appropriate translation of medical and Aboriginal health concepts. To evaluate patient "competence" and capacity to understand diagnostic and treatment information, it is often necessary to use an interpreter. However, using a language intermediary, such as a medical interpreter, a family member or patient advocate, may also introduce the translator's personal explanatory framework and agenda into the consultation. This may occur without the awareness of either the client or clinician. The requirement that patients be informed about proposed treatments ultimately may require interpreters to reconcile fundamentally different, and sometimes incompatible, concepts of illness and healing. The legal expectation that patients will be placed in situations in which they are autonomous may also be hard to achieve in situations where patients are transported from northern communities without access to family support systems and without an adequate knowledge of the workings of the urban health care system.

The final significant problem in cross-cultural consent decisions involves cultural differences in patients' and health providers' understandings of the clinician-patient relationship. Relationships with healers in Aboriginal cultures emphasize generalized trust in the practitioners' guardianship of the patient, rather than the need for agreement about treatment details. A culturally valid expression of trust in a healer may not meet the current legal criteria for informed consent.

The Interpreters' Role

Current research has not systematically examined the effect which intermediaries, such as interpreters, family members or advocates, have upon consent negotiation. From our observational study of the work of Cree, Ojibway, and Island Lake language-speaking interpreters it is apparent that the negotiation of consent agreements provided a clear illustration of the impact of alternative linguistic and cultural reference frames. The cases also highlighted the differences in access to knowledge and power among clinicians and Aboriginal patients.

Despite emphasis in the communication literature on the role of interpreters in "objective" language translation, we observed that medical interpreters and family members sometimes introduced their personal explanatory frameworks. In Winnipeg hospitals, where clinicians knew little of the patient's home environment, interpreters were a key source of information about the client's previous medical care, family and home community and migration experience. The interpreters' capacity to introduce contextual information on the client's background and current hospital experience was observed to influence the outcome of consent negotiations.

To address both the more generalized issues associated with the roles of intermediaries in cross-cultural communication and the more specific issues raised by consent we will briefly summarize the contribution of social science perspectives to extending the analysis of consent decisions in the medical-legal and ethical literature.

Ethnomedical Perspectives on the Role of Intermediaries in Consent Negotiation

In the past three decades the clinician-client relationship has been the focus of significant theoretical work in the fields of medical anthropology and medical sociology (Lazarus 1988; Zola 1985; Waitzkin and Stoeckle 1976). In ethnomedical research, cultural barriers to effective client-clinician communication have been linked with non-compliance, client dissatisfaction and unequal access to care. Medical anthropology's approach to understanding cross-cultural, healer-client relationships has primarily involved attempts to document how client's and clinician's interpretations of illness and health diverge. Ethnomedicine has sought to define how personal and group models of illness are developed and articulated using the concept of explanatory models (Katon and Kleinman 1981).

In contrast to anthropologists' search for cultural models, medical sociologists have primarily focused on the dynamics of what happens or fails to happen in encounters between professionals and clients. Sociologists are concerned with the interaction process, with control mechanisms and with the impact of roles and the organizational structure of the medical institutions (Bloom and Summey 1978). Both anthropologists and sociologists have recently also begun to examine the impact of the broader environmental, sociopolitical and economic factors upon the dynamics of power in relationships between clients and care givers (Lazarus 1988; Waitzkin and Stoeckle 1976). In looking for ways of applying models from each discipline to the problem of understanding the roles of intermediaries in interpretation and cultural advocacy we found that scholars from both disciplines seldom explicitly recognized that clinician-client relationships are frequently mediated by a third party; involved as an interpreter, advocate, family member or "culture broker."

Before describing the specific case of consent negotiation we will first briefly summarize the models of client-clinician interaction formulated by each discipline and then consider the potential application of the expanded model to documenting triadic, interpreter-mediated relationships.

Analysis of informed consent decisions involving clients and clinicians from different linguistic and cultural backgrounds provides a systematic opportunity to examine the impact of cultural reference frameworks. Negotiation of consent in cross-cultural encounters may also provide a more generalizable model for understanding the more overall processes of interpretation and mediation which occur in all clinician-patient interactions.

Medical anthropologists have developed the concept of explanatory models as a theoretical and methodological device to document culturally-based assumptions about illness and treatment. Kleinman has defined explanatory models as culturally-based "notions about an episode of sickness and its treatment that are employed by those engaged in clinical processes, whether patient or clinician" (Kleinman 1980: 12). Individual and shared explanatory models shape clients' and clinicians' understanding of disease etiology, symptomatology, pathophysiology, natural history and guide proposals for treatment (Helman 1985). Contemporary analysis of clinician-patient interaction stresses the use of explanatory models to document and reconcile the ways that all participants perceive disease entities and treatment options (Katon and Kleinman 1981; Gains and Hahn 1984).

In informed decision-making, the clinician is expected to elaborate treatment options and explain the patient's right to refuse treatment and offer information about the risks and benefits of alternative treatments. In consent decisions, clinicians frequently follow up diagnostic explanations with a description of other diagnostic and treatment options using biomedical terminology. To provide the basis for meaningful choice, the clinician or an intermediary must first translate biomedical terms and concepts into more accessible explanations. Initial translation of biomedical concepts into lay language may never take place, or may occur when questions from the client force the physician to expand and clarify their initial explanation (Tuckett and Williams 1984). In situations where interpreters or other intermediaries are present, translation of biomedical terminology into lay concepts may occur as part of the process of language and cultural interpretation (Kaufert and Koolage 1984). For optimal communication, explanations of treatment options should involve mediation between client's and clinician's explanatory frameworks for understanding the concepts of risk and benefit (Katon and Kleinman 1981).

Our observation of the negotiation of consent agreements involving Native patients revealed that clients were frequently presented with a limited subset of treatment or diagnostic options which the clinician priorized on the basis of his or her assessment of the best clinical option. Actual cases of true co-participatory decision-making in which all options were discussed and relative risks and benefits presented were seldom observed. These observations resonate with the wider critique of the explanatory model approach. Despite the strong appeal of ethnomedical approaches, explanatory model frameworks have been criticized in terms of their limited capacity to relate client and clinician beliefs to actual interaction patterns. Ethnomedical frameworks have also been criticized from a critical theory perspective emphasizing either political economy

(Young 1982; Taussig 1980) or deconstructionist perspectives (Scheper-Hughes and Lock 1987). These critiques suggest that people's interpretations of events and the meanings they assign to those events are structured by their historical participation in the social hierarchy. More directly, they may be influenced by their capacity to participate as individuals in the construction of ideologies which define power relationships. Official ideologies defining the structure of the northern and urban health care system influence both the access of the Aboriginal population to medical care, and also may limit the prospects for empowerment of individual Aboriginal clients. Critical theoretical approaches emphasize that individuals do not freely choose their beliefs and values from a cultural smorgasbord, but rather their "explanatory models" are social and ideological products of historical, economic, and social inequality. This dimension of inequality continues to characterize the relationships of Aboriginal people with social institutions, including the health care system (O'Neil 1989).

Interactionist Perspectives on the Role of Intermediaries

The second source of theoretical models for interpreting the impact of intermediaries in cross-cultural negotiation of informed consent is the body of research on doctor-patient interaction developed by medical sociologists. As critics such as Lazarus have emphasized, even modified anthropological models of cross-cultural communication may have limited utility because they lack the capacity to represent the interactive dimension of clinician-client relationships. Models focusing on social interaction in clinician-patient relationships have been developed by both medical sociologists (Bloom and Summey 1978) and medical anthropologists (Katon and Kleinman 1981; Lazarus 1988). These models provide an alternative perspective for examining the impact of language interpreters, cultural advocates and family members. As we have indicated, ethnomedical frameworks do not fully convey a sense of the interactive dynamics, power relationships or temporal sequence of decision making. In contrast, social interactionist frameworks for analyzing client-clinician encounters focus on the process of exchange. Interactionists seek to understand how actors influence each other's perception of the situation and actions (Lazarus 1988). Medical sociologists have used a symbolic interactionist framework to examine the relative power, potential for social control and differential access to information among the participants in the client-clinician relationship (Stimpson and Webb 1975; Tuckett et al. 1985). They have also more explicitly considered the influence of external political structures within the health care delivery system and society (Waitzkin and Stoeckle 1976). Asymmetry in clinician-patient relationships has been explained in terms of professional dominance relationships and clinical control over technology (Zola 1981). Within interactionist paradigms describing the doctor-patient relationship, inequalities in access of power means that the clinician is more often autonomous and the client more dependent (Bloom and Summey 1978). Although sociological and anthropological approaches to physician-patient interaction stress the need to redress power imbalances, (Katon and Kleinman 1981) co-participatory decision-making may be inherently alien to some culture's models of healer-client interaction (Lazarus 1988; Kaufert and O'Neil 1991).

Unfortunately, sociologists applying the interactionist framework have also not systematically examined the impact of intermediaries, such as interpreters, family members or advocates upon clinical communication. For example, a compendium summarizing the development of sociological analysis of doctor-patient interaction over two decades (Bloom and Summey 1978) includes no models which adequately deal with the role and functions of intermediaries in clinical communication. Rather the models of the doctor-patient relationship reviewed by Bloom and Summey in 1978 only acknowledge the role of family members performing translation or client advocacy functions (Bloom and Summey 1978). Intermediaries are most often represented as part of the patient's subcultural reference group, family and social network. Professional language interpreters are represented in sociological models of doctor-patient interaction as ancillary clinical staff. As such their roles are analyzed as part of the clinician's professional reference group. They are presumed to act primarily to facilitate the application of the clinician's interpretive framework and clinical agenda.

Our ethnographic research with Native interpreters in urban hospitals (Kaufert et al. 1985) and more systematic analysis of video-taped encounters with Inuit patients (O'Neil 1988) has revealed that interpreters perform gate-keeping functions in providing linguistic access. This role in translation and developing rapport appears, in urban hospital settings, to give the interpreter significant, but informal power in clinical communication. In urban hospital settings we found that the interpreter's power was also limited to the situational context of the immediate clinical encounter. The interpreter's power was acknowledged in informal expressions of respect from clinicians. However, the de facto power resulting from the interpreter's role as go between did not usually result in the elevation of the medical interpreter to the status of a health professional. Interpreters in Winnipeg hospitals continue to be paid at the level of a mid range clerical worker. Despite this lack of formal status and power, we observed that within the context of the actual clinical encounter the informal power and control exercised by the interpreter accrued directly from the clinical staff's lack of linguistic access to information about, and rapport with, Aboriginal patients. Many Indian and Inuit patients spoke no English and were flown out of northern communities without accompanying family members or other escorts. Without a linguistic intermediary the clinician was unable to initiate the basic communication necessary to diagnose and treat the person.

From our own observations of the work of Native medical interpreter-advocates in urban hospitals, Kaufert developed an interactionist model representing the role of intermediaries who mediate relationships between the clinician and the client (Kaufert 1990). Our research has suggested that the presence of interpreters and family members contributes an additional dimension to dyadic interaction between clients and clinicians (Kaufert and Koolage 1984). The interpreter's presence introduces a third participant with linguistic and cultural access to personal and professional information.

In cross-cultural situations the interpreter's power to mediate and priorize information occurs within a linguistic and cultural "black box" which both the patient and the clinician must access through the interpreter. Within this "black box" the interpreter can actively intervene on the patient's behalf to explain a wider range of treatment options or pause to clarify the client's rights or the interpreter-advocate may use their "insider" knowledge and personal rapport with the patient to reinforce the clinician's definition of appropriate treatment choices.

Kaufert's (1990) interactionist model of clinician-client interaction incorporates the role of the interpreter as an active participant. This model (shown in Figure 1) concentrates on the range of options which the interpreter has in controlling the flow of information between client and clinicians. The model emphasizes that the role of the interpreter is imbedded in the broader structure of medical organizations, paraprofessional groups and infrastructure of urban and remote Native communities. The model emphasizes that interpreters influence communication in a number of different ways (see Figure 1).

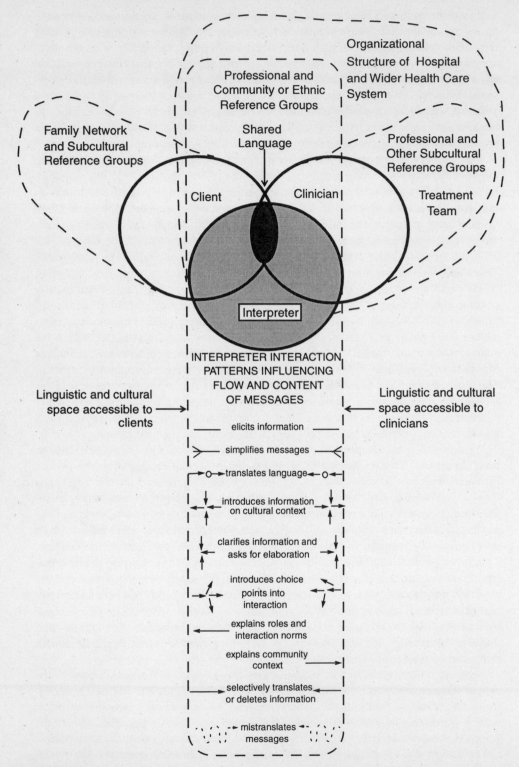

Figure 1
Interpreter interaction influencing information flow in clinician-client relationships

These include: (1) simplifying and clarifying messages and terminology; (2) expanding messages to include more contextual information; (3) failing to transmit information; (4) explaining the organization and social expectations of hospitals; (5) empowering the client through creating choice points; and (6) direct advocacy. The model also acknowledges that the interpreter may incorrectly or selectively translate messages.

In negotiating patient consent to treatment or diagnostic options, language translators and family members frequently added another level of interpretation in which the intermediary had the opportunity to introduce their own explanatory models or influence the level of information available to client and physician. Often, additional information provided by the interpreter incorporates information about the patient's previous experiences in the home and hospital which help to explain and contextualize the patient's narrative. Aboriginal patients' decisions then, were more often than not based on limited biomedical information combined with a broader personal ethnomedical and sociological understanding of the illness event. Unfortunately, few clinicians were aware of the cultural and socio-political construction of the consent decision, since it usually was negotiated in a Native language.

The experience of Native Canadians in urban hospitals provides an opportunity to examine consent decisions in cross-cultural interaction. Consent agreements bring into sharp relief the differences between biomedical and Native interpretations of cultural content and power relationships in clinician-client interaction. Our analysis of Native patient's experience in urban hospitals provides the opportunity to examine the impact of organizational, socio-political and economic factors upon consent agreements. Consent agreements involving Native clients provided a context for documenting the impact of intermediaries such as family members and language interpreters upon clinical communication.

Methods

The data base and methodological design for analysis of consent decisions were derived from a long term research program on medical interpretation in urban hospitals and health communication in Inuit communities of the Canadian Arctic (O'Neil 1988; Kaufert and Koolage 1984). The negotiation of informed consent in interactions between Native clients and clinicians was documented through recording case encounters in medical wards and outpatient clinics (Kaufert et al. 1984). Because of our focus on medical interpreters, the majority of observations were limited to consent decisions in which interpreters were used. However, some encounters were recorded in which family members, rather than a trained interpreter provided translation.

Field observations documented the work of eight Cree, Ojibway, and Island Lake language-speaking interpreters working in two Winnipeg teaching hospitals. About 25 cases involving consent agreements for surgery or invasive diagnostic tests were observed by the investigators and two research assistants who were fluent in Cree, Ojibway or Island languages. Field observations were followed-up with focused interviews with patients and attending medical or nursing staff. Half the consent proceedings were video-taped and translated into verbatim English text to facilitate more detailed analysis of the impact of language usage and sequence of interactions. Follow-up interviews allowed us to document the varied perceptions of the consent agreement from the standpoint of the interpreter, the client and the clinician. The impact of hospital organization and professional ideology among clinicians and medical administrators was documented through observing clinical staff meetings, case conferences, and medical rounds.

The remaining sections of this paper will be devoted to developing an analysis of a study of negotiation of a consent decision between Aboriginal patients, health professionals and medical interpreters. The case study facilitates examination of socio-cultural and structural influences on intercultural decision-making. It will be used to illustrate the contribution of ethnomedical approaches to understanding the problems of reconciling client and practitioner interpretations of illness and treatment alternatives. This case will also be used to examine the process of social interaction in consent negotiation within the broader sociopolitical context of power relationships experienced by Aboriginal people in the urban health care system.

Mediating Client and Physician Explanations of Invasive Diagnostic Procedures: A Case Example

The case documents the communication with an Aboriginal patient who was asked to consent to gastroscopic and colonscopic examinations. The 46-year-old Cree-speaking woman, was referred from a northern nursing station for further investigation of anaemia by a gastroenterologist in Winnipeg. A series of encounters were videotaped at each stage of the diagnostic workup. Several encounters involved the signing of formal consent agreements. In each encounter the physician worked with a Cree-speaking medical interpreter to explain diagnostic and treatment options and negotiate patient consent for examinations of the stomach, small and large intestine.

In the initial encounter, the physician attempted to evaluate the patient's understanding of her own problem and to explain his diagnostic model of the probable cause of anaemia. Specifically he attempted to move from discussing the client's understanding of anaemia (conceptualized by the patient in terms of weakness) to a more complex model linking the loss of blood to the presence of lesions caused by anti-inflammatory medication. Following a cursory explanation of the general diagnosis, the physician moved to a series of diagnostic questions about presence of blood in the patient's stool.

Doctor:	She's anaemic and pale, which means she must be losing blood.
Interpreter (Cree):	This is what he says about you. You are pale, you have no blood. (Cree term for anaemia connotes bloodless state.)
Doctor:	Has she had any bleeding from the bowel when she's had a bowel movement?
Interpreter (Cree):	When you have a bowel movement, do you notice any blood?
Patient (Cree):	I'm not sure.
Interpreter (Cree):	Is your stool ever black, or very light? What does it look like?
Patient (Cree):	Sometimes dark.

At this point the patient told the interpreter that she did not understand how her "weakness" (anaemia) was related to questions about gastrointestinal symptomatology in the physician's reference to dark stools. Without asking for additional explanation from the physician, the interpreter attempted to link the patient's understanding of her anaemia with the concept of blood loss.

Interpreter (Cree):	We want to know, he says, why it is that you are lacking blood. That's why he asked you what your stool looks like. Sometimes you lose your blood from there, when your stool is black.

In discussing the probable etiology of the woman's anaemia, the physician introduced a complex explanatory model which explained gastric or intestinal bleeding in terms of the possible side effects of anti-inflammatory medication for rheumatism. The patient again indicated that she did not understand why the questions about her experience with medication for rheumatism were relevant to the current diagnosis of problems of weakness and blood loss. The interpreter provided an unprompted explanation linking the line of questioning about the side effects of anti-inflammatory drugs with the concept of blood loss.

Interpreter (Cree):	He says that those pills you are taking for rheumatism, sometimes they cause you to bleed inside, or you will spit up blood. Not everyone has these effects. This is why he wants to know about your medication.

Following gastroscopy, the physician attempted to explain the results of the gastric studies and at the same time to extend the initial consent agreement to permit colonscopic examination of the lower bowel.

Doctor:	Everything looked good. There was no ulcer and no nasty disease in the stomach or the esophagus. No bleeding. You're still anemic so we still want to find out if there's any bleeding from the lower end.
Interpreter (Cree):	He says this about you: there's nothing visible in your stomach. Nothing, no sores, lumps, what they call "ulcers." Nothing from where you swallow. Nothing wrong that can be seen.
Patient:	(Nods, but makes no verbal response.)
Doctor:	We're going to put a small tube in from the colon. It's only this big. To have a look, to see if there's any abnormality. It won't take too long and it will be very quick and you shouldn't be uncomfortable with it at all. Okay?... So we'll go ahead and do that now while we can.
Interpreter (Cree):	He wants to see you over here from where your bowel movements come from. Something will be put there, like the first one (the tube you swallowed), but smaller. So you can be examined "down there." Maybe somewhere "down there," it'll be seen that you are losing blood from there. The reason why you are lacking blood. That's what he's looking for. The cause for your blood loss.

During the exchange the patient's willingness to extend the initial consent agreement to cover the investigation of the lower bowel is inferred from a nod and no real alternative was discussed by the physician. The patient was asked to initial the addition to the consent agreement, without formal translation of the English text.

Colonoscopic and radiological examination of the intestine revealed a benign polyp. The physician recommended that the polyp should be cauterized through a second colonoscopy and asked the patient to sign a consent form for the additional procedure. Although risks and benefits were not formally discussed the interpreter elaborated on the basic diagnostic information provided by the physician. The interpreter also introduced a more formal decision point at which the patient was asked to give her formal consent.

Doctor:	We X-rayed the bowel.
Interpreter (Cree):	And this is what they did this morning - when you were X-rayed. The pictures of the area you have bowel movements.
Patient (Cree):	Yes.
Doctor:	And that shows a polyp, a small benign tumor. And I have to take that out.
Interpreter (Cree):	This picture they took this morning. He saw it already. There's something growing there. About this size. And it has to be removed, because you might bleed from there.
Patient (Cree):	Yes.
Doctor:	Now I can take it out without an operation, by putting a tube inside the bowel, and putting a wire around it and burning the polyp off. That stops the bleeding, no need for an operation.
Interpreter (Cree):	He says they can put in a tube like before and burn off the growth.
Patient:	(Nods but makes no verbal response.)
Doctor:	If she wants to make the arrangements for the hospital admission she can come down and sign the consent form.
Interpreter (English):	Will there be complications?
Doctor:	There are a few complications but I think it would be difficult to explain them all.
Interpreter (Cree):	After this procedure has been done you won't be staying here at the hospital. You'll be able to go home on Saturday. It will be done on Friday, then you'll already be able to go home on Saturday. It won't be long. But it's entirely up to you.

In this exchange, the interpreter is providing more than a simple elaboration of the risks, benefits and rationale for the procedure. The physician assumes that his explanation of the reasons for doing the procedure will be sufficient to obtain the patient's consent. In addition the physician closes the exchange by asserting that it would be too difficult to explain all the possible complications. However, in both instances, the interpreter does not provide a literal translation of the physician's side comments, but attempts to assure the patient and justify the procedure through explanations addressing the patient's concern with the length of her stay and desire to return to her home community. The interpreter assures the patient, "You'll be able to go home on Saturday" emphasizing the expectation that the operation will be minor and she won't be separated from family and home for long. The interpreter's statement linking approval of the consent to the patient's early return to her community occurs in Cree and therefore is not accessible to the physician.

At the end of the encounter the physician included the consent agreement with the hospital admission protocol and assumed it would be signed with the other paper work. The interpreter provided a more direct opportunity for the patient to give or withhold consent.

Interpreter (Cree):	Do you want to have this procedure done? Will you consent to have this growth removed - burned? Do you consent to have it done?
Patient (Cree):	I don't know.
Interpreter: .	You know, if it's not removed it may bleed. It may cause problems.

Interpreter (English directed at physician):

	Dr _____, isn't it true that if it's not removed, it can bleed and she can become anemic?
Doctor:	That's correct, we feel that your anaemia may result from the bleeding of the polyp.
Interpreter (Cree):	If it's not removed, you may end up with cancer. You know? And you will not have an operation. It's harder when a person has an operation. You know? And [this procedure] that he's going to do will get it on time. Before it begins to bleed or starts to grow. You're lucky it's caught on time. And it will bother you when you have a bowel movement. This way there's no danger that this growth will bleed.
Patient (Cree):	I still don't know.
Interpreter (Cree):	Well if you want to come in for the procedure while you are here? It's all up to you to think about.

Again, the interpreter has assumed responsibility for providing a rationale for the procedure and explaining the potential benefits. Her explanations are also clearly based on her own medical knowledge, and her understanding of the patient's explanatory model. The fear of cancer in the Native community is linked to general understandings about the history of infectious disease epidemics that nearly destroyed Aboriginal society in North America. Cancer is increasingly viewed as the new "epidemic." The interpreter is using her knowledge of these fears to negotiate the patient's consent, but she is also using Cree models of negotiation emphasizing individual autonomy. Her final statement emphasizes her client's ultimate personal responsibility. "Its all up to you to think about."

At this point, the patient accompanied the interpreter and physician to the appointment desk and scheduled the colonscopy for the following day. After a brief summary of the text (which was printed in English) was provided by the interpreter, the patient signed the consent form. The formal act of signing the form was immediately subordinated to a discussion of specific arrangements for the client's discharge from hospital and travel arrangements for returning to the reserve community.

In this case, consent was negotiated by drawing on expressions of trust by the patient about her relationship with the interpreter. The physician initially assumed that little explanation was required for consent, and indicated his unwillingness to negotiate. Information sharing occurred gradually over the course of the encounter. The interpreter assumed the negotiator's role, based on shared cultural understanding of both biomedicine and Native culture. Throughout the sequence of interaction the interpreter worked to elicit and clarify both the client's and clinician's interpretation of the condition and the program of treatment. However, the interpreter's intervention introduced a third party into the clinician-client relationship. She directly influenced the course of the decision by independently introducing new information about illness and treatment *interpreter* consent agreements are rituals in which participants reconcile power imbalances + negotiate clinical trust.

options. She also imposed decision points where the patient could actually exercise her option to consent.

The patient's willingness to allow the interpreter to negotiate consent is also evident in her reluctance to ask the physician direct questions. In response to the interpreter's questions about her understanding, she repeats at several junctures, "I don't know." This provides a cue for the interpreter to introduce further information or elaborate relative risks. The final consent is passive, in the sense that the patient signs the forms without further resistance.

Power and Control in Consent Decisions Among Native Canadians

The case study demonstrates the role of interpreter-advocates in redressing cultural and structural constraints for Native people in consent negotiations in urban hospitals (Kaufert and Koolage 1984). In some urban hospitals interpreters have expanded their role beyond narrow language translation functions to assume advocacy roles which empower the client through providing information about the structure of the health care system and elaborating these treatment options.

However, in consent negotiations involving both Indian and Inuit patients, the presence of a language interpreter or patient advocate as an intermediary raises a number of ethical and sociopolitical issues. For example, the involvement of interpreter-advocates in the doctor-patient relationship may shift responsibility and initiative for disclosure from the professional to the intermediary. The translator may exercise control through selective interpretation of information provided by the client. The interpreter may also priorize and filter information about treatment options and associated risks or benefits. The interpreters' function of mediating and priorizing information occurs within a linguistic and cultural "black box." Within this box the interpreter may actively intervene on the patient's behalf, or use his or her cultural knowledge and personal rapport with the patient to reinforce the clinician's definition of appropriate treatment choices. Consideration of this variable by clinicians in obtaining informed consent is important.

In summary, sociocultural analysis of real interaction sequences in the negotiation of consent between clinician and client differs fundamentally from legal or ethical analysis of the marker decisions. For Native clients, agreements may reflect the emergence of trust relationships achieved through an extended, incremental process of exchange rather than a formal, final contract. Interactionist and ethnomedical approaches more clearly reveal the communication processes and power relations which are part of the process of translating and priorizing information. Our analysis of the role of Native medical interpreters in both case studies clearly indicates that dyadic clinician-client interaction is strongly influenced by intermediaries. Both confirm that translators, cultural brokers and personal advocates negotiate shared meanings and influence the balance of power in cross-cultural, clinical communication. As well as demarcating formal legal and ethical decision points, cross-cultural consent agreements also function as integrative rituals through which participants reconcile power imbalance and negotiate clinical trust.

Acknowledgements

The authors would like to acknowledge the special contribution of our colleagues and research associates including William Koolage, Margaret Lavallée, Ellen Haroun, Andrew Koster, and Charlene Ball. We wish to thank Jackie Linklater for her assistance in administering the research program and for help in preparing this manuscript. We also wish to thank Drs. Pat Kaufert, Barney Sneiderman, John Walker, Gareth Williams, and Brian Postl for their editorial assistance. Our initial study of hospital-based interpreters was financed by a grant from the Manitoba Health Research Foundation. Subsequent research on interpretation and health communication in Inuit communities was financed by a grant from National Health Research Programs Directorate of Health and Welfare Canada (Project No. 6607-1305-49).

References

Barber, B. 1978. *Informed Consent in Medical Therapy and Research.* New Brunswick, NJ: Rutgers University Press.

Bloom, S, and P Summey. 1978. Models of Doctor-Patient Relationship: A History of the Social System Concept. In E Gallagher ed. *The Doctor-Patient Relationship in Changing Health Science*, 17-42. Washington, DC: Department of Health Education and Welfare (PHEW Publication No. NIH 78-183).

Faulder, C. 1985. *Whose Body Is It? The Troubling Case of Informed Consent.* London: Virago Press.

Gains, A, and R Hahn eds. 1985. *Physicians of Western Medicine: Anthropological Approaches to Theory and Practice.* Dordrecht: Reidel.

Helman, CG. 1985. Communication in Primary Care: The Role of Patient and Practitioner Explanatory Models. *Social Science and Medicine* 20(9): 923–931.

Katon, W, and A Kleinman. 1981. Doctor-Patient Negotiation and Other Social Science Strategies in Patient Care. In L Eisenberg and A Kleinman eds. *The Relevance of Social Science for Medicine*, 253-282. Dordrecht: Reidel.

Kaufert, J. 1990. Sociological and Anthropological Perspectives on the Impact of Interpreters on Clinician-Client Communication. *Santé, Culture, Health* 7(2-3): 209–236.

Kaufert, J, and J O'Neil. 1991. Cultural Mediation of Dying and Grieving Among Native Patients in Urban Hospitals. In DA Counts and DR Counts eds. *Coping with the Final Tragedy: Cultural Variations in Dying and Grieving*, 231-251. Amittyville, NY: Baywood.

Kaufert, J, and W Koolage. 1984. Role Conflict among Culture Brokers: The Experience of Native Canadian Medical Interpreters. *Social Science and Medicine* 18(3): 283–286.

Kaufert, J, J O'Neil, and W Koolage. 1985. Culture Brokerage and Advocacy in Urban Hospitals: The Impact of Native Language Interpreters. *Santé Culture Health* 3(2): 2–9.

Kaufert, J, W Koolage, P Kaufert, and J O'Neil. 1984. The Use of "Trouble Case" Examples in Teaching the Impact of Sociocultural and Political Factors in Clinical Communication. *Medical Anthropology* 8(1): 36–45.

Kleinman, A. 1980. *Patients and Healers in the Context of Culture.* Berkeley: University of California Press.

Lautt, M. 1987. *Problems of Applying the Laws on Informal Consent: The Case of the Native Patient.* Unpublished Manuscript, Issues of Law and Bioethics, Faculty of Law, University of Manitoba, Winnipeg.

Lazarus, E. 1988. Theoretical Considerations for the Study of the Doctor-Patient Relationship. *Medical Anthropology Quarterly* 2(1): 34–59.

Meisel, A, L Roth, and C Lidz. 1977. Toward a Model of the Legal Doctrine of Informed Consent. *American Journal of Psychiatry* 1(34): 3.

O'Neil, J. 1989. The Cultural and Political Context of Patient Dissatisfaction in Cross-Cultural Clinical Encounters: A Canadian Inuit Study. *Medical Anthropology Quarterly* 3(4): 325–344.

O'Neil, J. 1988. Referrals to Traditional Healers: The Role of Medical Interpreters. In *Health Care Issues in the Canadian North.* Edmonton: Boreal Institute.

Scheper-Hughes, N, and M Lock. 1987. The Mindful Body: A Prolegomenon to Future Work in Medical Anthropology. *Medical Anthropology Quarterly* 1(1): 6–42.

Sharpe, G. 1979. *Options on Medical Consent.* A discussion paper prepared by Ontario International Committee on Medical Consent, Ontario Ministry of Health, Toronto.

Somerville, MA. 1981. Structuring the Issues in Informed Consent. *McGill Law Journal* 26: 740–754.

Stimpson, G, and B Webb. 1975. *Going to See the Doctor.* London: Routledge and Kegan Paul.

Taussig, M. 1980. Reification and Consciousness of the Patient. *Social Science and Medicine,* B14: 3–13.

Tuckett, D, and A Williams. 1984. Approaches to the Measurement of Explanation and Information - Giving in Medical Consultation: A Review of Empirical Studies. *Social Science and Medicine* 18(1): 571–580.

Waitzkin, H, and J Stoeckle. 1976. Information Control and the Micropolitics of Health Care: Summary of an Ongoing Research Project. *Social Science and Medicine* 10: 263–276.

While, WD. 1983. Informed Consent - Ambiguity in Theory and Practice. *Journal of Health Politics, Policy and Law* 8(1): 99–119.

Young, A. 1982. The Anthropology of Illness and Sickness. *Annual Review of Anthropology* 11: 257–285.

Zola, IK. 1985. Structural Constraints in the Doctor-Patient Relationship: The Case of Non-Compliance. In L Eisenberg and A Kleinman eds. *The Relevance of Social Science for Medicine,* 241-253. Dordrecht: Reidel.

8

Punctuality, Pain and Time-Orientation Among Sicilian-Canadians[*]

Sam Migliore

Introduction

Time is a key world-view universal (Kearney 1984). Although specific beliefs may vary from one society to another, all peoples have some conception of time. A review of scholarly literature indicates that this subject has received considerable attention. Studies of interest to social scientists include the works of: Eliade (1954); Evans-Pritchard (1939, 1940); Fortes (1970); Hall (1959); Hallowell (1937); Hallpike (1979); Helman (1987); Kearney (1984, 1972); Kluckhohn and Strodtbeck (1961); Leach (1961, 1976); Nilsson (1920); and others. Much of this attention has focused on time-orientation. More specifically, certain scholars have made use of the concepts 'past,' 'present,' and 'future' time-orientation as analytical devices in their attempt to interpret and explain the types of behavior they have observed (Kearney 1984; Hall 1959; Hallowell 1937; Kluckhohn and Strodtbeck 1961).

Mediterranean peoples in general, and southern Italians (including immigrants residing in North America) in particular, are often labeled as having a present time-orientation (Kearney 1984; Rozendal 1987; Sternbach and Tursky 1965; Zborowski 1952; Zborowski 1969). This conclusion is based on the following rationale:

...to many...Mediterranean peoples, and others, the future is seemingly unreal, uncertain, and intangible. What matters for them are events and conditions that they are immediately experiencing, now, in the present (Kearney 1984: 96).

This rationale, in turn, has been used as an explanation for diverse phenomena such as arriving late for appointments, seeking immediate relief from the sensation of 'pain,' and generally displaying a high degree of emotion and expression in illness behavior.

The conclusion that Italians (and others) are present time-oriented, however, leads to certain implications that may affect the type of medical treatment patients receive. First, Italians may be labeled as hypochondriacs who constantly complain and over-express the amount of pain they are actually experiencing (Helman 1984:

* Reprinted from *Social Science and Medicine,* Vol. 28, Sam Migliore, 'Punctuality, Pain and Time Orientation Among Sicilian-Canadians,' pp. 851–859, with permission from Elsevier Science Ltd, Oxford, England.

99-100). Second, Italians need not be provided with as much information concerning their complaints, because their primary interest is the relief of pain. Third, Italians cannot be trusted to adhere to an appointment schedule; nor can they be trusted to complete a treatment regimen once the pain has been effectively dealt with. The acceptance of the conclusion that Italians are present time-oriented, then, may lead to severe negative consequences for individual patients. Yet, to my knowledge, no systematic research has been conducted to verify this contention.

Without a systematic study of the issue, we are left with an unsubstantiated, and potentially dangerous, 'label' or 'stereotype' by which to identify an entire group of people and their world-view. This is particularly true when we consider that a number of well documented studies indicate that, with respect to the North American experience, Italian immigrants and their descendents have in many cases been very motivated, *future*-oriented, and successful in their efforts to achieve the goals they established for themselves (Kessner 1977; Migliore 1988; Nelli 1970; Nelli 1973; Radin 1970; Rolle 1968; Rolle 1972; Rolle 1980; Romanucci-Ross 1975). Romanucci-Ross (1975: 219), for example, goes as far as to suggest that early Italian immigrants to the American West displayed such a strong drive to succeed that they could be described as having a 'Protestant ethic-spirit of capitalism':

Activities of Italians in the West were so consonant with the ethos of the dominant white population there that Italian immigrants emerge as positively Puritan-ethic Anglo, even giving significant aid for the liberation of the West for our joint manifest Christian destiny. They have played this role extremely well in California, even managing to beat Max Weber to the West Coast.

Acceptance of the notion that Italians are present time-oriented is therefore, at best, *problematic*. Given this fact, it is disturbing to find that certain scholars and health care professionals continue to accept, adhere to, and/or promote this 'stereotype' (Rosendal 1987; Martinelli 1987; McMahon 1978; Rotunno and McGoldrick 1982). What is even more disturbing is that these individuals uncritically make use of the concept of time-orientation not as an analytical or interpretive device, but rather as a concrete, valid, and acceptable reflection of southern Italian world-view or value system.

Based on data collected among Sicilian-Canadians, I will present a preliminary statement challenging the notion that southern Italians have a present time-orientation. My findings indicate that Sicilian-Canadians are very much concerned about the 'future,' although the expression of this concern is often displayed in culturally specific terms that may be misread by health care professionals. For this reason, I suggest that further research is needed not only to determine whether southern Italians are 'present'- or 'future-oriented,' but also to determine the usefulness of these concepts in general. I believe, although it is well beyond the scope of this paper to prove, that the concepts themselves reflect an ethnocentric bias that should be avoided. The main focus of this paper is to provide alternative explanations for the following: (1) why Italians may arrive late for medical appointments; (2) why they may seek immediate relief from the sensation of pain; and, (3) why their illness behavior is often characterized by a high degree of emotion and expression. In order to accomplish this goal, I will examine Sicilian-Canadian conceptions of punctuality, and attempt to get at the *meaning* people attach to the experience of pain. Since 'punctuality' and 'reaction to pain' are often used as evidence that a specific group has a particular time-orientation, I believe it is necessary to examine both phenomena in order to clearly illustrate that the notion that southern Italians are present-oriented is untenable. In addition, an understanding of these two phenomena can benefit both health care providers and their patients. I will address the implications of my findings later in the paper.

Background

Over a period of several years, I have collected health-related information among Sicilian-Canadians residing in the Hamilton-Wentworth region of southern Ontario, Canada. There are currently more than 10,000 Sicilians residing in this region, and approximately 95% of these individuals were either born in, or can trace their ancestry to, a small area in South-central Sicily. The ethnographic data I will present and discuss was obtained through: participant observation; conversations with various members of the Sicilian-Canadian community; extended, open-ended interviews with key informants; and, the collection of case histories of individuals suffering from various complaints. Through this process, I was able to gain detailed, qualitative data concerning Sicilian-Canadian conceptions of health and illness.

Participant Observation

As a Sicilian-Canadian who has resided in the Hamilton Wentworth region of southern Ontario, I have participated actively in various family- and community-oriented activities. I began to formally engage in field research within the community in 1977, and to investigate health-related phenomena in the early 1980s. The bulk of the data relevant for this discussion was obtained between 1983 and 1986.

Through participant observation I have gained a great deal of background information concerning the community, and various aspects of Sicilian-Canadian world-view. This technique has also helped me gain an insight into the various ways that concepts such as 'nerves', 'evil eye', 'pain', and other idioms of distress can be utilized in both medical and nonmedical contexts. This insight provided the basis for formulating appropriate questions for my investigation.

Interviews

Although I spoke extensively with many members of the Sicilian-Canadian community, I interviewed informally 40 individuals concerning the nature of 'health' and 'illness.' This sample is composed of 28 females and 12 males. Four of the individuals I interviewed, three female and one male, are traditional healers who treat conditions such as evil eye, muscle injuries, and other complaints.

During the interviews, I asked people the following types of questions: What are *nierbi* (nerves)?; Are there different types of *nierbi*?; How are *nierbi* and pain related?; etc. The interviews themselves, however, were very unstructured. I made use of the preceding questions, as well as others, to give the interviews a degree of consistency. My primary aim was to ask very general questions, and then allow my informants to discuss what they thought was relevant for an investigation of 'health' and 'illness.'

Case Histories

In addition to asking people general health-related questions, I collected 45 case histories from individuals who had recently experienced some form of pain and suffering.

On a few occasions I was also fortunate to be at the right place at the right time, to witness a number of 'nerves'- and 'evil eye'-related episodes. Whenever possible I discussed specific illness episodes with both the victim(s) and significant others. This approach allowed me to gain an insight into not only the victim's perception of what had transpired, but also the views of other individuals who were directly or indirectly involved in the process. This case history material provides the basis for my discussion of Sicilian-Canadian illness behavior.

Although I speak of Sicilian-Canadians in general throughout the paper, the reader should be aware that the information I present was obtained primarily from Sicilian-born individuals, who came to Canada as adults, and are in the over 50 age range. For this reason the information presented in the paper should be viewed as a preliminary statement.

Looking to the Future

In contrast to the views expressed by other scholars (Rozendal 1987; Sternbach and Tursky 1965; Zborowski 1952; Zborowski 1969; Martinelli 1987; McMahon and Miller 1978; Rotunno and McGoldrick 1982), I would like to suggest that there is insufficient evidence to warrant a conclusion that Italians are present time-oriented. My findings indicate that Sicilian-Canadians are very concerned about their *future* and the *future* well-being of their families. In fact, many Sicilian-Canadian beliefs and practices reflect this concern.

Religious Beliefs and Activities

Sicilian-Canadians are predominantly Roman Catholic. This brand of Christianity is explicitly future-oriented. Roman Catholicism is goal directed; the faithful attempt to live the type of lifestyle that is pleasing to God, and that will bring them closer to God not only in this life-time but also in the eternal afterlife. More specifically, adherence to Roman Catholic ideals is rewarded with eternal bliss in heaven, while failing to meet these ideals may lead to eternal damnation. Although not all Sicilian-Canadians may adhere to, or value, these ideals, I find that they are of particular importance to the aged, and to female members of the community.

Honor and Shame

In 1954, Julian A. Pitt-Rivers (1954; see also Pitt-Rivers 1966; Pitt-Rivers 1977) presented a discussion of the Andalusian moral or value system in terms of honor and shame. This early discussion of the topic has influenced the work of most, if not all, mediterraneanists who deal with the phenomenon. Pitts-Rivers (1966: 21; Pitt-Rivers 1977: 1) defines 'honor' as not only the 'value of a person in his own eyes, but also in the eyes of his society.' Honor, then, is intimately linked to an individual's *reputation*. Today, although scholars may argue over specific points (Blok 1981; Davis 1969; Davis 1977; Herzfeld 1980; Herzfeld 1984), honor and shame are key concepts in the study of moral systems of societies throughout the circum-Mediterranean region.

Among Sicilians honor and shame are interrelated and complementary qualities. An individual's honor is a reflection of his or her reputation within the community. This reputation is based on both moral and economic factors. In order to maintain a good reputation, the individual must live up to local expectations. Honor, then, is a positive quality. Shame, at least in certain respects, is also a positive quality. A person who has *shame* does not act in a *shameful* way. It is a quality that enables individuals to regulate their own behavior, and thereby maintain their honor. A person who has both honor and shame commands respect.

An individual's reputation influences how he or she is able to interact with other members of the community. Engaging in what the community regards as 'shameful' behavior may have severe ramifications. The individual, for example, may be subjected to negative sanctions such as vicious gossip, partial or total ostracism, and in certain cases violence. These negative sanctions obviously have an immediate effect on the individual. More importantly, however, are the long term effects these sanctions may have for both the actual individual who committed the 'shameful' act and his or her entire family. It has severe implications for the future. The following hypothetical example, based on conversations with informants, clearly illustrates this point:

If a man allows himself to become a cuckold and does not take action to avenge the insult, he suffers an immediate loss of honor. He will not receive the same degree of respect that others displayed toward him in the past. In addition, it affects his ability to make suitable marriage arrangements for his children; his descendents will be referred to not only by their own name but also by a qualifier such as son- or grandson- of the cuckold; he and his family may no longer be viewed as suitable business partners; etc.

By maintaining a 'good' reputation within the community, Sicilians are taking positive action towards ensuring that both they and their family will have continued success, or at least avoiding the effects of negative sanctions in the future.

Immigration

Until very recently, Sicilian history has been characterized by successive waves of foreign invasion, domination, and exploitation. This state of affairs created severe social and economic problems for the region. Sicily officially became an integral part of the newly united Italian state in 1861. The economic policies of the new government, however, favored the northern regions of Italy; unification did not improve conditions in the south. In response to these adverse economic and social conditions, many Sicilians chose out-migration. Initially people migrated to northern Italy and the other European countries. By 1900, the pattern changed; Sicilians began to travel to overseas destinations – including Canada.

The major wave of Italian immigration to Canada occurred after the Second World War. By 1981 there were approximately 750,000 Italians residing in Canada (Statistics Canada 1984). Although Canadian census figures do not distinguish between people from different regions of Italy, it is fair to say that a relatively high percentage of the Italians residing in Canada are of southern Italian or Sicilian background.

Sicily, then, has experienced an extraordinary rate of out-migration in the last 100 years. People emigrated out of the region in order to improve their socio-economic status. Sicilians-Canadians, however, quickly qualify this by adding that they left their homes and families, and faced many hardships, not only for their own benefit, but to improve their children's chances of achieving success. Here again Sicilians are looking to the future, and more importantly to their children's future.

Sortilegio

The means by which humans can affect 'future' events. Although the term sortilegio literally means 'to fortell the future,' at a very general level it refers to the various means by which human beings can affect or disrupt the natural course of events (Migliore 1983). See the classificatory system below (Migliore 1983: 6). Human beings can affect future events by either causing or alleviating the effects of misfortune. A brief discussion of evil eye beliefs and practices will illustrate this point.

The *evil eye* refers to the belief in the ability of the human eye to cause, or at least project, harm when it is directed by certain individuals towards others in anger, envy, or some other strong emotion. An individual may be exposed to an evil eye either intentionally or unintentionally. Once an individual is effectively exposed to the evil eye the natural course of events is disrupted. He or she experiences certain negative consequences immediately. More importantly, however, the individual's future well-being is called into question. In certain cases, for example, he or she may suffer long term consequences in the form of serious illness or bad luck if steps are not taken to relieve the effects of the evil eye. When a traditional healer performs the appropriate diagnostic and healing ritual(s), the natural course of events is restored. The victim's future well-being is no longer in question, although steps are often taken to help ensure that further exposure to the evil eye is avoided.

This brief discussion of the *evil eye*, and *sortilegio* in general, again illustrates that there is a tendency in certain Sicilian-Canadian beliefs to reflect a 'future', rather than 'present', time-orientation.

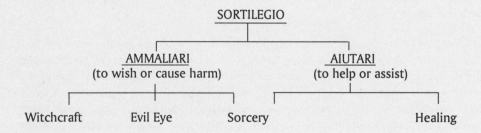

Popular Phrases and Proverbs

Many Sicilian-Canadian popular phrases and proverbs also reflect an explicit or implicit concern with the future, for example:

(a) 'The best time is the time to come.' This phrase is most often said in times of hardship or sorrow to consol the victim; it serves as a reminder for people to look to the future, rather than the problems of the moment.

(b) 'Maybe not today, maybe not tomorrow, but I fix.' This phrase reflects the fact that Sicilians can display a great deal of patience in their attempt to avenge a slight or an injury. The message, however, is clear; vengeance will take place in the future.

(c) 'Speak of 'ill', and 'good' will be the result.' The meaning behind this proverb is that an individual must conceal his or her present good fortune, in order to ensure continued success in the future. To boast about one's good health, prosperity, achievements, etc. is to invite the envy of others (Foster 1972). Sicilian-Canadians recognize envy (*mmidia*) as a potentially dangerous emotion that can activate various malevolent forces. By concealing or down playing the fact that he or she is in a state of good health, then, the individual is able to consciously or unconsciously play a role in avoiding future misfortune.

A concern with the 'future,' then, can be found in various Sicilian-Canadian beliefs, practices, and proverbs. When I asked people whether the past, present, or future is most important to them, they generally agreed that the 'future' was most important. One woman, for example, stated that:

... the past is something we have already gone through; it is something that is gone. If you had good times, they won't come back. If you had hard times, you don't want to remember. The present might be good or bad ... but, the future is most important; it is our hope, our aspirations. Whether things were good or bad in the past, we can have hope for the future ...

The discussion I have presented thus far calls into question the often accepted notion that southern Italians are primarily concerned with the 'present.' In fact, the preceding examples serve as evidence that the concept of 'present' time-orientation is not a useful analytical device for interpreting Sicilian-Canadian belief and action. More importantly, these examples clearly indicate that a 'present' time-orientation cannot be accepted as a concrete value inherent in Sicilian-Canadian, and possibly southern Italian, world-view. To continue to adhere to this notion is to maintain a false, and potentially dangerous, characterization of their world-view. I believe additional research is needed in order to arrive at an ethnographically valid interpretation(s) of the interrelationship between *time, value-orientation,* and *illness behavior.* Until this type of research is conducted, I suggest that it is not appropriate to explain phenomena such as 'arriving late for appointments' and 'seeking immediate relief from pain' in terms of a present time-orientation. In the following discussion I will provide alternative explanations for these phenomena.

Sicilian-Canadian Conceptions of Punctuality

According to Michael Kearney (1984: 96), many Anglo-Americans have a false stereotype of Mediterranean, Latin American, and certain other peoples as 'unreliable and oblivious to time.' Kearney suggests that this misunderstanding is based on the observation that these people are often late for appointments and slow in getting their jobs done. He proposes that in reality, these people simply have a different time-orientation; they are present-oriented, while Anglo-Americans are future-oriented. For Anglo-Americans appointments are real and tangible right from the moment they are made. In contrast Mediterranean peoples, Latin Americans, and others are primarily concerned with what is happening in the present moment, future appointments have little meaning.

In my view, Kearney is correct in suggesting that many Anglo-Americans have misinterpreted certain Mediterranean (Latin American, etc.) attitudes towards 'time' as signs that these people are 'unreliable and oblivious to time.' However, I disagree with his conclusion that Mediterranean peoples are present-oriented. I suggest that we must look for other reasons to explain why these people are often reported to be late for appointments.

In the case of Sicilian-Canadians, I would like to argue that they simply have a different conception of *punctuality.* Whereas Anglo-Americans regard the time set for appointments as very specific and precise, Sicilian-Canadians regard it as an approximation. If an individual arrives for an appointment within a certain 'range of time,' he or she is meeting cultural expectations. The following hypothetical example, based on the views expressed by various informants, will serve to illustrate this point:

Several families are invited for a Sunday lunch at a friend's home. They are asked to arrive at 1:00 p.m. No one, however, is actually expected to arrive at precisely one o'clock. There is a built in expectation that everyone will arrive within a certain range of time. As long as people arrive, for example, between noon and 1:30 p.m. they will not be considered late.

Some people, if they have a close relationship with the host(s), will rationalize that: if they are invited to attend lunch at 1:00 p.m. it means that the host will start preparing much earlier. It is only proper for them to arrive early so as to either help with the preparations or at least not keep the host waiting in the case that the preparations are completed early. For these reasons they arrive between 12:00 and 12:45 p.m.

Others, who do not have as close a relationship with the host(s), will rationalize that: although they were asked to arrive at 1:00 p.m., the host will probably not be ready at that time. They begin to think that they would only inconvenience their host and themselves by arriving at the appointed time. Rather than arrive early and be in the way, these people make a conscious effort to arrive 20-30 minutes late.

Since both the host and the guests are making decisions based on the same experiences, expectations, and conceptions of punctuality, arriving early or late for appointments is not a problem as long as everyone arrives within a certain 'range of time'– a range of time that is appropriate for the type of relationship that exists between the host(s) and the guests. Sicilian-Canadians will appear to be 'unreliable and oblivious to time' if, and only if, they are dealing with people who have different conceptions of punctuality.

The etiquette that applies in the context of hospitality, however, does not necessarily apply in other social contexts. With respect to work, medical appointments, and various other official appointments Sicilian-Canadians stress that it is best to arrive early and to wait patiently. The rules of punctuality tend to differ depending on the specific social situation. In the case of medical appointments, then, Sicilian-Canadians should be expected to arrive early rather than late. Yet, my observation is that many Sicilian-Canadians do indeed arrive late for these appointments. I would like to suggest that this occurs as a result of people adjusting their notions of punctuality to meet the *reality* of the 'waiting room' experience.

The Sicilian-Canadian individuals I have worked with seek medical assistance from Italian-speaking doctors. These Italian-speaking doctors, however, generally do not share the same values and beliefs as their Sicilian-Canadian patients. When the patients arrive for their scheduled appointments, the receptionist records their names and asks them to be seated. Patients soon realize that arriving early will mean waiting for an hour or more before they actually see the doctor. This is due, at least in part, to the fact that many people seek the services of a relatively small number of Italian-speaking doctors. Rather than seek assistance from non-Italians, Sicilian-Canadians attempt to adjust to the situation in the following ways:

(1) Certain individuals simply arrive late for the appointment, in order to avoid the long wait. This type of adjustment, however, tends to irritate the receptionist who now has to juggle the appointment schedule.

(2) A number of individuals continue to arrive either early or on time for their appointments. These individuals do not appreciate having to wait for an extended period of time, but they have accepted the situation. One individual, for example, had this to say about the problem:

I come to see the doctor and I have to wait. If I don't need to see the doctor, I wouldn't come here. It's like going to church. You sit through a long ceremony, and then you get in to see the doctor; he gives you the communion and a quick blessing and you go home.

One of the reasons people continue to arrive early for their appointments is that the 'waiting room' experience is not entirely a waste of time. While waiting to see the doctor people often meet friends and acquaintances in the reception area. This gives them a chance to socialize. Although the actual visit with the doctor may be short and unsatisfying, people gain some satisfaction from communicating their problems to other victims of misfortune.

(3) Some people arrive early and follow the typical pattern of registering their names with the receptionist. These individuals, however, refuse to wait in the reception area; instead, they quietly leave the office and either visit friends or go shopping. After a period of time, they return to check if their names have been called. This type of adjustment often results in conflict between the patient and the receptionist, and sometimes between patients.

(4) A small number of individuals have adjusted to the situation by simply not making appointments. These individuals reason that the receptionist must leave a block of time free, approximately 20-30 minutes, prior to the doctor's scheduled lunch break. They also reason that the doctor will not take a lunch break until all the patients in the 'waiting room' have been examined. By arriving during this time period, these individuals feel that they will be able to see the doctor within a relatively short period of time. This plan of action, however, may again lead to conflict between the receptionist and the patient. In addition the patient takes the risk of having an unsatisfying and rushed visit with the doctor.

In summary, 'arriving late for appointments' should not be construed as evidence that Sicilian-Canadians are: (1) 'unreliable and oblivious to time'; nor, (2) 'present time-oriented.' Arriving late for appointments must be understood within the context of Sicilian-Canadian conceptions of *punctuality*. Health care professionals must realize that the reality of the 'waiting room' situation leads people to make use of their conceptions of punctuality to arrive at some type of adjustment to what they perceive as a problem. Health care professionals must also realize that the situation is complicated further when Sicilian-Canadian patients are referred to non-Italian specialists who share even fewer values and beliefs with the patient.

Pain as Symbol

The sensation of pain has biological significance. It serves as an early warning signal that enables an organism to take action against environmental factors threatening its well-being (Zborowski 1969: 24-25). To a certain extent the reaction to pain is a biological reflex activity. Subjective 'feelings,' however, are also associated with the pain experience. Reich (1987: 117) defines pain as: "... the stimulation of some part of the body which the mind perceives as an injury or threat of injury to that portion of the body or to the self as a whole." These subjective feelings are influenced by *culture*.

Mark Zborowski's (1952; 1969) pioneering work on the cultural components of the pain experience is still widely acknowledged and accepted. In these reports, Zborowski (1969: 47) argues that: "... time orientation has an important bearing on people's attitudes toward pain." He then examines the interrelationship between time-orientation and pain among hospital patients of Irish, Italian, Jewish, and Old-American origins in New York City. With respect to the Italian-Americans, he concludes that they are present-oriented.

Zborowski (1969: 46-47) arrived at this view for two primary reasons: (1) the Italian-Americans seemed to be much more concerned with the immediacy of the pain sensation, rather than "its implications for the future"; and, (2) they were "more preoccupied with its relief ... than with the cure of the condition of which the pain is a symptom." More recently, certain writers have either accepted this view, or they have arrived at a very similar conclusion (Rozendal 1987; Sternbach and Tursky 1965; Martinelli 1987; McMahon and Miller 1978; Rotunno and McGoldrick 1982).

I would like to argue that Italians, or at least Sicilian-Canadians, are concerned about the implications of the pain sensation for their future. Although they may react directly to the sensation of pain and seek its immediate relief, Sicilian-Canadians do not react in this way because they have a present time-orientation. In my view, the feelings of anxiety and apprehension they experience over the possible implications of the pain sensation are not directly expressed, but rather collapsed together so that the pain sensation itself symbolizes the fact that their future well-being – both physical and social – is in question. Once the individual receives relief from his or her pain, and reassurance and support from family and friends, the future begins to look much brighter.

For Sicilian-Canadians, an individual's health is the key to his or her future. The proverb stating that 'the best time is the time to come,' for example, is usually qualified with the following remark: 'as long as there is health.' The absence of pain, in turn, is one of the more important indicators of health. Pain serves as a symbol that the person's future well-being is in danger, and it evokes various non-verbalized feelings of anxiety about the future. This anxiety, however, is expressed in terms of illness behavior associated with the pain sensation itself. At one level of analysis, then, the dramatization of the pain experience serves as an *idiom of distress* to convey the following messages: (1) I am suffering; (2) the suffering may have physical and social consequences for my future well-being; and (3) I need assistance and reassurance.

By actively complaining and dramatizing the pain, the individual is seeking reassurance that his or her lifestyle will not be affected adversely and that various social relationships will remain intact. This reassurance is obtained in two ways. First, it is provided by medical practitioners, or others, who take action to relieve the pain. This reassures the individual that his or her health is being restored. Second, the individual's family and friends – through their constant and consistent visiting – provide reassurance that his or her interactions with others will continue, relatively unaffected, by the temporary illness episode. The following case history will serve to illustrate these points.

The Case of Pina and the Heart Pain

Zia Pina is approximately 55 years old. Her husband, Zio Leno is roughly 62 years old, and their two teenaged daughters Rosa and Pinetta are aged 17 and 14 respectively. Zia Pina, Zio Leno and Rosa were all born in Sicily. They arrived in Canada when Rosa was approximately 2 years old.

One Saturday evening, Rosa went out with her girlfriends. She was to return home by 10:30 p.m. From the moment Rosa left home I began to worry about her. I tried to work around the house, but I couldn't complete anything. I tried to watch some television, but I couldn't keep my mind on the program. My husband seemed very calm. He reasoned that Rosa had gone to school dances before, and that everything had always been fine. He wasn't sure why I was so worried today. He said that I was starting to make him anxious too.

Rosa did not arrive home at 10:30 p.m. I became very upset; I wanted to call the police. I was worried that something had happened to her: "maybe she was in a car accident"; or, "maybe she was abducted." I wasn't sure what to think. Rosa had not been late before. I just knew something was wrong; I had been feeling it all evening, that's why I had been so worried. Leno was also concerned, but he convinced me to wait for a little while longer.

When Rosa had not returned by 11:00 p.m., Leno was not only concerned, he was angry. He said: "Rosa better have a good excuse, or she's in trouble." He would teach her a lesson; he would never let her go to dances again. At this point, I began to phone the parents of the other girls. The response was that the other girls had been home for the last 30 minutes, and that Rosa should have been home by now. I was concerned, upset, and angry. I kept thinking: "Should I call the police?"

Rosa arrived home at about 11:15 p.m. Both my husband and I were glad to see her, but we were also very upset. We had harsh words for Rosa. We demanded an explanation. We also threatened not to let her out for dances with friends again. Rosa tried to defend herself, and began to argue with us. She told us that she was old enough to take care of herself. She said she was late because she had missed the bus, and that at that time of the evening the buses were slow and infrequent. She stressed that she had done nothing wrong. Her friends had arrived home earlier because they lived a short walk from the school. That night we were all upset, and everyone went to bed upset.

The next day everyone was very quiet. There was no arguing, and there was no discussion of what had happened the previous night. Leno spent most of the day outside in his garden. I spent most of the day completing various chores. In the evening, we all sat together to watch television, that's when my problems began. Initially I experienced difficulty breathing. Then I felt this strong duluri [pain] in my chest. The pain was so intense that I began to make loud lamenting sounds – Aii Aii. [This type of lament is a characteristic Sicilian-Canadian way of expressing pain.] Within a short period of time I began to scream, the pain was in my heart. I felt as if I was about to die.

Leno and Rosa helped me to bed, while Pinetta ran for water. They sprinkled cold water on my face, but I was delirious and in extreme pain. I kept repeating that I was having a heart attack. I wanted someone to call for an ambulance. Leno tried to get me to drink some water and calm down, but I just had to get to the hospital immediately. I told them: "Do you want me to die!" Finally Rosa phoned the ambulance service, and I was taken to the hospital.

The examining doctor tried to ask me questions but I was in too much pain. He gave me an injection. I don't know what type of injection I received but it seemed to ease the pain. I spent about one hour in the hospital. The doctor mentioned something about 'stress' and 'general weakness.' My heart was strong. The doctor suggested that I visit my family physician in the next few days.

I spent the rest of the evening, and the next day, in bed. I felt very weak. But my family helped me, they helped me whenever I needed assistance.

My sister and brother came, with their families, to visit me as soon as they heard of my sickness. They all came into my bedroom to see me and to ask about the problem. Later, while the men played cards in the kitchen and the kids watched television, all the women – me, my sister, my sister-in-law – stayed in the bedroom. We talked about the problem. We decided that I didn't have a heart attack; if I had had a heart attack they would have kept me in the hospital and I would have been in real bad shape. It must have been 'nerves.' I was upset and worried the night before. My 'nerves' started acting up and attacked my heart. I was lucky, it could have been more serious. People can die from 'nerves' attacking the heart.

My sister took care of washing all the dishes, cups, everything. Rosa also helped; she made coffee for everyone and tea for me.

The women started to bother Rosa. They said: "Do you want to kill your mother." "If you do that again, you're going to make her heart burst." Rosa tried to defend herself; she explained about the bus. But everyone, women and men, started saying that she should think about that ahead of time; she should catch the earlier bus. My brother told her if she missed the bus she should try to phone at least. Then Rosa got upset and left the room. Someone said: "These kids don't think of anyone else." But my sister-in-law told everyone to stop, and yelled to Rosa: "OK forget about everything, but next time try to phone." I asked everyone to calm down. They were starting to upset me again. After a while everyone went home.

At bed time Rosa told me that she just missed the bus, and that next time she would try to leave earlier or phone. We hugged and everyone went to bed.

The next day I felt better. I was able to do some things around the house, but I was still weak. Since I was feeling better, I decided not to go to see my family doctor.

In this case history two distinct, but complementary, idioms of distress are in operation. First, the expression of pain in itself serves as a means of communicating that things are not right. Zia Pina's pain is both *real*, and anxiety provoking. By dramatizing the pain she is feeling, Zia Pina communicates to the family that she is suffering and needs immediate assistance. The family responds positively to her cry for help. Their actions enable Zia Pina to seek and receive immediate medical attention. The concern and attention they display towards her confirms that the family is still healthy and united. Second, labeling the ailment as an attack of 'nerves' serves to focus attention on the misunderstanding of the previous evening. Zia Pina became ill because she had been extremely worried, upset, and angry; her emotions were out of balance. As a result of this disequilibrium, Zia Pina's 'blood' was agitated and her 'nerves' began to tighten. The 'nerves' tightened in the area of her heart to produce a great deal of pain and suffering that left her very weak. The positive feedback Zia Pina received from both her immediate and extended family helped to move her back towards an equilibrium state. In order to avoid further complications and possible future attacks, however, Zia Pina would need continued support in the future. By agreeing to at least phone if she was going to be late, Rosa confirmed that Zia Pina could count on her for future support.

The case history, then, illustrates how *the expression of pain* can serve as an *idiom of distress*. It also illustrates the process by which significant others decode the vague message contained in the pain episode, and transform it into a culturally specific idiom that not only communicates that the individual is suffering, but also: (1) explains why he or she is experiencing the problem; and (2) what can be done to correct the problem. Illness behavior characterized by the seeking of attention and the immediate relief from pain should not be interpreted as an indication that Sicilian-Canadians have a present time-orientation. To make this type of interpretation would be to lose sight of the fact that the body is capable of conveying certain messages about the person's physical, emotional and social well-being (Kleinman 1986; Scheper-Hughes and Lock 1987).

Summary and Implications

In the past, scholars made use of the concept of 'present' time-orientation as an analytic or interpretive device to gain an understanding of certain behavior commonly attributed to southern Italians. More specifically, 'present' time-orientation became an acceptable abstract device to explain phenomena such as: 'arriving late for appointments'; 'seeking immediate relief from pain'; and, 'dramatizing the pain experience.' Over the years, however, the concept was uncritically transformed from an abstract interpretive device into a concrete value characteristic of southern Italian world-view. In my view, the notion that southern Italians (including immigrants residing in North America), and possibly other peoples, are 'present'-oriented is both unsubstantiated and untenable. My findings indicate that various Sicilian-Canadian beliefs, practices, and proverbs reflect a strong concern for the future well-being of individuals and families. I suggest that there is a need for systematic research to objectively reevaluate the evidence. Scholars must reexamine the abstract models they create to interpret the value system(s) of other peoples, while health care professionals must be more critical and responsible in their use of ethnographic materials. Labeling an entire group of people as 'past,' 'present,' or 'future' time-oriented does little more than generate stereotypes that will benefit neither health care providers nor their patients. In the case of medical attention, these stereotypes may in fact have negative consequences for everyone involved.

With respect to the focus of this paper, I suggest that there is no need to rely on the notion of 'present time-orientation' to explain the diverse phenomena outlined above. Valid alternative explanations are possible. First, Sicilian-Canadians often arrive late for appointments with medical professionals as a result of two interrelated factors: (1) they do not share our conception of punctuality; and, (2) they manipulate their conception of punctuality in order to adjust to the reality of the 'waiting room' experience. Second, the dramatization of the pain experience serves as a communicative device. It serves as an idiom of distress. For Sicilian-Canadians, 'pain' operates as a symbol that the individual's future well-being is in question.

Preliminary Implications

Hospital personnel emphasize that patients need their rest, and often complain that Italians tend to over-visit and to over-stay each visit. The visiting process, however, is often essential because it allows family and friends to demonstrate that they are committed in their relationship to the patient. This reassures the patient concerning his or her social well-being in the future. In addition, the visiting process provides people with an opportunity to discuss the various aspects of the problem, to label the complaint, and establish a plan of action to deal with the dimensions of the problem that are not handled by health care professionals.

Although Italians may appear to be solely interested in obtaining relief from the immediate sensation of pain, medical practitioners must remember that this is only the first step towards providing the individual with reassurance and support concerning his or her well-being. If additional reassurance is not provided, and the pain were to resurface, it may breed discontent or disillusionment, and eventually lead to the use of alternative healing techniques.

Sicilian-Canadians may indeed arrive late for appointments scheduled with various medical professionals. This, however, should not be interpreted as evidence that Sicilian-Canadians are not concerned about the ailment and its implications for their future well-being. Instead, it must be understood within the context of both Sicilian-Canadian conceptions of punctuality, and, Sicilian-Canadian interpretation of, and interaction with, 'waiting room' culture. In dealing with Sicilian-Canadians, then, medical professionals must distinguish between what they perceive as tardiness on the one hand, and the patient's genuine concern with the health problem on the other.

Finally, the constant complaining and dramatizing of the pain experience should not be interpreted as evidence that a Sicilian-Canadian patient is displaying hypochondriacal behavior. This type of illness behavior is a culturally appropriate and acceptable way of communicating distress to others.

In closing, I would like to suggest that an understanding of Sicilian-Canadian conceptions of time and health/illness is necessary to avoid various misunderstandings – misunderstandings that could potentially generate stress and anxiety for the patients, and frustration for health care providers.

References

Blok, A. 1981. Rams and Billy-goats: A Key to the Mediterranean Code of Honor. *Man (N.S.)* 16: 427–440.

Davis, J. 1977. *People of the Mediterranean: An Essay in Comparative Social Anthropology.* London: Routledge and Kegan Paul.

Davis, J. 1969. Honor and Family in Pisticci. *Proceedings of the Royal Institute of Great Britain and Ireland,* 69–81.

Eliade, M. 1954. *The Myth of the Eternal Return.* Princeton, NJ: Princeton University Press.

Evans-Pritchard, EE. 1940. *The Nuer.* Oxford: Oxford University Press.

Evans-Pritchard, EE. 1939. Nuer time-reckoning. *Africa* 12: 109–126.

Fortes, M. 1970. *Time and Social Structure and Other Essays.* London School of Economics Monographs on Social Anthropology, No. 40. London: Athlone Press.

Foster, GM. 1972. The Anatomy of Envy: A Study in Symbolic Behavior. *Current Anthropology* 13: 165–202.

Hall, ET. 1959. *The Silent Language.* Garden City, NY: Doubleday.

Hallowell, AI. 1937. Temperal Orientation in Western Civilization and in a Preliterate Society. *American Anthropology* 39: 647–670.

Hallpike, CR. 1979. *The Foundations of Primitive Thought.* Oxford: Clarendon Press.

Helman, C. 1987. Heart Disease and the Cultural Construction of Time: The Type A Behavior Pattern as a Western Culture-Bound Syndrome. *Social Science and Medicine* 25: 969–979.

Helman, C. 1984. *Culture Health and Illness.* Bristol: Wright.

Herzfeld, M. 1984. The Horns of the Mediterraneanist Dilemma: A Hardening of the Categories. *American Ethnologist* 11: 439–454.

Herzfeld, M. 1980. Honor and Shame: Problems in the Comparative Analysis of Moral Systems. *Man (N.S.)* 15: 339–351.

Kearney, M. 1984. *World View.* Novato, Calif: Chandler & Sharp.

Kearney, M. 1972. *The Winds of Ixtepeji: World View and Society in a Zapotec Town.* New York: Holt, Rinehart & Winston.

Kessner, T. 1977. *The Golden Door: Italians and Jewish Immigrant Mobility in New York City, 1880-1915.* New York: Oxford University Press.

Kleinman, A. 1986. *Social Origins of Distress and Disease: Depression, Neurasthenia, and Pain in Modern China.* New Haven, Conn: Yale University Press.

Kluckhohn, F, and FL Strodtbeck. 1961. *Variations in Value Orientations.* Evanston, Ill: Row, Peterson.

Leach, E. 1976. *Culture and Communication.* London: Cambridge University Press.

Leach, E. 1961. *Rethinking Anthropology.* New York: Humanities Press.

Martinelli, AM. 1987. Pain and Ethnicity: How People of Different Cultures Experience Pain. *AORN Journal* 46: 273–281.

McMahon, MA, and P Miller. 1978. Pain Response: The Influence of Psycho-Social-Cultural Factors. *Nursing Forum* 17: 58–71.

Migliore, S. 1988. Religious Symbols and Cultural Identity: A Sicilian-Canadian Example. *Canadian Ethnic Studies* 20: 78–94.

Migliore, S. 1983. Evil Eye or Delusions: on the "Consistency" of Folk Models. *Medical Anthropology Quarterly* 14: 4–9.

Nelli, HS. 1983. *From Immigrants to Ethnics: The Italian Americans.* New York: Oxford University Press.

Nelli, HS. 1970. *Italians in Chicago, 1880-1930: A Study in Ethnic Mobility.* New York: Oxford University Press.

Nilsson, MP. 1920. *Primitive Time-Reckoning.* Lund: Gleerup.

Pitt-Rivers, JA. 1977. *The Fate of Sheechem or the Politics of Sex; Essays in the Anthropology of the Mediterranean.* Cambridge: University of Cambridge Press.

Pitt-Rivers, JA. 1966. Honor and Social Status. In JG Peristiany ed. *Honor and Shame: The Values of Mediterranean Society,* 21–77. Chicago: University of Chicago Press.

Pitt-Rivers, JA. 1954. *The People of the Sierra.* Chicago: University of Chicago Press.

Radin, P. 1970. *The Italians of San Francisco: Their Adjustment and Acculturation.* Originally published in 1935. San Francisco: R & E Research Associates.

Reich, WT. 1987. Models of Pain and Suffering: Foundations for an Ethic of Compassion. *Acta Neurochirurgica Supplementum* 38: 117–122.

Rolle, AF. 1980. *The Italian Americans: Troubled Roots.* New York: The Free Press.

Rolle, AF. 1972. *The American Italians: Their History and Culture.* Belmont, Calif: Wadsworth.

Rolle, AF. 1968. *The Immigrant Upraised: Italian Adventures and Colonists in an Expanding America.* Norman, Okla: University of Oklahoma Press.

Romanucci-Ross, L. 1975. Italian Ethnic Identity and its Transformations. In G DeVos and L Romanucci-Ross eds. *Ethnic Identity: Cultural Continuities and Change,* 198–226. Chicago: University of Chicago Press.

Rotunno, M, and M McGoldrick. 1982. Italian Families. In M McGoldrick, JK Pearce and J Giordano eds. *Ethnicity and Family Therapy,* 340–363. New York: The Guilford Press.

Rozendal, N. 1987. Understanding Italian American Cultural Norms. *Journal of Psychosocial Nursing and Mental Health Services* 25: 29–33.

Scheper-Hughes, N, and MM Lock. 1987. The Mindful Body: A Prolegomenon to Future Work in Medical Anthropology. *Medical Anthropology Quarterly (N.S.)* 1: 6–41.

Statistics Canada. 1984. *Census of Canada, 1981.* Ottawa: Queen's Printer and Controller of Stationary.

Sternbach, RA, and B Tursky. 1965. Ethnic Differences Among Housewives in Psychophysical and Skin Potential Responses to Electric Shock. *Psychophysiology* 1: 241–246.

Zborowski, M. 1969. *People in Pain.* San Francisco: Jossey-Bass.

Zborowski, M. 1952. Cultural Components in Response to Pain. *Journal of Social Issues* 8: 16–30.

9

Women's Perspectives on Chronic Illness: Ethnicity, Ideology and Restructuring of Life*

Joan M. Anderson, Connie Blue and Annie Lau

When you get up in the morning without a health problem you get up and you look at your day and you see your day stretching ahead of you ... What I see, is my day stretching ahead of me with blocks ... I see headstones when I am in bad mood ... and I see these blocks every couple of hours; either I have to eat, or I have to test or I have to do something ... So that for me is the adjustment there. That was hard to do. It's still not easy to do after this length of time ... This is not my choice ... I'm having to do something that is not my choice. (Anglo-Canadian)

So it did wreck my career. It wrecked my self-image of who I was a lot, too, to think of yourself as a sicko basically ... So it's the same as having cancer ... Well you live with it for so long and then you die. (Anglo-Canadian)

Diabetes is not a serious disease, it is only long-term. Since I have the disease, I have to face it, and I have to deal with it. Especially now that I have a baby, everybody is concerned about me, then I am not scared now. But I feel it's very troublesome ... It's troublesome because initially, in a few days in the hospital, I was worried about my job, you know I have a job. (Chinese)

Nobody ever explained to me what diabetes is about. The doctors said high blood sugar. And that's it, high blood sugar ... I'm just scared. I heard diabetes will cause stroke or the person will become paralyzed, but I can't look so far ahead. (Chinese)

Expressions of illness are multivocal. Yet, these extracts from interviews with Chinese and Anglo-Canadian women reflect one common feature of the experience of diabetes; they exemplify how chronic illness not only disrupts the fabric of daily life, but also how self is redefined, and how new images are produced. Bury contends "that illness, and especially chronic illness, is precisely that kind of experience where the structures of everyday life and the forms of knowledge which underpin them are disrupted" (Bury 1982: 169). This disruption calls for a major restructuring of self – the perception of who one is, and what one is able to do; in other words, the individual has "to reconstruct a sense of order from the fragmentation produced by chronic illness" (Williams 1984: 177).

* Reprinted from *Social Science and Medicine*, Vol. 33, Joan M. Anderson, Connie Blue and Annie Lau, 'Women's Perspectives on Chronic Illness: Ethnicity, Ideology and Restructuring of Life,' pp. 101-113, 1991, with permission from Elsevier Science Ltd., Oxford, England.

Restructuring of life in the face of chronic illness is not a static phenomenon that takes place once and for all. Rather, it is an ongoing process that is reflexively shaped by the ups and downs not only of the illness course, but also by the events that make up the furniture of everyday life – getting and keeping a job, making ends meet, forming new relationships and the like. The meaning and experience of illness is nested in a complex personal, socioeconomic and political nexus (Kleinman 1986; Kleinman 1987).

In this paper, we will examine the context in which the process of restructuring is located when a woman's life is disrupted by a chronic illness. We take the perspective that local lives are inextricably linked to a set of social relations in the larger social organization. This analysis is the product of a three year study examining how Chinese and White women living with diabetes construct their chronic illness, and the circumstances shaping their illness experiences. This study continues a line of research on the health of women from different ethnocultural groups (Anderson 1985; 1987; 1988).

There is growing literature to support the notion that women's experiences cannot be subsumed under those of men, as there are specific issues, e.g. women's roles inside and outside the home, which influence a woman's experience of illness (Anderson 1985; 1987; Sorensen et al. 1985; Verbrugge 1985). Furthermore, there is increasing evidence that men and women use health care resources differently. For example, one study, comparing how men and women use the same health care system, found that "men of higher social classes were more likely to use medical care, whereas, among women, those in higher social classes were more likely to use lay consultants" (Meininger 1986: 291).

We have felt the urgent need to inquire into the lives of women who, as well as living with a chronic illness, must also deal with uprooting from their homelands and resettling in a new country that is quite different from their home country in terms of language and culture. Over the past few decades, there has been a marked increase of people immigrating to Canada from Asian countries. In 1986, India, Vietnam and Hong Kong were among the top four source countries of landed immigrants to Canada (Canada Employment and Immigration 1986). According to the 1986 census, in one regional district in Greater Vancouver, Canada, Chinese was the most common mother tongue among the nonofficial languages (Statistics Canada 1986a).

About fifty percent of the recent immigrants from Asia are women (Canada Employment and Immigration 1986). Not only do some of these women face difficulties different from those of men, but also from mainstream Canadian women as well, as many immigrant women from Third World countries do not speak English, and do not have skills suitable for Canada's labour market. It would seem, therefore, that different issues could surface in illness management among mainstream Anglo-Canadian women and immigrant women, as the material circumstances of their lives are different. As Meleis, Norbeck, Laffrey, Solomon and Miller have pointed out, "While women in high-status occupations tend to balance their role stressors with satisfactions such as freedom and status ... women in low-status occupations may not have the same advantages" (Meleis et al. 1989: 320).

Theoretical and Methodological Perspective

This inquiry into women's existential responses to illness begins from the standpoint of women (Pirie 1988; Smith 1975; 1979; 1986; Oakley 1981; Stanley and Wise 1983) and proceeds to elucidate the context in which personal meanings are nested. Following the line of analysis derived from Smith (Smith 1979; 1986), we ask how women's experiences of illness are organized, how they are determined, and what the social relations are that generate them, and develop an inquiry "which explores the everyday world not in itself but as it is articulated to the social relations of the larger social and economic process" (Smith 1986: 6). Smith has used the term 'institutional ethnography' to describe the research strategy she has proposed. "Rather than defining issues and problems as they have been established as currency in the discipline," she tells us, "the aim is to explicate the actual social processes and practices organizing people's everyday experience" (Smith 1986: 6). This approach is not concerned exclusively with the world of women's experiences. Rather, the search is for a method "which provides for subjects' means of grasping the social relations organizing the worlds of their experience ... institutional analysis ... offers a means of exploring and making public the social ground and organization of our common and diverging experience" (Smith 1986: 6-7), and therefore directs us to analyze the material conditions that shape the experiencing of illness.

A central argument here is that both Chinese and Anglo-Canadian women experience a restructuring of their lives in chronic illness; however, the issues are usually different for both groups of women, and must be understood within the socioeconomic and political context of women's lives. While the social circumstances of the lives of many women produce a set of conditions that impinge upon illness management, some Chinese women are at a special disadvantage in having their health care needs met. The conditions under which they work are often a deterrent to illness management. Furthermore, immigrant women, especially those who are non-English speaking, are excluded from the forms of thought that organize how health care services are delivered.

We argue that, within the local context of illness management, the vocabularies of the larger social organization are reproduced in micro level interactions between women and health professionals through a set of ideologies that structure health care delivery. The notion of ideology, derived from Smith, is used to refer to the ideas and images that are produced within the society "for others to use, to analyse, to understand, and to interpret their social relations, what is happening, the world that they experience and act in" (Smith 1975: 355). These ideas and images are interwoven in a complex fabric of social, economic and political processes. There is a dialectical relationship, then, between individual meanings and the wider social organization, that is mediated through the health care encounter.

One of the most powerful ideologies that underscores the organization of health care delivery services today, is the ideology of self-care. Of special interest in this analysis is the way in which the 'ideology of self-care' structures health care delivery, and how this, in turn, impinges on women's restructuring of life. The self-care movement has gained momentum since the 1970's and has been discussed in government documents (Epp 1986), and a number of professional articles and books (Steiger and Lipson 1985; Canadian Nurses Association 1988; Graham and Schubert 1985; Orem 1985). A basic premise of this movement is that individuals are empowered through self-care; by taking more control over their lives, they come to rely less on health professionals. It is one way, then, of erroding professional dominance. As Steiger and Lipson have noted, "The basic premise of self-care is that individuals have the ability to influence their health and to participate in their health care. Self-care is defined ... as those activities initiated or performed by an individual, family, or community to achieve, maintain, or promote maximum health potential" (Steiger and Lipson 1988: vii).

However, there is another side to the self-care movement which cannot be ignored, and that is pivotal to this analysis. Self-care is not an isolated ideology, but mirrors the ideology of individualism in the capitalist state; individual responsibility for self and individual ability to chart the course of ones life underpin this movement. Illness management is often reduced to individual capabilities, divorcing the personal from the complex sociopolitical, cultural and economic context. Within this reductionist framework, 'culture' and 'ethnicity' may be treated as concrete characteristics, as 'variables,' that determine why a person may or may not comply with 'self-care.'

We take a different tack in this analysis. We argue that treating 'culture' as static, as an 'objective fact' that determines illness meanings and the restructuring of life, glosses the harsh reality of poverty and oppression. Culture, as Brittan and Maynard remind us, does not have "a 'free-floating' reality independent of any structural constraints" (Brittan and Maynard 1984: 20). There is, therefore, the need to conduct empirical work that will illuminate the contextual features of the illness experience, and bring to explicit clarity the sources of oppression of the socially disadvantaged.

The Study

Methods of Data Collection and Analysis

Personnel from selected health care and community agencies agreed to circulate a letter to potential participants describing the research, and informing them of the voluntary nature of their participation and their rights as research subjects. The letter was written in the women's native language, and accompanied by a reply sheet, so that they could contact us if they so choose. Thirty women (15 Anglo-Canadian, and 15 Chinese), were recruited through this process. Those who agreed to participate were asked to give written consent in the language of their choice (English or Chinese).

One of the limitations of this process of selecting women was the exclusion of those who were not in contact with health care providers or other community personnel – quite probably, the very women whose voices need most to be heard. We pondered this problem but could not find an acceptable solution. We recognized that the strategies available to us for recruiting women, would of necessity exclude those isolated from Western health care and community agencies.

Data collection. Our discussions with women were guided by an interview schedule constructed in consultation with two health care providers, and a woman with diabetes. Questions covered various aspects of women's lives, such as beliefs about illness, the effect of the illness on social relationships, perceptions of relationships with health professionals, help-seeking patterns, and daily management of diabetes. However, we must stress that this interview guide was used as just that – a general guide; the discussions were flexible enough to allow women to speak of their experience of living with a chronic illness, and to discuss the areas that were paramount in their lives. In other words, women were encouraged to 'tell their story.' Women allowed us to audiotape record our conversations with them. Sociodemographic data were also obtained to help construct a profile of the women.

Sequential interviews were done over a two year period to give us a longitudinal perspective on what it was like to live with a chronic illness and how this illness changed over time. Although we had intended to conduct three interviews with each woman, the number of interviews varied to accommodate a woman's life circumstances. Due to time constraints, and migration to another part of Canada, three women were interviewed only once. Another woman died of complications from diabetes after the first interview. All the other women were interviewed at least twice. A third interview was done with eleven Anglo-Canadian and seven Chinese women; and a fourth with two women for the purpose of clarifying the meaning of some of the data obtained from them. With the exception of two women, one of whom was interviewed in the research office and another in the restaurant that she owns, women were interviewed in their homes. Each interview lasted for one to two hours.

The interviewing was shared among the three of us (two of us are immigrant women, and one of us speaks Cantonese). Another Cantonese speaking woman assisted during the first year of the study. Interviews with the Chinese women were conducted in Cantonese, and translated into English. Interviews were then transcribed by a typist, and the data organized with a computer program, the Ethnograph (Seidel et al. 1988), to facilitate data analysis.

Data analysis. Data collection and data analysis proceeded simultaneously. As tapes were transcribed, we identified topics from the transcript materials by reviewing each line of the transcript. From these initial topics, a set of broader analytic categories were devised. Each category usually incorporated a number of topics that reflected the women's experience of illness. For example, topics like reorganizing work schedules, changing jobs, changing dietary patterns, were included in the analytic category of "restructuring of life." The analytic categories were neither mutually exclusive, nor were they seen as the 'hard facts' about women's experiences of illness. We were not attempting to tabulate the categories, but rather to examine recurrent patterns and processes in women's lives.

Sociodemographic Characteristics of Women

The two tables that are included provide a summary of the sociodemographic data from 15 Anglo-Canadian and 12 Chinese women. (Three of the Chinese women were not available for a second interview to obtain these data.) The sociodemographic data (see Table 1) are provided only to give a sense of who the women were. It is not intended that statistical inferences be drawn from them.

TABLE 1
Comparative sociodemographic characteristics

	Caucasian		Chinese	
	n=15	%	n=12	%
Age of Women				
Under 25	0		0	
26-34	4	26.66	0	
35-39	3	20.00	2	16.66
40-44	1	6.66	2	16.66
45-49	2	13.33	0	
50-54	3	20.00	2	16.66
55-60	0		2	16.66
60 and over	2	13.33	4	33.33

Continued on next page

Table 1 - *continued*

	Caucasian n=15	%	Chinese n=12	%
Language spoken				
English (primary language)	15	100.00	0	
English/Cantonese	0		2	16.66
Cantonese only	0		10	83.33
Education				
None	0		0	
Grades 1-7	0		6	50.00
Grades 8-10	0		5	41.66
Grades 11-12	3	20.00	0	
Post secondary	7	46.66	0	
University	5	33.33	1	8.33
Occupation				
Unskilled	0		3	25.00
Skilled blue collar	0		3	25.00
Professional/semi prof./				
white collar	11	73.33	1	8.33
Homemaker/retired	4	26.66	5	41.66
Employment status				
Unemployed	2	13.33	0	
Part-time	2	13.33	2	16.66
Full-time	7	46.66	5	41.66
Homemaker/retired	4	26.66	5	41.66
Marital status				
Never married	6	40.00	0	
With partner	7	46.66	8	66.66
Separated	0		0	
Divorced	2	13.33	0	
Widowed	0		4	33.33
Living arrangements				
Living alone	8	53.33	1	8.33
Nuclear family	6	40.00	6	50.00
Extended family	1	6.66	3	25.00
Widowed (living with				
adult children)	0		2	16.66
Family income				
Under 9999	2	13.33	1	8.33
10,000-14,999	0		1	8.33
15,000-19,999	2	13.33	0	
20,000-24,999	1	6.66	3	25.00
25,000-29,999	2	13.33	1	8.33
30,000-39,999	3	20.00	3	25.00
40,000 and over	5	33.33	3	25.00
Length of time in Canada				
Born	13	86.66	0	
2 yr or less	0		3	25.00
3-5 yr	0		1	8.33
6-8 yr	0		1	8.33
9-11 yr	0		1	8.33
12 yr or more	2	13.33	6	50.00

Prior to starting the study, we had intended to match the Chinese and Anglo-Canadian women on the basis of education and occupation; however, it was difficult to find Chinese immigrant women who were at a level similar to that of the Anglo-Canadian women. The differences between the two groups of women are not seen as a shortcoming of the study, as the focus is on the contextual features of the illness experience. That it was difficult to find Chinese women of a similar educational and occupational level to Anglo-Canadian women, speaks to the reality of the lives of many immigrant women. This will be taken up in the analysis of the qualitative data.

All the Chinese women, with the exception of one who had immigrated from Malaysia, were first generation immigrants from mainland China and Hong Kong. All spoke Cantonese; only two spoke English as well. Even though the majority had lived in Canada for more than nine years, they had difficulty learning English. This is not unusual. Several studies including an earlier study by one of us (Anderson and Lynam, 1988), document that many immigrant women have little time to take English language classes. They work long hours in the paid workforce; on top of this, they must do the housework and mind children. Some also have to look after aging parents and in-laws. Gannage, in her study of women garment workers, found that, "their double day of labour at work and at home made it difficult for immigrant women to obtain the language training that their male counterparts were able to obtain" (Gannage 1986: 196). Furthermore, some women are illiterate in their native language and so have difficulty learning English (Anderson and Lynam 1988).

These are the same reasons that the women in this present study gave for not being able to learn English. It's not surprising then, that the Chinese women were clustered in the lower echelons of the workforce – they did not have the opportunity to move out of these jobs, as they could not speak English.

Of the 15 White women, 13 were born in Canada of Anglo-Canadian descent. One woman had immigrated from England and another from continental Europe. Both of these women had resided in Canada for more than 12 years. All the White women spoke fluent English. The White women had a higher level of education than the Chinese women, and were mostly in professional or semiprofessional jobs.

Family income levels, though fairly similar for both groups of women, should be interpreted with caution. The White women, unlike their Chinese counterparts who lived mostly in extended families, were either alone or in a nuclear family. Also, widowed Chinese women tended to live with their adult children. Therefore, as a general rule, there were more wage earners per household in the Chinese family than in the White family.

The majority of the women in both groups had lived with diabetes for more than nine years (Table 2). All were required to take insulin injections or oral hypoglycemic medications. Fourteen of the 15 Anglo-Canadian women took insulin injections, as compared to 6 of the 12 Chinese women.

The Process of Interpreting the Qualitative Data

As we examined the ways in which women managed diabetes, it was evident that the Chinese and White women differed in several respects, such as, in their blood glucose monitoring patterns, help seeking patterns, pathways of medical treatment, and the like. In our initial analysis of the data, we tended to see the differences in how life was restructured and illness managed as attributable to a woman's ethnicity, and started to examine the symbolic meanings surrounding injections, loss of blood, and the like, that might have explained the preferences of the Chinese women. We also paid attention to the herbal remedies that the Chinese women used, and saw these practices as one way of getting a handle on the data so as to describe the cultural differences between the two groups of women. We found, for example, that 9 of 12 Chinese women had used a combination of Western medicine and Chinese herbal medicine (see Table 2). This was seen as informing us of the cultural differences between Chinese and White women. However, in further discussion with Chinese women, we found that some did not see themselves as using "herbal medicines." Rather, the herbs that they used were viewed as 'tonics' or dietary supplements (e.g., pig's pancreas soup, ginseng, pearl barley, squash) to give strength. (Similarly, the White women took vitamins to give strength.) In the words of two Chinese women:

I'm taking ginseng. Ginseng is not really medicine, it's only tonic, and it would boost up your health.

American ginseng is not medicine neither. Everyone can drink it. Let's say if you want to have your skin nice and smooth, you probably drink a little bit, then your acnes would disappear.

TABLE 2
Details of management of diabetes for women in the study

	Caucasian n=15	%	Chinese n=12	%
Length of time since diagnosis				
Less than 1 yr	0		0	
1-3 yr	2	13.33	2	16.66
4-6 yr	1	6.66	1	8.33
7-9 yr	4	26.66	2	16.66
More than 9 yr	8	53.33	7	58.33
Health care services utilized				
Traditional Chinese only	0		0	
Physician/clinic				
(Western Bio-medical)	15	100.00	3	25.00
Combination trad.				
Chinese/Western	0		9	75.00
Type of medication				
Insulin injections	14	93.33	6	50.00
Oral hypoglycemics	1	6.66	6	50.00

Even those who viewed herbs as 'medicines' rather than 'tonics,' deliberately avoided replacing Western medicine with Chinese herbal remedies. As this woman explained:

I had taken quite a bit of herbal medicine in the past, but now I don't dare to do it because I'm on insulin injections and I don't want to get the Chinese medicine mixed up with insulin in my body. They may not be compatible.

Another Chinese woman who tried to use both Chinese and Western medicine stated that:

Now since I am on Western medication, I am still taking Chinese medicine, the pig's pancreas soup. Anyways, the pig's pancreas soup with the herbal medicine in it is quite ordinary. I still can't be sure how effective it is. If you tell me just go on with the Chinese medicine, not to take care of my diet, not to take the Western medicine, I don't think it will work. I believe it cannot be done.

We found that when a woman was advised by the Western trained physician to discontinue the use of Chinese herbs, she usually complied, as this woman's account suggests:

The doctor told me that the more Chinese herbal stuff you take, the worse you would become. The doctor said that I must go on insulin injections, and eating Chinese herbal soup is useless. He said that eating the Chinese herbal stuff would harm a body. Actually, initially, I did try some Chinese herbs. I went to see a Chinese herbalist in Chinatown and told him that I had a bit of high blood sugar, so he gave me some Chinese herbs and I cook it up and made some soup to drink, but it's useless. And I have to go on insulin injections, and insulin injections will work for me. The doctor said nothing will work, only insulin will work for my body.

The fact is, herbal remedies did not get in the way of using western medicines. When hypoglycemic medications were prescribed, the woman administered them when she received clear instructions. When it was essential for a Chinese woman to monitor her blood glucose level, she did so if she had the resources, and if she understood how. Furthermore, some Chinese women subscribed wholeheartedly to the Western biomedical model. One woman, a former nurses' aide in Hong Kong, managed her illness and restructured her life in a way similar to that of the White women. Length of time in Canada did not seem to be crucial to how a woman managed. A woman who had been in Canada for less than a year displayed a similar pattern of managing illness to the women who had been in Canada for longer. Women showed a certain pragmatism in dealing with diabetes; they were receptive to what western medicine had to offer.

How a woman managed illness then, was not reducible to her 'ethnicity.' In fact, what could be interpreted as 'ethnic differences' could also be interpreted in the context of material existence, anchored in class relations and the ideologies which are reflected in these relations. For example, failure to monitor her blood sugar level could be interpreted in the context of her beliefs about loss of blood. However, some women didn't monitor their blood sugar level because instructions weren't clear, and/or they did not have the money to buy a glucometer. Although expected by health professionals to assume responsibility for their self-care, they were without the resources to do so.

In forwarding this perspective we want to draw attention to the complex set of circumstances that surround the experiencing of illness. Cultural meanings are not static, but are constructed and reconstructed in ongoing human interactions, and have to be understood within the sociopolitical and economic context. The ongoing reconstruction of illness meanings, and the subsequent restructuring of life, are contingent upon the mediating circumstances of everyday life. There is a dialectical relationship between the medicocultural and social contexts, and daily experiences.

In the following section we draw upon two case histories, one from a middle class White woman, and the other from a working class Chinese woman, to illuminate the context in which illness is experienced, and how life is restructured. We want to highlight the issues that were paramount in each woman's life, as she went about the task of reorganizing her life to live with diabetes. We use these case histories because they typify the life circumstances of the two groups of women we interviewed, and how the situations under which women lived influenced the process of restructuring of their lives to accommodate a chronic illness. The following are the kinds of data we were confronted with and had to make sense of. What interpretations can we bring to them?

The Case of Jane, a 48-Year-Old English-Speaking Woman with Diabetes

Jane lives with her husband in their own home in a 'middle-class' suburb. They have no children. The family is of comfortable means, with an income of well over $40,000 per year. Her husband is a businessman, and she has a University education.

She was diagnosed as having diabetes seven years ago. This is how she described the onset of symptoms, and her recognition that this could be diabetes:

I had to go to the bathroom a lot and I was drinking a lot and I was still working, too, at a full time job ..., even people there were saying to me, 'oh, you look terrible.' And I had black circles under my eyes, and I said, 'ya, I've made a doctor's appointment.' So I went to this doctor – and this is just in the span of about a week – went to the doctor and I said to my doctor, I said, this is what's happening. I'm urinating. I'm losing weight ... I think I have diabetes. So he said, 'we'll test it', and he did the urine testing and indeed showed that my blood sugars were all over the norm, and he sent me to the lab, and that confirmed it; I went the following day and the blood test confirmed it. Indeed I had diabetes.

Although the diagnosis of diabetes came as a complete shock to her, in her words:

I knew I had to do something about it ... I was very persistent, went to the doctor every week, and had a blood test done, and he put me on pills and it didn't work, the blood sugars just don't come down low enough. I even begged him, I said, 'please put me on insulin.'

Soon after this, she was briefly hospitalized to stabilize her diabetes, and to get established on insulin therapy.

Prior to the onset of diabetes, she exercised regularly, ate three well balanced meals a day, and had quit smoking. In spite of what might seem a 'healthy lifestyle' by the standards of health professionals, diabetes meant a total restructuring of her life. She had to adjust her daily time schedule to monitor her blood sugar. Furthermore, she had to forego outings for late night snacks, which was something she had enjoyed before the onset of diabetes. Consequently, her lifestyle became highly regimented:

The blood testing, I think, is the biggest thing. Getting up in the morning at a certain time. Also, actually having it in my head that I have to do exercises – even if I did it already before – but I feel the importance of it is much greater now. I have to see doctors, which I used to go once a year for a check-up, and that was it. Now I have to go regularly, and I go every three months.

She started to find her job stressful; furthermore, her work got in the way of managing the diabetes:

What got in the way, is that I had to eat on time – my lunch – and I felt that with the interruptions that I was having in my job, I couldn't handle that. I also had trouble with always checking my blood sugars when I wanted to do it because the demands of the job were such that it got in the way, and so I was really stressed out about that, and discussed it with my husband ... and we decided that I would leave this job and look for something else. Maybe don't work at all, but that wasn't right for me either. I wanted to do something and be active. I was doing a lot of volunteer work, too.

Being able to leave a job she no longer found satisfying, gave her a sense of power over her life. In her words:

That's why it also felt like a weight off my shoulders when I had made the actual decision to resign from that job, because that gave me power again. Hey, I was capable of doing it after having been in a job for 15 years, I was capable of saying "stuff it." (laughs)

Support from her husband helped her to make the job change:

And then it wasn't financially necessary for me ... I don't know what would've happened, I probably would have coped with it if I had been on my own ... You know, I know from deep down that I can be very innovative, too, so that I'm sure I would have come up with a solution, but I had the support that I didn't have to do that kind of work.

It was clear that she had the resources that made changing her job possible. The job she later found was not as well paid, but it was emotionally gratifying, and provided the flexibility so she could manage her diabetes.

This is not to say that she did not encounter discrimination in the workplace. On one occasion, a prospective employer, on finding out that she had diabetes, told her she was unsuitable for the job. She contemplated challenging the employer, but decided against it. From this experience, she learned to "put the diabetes in a little different way," meaning that she did not immediately tell a prospective employer about her diabetes.

Jane feels no pressure about managing diabetes in her present job. Her coworkers know that she has diabetes, and are well informed about her management in case of an emergency. "Quality of life" is important to her:

Jane: For me ... I like to be having a quality of life that will take me probably into the time that I get to 80, you know. I am not ready to go at the moment.

Interviewer: So in other words then, for you it's very important that you structure your life so that the management is an integral part of it?

Jane: Correct ... yeah, yeah, yeah. I really feel very clear on that, that this is important for me.

The priorities in her life were not determined by the need to earn a living, but by her attentiveness to the demands that diabetes placed on her time.

Jane described health professionals as very supportive. Furthermore, she knew how to get what she needed. She asked for consultations with specialists when she believed they were necessary, and insisted on getting them, even if the family physician didn't agree. She expressed satisfaction with her care, and described her physician in the following way:

I find him very supportive. He wants to do all kinds of tests to find out if this body is functioning the way it should, and also when I went through this, 'Should I resign from my job? Should I not?' I expressed that with him, and I got that he was listening to me. I also get that he wants the best for me. And yeah ... even going to a specialist – I go to an ophthalmologist and he keeps saying, "I want to see you back next year."

She believes that her physician learns from her, and she from him; there is reciprocity in the relationship. He is interested in finding out about her life, so that together they can plan the best possible care for her.

She has access to the literature on diabetes through libraries, bookstores, the diabetes association, and support groups. She is involved in volunteer work. She runs a support group for people with diabetes, and states that one of the reasons she is so involved with the support group is "because I know that it does a lot for me, too, by putting myself out."

She is well informed about complications of the disease, but feels that with good management, she will live to a ripe old age. She believes that the management of her illness is her responsibility, and does not feel that she has to rely on health professionals for the answers.

For Jane, life has its ups and downs, but she feels that she has the resources to meet the challenges as they come along – a husband whom she finds supportive, a job that she now enjoys, and health professionals with whom she can communicate. She also believes that her biggest asset is her 'inner strength,' and her self knowledge. On a recent visit, she discussed retirement plans, and she and her husband look forward to an old age with a secure pension, and all the other comforts of a 'good' middle class life.

To the health care professional, Jane may very well represent the 'model' patient. She is well informed about diabetes, and puts her illness first. She believes very strongly in self-care and individual responsibility for self, and has the financial means to organize her life so that she can, indeed, 'put the diabetes first.' She is immersed in the ideology to which health professionals subscribe. What most health professionals may overlook, however, is that the material circumstances of her life are such, that she has the resources available to follow their prescriptions.

In presenting this case history, we do not mean to imply that all White, English speaking women experience diabetes in a similar way. Rather, we would argue that in analyzing women's experiences we must look at the social circumstances of their lives, and the context in which these experiences are embedded. Depending on their life circumstances, some Anglo-Canadian women may identify more closely with May, the Chinese woman whose case history follows.

May, a 39-Year-Old Cantonese-Speaking Woman with Diabetes

When we first visited May, a 39-year-old married woman, she had been in Canada for less than 2 years, and worked full-time in a factory. Her husband also held a full-time blue collar job. Their combined annual income was $22,000. They both completed junior high school in Hong Kong. They were renting a basement suite, and May was expecting her first child.

We kept in contact with her until after the birth of her child. We therefore gained insight into the circumstances that structured her experience of illness over time: her work situation, the economic conditions under which she lived, her marginal position in Canadian society – all of which shaped her experience and management of illness.

These interviews also revealed that although women are expected to manage self-care for chronic health conditions like diabetes, there is little help to enable them to do so. In fact, it seemed that, despite difficulties, May was able to get the help she needed during her pregnancy. However, from her account, this was not the case after the birth of her child. Perhaps this informs us not only of the priorities within the health care delivery system, and how chronic illness is viewed, but also of how relationships with health care providers structure the experiencing and management of illness. For, as we will see, the difficulties May experienced in managing diabetes were exacerbated by the withdrawal of professional assistance.

May was diagnosed with diabetes about five years ago when she went for a physical examination for the purpose of migrating to Canada from Hong Kong. She had not realized she had diabetes:

Before coming here I didn't realize I had diabetes, because my work was so busy. Only occasionally I found that I had blurry vision, then I thought perhaps because I was too tired from work, or I was too nervous because of pressure from work and society.

May's physician in Hong Kong prescribed hypoglycemic pills, and she brought a few months supply of the medication when she came to Canada. As she put it:

I have my pills all from Hong Kong. I have brought a few months supply of medication from Hong Kong. Then I asked my friends to send from Hong Kong to Canada because I was afraid that they wouldn't have the type of medications I need here. And then I went to see my family doctor and he prescribed some pills for me. After I ran out of the pills, the ones brought from Hong Kong – I didn't want to bother my friend anymore – so I just have the medications prescribed by my family doctor.

Shortly after she arrived in Canada, she became pregnant, and stopped taking the hypoglycemic pills prescribed by her family physician in Canada. When asked why, she explained:

Because I was pregnant, and when I am pregnant, I was told I was not supposed to take pills. The doctor told me not to take any more diabetic pills, because the pill would affect the fetus, so I stopped taking the diabetic pill. I didn't take the pill for the period of after the first appointment, waiting for the next appointment, for check-up, so it's about a few weeks of time ... Also, I wasn't too sure about what food I should be taking or what food I should be avoiding. The only sure thing I knew, I don't understand how to control my diet. After the doctor got my physical report, I was sent to the hospital for more than 10 days.

Through an active referral process, she obtained the services of a specialist in the maternity hospital. The reason for going to the hospital was, in her words, "my diabetes was pretty bad." During her hospitalization, insulin injections were prescribed, and she was taught how to give them. At first she was "scared" of giving the injections:

To start with I was scared, because I have no such training. Also, I have no medical knowledge or nursing knowledge ... I didn't have enough guts to jab myself because it's my own flesh.

She had to remain in hospital for 10 days to become proficient in administering the injections. A major worry for her at this time was that she had to take time off from work:

It's troublesome because initially, in a few days in the hospital, I was worried about my job ... I have a job. Originally, I just thought I had to stay in the hospital for a few days to have my blood sugar lowered, and I never thought I had to have injections. Then, they told me that I had to go on injections and they wouldn't let me go until they feel I'm confident with the needles. I waited to get out day after day, but I still have to stay in the hospital ... I couldn't take too much time from my work because the factory is busy. That's why I felt quite frustrated, and I thought it's quite troublesome to have this kind of disease. On the whole, I'm an easy going person, but I do worry about my work, and feel quite frustrated about the time, which is quite time-consuming on everything. But since I have this illness, there is no choice, especially I have a baby now.

Added to the worry about her work, she had to deal with the language problem:

I think the worst thing is language barrier, especially in the hospital. Language problem is the most serious problem. For example, in my case, I just don't speak very much English. I just know a few words. What the other people say in the hospital I wouldn't understand, and I think that's the most serious problem I have ... The problem with language barrier imposed quite a lot of trouble for me. I wanted to tell them something, and sometimes they wanted to tell me something, but we cannot talk to each other. Sometimes, for simple questions I just understood half of it maybe. Usually I did not want to answer because I did not want to have any mistakes happen, like I didn't want to have the wrong pills or I didn't want to pretend that I understand and so I got the wrong information.

May's difficulty in communicating her needs should not be interpreted as insensitivity on the part of hospital personnel. Rather, they too had to deal with a structure that did not provide adequate interpreter services. As May put it:

The nurses are very good. They taught me how to do my injections ... Sometimes they even taught me English. If you don't understand English they would teach you slowly and they never laughed at me ... The nurses are very patient with teaching me. They spent a lot of time on me.

Following her hospitalization, she was required to have regular medical follow-ups. Not only did this mean taking more time off from work, but additional issues like finding interpreter services, and arranging transportation had to be dealt with. Her words speak poignantly to the situation that the new immigrant faces:

I see specialists three weeks out of four weeks in the month. I find it very troublesome to have all these medical follow-ups, because of my language problem. I have to go to see these doctors with an interpreter; usually it's my sister, and she has to work, but she works in the evening, so I usually take Wednesday off. Also I don't know how to get to [Name of] Hospital by bus. So far I just know how to take the bus to work, to Chinatown and how to go home – that's it. I think it's okay to have trouble myself, but it's really bad and tough to give trouble to somebody else, like you know, I have to take my sister along to see a doctor, and I'm giving her quite a bit of trouble and it's really troublesome ...

I have to adjust to everything. Everything is new to me here. This is a big change for me. The only thing I could do is to take time slowly to adjust to the environment, and you have to face the reality ... here, everything is so far away, it's not easy to get to [name of] Hospital, so I think it's best for me to go with someone the next day. Since I don't know the way, and also I don't understand English.

The daily adjustment to a new society became interwoven into chronic illness management. Everyday routines like getting around a city that mainstream Canadians take for granted, were matters of paramount concern for May. But these were not her only concerns; she had to find ways of balancing work with diabetes management.

She feared that the diagnosis of diabetes would jeopardize her job, and felt the need to devise ways to manage her treatment, so as to conceal her condition from coworkers. Monitoring of her blood sugar level with a glucometer needed special precautions:

I never let them know I have diabetes. I just use a plastic bag to put the glucometer machine in, and take the bag into the washroom to do my own blood tests. I don't want people to know about this. If the factory knows that I am using their time to do my blood tests, that wouldn't be very good.

She went on to describe how scared she was when hospital personnel contacted her at the factory, as this could have alerted her employer to her diabetes. Even though her employers were willing to give her time off from work to keep medical appointments, she wanted to make sure that she remained in their good graces, by putting in overtime even in the sixth month of her pregnancy to make up for lost time:

I'm willing to do some overtime for them, even though I am not feeling that great. That's why I'm working six days a week – Saturday is overtime day – and also every day I work one extra hour – one hour overtime, because they are really on a tight schedule. And also I am taking Wednesday off for appointments and I am really owing them one day, that's not good. That's why I am willing to work overtime for them.

There were pragmatic reasons for being worried about her job. Strapped for funds, she was afraid of being fired. She had no labour union to protect her, and had to depend on the goodwill of her employers. She feared they would see diabetes as affecting her productivity, and find someone else to replace her.

During her pregnancy, concern for the well-being of the baby prompted her to follow the prescribed diet, even though it was difficult. She monitored her blood sugar levels faithfully, and also took the insulin injections regularly. Her stay in the hospital seemed to help her get a handle on her management.

However, she said that after the birth of the child, health professionals did not explain the changes in her management, for example, the switch from insulin injections to oral medications. She did not have a clear understanding of how to proceed, and felt she was left to figure things out. In her words:

They were very serious and aggressive about strict monitoring and treatment during my pregnancy but after the delivery, I was left on my own. Maybe it's their arena of responsibility to monitor me during the pregnancy. Now, after the baby was born, it's my own responsibility. The specialists have finished their work.

The specialist referred her back to her family physician. Although he spoke Cantonese, she did not feel at ease to ask questions about her diabetic management, nor did she feel that information was forthcoming from him. Not only did she have difficulty communicating with the English-speaking health care providers, but she also had difficulty communicating with the Cantonese-speaking physician.

May was asked to return the glucometer that was on loan to her from the hospital where she received care during her pregnancy. She could not afford to buy one, and did not know how else to get it. Furthermore, she was not sure whether she needed to continue to monitor her blood sugar level, because no one had explained monitoring procedures after the delivery. Since she felt that she had to monitor her sugar level somehow, she now tests her urine regularly, without being sure of the accuracy of the tests. From what she has to say, it would seem that health professionals expect her to manage her self-care, yet she does not have the knowledge and material resources to do so effectively.

She now feels that it is hard to manage her diabetes, take care of her child, do the housework, and hold down a job outside of the home for 6 days a week. Taking time to manage a diet seems beyond the realm of possibility at the moment. The economic circumstances of the family are such that she needs to work outside of the home for 6 days a week to provide for the family's basic needs. In addition to the ambiguities surrounding the management of her illness, the material circumstances of her life are such that survival takes precedence over illness management. Her own words provide a powerful account of her life situation:

Every morning I get up at about 6:30 to feed the baby. Then I go to work, and then I come home after work. So as I finish everything, cooking and bathing the baby, that would be 9 o'clock. I really don't know. I just have no feelings. It's so busy. Usually, I don't get to sit down until about 9 o'clock.

Discussion

Restructuring in the Social Context

These case histories from a Caucasian woman of comfortable means and a Chinese woman who works in a factory for six days a week to make ends meet, have been used to exemplify how the restructuring of life in the face of chronic illness has to be viewed within the total circumstances of a woman's life. The styles of managing illness that are often attributed to 'ethnic differences,' have also to be understood in terms of class relations in society, and how social processes organize the experiencing of illness.

In this section we will focus on two areas that seem to warrant discussion. First, the material circumstances of each woman's life will be examined. Then, the ideology of self-care that structures health care delivery will be discussed. This ideology, located within the larger social system, is reproduced in interactions between health care providers and patients, and organizes how women experience illness, and how they restructure their lives.

Restructuring, and the material circumstances of women's lives. The picture that emerges from the case histories is that both women were deeply concerned about diabetes, and wanted to manage it in the most effective way. What is striking, however, is that the energies of the working class Chinese woman were consumed with trying to survive in a new country. The demands of her life were such that it was difficult for her to manage her diabetes. In the workplace, she felt the need to keep her diabetes a secret out of fear of losing her job. Monitoring of blood sugar levels had to be done with this in mind. Yet, even though her work environment was not congenial to the management of her diabetes, reorganizing work to accommodate diabetes was not an option for her. Strapped for funds, and not having the skills that make one mobile in Canada's labour market, she had to stay in the job she had. There were limits then, to the extent to which she could restructure her life to accommodate diabetes.

The plight of non-English-speaking immigrant women in the labour force is well documented in the literature (Anderson and Lynam 1988; Gannage 1986; Arnopoulos 1979; Ng and Ramirez 1981). As Ng and Ramirez point out,

They [immigrant women] form a 'captive labour pool' with no possibility for advancement or for gaining better working conditions ... Immigrant women are usually restricted to jobs which have no benefits or permanency, such as domestic and janitorial work, the lowest strata of factory work, and unskilled restaurant work ... And immigrant women have to rely on good personal relations with their employers to keep their jobs and negotiate pay increases, etc. Unless they work from 12 to 16 hours a day, there is little chance that they could make enough money to maintain themselves and their children (Ng and Ramirez 1981: 48).

Complex factors influence how a woman manages her illness, not least among them are historical factors that shape the non-English-speaking immigrant woman's experience in Canada, and her class position in Canada's labour market. Recent perspectives in Marxist analysis focus on class as a set of historical relationships which is not reducible to social and economic indicators. Class experience is profoundly shaped by relations of production (Ng 1988; Marx and Engels 1965). Immigrants are most likely to be found in those occupations linked to the expansion and accumulation of capital. Li points out: "Throughout the history of Canada, various racial groups have been used en masse as labourers to fill menial jobs at different junctures of capitalist development" (Li 1988: 48). Many of these jobs are without labour market protection.

As we have seen from the case history of Jane, women fluent in English, and who have the skills for mobility in Canada's labour market, could usually afford to change their job to accommodate the management of diabetes. This is not to say that these women did not experience labour market discrimination. However, more options were open to them; they also knew their rights, and could speak out.

The women in the study all understood the importance of looking after themselves, so it would seem that it was not a woman's 'beliefs' as such that impinged upon her management. Rather, the conditions of a woman's work profoundly shaped the illness experience. Consequently, May's difficulty in carrying out procedures like 'following the right diet,' and monitoring her blood sugar should be understood in the context of what constitutes the reality of the lives of working class women, who must not only labour in the home, but must also labour outside of the home for low pay, in jobs that are unprotected by collective agreements.

The necessity for May to work full time – and overtime, and her feeling of responsibility for housework and child care, left little time for her to look after herself. Poverty and lifestyle circumstances seemed to be the major deterrents to the management of her diabetes. Furthermore, being in contact with health professionals did not guarantee her the help she needed to manage diabetes, and so we must ask why.

Restructuring of life, the ideology of self-care, and relationships with health professionals. Included in Canada's health care system "has been a program of pre-paid health services which substantially removes financial barriers to medical and hospital care" (Lalonde 1978: 5). Although each province in Canada operates its own plan, the ten provinces have many common features; each province must meet certain federal standards, including comprehensive coverage and universality. Comprehensive coverage means that, "Insured benefits must include at least all medically required services rendered by a physician...," and universality means that "insured services must be furnished to all insured residents with uniform terms and conditions" (Soderstrom 1978: 132–133). In theory, then, both the middle class woman and the working class woman described earlier have access to equal health care services. It is clear, however, that the women's needs were not equally met. Although the barriers to health care might not have been financial (given that each woman had access to the health insurance scheme in the province), other issues seemed to impinge on health care access.

A number of factors seemed to stand in the way of the Chinese woman from getting the help she needed. First, there was the difficulty of communicating her needs, since the majority of health professionals whom she encountered spoke only English. Her lack of English language skills also excluded her from the ongoing discourse within the society, and the dominant forms of thought that the English speaking women had access to; for example, the popular literature about diabetes, libraries, the media, and the like. In other words, the non-English-speaking immigrant woman is marginal to the flow of daily life through which the background notions about health and illness management are constructed.

Lack of English language skills is not the only obstacle that women face. As we saw in May's case, although under the care of a family physician who spoke Cantonese, she was ill at ease asking questions and, from her report, he did not volunteer information. Clearly, speaking a similar language does not guarantee communication. Twaddle observes that:

Not only does the patient have to cope with the disabilities and discomforts of diseases, the strangeness of alien organizations, and the economic problems of sickness, but (s)he must also bridge a widening gulf of social class as well. From the patient side the physician is increasingly an awesome figure who represents people in the community who are otherwise unapproachable. From the physician's side it is increasingly difficult to grasp, much less understand or appreciate, the circumstances of the patient, particularly the degree to which the patient is constrained by a lack of resources needed to cope with symptoms, follow treatment regimens, etc. With class-linked differences in language and culture, simple communication cannot be taken for granted (Twaddle 1982: 338–339).

Shared meanings between patients and professionals cannot be assumed even when both speak a similar language, as the life circumstances of the patient may not be readily understood by the health professional. This lack of understanding of the social circumstances of people's lives is situated in the complex arena of class relationships, and the ideologies that structure the medical discourse which, as we will point out later, are inextricably intertwined with these relationships.

Comaroff has argued that:

In the terms of formal medical aetiology, illness is explained predominantly as the result of the interaction of 'pathogens' and 'host' ... These aetiological models entail a specific image of man – and a tacit ideology. For they connote a view of disease as an asocial, amoral process, and a view of man as the decontextualised 'host' to a set of unmediated natural processes, which call for technical intervention (Comaroff 1982: 59).

This orientation obscures "the extent to which health and illness depend upon socially determined ways of life" (Bolaria 1988: 538), hence the situations that people face in their everyday lives that influence their experiencing of illness are outside of the medical discourse. It is not surprising, then, that May found no common ground for communication with physicians, especially after the birth of her child. Dealing with 'diabetes in pregnancy,' requires, from the biomedical perspective, 'scientific knowledge' and technological interventions – well within biomedicine's mandate. After the birth of her child, these interventions were no longer needed. May summed it up well when she said, "The specialists have finished their work."

After the birth of her child she was left to deal with the daily routines of diabetes management within the context of her life situation. Trying to survive and to make ends meet were foremost in her mind. It was clear that in her ongoing daily life 'the biomedical entity – the disease' was inseparable from the socioeconomic and political context; each aspect of her life was inextricably intertwined with the other. Yet, the social context of everyday life is separated from the 'biomedical entity' in the medical discourse. This is not to say that she received the help that she needed with the 'disease' management. From her report it would seem that this was not the case.

In analyzing the two case histories, it appears that the gulf that separated the physician and patient was not as great in the case of middle class women. Jane, and other middle class women like her, seemed to share common meanings with health professionals – there seemed to be more of a common ground between them. As we spoke with these women, it became apparent that they had access to the information that health care providers produce about diabetes (e.g., pamphlets, literature, lectures, and the like); the perspectives that they held about diabetes management were therefore quite similar to those of health care providers. In a chronic illness such as diabetes, the concept of self-care, for example, is widely acclaimed among health professionals. For the most part, the Anglo-Canadian women whom we spoke with, as well as patients writing about diabetes management also shared this notion [see for example, Sims

1986], highlighting the fact that the highly literate, English-speaking woman, and health care providers have access to similar forms of thought about illness and its management. These forms of thought are not static, but are constructed and reconstructed in ongoing dialogue between health care providers and patients.

It can be further argued that the consensus between health care providers and patients should not be understood only as it pertains to the 'professional discourse,' but that this discourse is embedded in the dominant ideas of mainstream Western society. Self-care is not an isolated ideology, but is consistent, as both Bolaria 1988 and Li 1988 point out, with "the basic tenets of bourgeois individualism and freedom of choice which have been with us for some time" (Bolaria 1988: 538). "Individual effort alone is responsible for success, and ... inner qualities, as epitomized in Puritanism, are the keys to achievements. In contrast, social failures are believed to result from the personal weaknesses of individuals who fail to respond to opportunities" (Li 1988: 5). Not only do these notions organize everyday life experiences, but also how resources are allocated within the society.

It is against this background that the scientific discourse of biomedicine is constructed. This discourse is grounded in a set of assumptions that are culturally located. It should be clear that what is being argued is not that biomedicine is 'unscientific' but that medicine, like science, is essentially a social enterprise (Lock and Gordon 1988; Wright and Treacher 1982).

Dominant ideologies are interwoven into, and are reproduced in ongoing social interactions; they are used to assess how well one is doing. For example, tacit knowledge about the value of 'inner strength' and 'taking responsibility for self,' provide the background for interactions in the patient-practitioner encounter. Women who are excluded from the discourse of the dominant society do not have access to these mainstream forms of thought, and the vocabularies that enable them to present themselves as 'competent members of the culture.' So, not only does the ideology organize the expectations that practitioners have of patients, but also it enables patients to incorporate the professional corpus of knowledge, and to meet the expectations of professionals. 'The state' then, is not an apparatus that functions apart from individuals and institutions (Ng 1988) like the health care system, to produce and maintain ideologies such as self-care, but the discourses of daily life including the professional discourse are instances of how the state works – there is a dialectical relationship amongst the different arenas of health care; patients, practitioners, and policy makers, through which ideas are constructed and maintained.

But not only is the immigrant woman excluded from the discourse of the mainstream; she is also confronted with the paradox of the ideology of self-care. On the one hand, she is expected to take responsibility for carrying out her care. On the other hand, she does not have access to the resources that would allow her to do so. In fact, the notion of 'taking responsibility' seems to imply that she should provide what is needed to facilitate her care. This is not to say that women do not want to take responsibility for their care. The Chinese women with whom we spoke wanted to be self-reliant. However, the barriers to their 'self-care' went unrecognized. The following is an instance of this situation.

In the region where this study was conducted, the Chinese are the second largest ethnic group (Statistics Canada 1986b). Yet, at the time this study was done, there were no interpreter services in institutions from which women sought health care. Being able to understand what health professionals had to tell them was seen as a woman's responsibility. Consequently, women had to rely either on family members to interpret for them, or hospital staff who were neither trained for this role, nor paid to perform this service. In many instances women left the health care encounter without having their questions answered, and without a clear understanding of what they were supposed to do.

Those who allocate the resources did not seem to understand the complexity of the process of adequate interpretation, nor did they seem to comprehend the life circumstances of poor immigrants. They seemed unable to grasp the fact that many immigrants cannot afford to take time off from work to provide interpreter services for their relatives. Unlike people in 'middle class jobs' with fringe benefits, if people in jobs without such benefits do not go to work, they do not get paid.

But it is not just interpreter services that are lacking. May had difficulty getting the equipment that would help her monitor her blood glucose level. She had the use of a glucometer during her pregnancy but had to return it after the birth of her child. She could not afford to buy one, nor did she known how else to acquire it. She did not know how the system worked. Furthermore, she was not informed of other ways of testing her blood sugar level. So, while people are expected to manage their care, the resources that would enable them to do so are not in place. Those of economic means can acquire what is necessary for managing their care; however, the socially disadvantaged are excluded by virtue of the distribution of resources. Ironically, such patients are usually seen by health professionals as 'noncompliant,' or 'difficult,' or a 'problem,' or as not motivated to take responsibility for 'self-care.'

Restructuring of life to accommodate a chronic illness does not take place in a vacuum independent of the social context. The disruption of life, and the search for new meanings, are enmeshed in the ideological frameworks that permeate the health care system. What may be seen as being due to the patient's ethnic background, for example, lack of understanding of illness management, has therefore to be analyzed within the structures of the health care system, and the ways in which resources are allocated within the health sector. The lack of recognition of the social context of illness conceals unequal class relationships (Li 1988), and institutionalized inequities in society, and result in the exclusion of those who are most in need of care. Therefore, the very ideology that promotes self-care, excludes the possibility of self-care by the socially disadvantaged.

Conclusion

This inquiry into the existential experiencing of illness, raises issues that pertain not only to the management of chronic illness in everyday life, but also to how ethnic categories are generated. The viewpoint is taken that ethnic categories are embedded in a set of social relations, and are constructed in ongoing interactions among people. In this discussion 'ethnicity' is not seen as an 'objective fact' that determines illness meanings and patterns of restructuring of life. In other words, culture and ethnicity are not viewed as static determinants of behaviour; individuals are not seen as following pregiven scripts that dictate their beliefs about illness and its management. Treating culture as static, and glossing over the process by which 'cultural' or 'health beliefs' are constructed and maintained, exempt health professionals from holding up to scrutiny the grounds of their practice, and how their interactions with clients contribute not only to the structuring of ethnic categories, but also to people's experiencing of illness.

Our analysis derives from the perspective that culture and ethnicity are socially organized, and socially produced in the context of everyday social interaction. What may be interpreted as due to ethnic differences in illness management, can also be understood as a product of the social divisions that occur in the modern state. Li argues that "race and ethnicity are not social classes *per se*, although under certain circumstances race and class may overlap to generate a class structure along racial lines" (Li 1988: 48). The Chinese women in this study who were without English language and other skills needed for an advanced labour market, were concentrated in menial jobs. The structuring of illness management was a product of their situation. Not monitoring blood sugar levels, and not divulging their illness to coworkers and employers, are pragmatic ways of dealing with their tenuous position in the labour market.

What is obvious from this study is that women from the same ethnic category did not always share similar cultural meanings about illness, nor did they manage chronic illness in the same way. The process of restructuring of life is situated within a complex nexus of economic circumstances; hopes, aspirations and fears; support or lack of it from friends, family, and employers; relationships with health professionals, and the like.

As the multiethnic population of Canada increases, a trend in health care is to examine ways of delivering culturally sensitive care to people from different ethnocultural groups. While this move is highly commendable, caution needs to be exercised to avoid viewing ethnic categories as givens, 'out there,' in the 'real world,' waiting to be described. Such a perspective heightens the risk of ethnic stereotyping, and exacerbating the problems that people already face. A different stance is required that holds up for questioning the institutionalized practices within the society that perpetuate a life of poverty and oppression amongst people who enter Canada (and other Western nations) as immigrants, without the skills necessary for the labour market in highly industrialized Western nations.

Delivering culturally sensitive health care then, does not imply a cataloguing of assumed beliefs of people from different groups, and basing the provision of health care on these assumptions. There is a need to examine the context in which belief systems are constructed, and the social inequity within the society that impinges upon illness management. The trend toward individualizing social problems, and shifting the responsibility for caretaking from the state to the individual obscures the barriers to adequate health care for the socially disadvantaged. Strategies of managing illness that may not conform to the expectations of health professionals are often labelled as 'noncompliant,' with the connotation that this is deviant behaviour, idiosyncratic to the individual, and in need of correction; in some instances, noncompliance is seen as the result of 'ethnic beliefs.' What fails to be recognized is that what is construed as 'noncompliance' is a function of socioeconomic-political factors, and the medicocentric approaches to health care delivery.

A critical component of delivering culturally sensitive health care is the reflexive grasping of the ideologies that shape the practices of health professionals, and the comprehension of the ideologic basis of theorizing. Ideologies like self-care are, for the most part, not recognized as such by health professionals. Instead they are seen as innovative theories, indicating 'progress' in the strategies for the delivery of health care.

Health professionals speak from their position in the social structure, and reflect the dominant societal ideologies which sustain their position of dominance in relation to patients. Holding up to scrutiny the grounds of their own practice, and questioning the basis of theorizing, will require a new political and social consciousness amongst health care professionals, and a shift from the ethnocentric perspective of professionalism to the search for social justice in a society where resources are unequally distributed.

Acknowledgements

This research was supported by a grant from the British Columbia Health Care Research Foundation, and a Research Scholar Award from Health and Welfare Canada, held by Anderson. We wish to thank the anonymous reviewers for their helpful comments which guided us in the revision of an earlier draft of this paper. We gratefully acknowledge the assistance of the following people: the agency personnel for recruitment of the women, Mayeeta Leung for doing some of the interviews during the first year of the study, Marie Bennett for typing the transcripts, and Denise Beaupre for helping with the final preparation of this manuscript. We are indebted to the women who gave so generously of their time, and who allowed us the privilege to enter into their lives.

The views expressed in this paper do not necessarily reflect those of the funding agencies. We alone must remain responsible for whatever shortcomings are present.

References

Anderson, JM. 1985. Perspectives on the Health of Immigrant Women: A Feminist Analysis. *Advanced Nursing Science* 8(1): 61–76.

Anderson, JM. 1987. Migration and Health: Perspectives on Immigrant Women. *Sociology of Health and Illness* 9(4): 410–438.

Anderson, JM, and J Lynam. 1988. Immigrant Women: Issues in Health Care. *Multicultural Health Bulletin IV* 3: 3–5.

Arnopoulos, S. 1979. *Problems of Immigrant Women in the Canadian Labour Force.* Ottawa: Canadian Advisory Council on the Status of Women.

Bolaria, BS. 1988. The Politics and Ideology of Self-Care and Lifestyles. In BS Bolaria and HD Dickinson eds. *Sociology of Health Care in Canada.* Toronto: Harcourt Brace Jovanovich.

Brittan, A and M Maynard. 1984. *Sexism, Racism and Oppression.* Oxford: Basil Blackwell Publishers.

Bury, M. 1982. Chronic Illness as Biographical Disruption. *Sociology of Health and Illness* 4(2): 167–182.

Canada Employment and Immigration. 1986. *Immigration Statistics.* Ottawa: Minister of Supply and Services.

Canadian Nurses Association. 1988. *Health For All Canadians: A Call for Health-Care Reform.* Ottawa: CNA Publishing.

Comaroff, J. 1982. Medicine: Symbol and Ideology. In P Wright and A Treacher eds. *The Problem of Medical Knowledge: Examining the Social Construction of Medicine.* Edinburgh: Edinburgh University Press.

Eichler, M. 1985. And the Work Never Ends: Feminist Contributions. *Canadian Review of Sociology and Anthropology* 22(5): 619–644.

Epp, J. 1986. *Achieving Health for All: A Framework for Health Promotion.* Ottawa: Minister of Supply and Services.

Gannagé, C. 1986. *Double Day, Double Bind: Women Garment Workers.* Toronto: The Women's Press.

Graham, O and W Schubert. 1985. A Model for Developing and Pre-Testing a Multi-Media Teaching Program to Enhance the Self-Care Behavior of Diabetes Insipidus Patients. *Patient Education and Counseling* 7: 53–64.

Kleinman, A. 1986. *Social Origins of Distress and Disease: Depression, Neurasthenia and Pain in Modern China.* New Haven CT: Yale University Press.

Kleinman, A. 1987. Illness Meanings and Illness Behaviour. In S McHugh and M Vallis, eds. *Illness Behavior: A Multidisciplinary Model.* New York: Plenum Press.

Lalonde, M. 1978. *A New Perspective on the Health of Canadians.* Ottawa: Minister of Supply and Services.

Li, P. 1988. *Ethnic Inequality in a Class Society.* Toronto: Wall and Thompson.

Lock, M and D Gordon eds. 1988. *Biomedicine Examined.* Dordrecht/Boston: Kluwer Academic Publishers.

Marx, K and F Engels. 1965. *The German Ideology.* S Ryazanskaya ed. London: Lawrence and Wishart.

Meininger, J. 1986. Sex Differences in Factors Associated With Use of Medical Care and Alternative Illness Behaviors. *Social Science and Medicine* 22(3): 285–292.

Meleis, A, J Norbeck, S Laffrey, M Solomon, and L Miller. 1989. Stress, Satisfaction, and Coping: A Study of Women Clerical Workers. *Health Care Women's International* 10: 319–334.

Ng, R. 1988. *The Politics of Community Services: Immigrant Women, Class and State.* Toronto: Garamond Press.

Ng, R and J Ramirez. 1981. *Immigrant Housewives in Canada.* Toronto: The Immigrant Women's Centre.

Oakley, A. 1981. Interviewing Women: A Contradiction in Terms. In H Roberts ed. *Doing Feminist Research.* London: Routledge and Kegan Paul.

Orem, DE. 1985. *Nursing: Concepts of Practice,* 3rd ed. New York: McGraw-Hill.

Pirie, M. 1988. Women and the Illness Role: Rethinking Feminist Theory. *Canadian Review of Sociology and Anthropology* 25(4): 628–648.

Seidel, J, R Kjolseth, and E Seymour. 1988. *The Ethnograph: A User's Guide (version 3.0).* Colorado: Qualis Research Associates.

Sims, D. 1986. Diabetes Patient Education: A Consumer View. *The Diabetes Educator* 12(2): 122–125.

Smith, DE. 1975. An Analysis of Ideological Structures and How Women are Excluded: Considerations for Academic Women. *Canadian Review of Sociology and Anthropology* 12(4)Part 1: 353–369.

Smith, DE. 1979. A Sociology for Women. In J Sherman and E Beck eds. *The Prism of Sex: Essays in the Sociology of Knowledge.* Madison: University of Wisconsin Press.

Smith, DE. 1986. Institutional Ethonography: A Feminist Method. *Resources for Feminist Research* 15(1): 6–13.

Soderstrom, L. 1978. *The Canadian Health System.* London: Croom Helm.

Sorensen, G, P Pirie, A Folsom, R Luepker, and D Jacobs. 1985. Sex Differences in the Relationship Between Work and Health: The Minnesota Heart Survey. *Journal of Health and Social Behavior* 26: 379–394.

Stanley, L and S Wise. 1983. *Breaking Out: Feminist Consciousness and Feminist Research.* London: Routledge and Kegan Paul.

Statistics Canada. 1986a. *Census Divisions and Subdivision, B.C.* Ottawa: Minister of Supply and Services.

Statistics Canada. 1986b. *Census Tracts Vancouver.* Ottawa: Minister of Supply and Services.

Steiger, N and J Lipson. 1985. *Self-care Nursing: Theory and Practice.* Maryland: Brady Communications.

Twaddle, AC. 1982. From Medical Sociology to the Sociology of Health: Some Changing Concerns in the Sociological Study of Sickness and Treatment. In T Bottomore, S Nowak and M Sokolwska eds. *Sociology: The State of the Art.* London: Sage.

Verbrugge, L. 1985. Gender and Health: An Update on Hypotheses and Evidence. *Journal of Health and Social Behavior* 26: 156–182.

Williams, G. 1984. TheGgenesis of Chronic Illness: Narrative Re-construction. *Sociology of Health and Illness* 6(2): 175–200.

Wright, P and A Treacher eds. 1982. *The Problem of Medical Knowledge: Examining the Social Construction of Medicine.* Edinburgh: Edinburgh University Press.

10

"What are Women for?": Cultural Constructions of Menopausal Women in Japan and Canada*

Patricia A. Kaufert, Margaret Lock

If they live long enough, all women eventually stop menstruating. By this criterion, menopause is universal. Yet the timing of even basic physiological changes depends on such factors as women's access to food (starving women do not menstruate) or their access to gynecological surgery (protection against a surgical menopause is one of the paradoxical benefits of inadequate medical care for women). These are extreme examples, but they serve to demonstrate that becoming menopausal is also the product of social rather than simply biological processes.

The subject of this chapter is not menopause per se, but the menopausal woman: more precisely, the menopausal woman in Japan and in Canada. The material comes from studies we have conducted separately but are linked by our interest in menopause, an agreement to match methods and design, and the decision to collaborate on the analysis of common data. Having created one of the very few opportunities for comparative research on menopause, we will be obliged to deal with such issues as differences in menopausal symptoms, in attitudes toward menopause, in rates of hysterectomy, and in the prescription of hormone therapy. Here, however, we want to compare the ways in which Canadian and Japanese women, and their physicians, select, organize, and interpret the bundle of physiological changes that occur in women as they age. For we see in menopause a unique opportunity for exploring how differences in class and culture, in economic and political power, find their expression through the bodies of women.

Our objective in this chapter is to explore the relationship between social reality (the diverse realities lived by women who are menopausal) and cultural construct ("the menopausal woman," a unitary construct created in part by the medical profession). Differences in the medical construction of the menopausal woman in Japan and Canada can be related to different histories and traditions in medicine. Yet, as we will also show, these quasi-medical, quasi-public representations of the menopausal woman have less to do with medical science's past than with the present and future political and economic structure of the two societies. Both in Japan and Canada, the menopausal woman is viewed as a medical and social problem; and the implicit question is What is to be done with women as they age?

* Reprinted from Patricia A. Kaufert and Margaret Lock, "'What are Women for?': Cultural Constructions of Menopausal Women in Japan and Canada' in *In Her Prime*, 2nd ed., edited by V. Kerns and J.K. Brown, University of Illinois Press, 1992.

Research Strategies

The comparative material that we will discuss comes from studies carried out in Japan and Canada in the 1980s, using a variety of research methods. The most structured data come from two surveys, one conducted in and around Kyoto, Japan, in 1983-84 and the other in Manitoba, Canada, in 1980-81. The Canadian survey was larger, involving 2,500 respondents, while the Japanese survey data come from about half that number of women (n = 1,326). The age band of the Canadian respondents was also wider (forty to fifty-nine years) than that of the Japanese (forty-five to fifty-five years). In other respects, however, the two surveys are very similar. Both surveys selected their study populations from general population sources and both included urban and rural women. Self-completed questionnaires were used in both surveys. The questionnaire completed by Japanese women included many questions directly translated from the earlier Canadian survey. Other questions, while dealing with the same topic area, were adapted to the Japanese context: for example, a section on medical care was extended to include questions on the use of Japanese traditional medical practitioners and medicines. In addition to the survey, the Japanese study included a series of in-depth interviews with fifteen gynecologists and fifteen family practitioners. Both studies included a set of in-depth interviews with women at, or close to, the age of menopause.

Other material comes from reviews of the North American and Japanese clinical and epidemiological research literature on menopause. The works reviewed also include those directed to a general audience: articles on menopause and the menopausal woman published in newspapers, magazines, and paperback books. Often written by physicians, these articles are not constrained by the rules of scientific presentation that prevail in the professional literature. Their mix of medical information with social and moral commentary provides a rich source of material on the ways in which Canadian and Japanese physicians construe the menopausal woman and visualize the processes of her body.

Finally, extended fieldwork in Canada and Japan has given us the opportunity to meet the variety of experts who act as interpreters of the menopausal woman. They include practicing physicians, clinical researchers, epidemiologists, psychologists, feminist filmmakers, journalists interested in women's health, and the occasional sociologist or anthropologist. Through their work and through their writing, these experts are all variously engaged in a discourse on the menopausal woman. They would become her architects, imposing their definition of who she is and how she is to recognize herself.

It is with their products, their constructions of the menopausal woman that the first part of this chapter is concerned. The second part, which draws on demographic data from our surveys, shows the diversity among women who are menopausal: diversity in their life circumstances and in their self-definitions. The final section addresses some questions about the menopausal woman, the economic order, and the political self.

The Menopausal Woman as a Medical Construct

Most women know the script laid out in their particular society for the woman in midlife, including what symptoms she should expect from her body. Greek women, for example, expect hot flushes, while Mayan women do not (Beyene 1989). Women will know not only the repertoire of menopausal symptoms, but also the repertoire of behavior considered appropriate for a woman who is menopausal. Women in California are told that a loss in libido is a medical problem to be treated by hormone therapy, whereas a Bengali woman in India knows very well that sexual activity is inappropriate for the postmenopausal woman (see Vatuk, this volume).

Both the denial and the affirmation of sexuality are social phenomena, but for the California woman the responses of her body have been transformed into a medical problem to be medically managed. It is her physician who will tell her that the continuation of sexual activity is "normal," but that to lose the desire for sex is an expression of a disease state, the menopause, which is to be managed by hormone therapy. Just as obstetricians and pediatricians would define how women should feel and behave when becoming mothers, gynecologists and psychiatrists tell women what it is to be menopausal. What they say, however, varies from one society to another and from one period of time to another.

The Menopausal Woman in Japan

The medical literature on menopause read by Japanese physicians is not dissimilar to that read by their Canadian counterparts. Occasional traces of the influence in Japan of late nineteenth-century German medical thinking still linger in the long lists of menopausal symptoms. The main sources of clinical and epidemiological information, however, are often the same American and European studies that are quoted and read by Canadian gynecologists. When referring to physiology, the answers to such questions as Why do some women get symptoms and others not? are often essentially the same whether the physician is Canadian or Japanese. Many Japanese physicians will then go on to emphasize that the instability in the autonomic nervous system is implicated, in addition to falling estrogen levels, as casual of menopausal symptomology. The emphasis given to the autonomic nervous system in Japanese medical discourse is largely due to the cultural proclivity for using models in which theories of balance and harmony are central (Lock et al. 1988). If the question is repeated, however, answers may become quite different.

At the level of patient as person, physicians draw on a potent mix of psychological theorizing about the nature of women with political statements on their proper role (or rather lack of role) that are particular to each society. To explain why Japanese physicians, for example, adopt a somewhat censorious stance toward their menopausal patients requires an understanding of relationships of class, gender, and power in Japanese society.

Discussing the faults of the middle-class, middle-aged homemaker has become one of the preoccupations of the popular media in Japan. The topic of numerous quasi-medical, quasi-psychological articles, she is castigated for selfishness, individualism, and lack of discipline (Ikemi and Ikemi 1982; Kyutoku 1979). She is described as deficient in the strength and willpower once characteristic of the traditional Japanese woman. She is blamed for becoming the victim of an assortment of new diseases, including "the kitchen syndrome," "apartment living neurosis," and the "menopausal syndrome" (Lock 1986a).

The "menopausal syndrome" has now achieved status as a formal medical category in Japan and is discussed in the medical scientific journals. In the popular media and in less formal discussions, however, physicians attribute vulnerability less to hormonal than to moral factors.

Menopausal syndrome is described as a luxury disease (zeitakubyo), a problem which occurs in women with too much time on their hands, who are selfish and concerned only with their own pleasures. Women like this are said to lack a real identity (which is bound up inextricably with one's social role (Lebra 1976)); they have no sense of self (jibun ga nai), and are deficient in the willpower, positive attitude, and endurance that were characteristic of their mothers (Lock 1986a).

A few of the physicians interviewed in the study were sympathetic toward their meno-pausal patients rather than condemnatory. They discussed the plight (as they saw it) of women with nothing to do, closeted in small apartments, lacking meaningful occupa-tion. Those physicians who were sympathetic were more likely to say that they offered counseling to their menopausal patients, although even this is normally little more than advice on the value of cultivating hobbies (Lock 1988). They prescribe herbal teas, but are much less likely than Canadian physicians to offer psychotropics and hormones.

The moralistic stance toward women complaining of menopausal symptoms can be traced back to the ideal codes of behavior for women in Japanese society. The behavior and discipline expected of women is based originally on rules laid down in the feudal period for the wives of samurai. The *sengyo shufu*, a term that can be glossed as a "pro-fessional homemaker" is the modern form of the "good wife/wise mother" (*ryosai kenbo*), the "correct woman" of the Meiji period. Somewhat adapted to suit postwar Japan, the good wife/wise mother remains the epitome of the Japanese woman.

The samurai valued discipline, submission and unquestioning obedience not only of themselves but of their wives and children. According to their Confucian-influenced code, a woman should be patient, submissive, diligent, even-tempered, compliant and gentle. Her life should be devoted to the care of her husband, her children, and her par-ents-in-law. Her concern should not be for herself but always for these others. Domestic skills and an orderly household were to be valued as an expression not just of compe-tence as a woman but of virtue. The body also became an expression of virtue. Inner discipline, for example, was reflected in a body language based on good posture, a neat appearance, elegance in the handling of objects, graceful manners. A virtuous body was considered healthy and, hence, sickness in a woman revealed a lack of discipline and of balance. According to this code, a woman was blamed both for allowing her body to become ill and for failing through illness in her responsibility to others. The moral roots of negative attitudes toward the woman complaining of menopausal symp-toms can be traced in part to this idea of the good woman holding mastery over her own body.

There is another explanation, however, that has less to do with traditional codes for womanly behavior and more with the role assigned to women in modern Japanese soci-ety. This explanation depends on the answers to a question that is partly political and partly philosophical: What are women for? In the Meiji period, the answers to this question could be framed in terms of the responsibilities of the wives of samurai living within a large traditional household. After the war, many samurai values became part of the code by which the newly emerging middle class was to live. Unlike the samurai wife, however, the modern homemaker is expected to reside in a small apartment with a husband and no more than two children. The hard work, perseverance, and discipline, which were central to the traditional code for womanly behavior, are now to be fun-neled into the work of raising and educating children in the context of the nuclear fam-ily. The modern version of the good wife/wise mother is responsible for the success (and survival) of children within the highly structured, highly competitive system of contemporary Japanese education. (A reversed image, the woman-as-bad-mother, is blamed for children who fail or who are destroyed by the system; see Lock 1986b.)

In modern Japan, a woman is above all else "for" the education and training of children. She is responsible for inculcating the virtues seen as essential to the Japanese workplace: loyalty, discipline, and perseverance. In this interpretation of her role, the Japanese woman is essential to the maintenance and reproduction of modern society. The dilemma is that raising children is a time-limited function. Japanese families are small, and childbearing is completed relatively early. The highly active, intensive involvement of a mother in her children's education is practically over by the time most women reach menopause.

The professional homemaker is not expected to go out to work, and she cannot take up a role in public life. Neither of these options is compatible with the essentially domestic locus of the image of the good wife/wise mother. At the same time, she cannot continue to play a role designed for the period of life when her children were young. Neither the Japanese husband nor the Japanese adolescent is expected to spend much time at home. A woman should not remain overcommitted to being the good housewife, overzealous of the order of her household, or overly protective of her children. Such women are described by physicians as neurotic, blamed for their lack of balance and control (Lock 1988).

Left without an occupation and living in a society that values perseverance, hard work, and discipline, the menopausal woman is anomalous. Anomalous social categories are always troublesome, but particularly when they are a product of social changes toward which many are ambivalent. By attaching the menopausal syndrome to the leisure and lack of social responsibility, the Japanese physician engages in victim blaming. Lacking any legitimate outlet for the traditional virtues of self-sacrifice, hard work, and devotion to the family, the menopausal patient is described as selfish, idle, individualistic. Most important, she is told that she has brought her own troubles, her menopausal syndrome, upon her own head. The implications of modernization are displaced onto the body of the woman.

This portrait of the menopausal woman is not simply a product of the medical or the male imagination. The interviews with Japanese women in midlife revealed that many of them agreed to its essential lineaments. Yet, when we analyzed the data from the Japanese survey, reports of stress were more common among women living in multigenerational households than those in single-family homes. Women living only with their husbands and children were more likely to say that they were satisfied with their lives, less likely to report the symptoms associated with menopause than women living with other kin. Whatever the leisure now available, and whatever the moral stance of the wider society toward this leisure, the women themselves appeared to enjoy and be content with their lives.

The Menopausal Woman in Canada

Much of the European and North American literature on menopause shares an assumption that women are defined (and define themselves) by their relationships with others. For the adult woman, the most significant of these others are her husband and children. This echoes the Japanese idea of a woman's sense of self being contingent on her social identity as a wife and as a mother (Lebra 1984). North American physicians are told that the loss or diminution of these relationships threatens psychological well-being and that this explains the depression of their menopausal patients. The appropriate

Menopause = natural end - partial death
Does society think the same about menopause as it does about osteoporosis & ♡ disease?

medical response, they are also told, is some mixture of counseling, psychotropics, and hormone replacement therapy.

The casual stereotype of the menopausal woman is a depressed homemaker: her children are leaving home while her husband is at best preoccupied with work and at worst divorcing a wife he no longer finds sexually attractive. In her lack of meaningful occupation, she is reminiscent of the Japanese professional homemaker except that she is to be pitied rather than condemned. Depressed and depressing, suffering a multiplicity of losses, the menopausal woman makes a sad and forlorn image.

This view of the menopausal women owes something still to the influence of Freud. In Freudian logic, the meaning of a woman's life is based on her ability to bear children; hence, once she loses this capacity it follows that her life has lost its purpose. Helene Deutsch, who was largely responsible for framing a Freudian interpretation of menopause, described the menopausal patient as a being without hope. The best that could be offered was a form of palliative care; for with the end of her fertility, a woman "had reached her natural end – her partial death" (Deutsch 1945: 459).

Articles on the management of the menopausal patient still tend to remind physicians that the biological end of fertility at menopause coincides with the social ending of the mothering role. The menopausal patient is described as "neurotic, depressed, unable to cope with emotional crisis such as children leaving home, and constantly subject to vague complaints and gynecological disorders" (Roberts 1984). This caricature of the physician's view of the menopausal patient is British, but might as well be Canadian. It might also be Japanese for there are echoes in this of the description of the menopausal patient offered by a Tokyo physician: "These women have no *ikigai* (purpose in life). They have free time but can't think of anything to do, so they get a psychosomatic reaction. They can't complain openly so they use 'organ language' [said in English]" (cited in Lock 1988). Whether Japanese or Canadian, this image of the menopausal woman is a powerful one, suggesting that it may reflect attitudes toward women, women's roles, and the impact of aging on women, attitudes that are widely held in both societies.

Freud is now being replaced, and a new version of the menopausal woman has emerged gradually in North America over the past ten to fifteen years. Medicine has defined menopause as a deficiency condition (akin to diabetes or anemia) and a risk factor for the chronic diseases of old age. Osteoporosis and cardiovascular diseases are highlighted as the major killers, but incontinence and atrophic vaginitis are thrown in for good measure. Menopause becomes not only a threat to the lives of women but strikes at the root of their identity as continent, sexually active, mature adults.

Regardless of whether one thinks in terms of the burden of suffering and pain to the woman or the burden of cost to society, osteoporosis and heart disease are not trivial conditions. The message being put out in the medical literature, both the professional and popular varieties, is that the middle years, the menopausal years, represent the period in a woman's life when she can make the changes necessary to their prevention or delay. By changing her diet, exercising, giving up alcohol and cigarettes, and above all else by taking her hormones, a woman may ensure her own survival into a healthy old age. Her choice is between an old, diseased, and broken body or a fit and vigorous one.

Corresponding to the activist approach to the physiological tasks of midlife, the psychological literature lays out a series of actions to ward off the consequences of menopause for mental well-being. A dismal listing of the events to be expected by women is still customary in the literature on midlife. A book published only in 1989 carries the

Diff views toward g overtim.

ominous title *Midlife Loss* (Kalish 1989). Its chapters have titles such as "Stress and Loss in Middle Age," "Divorce at Midlife," "Death of a Spouse," and "Job Loss in Middle Age." The subtitle of this book, however, is "Coping Strategies," and the chapters are written from what is described as a "developmental perspective." Rather than stoic endurance breaking down into depression, the key words are "challenge," "liberation," "growth," "development," "joy," "excitement."

Replacing Freud, the intellectual father figure among these current writers seems to be Jung. They quote Jung's argument that the second major phase of psychological development begins after forty years of age. Like Jung, they present the development of the maturing self as both work and moral obligation. They share his concern over the risks of stagnation, of clinging to the past. Describing the neuroses of midlife among women, Jung wrote: "They cling to the illusion of youth or to their children, hoping to salvage in this way a last scrap of youth. One sees it especially in mothers, who find their sole meaning in their children and imagine they will sink into a bottomless void when they have to give them up" (Jung 1954: 114). Allowing oneself to stagnate is a sign of a lack of spiritual will. In its own way, the developmental approach to midlife is as much about virtue and the moral imperatives for women as any samurai code.

Rather than Jung, the new ideas about the woman in midlife might also be traced to the impact of the women's movement and feminist scholarship. The following quotation, for example, comes from an essay included in one of the collections of papers on women in midlife published in the 1980s:

Although a woman may have enacted only her family roles to the exclusion of all others in early adulthood, at midlife as family demands slack off, she is capable of launching a delayed career in spheres other than the family. At this point in her life course, a woman may complete an education or begin one, train for a new job or seek promotion, join a volunteer association or found one. A midlife woman is much more than her familial roles, more than just a mother (Long and Porter 1984: 140).

The energetic, forceful, competent woman of this description is more attractive than the depressed and depressing homemaker. She is also very different from the Japanese image of the aging homemaker: idle, selfish, expressing her distress through "organ language." Appealing though she may be, the feminist version of the woman in midlife is equally a construct, an abstraction from the diverse realities of women's lives.

The Demography of Midlife

Our survey data reveal significant differences among Japanese or Canadian women at midlife, as well as cross-national variation or differences between them. The respondents vary in terms of marital status, reproductive history, family size, household structure, educational background, occupation and class. Among Canadian women, there are also differences in ethnicity, language, national origins, and cultural identity.

The Japanese survey included three quite distinct groups: women living in the suburbs of Kobe (a mainly middle-class area), women employed as factory workers in and around Kyoto (working in large, modern plants or in small, traditional silkweaving enterprises), and women living and working in rural areas. This rural sample included women from the rich farming areas of Nagano and women from fishing villages in Shikoku. Finally, a few questionnaires were completed by women working in service and entertainment sectors in Kyoto. Questionnaires were distributed to 1,738 women;

1,328 were returned, giving a response rate of 76%; 1,316 were used to draw conclusions.

The Canadian study is based on a single sample selected from a listing of all Manitoban women, aged forty to fifty-nine, registered with the provincial health insurance system. (Coverage is almost universal for residents in Manitoba.) Completed questionnaires were received from 2,500 women, a response rate of 68%. For purposes of comparison with the Japanese survey, only the 1,326 women who were from forty-five to fifty-five are included.

The product of these two surveys is a long list of responses by Canadian and Japanese women to the same questions on health, medical care, menopause, medications, or other such matters. We have selected only very simple and standard demographic data for use in this chapter. Our purpose is not to set up any elaborate statistical comparisons; rather, we want to use these data initially as a series of clues, or stimuli, to thinking about the diversity among women at midlife, whether Japanese or Canadian.

Some direct comparisons can be made, such as the number of women who are married or have children. Measurement levels are often not the same, however. Educational data, for example, are not comparable; these same data are invaluable as a reminder of a critical difference among Japanese women and between them and Canadian women of the same age group. Reading the Japanese educational data reveals a sharp break in educational background between women born before and after 1933. This timing suggests that the split in these data is most probably a function of age at the beginning and end of World War II. The age band of the women included in the study is deceptively narrow. The assumption that they may be treated as a single cohort seems eminently reasonable. The educational data serve as a clue to a diversity born of the historical contest of the lives of these women. Memories of the traditional household and the role of the traditional woman within that household will be vivid for the older of these women, but hearsay for those born too recently to remember the prewar years. The older women also remember much more clearly than the younger ones the hardships and poverty associated with the years of war and occupation.

The war had effects on the lives of Canadians, but without creating the same degree of discontinuity for the women born in Canada. The diversity among these women is less a matter of time than place, insofar as the latter is related to ethnicity, language, and cultural identities. Among the Canadian women, while only 13% were born somewhere other than Canada, 51% said that their mothers and 66% that their fathers were not Canadian born. While 90% spoke English most of the time, 53% were in the habit of using a second language. The most common were Ukrainian (12%), German (11%), and French (5%), but the list includes twenty-two languages other than English. Admittedly, languages spoken and places of birth are crude, simplistic indicators; nevertheless, these data are corrective against any assumption of cultural homogeneity. There may be as many variations on what it is to be a woman in midlife as there are languages spoken.

Occupational data reflect the ways in which women in midlife spend their time, earn money, have access to a support group other than their family, have identities other than as wives or mothers, are powerless or have acquired some control in their lives. The same data also indicate something of the position of women within the macroeconomic and political structures of their society. The rapid increase since the sixties in the proportion of married women in the Canadian labor force is an economic statistic but the women who took part in the Canadian survey had lived this trend within their own lives. Women of their generation went into the labor force as their children started school, and most had remained there. In 1980-81, 55% of the respondents were currently employed. They worked in shops, offices, hospitals, schools, factories, banks and universities. The occupations they listed were those standard for Canadian women: nurses, teachers, social workers, sales clerks and clerical workers.

The single Canadian sample is a cross-section of women in midlife in the provincial population, but the three Japanese samples of women were selected from backgrounds chosen partly because of anticipated differences in occupation. In the Kyoto sample all respondents were factory workers. The Kobe sample was selected from a middle-class residential district, partly with the expectation that the majority of middle-class, middle-aged women would not work. The rural sample was chosen on the assumption that the majority of these wives of farmers and fishers would be engaged, much as the traditional Japanese woman, in working within and for the family as an economic unit.

By and large, the expectations about the occupational profile of these samples were confirmed, but not exactly. Only approximately a third of the women living in Kobe, for example, chose to describe themselves as *sengyo shufu*, a professional homemaker. Almost a quarter of the women from the farm and fishing communities, however, chose this term as their own designation. Another quarter of the rural women described themselves as working in a family business, as was expected, but so did slightly more than an eighth of the women living in Kobe. Other rural women said that they worked in manufacturing. While possibly a reference to the traditional processing of food or other products, small-scale modern factories do exist in the villages and do use women in their labor force.

Deciphering the occupational data is sometimes difficult, due partly to conventions of nomenclature, partly to issues of occupational law in Japan, and partly to the structure of the Japanese labor force and the position of women in that force. The use of the term *teacher* is a good example. A woman describing herself as a teacher might work in the formal school system or simply run a few classes in one of the traditional arts from within her own home. A question on the number of hours worked indicated that employment was often a matter of a handful of hours a week, particularly for the women from Kobe. Only slightly over a quarter of all the women in the study described themselves as working full-time outside the home, and almost half were in the sample of factory workers. But women in the factory sample also used part-time less as a descriptor of the number of hours they worked than of their legal status as workers. (Under Japanese labor law the rights and pay of part-time workers are much less than those of a full-time worker. Most women in blue-collar jobs are hired in the category of part-time worker, although they may be working more than forty hours a week (Cook and Hayashi 1980).)

At one level, the description of her work as part-time or freelance or piecework is simply information on how a particular woman divides her time between home and workplace. At another level, the cumulation of these data across all the women taking part in the survey is a source of insight into the relatively tenuous involvement of women in this age group within the Japanese labor force. Part-time and piecework is inherently more unstable than full-time employment and more subject to economic fluctuation. Another clue lies in relative absence of Japanese women working in the arenas that offer some degree of security, higher income, and career mobility to their Canadian counterparts. Using the Canadian occupational classification system, only 63 Japanese women relative to 225 Canadian could be classified as working in administration, teaching, social work, or the health professions. Like the educational or language data, occupational data are also crude and simplistic. Nevertheless, the overall impression of midlife women being marginalized to the fringes of the Japanese labor force economy is probably correct.

The proportion of married women is almost identical (85% in Canada and 86% in Japan) and the proportion of divorced and separated women is only marginally higher in Canada (6% relative to 3%). Canadian women are slightly more likely to have had children, but the proportion of childless women is marginal in both societies (5% relative to 9% among the Japanese women). The most striking difference between the Canadian and the Japanese data is in the number of children born by each woman. Among women with children, less than a third of the Canadians but approximately two-thirds of the Japanese women had one or two children. Approximately a tenth of these Canadian women had five or more children, but slightly less than a tenth of the Japanese women had four or more. The number of children in the Japanese survey ranged from one to seven, but from one to thirteen in the Canadian data. By the age of thirty-three, almost three-quarters of the Japanese women had given birth to their last child relative to approximately two-thirds of Canadian women.

If nothing else, these few statistics reflect a very critical difference in the relationship of these Japanese and Canadian women to the fertility and reproductive powers of their bodies. Yet, the difference in the number of children has only a relatively slight impact on the percentage of women who at this stage in their lives still have children living in the home. Only 30% of the women in the Japanese survey and 25% of the Canadian women live in homes without children. Apart from the presence of children, however, the structure of households is often quite different (see Table 1). Among the Canadian women, the majority (82%) live with only their husband, only their children, or with their husband and children; the corresponding figure for the Japanese is 59%. The difference lies not in the number of women who live in the same household as their parents (these figures are almost the same), but in the number who live with their parents-in-law: only 4 women in the Canadian survey, but 287 women in the Japanese data.

The purpose in presenting these data is partly to demonstrate the diversity of women's lives. Certainly, each study includes women who can be classified as middle-class urban homemakers who are not working, whose children have grown, and whose leisure has presumably increased. They seem more often content than depressed, but the demographic profile at least fits the portrait of the menopausal woman found in both medical literatures. There are also women in the Canadian sample who represent the new woman in midlife engaged in her career, active in political and community affairs, possibly liberated from an old marriage, certainly free from the daily care of young children.

"Career women" are very rare in the Japanese sample. Most young Japanese women work, but more than 40% leave the work force permanently with the birth of their first child. There are important class differences, however. White-collar and professional women (those who might become career women in the North American sense) are under considerable pressure to comply with the customary withdrawal from the labor force, whereas women working in blue-collar occupations are sought after as a part-time, relatively cheap, source of labor. These women are invisible, however, when the woman in midlife is publicly discussed.

TABLE 1

Household structure for Canadian and Japanese women (percentages)

	Household Structure	
	Canadian (n = 1,326)	Japanese (n = 1,316)
Woman living		
Alone	4.3	4.2
With husband only	27.3	14.3
With children only	6.3	5.2
Husband and children	50.3	39.5
Parent only	.8	.4
Parent and husband	.2	.6
Parent and children	.2	.4
Parent, husband, and children	.9	.8
Parent-in-law and husband	.1	2.7
Parent-in-law, husband, and children	.2	10.3
Other relative	.5	.2
Other relative and husband	1.3	2.0
Other relative and children	.7	.5
Other relative, husband, and children	3.0	3.7
Other relative and parent	.4	.9
Other relative, husband, and parent	.5	.4
Other relative, parent, and children	.1	.5
Other relative, parent, husband and children	.8	.9
Parent-in-law only	0	.5
Parent-in-law and children	0	1.0
Parent-in-law and other relatives	0	.1
Parent-in-law, husband, and other relatives	0	1.3
Parent-in-law, children, and other relatives	0	.5
Parent-in-law, husband, children, and other relatives	0	5.5
Unknown	2.1	3.6

Talking with Japanese women of the middle class, it was clear that many believe that the work of running a household and raising children is of outstanding importance. Describing the punishing working routines endured by most Japanese men, many also said that they were not attracted by the idea of full-time employment, even when the choice was available. There are signs of change, however. The divorce rate among middle-aged women is rising. A few career women, again in the North American sense of that term, are emerging. There are other signs of unrest, including a small but active feminist movement.

The portraits of woman in midlife that are found in the medical literature of either society, while having their roots in the lives of real people, are simplified and decontextualized. The Japanese professional homemaker undoubtedly exists, although she is not necessarily depressed. She is also, however, a minority figure in the sense that whatever they may have thought of the popular model of woman as homemaker, the label was not chosen for themselves by the majority of women in either the Kobe, Kyoto, or the rural sample.

Profits, Loss, and Fear of the Old Woman

A cynical explanation for the new emphasis on menopause and hormones, the problems (physical and psychological) of the middle-aging body, the creation of middlescence, is that the medical marketplace senses a potential profit. Money is being made in North America (including Canada) by selling hormones, running exercise workshops, testing for osteoporosis. As the baby-boom generation ages, profits will increase. Obstetrician-gynecologists in both Canada and Japan find in the menopausal woman a convenient new source of patients. Their problem is to convince women that menopause requires the care of a physician. The barrage of propaganda presenting menopause as a disease in need of treatment can be interpreted as advertising, a promotion to attract new consumers.

While there is probably some element of truth to an explanation based on medical profit, it is not sufficient. Predictions based on the economic costs to society of the aging woman are more powerful and far more political in character. Fear of an aging population, more particularly fear of an aging population of women, is widespread in both Canada and Japan. Looking at the Canadian data, projections from Statistics Canada describe a demographic profile for the year 2000 in which there will be 134 women for every 100 men in the sixty-five to seventy-nine age group and 218 women for every 100 men in the eighty and over age group. In the year 2000 in Japan, there will be 136 women for every 100 men over the age of sixty-five (Japan Statistical Association 1987).

Describing what she terms as the crisis approach to aging, McDaniel writes: "The contemporary fear is that the growth in the older population will outrun the ability of society to provide pensions and health care" (1986: 26). Canadian policymakers present a future image in which the health-care system is overburdened by sick, passive, dependent old women. The economic appeal of estrogen therapy and lifestyle modification lies in the promise that money will be saved by delaying or preventing high-cost conditions, such as hip fractures, by exercise, diet, hormone therapy. The message to women emphasizes individualism, responsibility, remaining autonomous, not being dependent on others.

Within the last five or six years, there is much talk in Canada – both formal academic talk published in journals and supported by research grants and informal talk between friends – about the problems of the caretaker generation, the women in midlife. Much of the official talk about women in midlife in Japan, however, deals with their neglect of obligations, their failure to serve as caretakers. At first sight, these two positions seem incompatible with the actual data. In this study at least, Japanese women are far more likely to be heavily involved in caretaking than Canadian women. The issue, of course, is not the numbers but their interpretation; a figure high from a North American perspective may be low from a Japanese viewpoint.

The explanation for an apparent discrepancy between the two societies can be tracked partly to differences in ideas about women and their place in the scheme of the political and moral order. The time Jung would have a woman spend on the development of self becomes idleness and a loss of self-discipline in the samurai code. But there is another explanation rooted in the place of women within the economic system: Canadian women are integrated into the economy of the workplace to a greater extent than the Japanese woman in midlife. Their labor power is essential to some sectors of the Canadian economy (the health-care system has long been propped up by the low wages of women workers), but so also is their earning capacity. The economy is set up on the assumption that most families will have two paychecks to buy not only their basic needs but also the array of unnecessary goods and services for sale. Canadian women have expressed the fear that the politicians may force them into a caretaking role for the old and the sick. They see this as another trap, akin to the trap of mother-hood, into which they may fall. But as the population ages, it is doubtful that the econ-omy could withstand the loss of too many women from the labor force, taking away their earning capacity and their capacity to pay taxes.

Faced with the same problem of an aging population, the alternative chosen in Japan is not to delay the burden on society but to deny that care of the old is a burden to be assumed by society. The shortage of nursing homes and ambulatory care facilities in Japan reflects this attitude on the part of government (Kiefer 1987). Rather than the government shifting resources from industrial to social services, the public message is that the care of the aged is a burden that should continue as the responsibility of women, just as it was in the years before the war. By this interpretation, the refusal to provide a meaningful place in the labor market to women ensures that they cannot escape the burden of caring for the old.

Menopause, Medicalization, and the Politics of Being an Aging Woman

Ironically, the attempt to medicalize menopause, sponsored by some members of the Japanese medical profession, is having a consciousness-raising effect among Japanese women. Meetings arranged to discuss the health problems of middle age may turn into "a forum for debate about family relationships, social roles, and even politics" (Lock 1988). To a greater extent than in Japan, the North American medical profession has inflated menopause into an event of critical medical significance. By the same process, however, the consciousness of women in midlife has also been heightened. A Canadian newsletter, focused initially on menopause, has broadened its mandate to encompass not only the health but other problems of women in midlife. Media discussion of the problems of menopause have fostered the emergence of support groups and the organi-zation of information sessions for menopausal women. Such meetings shift easily from the discussion of estrogens and exercise into a critical exploration of the stereotype of the menopausal woman. Concern over osteoporosis may turn into a discussion of the economic pitfalls of aging or a questioning of the responsibilities of women toward their children, their husband, their parents. Shared identity as menopausal women may yet create an alliance among Japanese women and refusal to become sole caretakers of the old. They may demand more help, more sharing of the burden, more access for themselves and for the old to the resources of society. Canadian women may do the same, demanding not hormones, but the resources to maintain health in old age, includ-ing an adequate income, decent housing, security, and a health-care system responsive to their needs. In sum, consciousness of the menopausal body may lead into conscious-ness of the political self.

References

Beyene, Y. 1989. *From Menarche to Menopause.* New York: State University of New York Press.

Cook, AH, and H Hayashi. 1980. *Working Women in Japan: Discrimination, Resistance and Reform.* Cornell International Industrial and Labor Relations Report, No. 10. Ithaca: New York State School of Industrial and Labor Relations.

Deutsch, H. 1945. *The Psychology of Women, Vol. 2.* New York: Grune and Stratton.

Ikemi, Y, and A Ikemi. 1982. Some Psychosomatic Disorders in Japan in a Cultural Perspective. *Journal of Psychotherapy and Psychosomatics* 38: 231–38.

Japan Statistical Association. 1987. *Japan Statistical Yearbook.* Tokyo: Japan Statistical Association.

Jung, CC. 1954. On the Psychology of the Unconscious. In RFC Hull, *Two Essays on Analytical Psychology*, Vol 7. New York: Pantheon.

Kalish, R ed. 1989. *Midlife Loss.* Newbury Park, Calif: Sage Publications.

Kiefer, CW. 1987. Care of the Aged in Japan. In E Norbeck and M Lock eds. *Health, Illness, and Medical Care in Japan: Cultural and Social Dimensions,* 89–109. Honolulu: University of Hawaii Press.

Kyutoku, S. 1979. *Bogenbyo.* Tokyo: Sanmaku Shuppan.

Lebra, TS. 1976. *Japanese Patterns of Behavior.* Honolulu: University of Hawaii Press.

Lebra, TS. 1984. *Japanese Women: Constraint and Fulfillment.* Honolulu: University of Hawaii Press.

Lock, M. 1986a. Ambiguities of Aging: Japanese Experience and Perceptions of Menopause. *Culture, Medicine and Psychiatry* 10: 23–47.

Lock, M. 1986b. Plea for Acceptance: School Refusal Syndrome in Japan. *Social Science and Medicine* 23: 99–112.

Lock, M. 1988. New Japanese Mythologies: Faltering Discipline and the Ailing Housewife. *American Ethnologist* 15(1): 43–61.

Lock, M, PA Kaufert, and P Gilbert. 1988. Cultural Construction of the Menopausal Syndrome: The Japanese Case. *Maturitas* 10: 317–22.

Long, J, and KL Porter. 1984. Multiple Roles of Midlife Women: A Case for New Directions in Theory, Research and Policy. In C Baruch and J Brooks-Gunn eds. *Women in Midlife*, 109–59. New York: Plenum Press.

McDaniel, SA. 1986. *Canada's Aging Population.* Toronto: Butterworths.

Roberts, H. 1984. *Patient Patients: Women and Their Doctors.* London: Pandora.

Roy, M. 1985. *Bengali Women.* Chicago: University of Chicago Press.

11

Role Strains And Tranquillizer Use[*]

Ruth Cooperstock and Henry L. Lennard

Over the past fifteen years minor tranquillizers, particularly the benzodiazepines, have become a part of the armament of physicians as well as an accepted component of the lives of large segments of our population. Social critics and sociologists (Lennard et al. 1971; Stimson 1975: 265-67; Illich 1976) have described the ways in which these drugs, termed "antianxiety agents," have become identified as solutions to "problems of living." Consistent with this analysis, the preparations acting on the central nervous system, of which the benzodiazepines comprise an increasing part, are those most likely to be prescribed for long-term use (Dunnell and Cartwright 1972).

In an extensive study of prescribed drug use in Oxfordshire (Skegg et al. 1977), psychotropics accounted for almost one-fifth of all prescriptions, with almost 10 percent of the males and 21 percent of the females receiving at least one psychotropic prescription during the year. Canadian investigators found 13.7 percent of all adults reporting use of minor tranquillizers within the past twelve months (Smart and Goodstadt 1976) while another study found 8.8 percent of a community sample claim use of a sedative/hypnotic in the past 48 hours (Chaiton et al. 1976: 114). Over a recent nineteen-month period in Saskatchewan, it was found that one in every seven over the age of 19 received a prescription for diazepam alone (the generic term for Valium) (Harding et al. 1978). In all of these studies, it is clear that prescribing is not random within populations. Women consistently receive twice the proportion of prescriptions for tranquillizers as do men (Cooperstock and Parnell 1976: 115). Additionally, women in the middle and late years are at highest risk. Skegg et al. (1977) report that 33 percent of women aged 45 to 59 received at least one psychotropic prescription in a year while 12.9 percent of these women received at least five such prescriptions over the year; among women 75 and over, 20.2 percent received this number. Although it has been well established that those using psychotropic drugs also report numerous somatic disorders this cannot account for the disproportionate use among women.

Prescriptions in general serve important symbolic functions for both physician and patient (Balint 1964; Bush 1977) but prescriptions for psychotropic drugs must be viewed as a special case. The acceptance of these agents for long-term use cannot be viewed as simply the result of vigorous promotion by the pharmaceutical

* Reprinted from Ruth Cooperstock and Henry L. Lennard, 'Role Strains and Tranquillizer Use,' in *Health and Canadian Society: Sociological Perspectives*, 1st and 2nd editions, edited by David Coburn, Carl D'Arcy, George Torrance, and Peter New, with permission from Fitzhenry & Whiteside, Toronto.

industry. Rather, this acceptance has coincided with changes in the nature of "illness" as presented to physicians today, with the precedence taken by chronic and ill-defined illnesses, and with the enormous growth of the pharmaceutical industry and the grateful utilization by the medical profession of the new and often lifesaving drugs developed in the past twenty-five years. Ironically, some of the very factors that altered the nature of presenting complaints have reinforced and strengthened the physician's belief in the biomedical model of illness. Engel (1977: 196) has described this belief system as the dominant model of disease today, assuming disease to be fully accounted for by "deviation from the norm of measurable biological variables." He further points out that this "leaves no room within its framework for the social, psychological, and behavioural dimensions of illness." Given this belief system, the prescription of a tranquillizing drug is often the outcome of a negotiation whereby problems and distress arising in a variety of life situations are defined as psychological "symptoms" of disease. This negotiation results in the labelling and definition of the problem as a medical one, requiring health-care resources and, frequently, continued medication. Needless to say, the biomedical model also finds the locus of illness in the individual, thus requiring individual treatment.

Engel proposes a "biopsychosocial" model of illness in which the physician must "weigh the relative contributions of social and psychological factors as well as of biological factors implicated in the patient's dysphoria and dysfunction as well as in this decision to accept or not accept patienthood and with it the responsibility to cooperate in his own health care" (1977: 1,966). Expanded in this way, for example, the problem of patient "compliance" with drug regimes could never again be viewed as simple patient unwillingness to accept the greater knowledge of the physician regarding the appropriate treatment of his bodily systems. Thus, the very notion of compliance would be altered to one of therapeutic co-operation or alliance.

What consequences ensue from use of these drugs? What functions do they serve for the individual? For the families and intimates of users? When sizable segments of the population ingest any drug, particularly one acting on the central nervous system and mood, it becomes necessary to examine the ways in which human interaction may be altered, and the range of functions served by the drugs. This chapter will report data from a study of the social and behavioural consequences and meaning of tranquillizer use conducted in Toronto in the spring of 1977. It will not deal with the physical effects of use reported (effects on motor skills, perception, cognition and mood) but rather with those functions, both negative and positive, that relate to the use of tranquillizers as a means of maintaining a given social role as expressed by the informants. Numerous drugs in use today do effect mood and hence would have an effect on relationships, self-image, and so forth (the steroids are an obvious example), but no others merit such close attention as the tranquillizers because of the extent of their use and because of their wide and increasing range of indications for use.

Studies of the effects of tranquillizers have tended to be either clinical (Greenblatt and Shader 1974; Preskorn and Denner 1977: 237), pharmacological (Kleinknecht and Donaldson 1975; Sellers 1978: 118) or based on surveys using prestructured questions (Uhlenhuth et al. 1978). No previous work has focussed on the perceptions of the drug's effects as viewed by the user. The decision was thus made to bring together groups of individuals to discuss, as freely as possible, the meaning they attribute to their use. Both authors were present at each group; the discussions, which were tape-recorded, lasted approximately two hours and were later transcribed. The approach selected was most akin to a natural history study of population – spontaneity, group interaction and discussion were permitted and encouraged, and there was minimal participation on the part of the investigators. An attempt was made to create a value-free atmosphere in the groups by opening discussion with a short statement of the investigators' interest in "any aspect of the drug that you were aware of, physical, emotional, social – its effect on your work, relationships, etc." The informants were thus made aware that the investigators' interests extended beyond the purely physiological. The informants had all responded to a newspaper announcement asking for volunteers who were now using, or who ever had used, tranquillizers and who would be interested in discussing the consequences of their use. Only those whose primary drug was a benzodiazepine (in all cases diazepam, chlordiazepoxide or Librax) were included.

The data are based on 14 group interviews with 68 participants and an additional 24 lengthy letters from individuals who could not participate in the groups but who wanted to offer their experiences. The groups ranged in size from two to eight people. Consistent with general tranquillizer consumption figures our volunteers were predominantly female (76 percent) and their mean age was 46 with a range from 23 to 74. Because of the exploratory nature of this study, the investigators chose to attract a population of articulate individuals, and this is reflected in the high educational attainment of the group.[1] Seventy-six percent had either university or postsecondary technical training. Sixty-six percent were married, 14 percent single, and the remaining 20 percent were separated, divorced or widowed. The majority were in the labour force (58 percent), 25 percent described themselves as housewives, 14 percent were either retired, disabled or not working and 2 percent were students. Of those working outside the home, the majority were in professional or managerial occupations.

Both the high educational and occupational attainment of the sample and the method used to solicit volunteers prevent direct application of the findings to the Canadian population as a whole. The informants did, however, match the characteristics of the general tranquillizer user in terms of sex and age. It must be emphasized that this method of sample selection was deliberately chosen because of the richness of the data required and because, in this exploratory study, the authors saw greater heuristic value emerging from this method than from more traditional sampling designs.

In each group, following the few opening remarks already mentioned, the investigators suggested that the members take turns giving a short history of their drug use, including the reasons for starting, the name of the drug, the amount, typical dosage and the length of time that they used the drug (66 were still using it either regularly or intermittently).

Only three individuals did not receive their tranquillizers from a physician, although all had gotten them from this source initially. Only one person had used the drug for less than a month, 8 percent had used it from one month to a year, 24 percent from one year to four years and 67 percent had used tranquillizers anywhere from four to eighteen years. Thus the informants were clearly long-term users, although their use patterns were close to the usual recommended daily dose of the drugs studied (the mean daily dose of diazepam reported was 16.2 mg).

The initial reasons for use varied widely, with 53 percent citing a somatic problem, although a high proportion of these commented on social stress as related to the disorder, 30 percent attributing use to social stresses only, and 19 percent to internal tensions. Continued use, however, was most often discussed in terms of "permitting" the informants to maintain themselves in a role or roles that they found difficult or intolerable without the drug.[2]

As might be expected of a predominantly female population, the most common roles mentioned related to the traditional ones of wife, mother, houseworker. As will be shown, these were typically discussed in relation to conflict over ability to perform the role or to adapt to its demands. Among males, discussion tended to relate to conflict regarding work performance or, more typically, the need to contain somatic symptoms in order to perform an occupational role. Difficulties in adapting to the role of the newly separated or widowed were also reported. Another conflict experienced by more than a few informants was that of the patient role itself.

Before proceeding, some mention should be made of the sex composition of the groups and the impact of this on the discussions. Five of the groups were composed only of females; nine groups contained one or more males. The groups were organized solely on the basis of convenience. Striking differences existed between the two types of groups, even though one of the investigators was male. Conforming to traditional roles and consistent with other studies (Phillips and Segal 1969: 34), the men tend to speak less of social and emotional problems than the women, instead putting greater emphasis on reports of somatic problems and side effects of the drugs. Again, as shown in other work (Ruble and Higgins 1976: 32), the mixed groups, even those with only one male member, tended to follow the lead of the male and focus less on problems of role strains and interpersonal relations than did the all-female groups who typically moved rapidly into discussion of social strains. Since there were no all-male groups, it is impossible to know how these would have evolved.

The following discussion will deal with the ways tranquillizing drugs helped to maintain female informants in the traditional female role of wife and homemaker. This will be followed by illustrations of the conflicts expressed in fulfilling the maternal role.

In a recent symposium on Valium (Hollister 1977: 18), the chairman, attempting to demonstrate the usefulness of the benzodiazepines, stated, "We hear much about the adverse effects of the drugs and their costs, while we hear little in terms of how many divorces Valium may prevent." The chairman here has clearly identified an important function of these drugs as expressed by our informants, i.e., to sustain strained social systems. Significantly, these strains within family groups were mentioned as resulting in drug use by female rather than male informants. The chairman's remark was consistent with the culturally accepted view that it is the role of the wife to control the tensions created by a difficult marriage, and, implicit in his comment, is the notion that drug use is justified in order to accomplish this. Valium as an aid in the maintenance of nurturing, caring role is seen in the following quote:

In the summertime I virtually live on them because we have a boat. And I can't sleep on the boat. My husband doesn't swim and I am up like this (indicating tension) all the time ... It's the only way I can get to be nice the next day to all those people we have floating around this boat all the time, preparing meals for them.

There were clear expressions of anger and resentment directed at their spouses by a number of women, at the same time as they saw no alternative to continued occupancy of the traditional wife-homemaker role. This anger may well reflect the greater sense of powerlessness felt by women than men (Olson 1969: 31). For example, a woman with four teenagers said:

I take it to protect the family from my irritability because the kids are kids. I don't think it's fair for me to start yelling at them because their normal activity is bothering me. My husband says I overreact ... I'm an emotional person, more so than my husband who's an engineer and very calm and logical – he thinks ... But I suppose I overreact, but because I overreact is no reason for the family to suffer from my irritability ... So I take Valium to keep me calm ... Peace and calm. That's what my husband wants because frankly the kids get on his nerves, too. But he will not take anything ... He blows his top ... He can bellow but I can't. And this I have resented over the years, but I've accepted it. I'm biding my time. One of these days I'm going to leave the whole kit and kaboodle and walk out on him. Then maybe I won't need any more Valium.

Other women spoke about adjusting their dosage in relation to family stresses; one said, "I need more on the weekends when my family is home."

Ginsberg (1976) has found that tranquillizer use may be particularly prevalent among women in situations of conflict. The following quotes exemplify just such conflicts:

Now I am in a situation which I cannot get out of. There is no way I will drop my responsibilities to my husband who is a very fine man, or my children. My husband's and my interests have gone different ways. The communication has diminished, but he's still a very good husband, and he's an excellent father to the children ... I can't leave them and because I can't leave them I'm sticking to the Valium. That's my escape.

I would like to be off in Australia somewhere, writing. You know, do only my work. But having to stop the writing to get the supper on, it irritates me. And there are so many irritations during the day. But I cannot change the situation because of my family.

This informant was the only woman expressing this type of conflict who worked, and, significantly, her writing was done at home and earned her no income. These women quoted above were all middle class, well educated, had been employed prior to marriage or child rearing and, at the time of drug use, were all economically dependent on their husbands. Again, a sense of powerlessness pervades these quotes. Bahr (1974), reviewing the literature, points out that a wife's power in the family relationship tends to increase when she is employed.

Oakley (1974) identifies the features of the housewife's role as being: 1) exclusively filled by women; 2) identified with economic dependence; 3) involved with maintaining a status as nonworking; and 4) of higher priority than other roles. The following quote is an example of a family in which the husband rigidly adheres to the view of the housewife role as having priority over all others. The wife, while attempting to fulfil the role, is nonetheless incapable of accepting or finding gratification from it.

But the problem started with marriage, where I have your English background with the stoicism. And I married a husband who was very open and out-going and for instance would sit down to dinner ... and say, "Am I supposed to eat this shit?" And I didn't know how to react to it. I cried a lot, and he was very verbal in his criticisms ... And then I went for two years without pregnancy so I was treated for infertility, after which I had ten pregnancies and four live children in four and a half years ... I was alternately feeling suicidal and yet feeling responsible to these four lovely little kids ... And I am constantly in conflict, because I'd like to get a job. And I'm into so many things because I am trying to compensate. You know at home there's nothing. There's my kids ...

You know if you tried to talk to him at this point (and said), "Guess what I did. Guess what I accomplished. Guess what happened today." He says, "I don't want to listen. You clean up the kitchen and then I'll listen." And this is terribly frustrating.

Another woman explained women's utilization of physicians' services by the fact that wives are not expected to make demands on their husbands. She said:

And the first thing a man will say to you when you're not feeling well, at least a husband, ... is "why don't you go to the doctor." Like, don't bother me that you are feeling sick, go see the doctor. So women do go running off.

Tranquillizers are also used to help individuals adapt to conflicts generated by intolerable behaviour in a spouse, in this case an alcoholic husband:

I started getting sick with stomach pains and I think I just couldn't cope at home anymore. I lived with an active alcoholic. ... I guess in 1969 it wasn't fashionable that you talk about your problems, especially when you have an alcohol problem. And I do have two children. (Subsequently it was found that the informant required major surgery.) I was in terrible shape after the operation because I knew the problem still existed at home and I was concerned about my children. The doctor gave me tranquillizers afterwards to cope and stop shaking whenever something came up ... When I found I got better (from the effects of the operation) and I learned about alcoholism and about my problem I looked for help myself. I joined Al-Anon (a group for the families of alcoholics) and I stopped taking the tranquillizers.

Many women reported initial tranquillizer use following the birth of children and the physical and emotional strains that frequently occur at this time. One informant described her inability to cope with her maternal role in the following way:

And then ... I realized that I'd better get some of this pressure off at some point, I was afraid I was going to kill my kids. I had one of those days and I just felt that something would snap. And I knew then that I needed something to detach myself from the pile-up of stress and pressure at that point. And it did; I felt very detached so that the next day the situation hadn't changed, but I felt very detached and able to cope without feeling so full of stress and tension. It was almost like I wasn't there. Probably a week's vacation away from the situation would have been just as valid a way of coping with the problem. I couldn't do that so I found that Valium did that ... And sort of the end of that week some of the pressures had gone down; like some of the problems with the children were sort of going together, as I got more hyper, they got more hyper. We were interacting and the pitch was getting higher and higher. And once I calmed down after the week, they calmed down.

She discontinued use at the end of the one-week period, finding that the drug had been extremely functional for this short-term alleviation of a strained situation but that long-term help came via attendance at marriage counselling, which was initiated soon after ceasing drug use. She says about this:

I have since discovered that a lot of the problems that I was bearing totally on myself weren't all mine, which I discovered in some very good marital counselling. So that has relieved it considerably.

Unlike the woman just quoted, other mothers of infants continued use over prolonged periods. These were women who expressed clearly conflicting attitudes regarding their maternal role. In the following example, these conflicts were initially triggered
by a difficult infant:

It turned out I couldn't have children so we adopted ... and with the adoption of the first child I
was deliriously happy ... And then I adopted a second child very quickly after the first, and she
was a holy terror. She screamed from the minute we brought her into the house and she never
stopped screaming. I was absolutely going around the bend and I called my G.P. and he
prescribed my first tranquillizers ... Maybe they should have given the kid the tranquillizers! I
don't know, or a shot of whiskey or something. But I had to learn how to cope with this screaming
and I felt very inadequate. I felt I was a lousy mother. I felt I didn't love her as much as I loved the
first and there was something wrong with me ... I think that was the start for me of really feeling
inadequate in the role of mother, and also feeling that basically I didn't really enjoy it that much.

Another informant suffered two postpartum depressions and used tranquillizers for
long periods following the birth of both her children. She began psychotherapy while
still using tranquillizers and, in the course of the therapy, recognized her dislike of the
role she had previously accepted as homemaker and mother. She said:

At the end of the therapy sessions I said one of the things I really wanted to do was to go back to
work part-time. I had taught student nurses and I really enjoyed that. And I felt that I really
needed to do something that gave me a good feeling about myself. And I've never really had that
as a mother or housekeeper. Like I'm always kind of wondering whether I'm doing the right thing
as a mother and I really don't know how to keep house, and don't feel very adequate in that
situation.

Following this statement, she was asked by another member of the group whether any
shift in her drug use occurred when she returned to work, to which she replied, "I could
cut right down and did." The reports of the effects of work by our informants are consistent with the general findings that employment tends to protect women from the
"sick role" (Nathanson 1975: 9; Brown and Harris 1978) as well as affecting drug use
(Cooperstock and Parnell 1976).

For the mother of older children, the time demands of the maternal role cause strains
expressed in the form of anger and resentment towards the spouse. For example:

Out at the cottage, even ... I have no escape. My husband wants to escape from the kids ... He
takes the sailboat out and disappears for three or four hours.

One informant used up to ten or twelve Valiums per day in order to nap in the afternoon and thus "escape" the feelings of guilt and responsibility she felt as a mother following her daughter's car accident:

My three children, I had raised them very carefully. I watched them every second – I mean they
were never on the beach alone. And the idea that she walked in front of a car with a boy, after a
party, and was nearly killed ... I just had to escape it every day when she was in the hospital and
during her rehabilitation period.

The severe strain of mothering two retarded children was the trigger for another informant, who said:

We found that our retarded children caused trouble in what had been a relatively happy marriage ... Most of us are overwhelmed by the physical care and emotional drain connected with caring for a handicapped child. The disappointment combined with the work is impossible for most of us to bear without help ... The hard work combined with the disappointment made me anxious and depressed.

Almost all the women quoted above described situations of extreme role strain, that is, inability to comply with traditional role expectations, in which they felt they lacked the "right" to express their dissatisfaction and preferences. They see husbands as having other "escape routes" when marital difficulties or obligations become burdensome. The issues addressed by almost all of these women are structural, and some were able to describe structural, as opposed to individual, remedies to their problems.

Tranquillizer use was also initiated as a response to the strain of adapting to a new role, whether related to loss through widowhood or through separation. The following quote illustrates the use of the drug to aid adaptation to sudden loss and the strains involved in an abrupt change from the traditional role of wife to that of separated and economically independent woman:

All of a sudden my husband decided he's going to be on his own. I thought we had a pretty good household. I liked being a mother and a housewife and wife. All of a sudden it's all over. My whole life crumbled all of a sudden; and I had to find a job. I can't change that quickly ... Instead of being able to discuss it rationally, his idea is to say nothing, absolutely nothing ... I asked what is the matter and he couldn't even tell me. This is when I blew it and went to a doctor.

The following description of use after the death of a spouse illustrates the function of the drug for this informant in easing his pain.

So then my wife passed away ... I was married for 35 years ... So I went to my doctor and said, "You know the situation. I need a little something to lean on for a few days." ... So he gave me Valium. It was 5 mg. He said, "Now take one after breakfast and one after supper." He gave me enough to do me for a month. You know what I mean, I was really upset. I couldn't face people, I couldn't do anything. So I was eating them like popcorn.

This informant, at the time of the group interview, was still using tranquillizers on a regular daily basis years after his wife's death.

Continuing use of tranquillizers can be viewed as an aid in adapting to an unsatisfactory role or as a means of coping with unresolved conflicts, but it also can be seen as a learned habitual mode of reacting to stresses as seen in the following:

I started taking them when my father died and I tapered off when I got married. I sort of tried to taper off because my husband wasn't too crazy about my taking them ... But after we were divorced I was worse than ever.

Although males occupy two major roles, an occupational one and a familial one as husband or head of household, the males in this sample tended to speak of their tranquillizer use in relation to only one of these roles – the occupational one. Significantly, sex-role research identifies competence as a dominant value in the male self-image (Fransella and Frost 1977). Most typically, male informants discussed the onset of somatic symptoms in relation to work stresses or new strains brought on by a change in jobs and the continued use of tranquillizing drugs as a means of controlling these symptoms. A number accepted that little change in their job status was possible, and, therefore, they saw no means other than drugs to alleviate the sometimes incapacitating symptoms. The most common symptom mentioned by the men was atrial fibrillation; others included dyspnea, colitis, muscle spasms, and so forth. Only two female informants mentioned occupational stresses as a factor in their drug use.

One informant, a minister, found his symptoms appearing following a change of jobs:

I changed jobs about 5 years ago from a preaching ... kind of job to a human relations job. It's competitive stuff. And about six months later I started having some ... psychosomatic induced dizziness, a sense of you're about to pass out. I fell enough that my colleagues took me off to a cardiac unit. And that went on. I was told there was nothing there but the fact is every day the dizziness was there and it was something to fight against.

He was placed on Valium to control his symptoms and continued on the drug for a number of years, varying the dose as necessary. While permitting him to carry on in his competitive job, the drug also affected his self-image. In his words:

When I do take Valium I'm conscious of being very quiet; I'm conscious of being the way I would like to be on my own, without drugs, but conscious of the fact that it's not me. And I really resent that. And I'd like to achieve that part without any tranquillizers.

A successful businessman summarized the functions served by Valium in his work. The drug, in this case, produced feelings of calm in situations that the informant found he couldn't control and hence produced stresses. He said he uses tranquillizers:

... if I know I am going into a meeting and I know that it's going to be something that has a lot of tension to it. Sometimes I look at the people and their styles in terms of how they are going to go through the meeting. And so I figure rather than put up with the nonsense of getting myself into an emotional twist I take one of these and I'm quite conscious, I'm in control of myself ... I find that I react less. ... I dislike ... making a decision and then going through this "if only" phase. I find that very frustrating. I prefer to look at the risks and the offsets, reach a decision and then put the whole damn thing behind us. If I know I'm going to be there with those types of people and we're going to be sitting on a mountain contemplating our navel for a long period of time I'll say, "O.K. I don't want to react to what they are saying." I take a diazepam.

Another male describes his use of tranquillizers as a means of reducing tensions related to his work that arose from his self-inflicted perfectionistic demands:

I'm overly conscientious, a perfectionist. I wouldn't dare go home thinking I'd made a mistake. I've got to be sure that I'm right. So that adds to my tension. And because my partners are careless that puts more onus on me.

A major use for tranquillizers is an adjunctive therapy for individuals with a wide array of chronic conditions (Greenblatt et al. 1975: 32; Blackwell 1973: 225). They are typically dispensed for two purposes: the first is prophylactic, to protect the person with a chronic illness from excessive stress that might have adverse effects on the course of the illness, and the second is to allay psycho-social reactions to the illness, prognosis or treatment.

Three of the informants suffered from dessiminated lupus erythematosus (a disease occurring predominantly in young women that attacks many internal organs, can be fatal and is difficult to diagnose), and all described long-term use of tranquillizing drugs, which they felt maintained them in a dependent patient role. Unlike the previous examples of role strains in relation to traditional roles, the frustration and anger expressed by these informants was related to the drug's use as a means of masking emotions and thus preventing the assumption of just such adult roles. One of these informants had spent the morning with a fellow lupus patient and describes the feelings of a person about to be discharged following long-term hospitalization and what she perceived to be the insensitivity of the health-care system in recognizing the difficulties encountered in rejecting the "sick role" (Parsons 1951):

And no one can understand what she's so upset about. She's going home. She should be in a high state. And like she said to me she was upset today. I said, "Oh I understand. Now you've got to face the world." She said, "Yes, before I was using my health as a crutch for not doing things. And now I'm going to be better, and I'm going home. But I have no friends, because I pushed them away in the past year. How do I make my life? I have nothing to go home to. I have my parents, I have my brothers and sisters. But I have nothing and no one to go home to. And I'm scared." I agreed with her wholeheartedly ... This is a very real problem. And I resent the doctors trying to cover it up with platitudes, "Oh, everything will be OK," which is ridiculous because it won't, or giving them the Valium which will put them into a very mellow type of mood. But that's not going to solve the problem one iota, it'll just postpone the problem. But it won't solve it.

The inability of a chronically ill person to view herself and be viewed as a mature adult is vividly illustrated in the following quote, as is the way in which tranquillizers, in her view, further prevent the adoption of an adult role:

But I want to go right back where I say they were using drugs to cover up my true feelings, because with as much anger and hate or anything I had in me I never voiced my anger to my husband or to his family or anyone whom it was obviously directed at. And consequently they knew I was upset, which I was with just cause. So they gave me Valium and the Serax and everything. But that did not solve the problem at all because they didn't even know I was angry with them. Then one day I blurted it out and they came back and grabbed and said, "Why didn't you tell me? We kept doing this to you because you never said anything. You left yourself wide open." Which was very true. You see, when you have chronic disease, many people tend to put you down. One beautiful statement they used to say to me was, "You were so lucky to have your George stick with you." This is a chronic one: you're so lucky he sticks with you. Consequently you have to be better than normal. You can't be the ordinary person who makes mistakes or does things wrong. You have to prove you're superhuman which is impossible. But you keep trying, you see, because you make these demands upon yourself. And when people make you angry, you figure, "Well I'm so lucky that they're still sticking with me." You're down about this low at that point so that you don't criticize. Even if they're out of line you never put them down or you never tell them off because you feel you're lucky to have this relationship, because since you're sick, you shouldn't have anything. Poor kid, but we don't want to cope with it. Consequently, and I'm not alone in this, we keep our true feelings submerged. But the anger is there, the hurt is there. And until you voice this hurt, until you listen to yourself, until you're honest enough with yourself and with them, it's never going to be corrected. I keep going back; using Valium or Serax or any of these things to hide them or mask them is not going to solve the problem at all.

It is clear from the above data that, in order to understand the functions served by these drugs, it is necessary to look beyond the medical model of disease to the structural factors creating the stresses, which bring many to the attention of the health-care system.

There has been no mention to this point of the image held by these informants of the prescribers of their drugs. A noteworthy finding was that considerably more anger was expressed by women than men towards their physicians. This may relate to a number of factors, including their greater difficulty in asserting themselves in relation to a male physician (Stephenson and Walker 1979), the awareness of differential prescribing to men and women as expressed by a number of informants (reflecting recent studies conducted by members of the medical profession: Milliren 1977: 18; Bass and Paul 1977; Dixon 1975: 24) and, at least as demonstrated in these groups, a greater awareness than the males of the structural, rather than individual, nature of the problems. Typifying this awareness is the following statement by a female informant:

I think the thing that upset me most about the way drugs were used with me was that in the early years when I was so obviously unhappy with what was happening in my life the solution to the doctors was so obviously a drug solution. And I had to push everybody I knew, including the doctors, except my psychiatrist who supported me all the way, that the solution for me was going to be really to quite radically change my life and not to make me comfortable with the life I was in.

Although some informants saw no alternative to their continued use of tranquillizers, others, particularly those who had already discontinued using them, discussed alternative solutions to their problems. These included both individual and structural solutions, such as yoga, relaxation exercises, strenuous exercise, consciousness raising and self-help groups, as well as paid full- or part-time employment and changes in marital relationships or type of employment. These also included new ways of viewing oneself and one's emotions, or at least the expression of one's emotions. A former alcoholic cross-addicted to tranquillizers repeatedly made the point that only through permitting oneself to "feel" could one change and thus remain drug free. In her words:

... it's my own personal feeling that as long as you keep taking drugs you're never going to feel what it is you're taking the drugs not to feel. So it's always going to be with you. It's going to be a continued problem throughout your life.

Conclusion

By utilizing a natural history approach to data gathering regarding the consequences of tranquillizer use, it becomes immediately obvious that the biomedical model of disease is inadequate to explain continuing use of these drugs. Although 53 percent of the informants claimed that their use began in relation to a somatic disorder, the majority recognized that their continuing use related to a variety of role strains. The most common strains and conflicts mentioned by female informants revolved around their traditional roles as wife, mother and homemaker while males tended to experience conflicts regarding their work or work performance. Some of those with chronic illnesses tended to discuss their use of tranquillizers as creating greater strains for them in their efforts to "normalize" their lives. The drug, by masking feelings, prevented the rejection of the undesirable "sick role" too often imposed by both the nature of their illness and their family members.

The data presented raises a wide variety of questions for the social scientist, the medical profession and our social institutions and legislators. A number of our middle-class informants found that they cease use during or after making structural changes in their lives. Are such alternatives open to all members of society? The poor? The elderly? If not, are tranquillizers to be accepted as adequate solutions to social stresses? These are clearly moral and ethical issues that transcend the bounds of the expertise of the medical profession and demand social, not medical, answers.

The data do, however, indicate a need for further studies of the physician-patient relationship. Little is now known of physicians' views of the prescribing of psychotropic drugs, particularly how they view continuing use. Are psychotropic drugs seen as necessary for continuous symptomatic relief? As the best of poor alternatives? To what extent are the sorts of social strains discussed by our informants known to their primary-care physicians?

Although the study did not intend to focus on the chronically ill, enough material was presented to suggest that use of tranquillizers by this large and growing population is again a means of resolving strains; in this case, the strains incurred by the individual's inability to perform a healthy "adult" role in the family. How applicable is this model to a range of chronic conditions? How common is this reaction among the chronically ill? Again, in relation to this group, our data raise the question of the desirability of psychotropic drugs as a solution. Clearly, there is a great need for continuing research to answer these questions and, additionally, to test programmatic alternatives.

Notes

1   The call for volunteers appeared in the Toronto Globe and Mail, a newspaper with a predominantly middle-class readership. However, the paper also has a national circulation, which resulted in calls and letters appearing from many parts of Ontario and Quebec.
2   Totals exceed one hundred because of multiple coding.

References

Bahr, S. 1974. Effects of Power and Division of Labor in the Family. In LW Hoffman and TI Nye eds. *Working Mothers*. London: Jossey-Bass.

Balint, M. 1964. *The Doctor, His Patient and the Illness*. Toronto: Pitman Medical.

Bass, M, and D Paul. 1977. *The Influence of Sex Tranquilizer Prescribing*. Paper presented at the North American Primary Care Research Group Meeting, Williamsburg, Virginia, March.

Blackwell, B. 1973. Psychotropic Drugs in Use Today: The Role of Diazepam in Medical Practice. *Journal of the American Medical Association* 225(13): 1,637–1,641.

Brown, G, and T Harris. 1978. *Social Origins of Depression*. London: Tavistock Publications.

Bush, PJ. 1977. Psychosocial Aspects of Medical Use. In AI Wertheinier and PJ Bush eds. *Perspectives on Medicines in Society*. Washington, DC: Drug Intelligence Publications.

Chaiton, A, WO Spitzer, RS Roberts, and T Delmore. 1976. Patterns of Medical Drug Use – A Community Focus. *Canadian Medical Association Journal* 114(1): 33–37.

Cooperstock, R, and P Parnell. 1976. Comment on Clancy and Gove. *American Journal of Sociology* 81: 1,455–1,458.

Dixon, AS. 1978. Drug Use in Family Practice: A Personal Study. *Canadian Family Physician* 24: 345–353.

Dunnell, K, and A Cartwright. 1972. *Medicine Takers, Prescribers and Hoarders*. London: Routledge and Kegan Paul.

Engel, GL. 1977. The Need for a New Medical Model. A Challenge for Biomedicine. *Science* 196(4,286): 129–136.

Fransella, F, and K Frost. 1977. *On Being A Woman*. London: Tavistock Publications.

Ginsberg, S. 1976. Women, Work and Conflict. In N Fonda and P Moss eds. *Mothers in Employment*. London: University of London Press.

Greenblatt, DJ, and RI Shader. 1974. *Benzodiazepines in Clinical Practice*. New York: Raven Press.

Greenblatt, DJ, RI Shader, and J Koch-Weser. 1975. Psychotropic Drug Use in the Boston Area. *Archives of General Psychiatry* 32(4): 518–521.

Harding, J, N Wolf, and G Chan. 1978. *A Socio-Demographic Profile of People Prescribed Mood Modifiers in Saskatchewan*. Alcoholism Commission of Saskatchewan, Research Division.

Hollister, E. 1977. Valium: A Discussion of Current Issues. *Psychosomatics* 18(1): 44–58.

Illich, I. 1976. *Limits to Medicine: Medical Nemesis. The Expropriation of Health*. London: Marion Press.

Kleinknecht, RA, and D Donaldson. 1975. A Review of the Effects of Diazepam on Cognitive and Psychomotor Performance. *Journal of Nervous and Mental Disease* 161(6): 399–411.

Lennard, HL, LJ Bernstein, and DC Ransom. 1971. *Mystification and Drug Misuse*. San Francisco: Jossey-Bass.

Milliren, JW. 1977. Some Contingencies Affecting the Utilization of Tranquillizers in Long-Term Care of the Elderly. *Journal of Health and Social Behavior* 18(2): 206–211.

Nathanson, C. 1975. Illness and the Feminine Role: A Theoretical Review. *Social Science and Medicine* 9(2): 57–62

Oakley, A. 1974. *Housewife*. London: Penguin Books.

Olson, A. 1969. The Measurement of Family Power by Self-Report and Behavioral Methods. *Journal of Marriage and the Family* 31(3): 545–550.

Parsons, T. 1951. *The Social System*. New York: Free Press.

Phillips, DL, and BE Segal. 1969. Sexual Status and Psychiatric Symptoms. *American Sociological Review* 34(1): 58–72.

Preskorn, SH, and LJ Denner. 1977. Benzodiazepines and Withdrawal Psychosis. *Journal of the American Medical Association* 237(1): 36–38.

Ruble, DN, and ET Higgins. 1976. Effects of Group Sex Composition on Self-Presentation and Sex-Typing. *Journal of Social Issues* 32(3): 125–132.

Sellers, EM. 1978. Clinical Pharmacology and Therapeutics of Benzodiazepines. *Canadian Medical Association Journal* 118: 1,533–1,538.

Skegg, DCG, R Doll, and J Perry. 1977. Use of Medicines in General Practice. *British Medical Journal* I (6,076): 1,561–1,573.

Smart, RG, and MS Goodstadt. 1976. *Alcohol and Drug Use Among Ontario Adults: Report of a Household Survey, 1976*. Toronto: Addiction Research Foundation Substudy No. 798.

Stephenson, PS, and GA Walker. 1979. The Psychiatrist-Woman Patient Relationship. *Canadian Psychiatric Association Journal* 24: 5–17.

Stimson, G. 1975. Women in a Doctored World. *New Society* 32(656): 265–267.

Uhlenhuth, EH, MB Balter, and RS Lipman. 1978. Minor Tranquilizers: Clinical Correlates of Use in an Urban Population. *Archives of General Psychiatry* 35(5): 650–655.

12

Self-Reported Sedative-Hypnotic Drug Use in Canada: An Update[*]

Nigel S.B. Rawson and Carl D'Arcy

Introduction

Physical and psychological symptoms of anxiety and disturbances of sleep patterns, both by themselves and as concomitants of physical and psychological illnesses, are among the most common conditions from which humans suffer. Consequently, it is not surprising that prescriptions for sedatives (minor tranquillizers) and hypnotics (sleeping pills) consistently outnumber those for many other types of drugs. This heavy consumption has been observed in many drug utilization studies performed in several countries in the last 30-40 years.

Some of these studies have been general reviews in which the utilization of different drug types has been evaluated (Anderson 1980; Aoki et al. 1983; Chaiton et al. 1976; Dixon 1978; George 1972; Kohn & White 1976; Quinn et al. 1992; Skoll et al. 1979; Tuominen 1988), but many have been concerned only with psychoactive drugs (e.g., Allgulander 1986, 1989; Anderson 1981; Archer & Benner 1980; Balter et al. 1974a, 1984; Baron & Fisher 1962; Blackburn et al. 1990; Blennow et al. 1994; Boethius & Westerholm 1977; Cafferata et al. 1983; Cooperstock 1971, 1976, 1978; Cooperstock & Sims 1971; Cummins et al. 1982; Dunbar et al. 1989; Fejer & Smart 1973; Flight et al. 1983; Frey et al. 1978; Greenblatt et al. 1975; Harris et al. 1977; Isacson & Haglund 1988; Johnson & McFarland 1993; Lapp et al. 1983; Marinier et al. 1985; Mellinger et al. 1978, 1984a, 1984b; Murray et al. 1981; O'Reilly & Rusnak 1990; Parish 1971; Parry et al. 1973; Pflanz et al. 1977; Pihl et al. 1982; Power et al. 1983; Riska & Klaukka 1984; Rosser 1980; Siciliani et al. 1985; Sketris et al. 1985; Smart & Goodstadt 1976; Swartz et al. 1991; Tamblyn et al. 1994; Thomson & Smith 1995; Uhlenhuth et al. 1978; van der Waals et al. 1993; Vázquez-Barquero et al. 1989; Wells et al. 1985; Weyerer & Dilling 1991; Wilcox 1977; Williams et al. 1982; Woods et al. 1987). Of the latter, some have focused on the psychiatric and medical conditions for which sedatives and hypnotics are usually prescribed (Allgulander 1989; Frey et al. 1978; Harris et al. 1977; Lapp et al. 1983; Mellinger et al. 1978, 1984b; Murray et al. 1981; O'Reilly & Rusnak 1990; Pihl et al. 1982; Siciliani et al. 1985; Weyerer & Dilling 1991; Williams et al. 1982), while others have assessed the misuse or abuse of these drugs (Allgulander 1986; Woods et al. 1987).

* This work is an updated and revised version of Rawson & D'Arcy (1991). The authors gratefully acknowledge the financial support of grants from Merck Frosst Canada Inc., the Medical Research Council of Canada, and the Department of Health, Province of Saskatchewan.

Another large and important group of studies have concentrated on the socioeconomic characteristics of patients taking sedative-hypnotics (Archer & Brenner 1980; Blennow et al. 1994; Cafferata et al. 1983; Cooperstock 1971, 1976, 1978; Cooperstock & Sims 1971; Cummins et al. 1982; Fejer & Smart 1973; Isacson & Haglund 1988; Marinier et al. 1985; Mellinger et al. 1984a; Parry et al. 1973; Pflanz et al. 1977; Riska & Klaukka 1984; Smart & Goodstadt 1976; Swartz et al. 1991; van der Waals et al. 1993; Vázquez-Barquero et al. 1989; Wells et al. 1985; Weyerer & Dilling 1991). The proportion of women taking these drugs has been found to be consistently larger than the corresponding proportion of men and, in almost all the studies, the proportion of individuals taking sedative-hypnotics increases with age. Indicators of poor psychological or physical health have also been shown to be positively correlated with increased use of these drugs.

In addition, socioeconomic characteristics, other than age and gender, have been found to be associated with sedative-hypnotic use; these include marital status (Archer & Brenner 1980; Blennow et al. 1994; Isacson & Haglund 1988; Riska & Klaukka 1984; Swartz et al. 1991), years of education (Allgulander 1989; Marinier et al. 1985; Pflanz et al. 1977; Smart & Goodstadt 1976; Swartz et al. 1991; Vázquez-Barquero et al. 1989; Wells et al. 1985), income (Allgulander 1989; Parry et al. 1973; Riska & Klaukka 1984; Smart & Goodstadt 1976; Wells et al. 1985), and employment status (Archer & Brenner 1980; Blennow et al. 1994; Isacson & Haglund 1988; Marinier et al. 1985, Riska & Klaukka 1984; Smart & Goodstadt 1976; Vázquez-Barquero et al. 1989). However, there has been a lack of consistency in the results concerning these latter variables. Some of the discordant results may be explained by differing societal features; for instance, in Sweden (Allgulander 1989), Finland (Riska & Klaukka 1984) and Canada (Smart & Goodstadt 1976), all countries with a universal health care system, higher rates of sedative-hypnotic use have been found to be associated with low income, but in the United States, which does not have universal health care coverage, increased usage of these drugs in higher income groups has been reported (Parry et al. 1973; Wells et al. 1985). Nevertheless, socioeconomic conditions alone cannot explain all the conflicting results; for example, researchers in Spain (Vázquez-Barquero et al. 1989), Sweden (Allgulander 1989), Quebec (Marinier et al. 1985) and the United States (Swartz et al. 1991; Wells et al. 1985) have found higher levels of use by individuals with a low educational status, whereas the results of studies carried out in West Germany (Pflanz et al. 1977) and Ontario (Smart & Goodstadt 1976) indicated increased usage by those with a higher educational status.

Only a small number of the utilization studies have been national surveys (Allgulander 1989; Anderson 1980; Cafferata et al. 1983; Cummins et al. 1982; Dunbar et al. 1989; Mellinger et al. 1978, 1984a, 1984b; Parry et al. 1973; Riska & Klaukka 1984; van der Waals et al. 1993) and even fewer have been international (Balter et al. 1974a, 1984; Kohn & White 1976). The majority have covered localized areas, e.g. community surveys of administrative areas (Archer & Brenner 1980; Blennow et al. 1994; Boethius & Westerholm 1977; Chaiton et al. 1976; Cooperstock 1971, 1976, 1978; Cooperstock & Sims 1971; Fejer & Smart 1973; Isacson & Haglund 1988; Lapp et al. 1983; Marinier et al. 1985; Murray et al. 1981; Pflanz et al. 1977; Pihl et al. 1982; Siciliani et al. 1985; Swartz et al. 1991; Uhlenhuth et al. 1978; Vázquez-Barquero et al. 1989; Wells et al. 1985; Weyerer & Dilling 1991) or surveys of patients using local hospitals (Flight et al. 1983; Frey et al. 1978; Greenblatt et al. 1975; O'Reilly & Rusnak 1990), general practices (Anderson 1981; Dixon 1978; Harris et al. 1977; Parish 1971; Rosser 1980; Sketris et al. 1985; Wilcox 1977; Williams et al. 1982) or health maintenance organizations (Baron & Fisher 1962; Johnson & McFarland 1993), and have, therefore, only been representative of utilization within the locale, which may or may not be representative of national usage.

This is the situation that exists in Canada. Most of the studies in this country have been concentrated in the large centres of Ontario and Quebec. One of the most significant contributors to the information about sedative-hypnotic use in Canada was the late Ruth Cooperstock, but even her important work (Cooperstock 1971, 1976, 1978; Cooperstock & Hill 1982; Cooperstock & Lennard 1978; Cooperstock & Parnell 1982; Cooperstock & Sims 1971), and that of her colleagues at the Addiction Research Foundation (e.g., Archer & Brenner 1980; Fejer & Smart 1973; Smart & Goodstadt 1976), is based primarily on surveys performed in and around Toronto. Work of a similarly localized nature has been done in other urban areas of Ontario and in a few other provinces (Anderson 1981; Chaiton et al. 1976; Dixon 1980; Frey et al. 1978; Lapp et al. 1983; Marinier et al. 1985; Pihl et al. 1982; Rosser 1980; Sketris et al. 1985). In addition, some utilization studies have been carried out at the provincial level in Quebec (Tamblyn et al. 1994), Manitoba (Aoki et al. 1983), Saskatchewan (Blackburn et al. 1990; Power, et al. 1983; Quinn et al. 1992; Skoll et al. 1979), and British Columbia (Thomson & Smith 1995; Tuominen 1988).

There has been, therefore, no systematic assessment of sedative-hypnotic utilization at the national level in Canada. We have tried to correct this deficit by using data from five large surveys undertaken over 22 years. Information on drug utilization from four areas in western Canada was included in an international study organized by the World Health Organization in 1968-9. Drug use data were also collected in four national Canadian surveys performed in 1978-9, 1985, 1989 and 1990. Information from all five surveys was available in the form of anonymous data files, which we have used to examine sedative-hypnotic use in Canada and to identify some socioeconomic and health care correlates of this use.

The Surveys

Some basic details of the five surveys are outlined in Table 1. The International Collaborative Study of Medical Care Utilization (ICS-MCU) was performed in 12 areas in seven countries in 1968-9; four of these areas were in Canada. The aims, methods and results of the study have been published in a large analytical report (Kohn & White 1976) and further details of the Canadian data have been reported by Josie (1973). The ICS-MCU attempted to measure and compare the use of hospitals, medicines, and physician and other services, as well as to assess the determinants of the use of health services using the Andersen (1968) model. Two questions relating to sedative-hypnotic use were included in the survey (Table 1). The answers were combined such that sedative-hypnotic use was coded "yes" if either answer was "yes" and "no" if both answers were "no"; otherwise, it was coded as "not known."

Ten years later, the Canada Health Survey (CHS) was carried out by Statistics Canada. The CHS was designed to provide information about the physical and psychological diseases and disabilities suffered by Canadians and the risks to which they are exposed by their lifestyle and environment (Health and Welfare Canada & Statistics Canada 1981). Data about Canadians' use of their health care system, including medicines, were also collected and, in particular, a question about sedative-hypnotic use was asked (Table 1). To take account of non-response biases, weighting factors were supplied so that the study results could be "weighted up" to the national population to provide unbiased estimates. We have used the appropriate weighting factor throughout our analyses.

TABLE 1
Basic details of the five surveys

Survey	Date	Area of Canada covered	Method used	Number of respondents	Overall response rate	Questions relating to sedative-hypnotic use asked in the survey
ICS-MCU[a]	June 1968-May 1969	Saskatoon, North Battleford & surrounding rural areas, Saskatchewan. Grande Prairie & environs, Alberta. 2 school districts (identified only as "Fraser" & "Jersey") in British Columbia.	Personal interview	16,319	96.4%	*Yesterday or the day before*, did you take or use: (1) any sleeping pills or medicines? (2) any tranquilizers or sedatives?
CHS[b]	July 1978-March 1979	Non-institutionalized population of the ten provinces, excluding Indian Reserves and remote areas.	Personal interview	31,668	86.5%	*Yesterday or the day before*, did you take any tranquilizers, medicine for the nerves or medicine to help you sleep?
HPS85[c]	June 1985	Non-institutionalized population of the ten provinces and the Yukon Territory aged 15 or more.	Telephone interview	11,339	>80%	*In the past 12 months*, have you used: (1) any sleeping pills? (2) any tranquilizers?
NADS[d]	March 1989	Non-institutionalized population of the ten provinces aged 15 or more.	Telephone interview	11,634	78.7%	*In the past 30 days*, did you take: (1) any tranquilizers? (2) any sleeping pills?
HPS90[e]	June 1990	Non-institutionalized population of the ten provinces aged 15 or more.	Telephone interview	13,792	78.0%	*In the past 12 months*, have you used: (1) any tranquilizers? (2) any sleeping pills?

[a]Kohn & White 1976; [b]Health and Welfare Canada & Statistics Canada 1981; [c]Health and Welfare Canada 1987; [d]Health and Welfare Canada 1990; [e]Stephens & Graham 1993.

In June 1985, Statistics Canada conducted the nationwide Health Promotion Survey (HPS85) (Health and Welfare Canada 1987). While the CHS determined the levels and demographic correlates of certain lifestyle behaviours and preventative health practices, the HPS85 was designed to provide a picture of Canadians' level of knowledge of, perceptions about, and attitudes toward those behaviours. The responses to two questions asked about sedative-hypnotic use were combined in the same way as those to the ICS-MCU questions (Table 1). A weighting factor was supplied to adjust the sample results to unbiased national population estimates. The weight was applied consistently.

The National Alcohol and Other Drugs Survey (NADS) was also carried out by Statistics Canada in March 1989 (Health and Welfare Canada 1990). The aim of the NADS was to document, describe and analyze the alcohol and other drug experiences of Canadians. Although the survey predominantly concerned alcohol and illicit drugs, there were questions about licit drug use, two of which asked about sedative-hypnotic use (Table 1). We combined the responses in the same way as those to the questions in the ICS-MCU and the HPS85. A weighting factor was also provided with these data and it was used in all our analyses.

A second Health Promotion Survey (HPS90) was conducted by Statistics Canada in June 1990 (Stephens & Graham 1993). Like its predecessor (HPS85), the HPS90 focused on Canadians' level of knowledge of, perceptions about, and attitudes towards those behaviours. The responses to the two questions about sedative-hypnotic use (Table 1) were combined as in the other surveys and the appropriate weighting factor was used throughout.

Since individuals aged less than 15 were excluded from the HPS85, the NADS and the HPS90, and relatively few children take sedatives or hypnotics anyway, we limited our analyses to persons over 14. Because three different time periods during which respondents were asked to recall their use of sedative-hypnotics were employed (48 hours in the ICS-MCU and the CHS, 30 days in the NADS and 12 months in the HPS85 and HPS90), the results are not strictly comparable. Nevertheless, health care and socioeconomic correlates of use of these drugs and their consistency across the surveys may be compared, even if the absolute values of the proportion of individuals reporting use cannot.

All analyses presented here are based on micro data tapes from each of the surveys. All computations were prepared by the authors and the responsibility for the use and interpretation of these data is entirely theirs.

Results

The overall proportion of individuals who reported sedative-hypnotic use within the previous 48 hours was 4.9% in the ICS-MCU and 6.1% in the CHS. In the HPS85 and the HPS90, the proportions reporting use within the previous 12 months was 11.9% and 10.7% respectively, while the rate of use within the previous 30 days in the NADS was 5.7%.

Gender and Age

The male and female rates of sedative-hypnotic use within the previous 48 hours were 2.9% and 6.8% in the ICS-MCU and 3.8% and 8.3% in the CHS. The proportions of males and females reporting use within the previous 12 months in the HPS85 were

8.8% and 15.0% and in the HPS90 were 8.6% and 12.7%, and the male and female rates of use within the previous 30 days in the NADS were 3.8% and 7.6%. The ratio of female to male usage ranged from 1.5:1 in the HPS90 to 2.3:1 in the ICS-MCU.

There was a clear trend of an increasing rate of sedative-hypnotic use with increasing age in all five surveys. Although there were slight deviations in the male results, this trend was apparent in both sexes (Figure 1) and was almost linear for women.

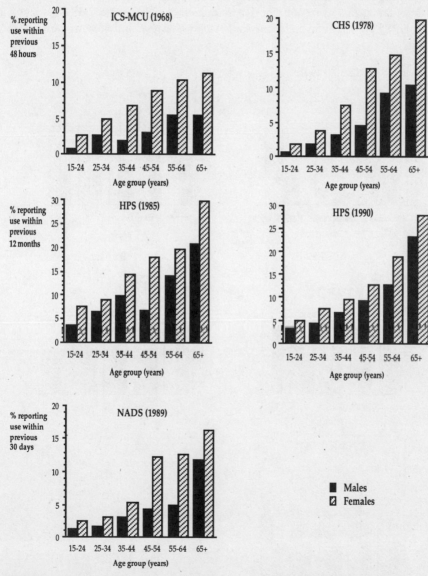

Figure 1
Sedative-hypnotic drug use by age and gender

Regional Variation

There was some variation in the rates of use between the areas in the ICS-MCU, the lowest being recorded in Grande Prairie and the highest in the British Columbia areas (Figure 2). In the Canadian surveys, the male rates of use were generally similar in all five regions. However, among the females, the highest rate of use was consistently recorded in Quebec and the lowest consistently recorded in the Prairie provinces. When the proportions of individuals reporting use in each region were subdivided by age, the reason for the high rate among Quebec females was found to be due to *very high* rates among elderly females (65 years or more) in that province: 27% in the CHS (48 hours), 44% in the HPS85 (12 months), 20% in the NADS (30 days), and 45% in the HPS90 (12 months).

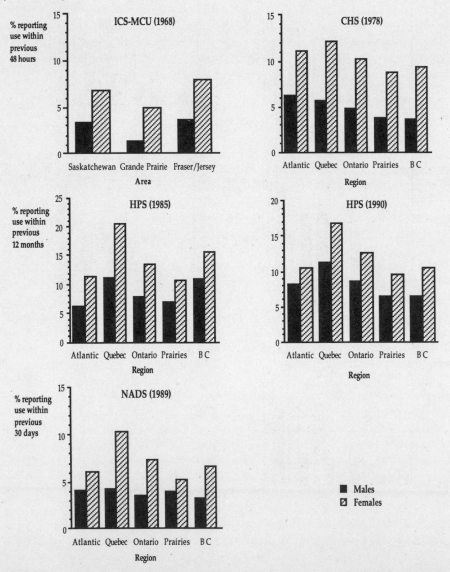

Figure 2
Sedative-hypnotic drug use by area and region

Marital Status

Table 2 shows that, in the different marital status categories, the lowest rates of use were recorded for single and unattached respondents and the highest for the divorced, separated or widowed. Over 90% of all single individuals were under the age of 45 and, therefore, the results were dominated by young single persons. When the rates of sedative-hypnotic use for the three marital status groups were subdivided by age, it was evident that the rate for single persons of either sex rapidly increased with age. Also, among those aged 65 years or more, the rate of use became increasingly similar *in all three marital status categories*; this was especially noticeable in the HPS90.

Education

Since educational status was not categorized consistently in the surveys, we grouped respondents into those whose education varied between none to secondary school graduation and those who pursued at least some post-secondary education (Table 3). There was generally higher use in the lower educated group.

Family Income

Family income was also not recorded in a consistent manner. In the ICS-MCU, it was grouped into seven categories, although the actual ranges used were unavailable; the two lower categories encompassed almost 30% of the respondents and the average rate of sedative-hypnotic use in this group was compared with the average of the other five categories (Table 4). In the CHS and HPS85, family income was recorded in quintile and Table 4 shows the rate of use by individuals in the lowest quintile compared with the corresponding average rate of the other four. Household income was recorded in eight categories in the NADS; just over 22% of the respondents had an income of less than $20,000 and the rate of use in this group was contrasted with that of individuals with an income of $20,000 or more (Table 4). Similarly, in the HPS90, household income was recorded in nine categories; just under 20% of the respondents had an income of less than $20,000 and the rate of use in this group was contrasted with that of individuals with an income of $20,000 or more. The rate of sedative-hypnotic use by the lower income groups was approximately twice that of the higher income groups in all five surveys.

Employment Status

Figure 3 shows the rate of sedative-hypnotic use by employment status. In the ICS-MCU, respondents were asked about their present employment status, whereas in the other surveys they were asked about their main activity during the previous 12 months. The "unemployed" category in Figure 3 includes those actively seeking work as well as those not seeking it, e.g. the chronically sick and housewives. In each survey, the highest rate of use was in the retired group and the lowest in the currently working group. However, the ratio of the rate of use by retired females to that for retired males has declined from 2:1 in the ICS-MCU and the CHS to 1:1 in the HPS90.

222 Self-Reported Sedative-Hypnotic Drug Use in Canada: An Update

TABLE 2

Proportions (%) reporting sedative-hypnotic drug use by marital status, age and gender

Survey	Marital Status	Males				Females			
		15-44	45-64	65+	All Ages	15-44	45-64	65+	All Ages
ICS-MCU (1968)	Single	0.8	3.4	3.2	1.1	2.4	11.1	13.8	3.3
previous	Married	2.1	4.0	5.8	3.4	5.2	8.9	11.6	7.0
48 hours	D / S / W	0.0	8.3	5.5	5.6	9.2	11.5	10.6	10.8
CHS (1978)	Single	1.4	9.3	12.2	2.0	1.7	11.7	23.9	3.2
previous	Married	1.7	6.2	9.6	4.2	4.3	12.4	16.2	7.9
48 hours	D / S / W	5.8	8.4	14.4	9.2	10.4	19.4	22.5	18.3
HPS (1985)	Single	5.0	13.1	17.8	5.7	9.3	18.6	24.8	10.6
previous	Married	6.7	8.9	22.5	9.5	9.8	16.0	28.1	13.4
12 months	D / S / W	14.7	20.0	15.6	16.5	17.3	29.4	32.4	27.7
NADS (1989)	Single	1.9	4.6	9.1	2.2	3.4	12.8	12.4	4.0
previous	Married	2.1	4.3	11.3	4.3	2.7	11.1	10.5	6.3
30 days	D / S / W	3.2	6.1	14.4	6.5	8.5	17.1	21.4	16.3
HPS (1990)	Single	5.2	12.7	23.7	6.0	7.0	11.6	25.8	7.9
previous	Married	4.5	10.2	22.9	9.0	7.2	15.0	28.3	12.0
12 months	D / S / W	7.3	13.9	25.6	14.5	13.2	18.6	27.7	21.4

D / S / W: Divorced, separated, or widowed.

TABLE 3

Proportions (%) reporting sedative-hypnotic drug use by educational status

Survey	Gender	Completion of secondary education or less	Beyond completion of secondary education
ICS-MCU (1968)	Male	2.6	3.9
previous 48 hours	Female	6.9	6.5
CHS (1978)	Male	4.4	2.4
previous 48 hours	Female	9.6	4.3
HPS (1985)	Male	8.8	8.9
previous 12 months	Female	16.3	12.5
NADS (1989)	Male	4.5	2.8
previous 30 days	Female	8.9	5.5
HPS (1990)	Male	9.7	6.8
previous 12 months	Female	13.6	10.8

TABLE 4

Proportions (%) reporting sedative-hypnotic drug use by family income group[a]

Survey	Gender	Lower income group	Higher income group	Ratio of rates
ICS-MCU (1968)	Male	4.1	2.4	1.7:1
previous 48 hours	Female	8.5	6.0	1.4:1
CHS (1978)	Male	7.5	3.3	2.3:1
previous 48 hours	Female	14.3	7.0	2.0:1
HPS (1985)	Male	18.8	8.7	2.2:1
previous 12 months	Female	21.0	11.4	1.8:1
NADS (1989)	Male	8.0	3.2	2.5:1
previous 30 days	Female	12.9	6.0	2.2:1
HPS (1990)	Male	15.3	7.2	2.1:1
previous 12 months	Female	19.5	10.4	1.9:1

[a] See text for definitions of income groups.

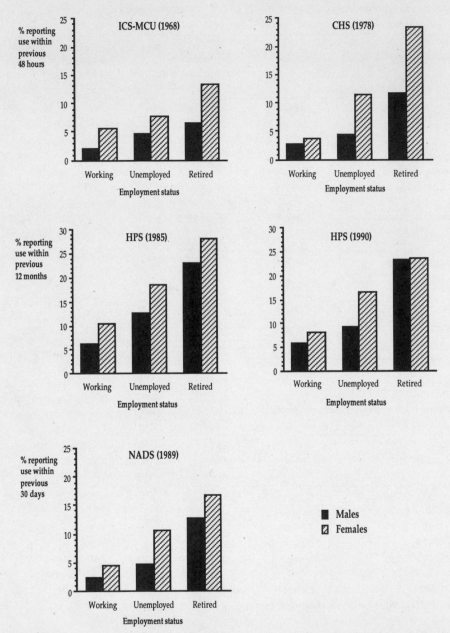

Figure 3
Sedative-hypnotic drug use by employment status

We also compared the proportion of females in employment reporting sedative-hypnotic use with the corresponding proportion for females whose main activity was keeping house (Figure 4). With the exception of the 25-34 years age group in the ICS-MCU and the 15-24 and 35-44 years age groups in the NADS, the rate of use reported by females who kept house was consistently higher than the rate reported by females in employment outside the home.

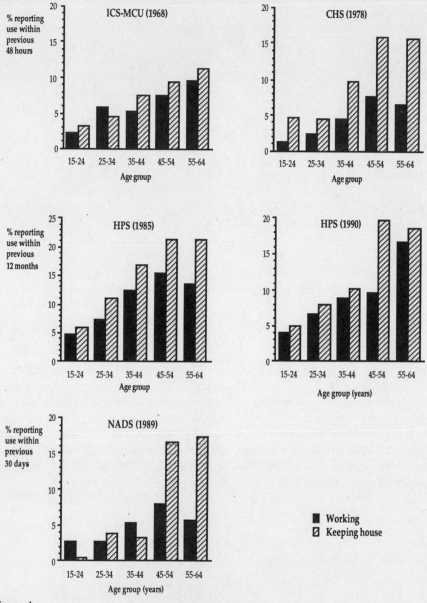

Figure 4
Sedative-hypnotic drug use reported by working and non-working women

Living Arrangements

In all five surveys, females who lived alone reported a higher rate of use than those who lived in a family environment (Table 5). There was no similar consistency among the male rates.

TABLE 5

Proportions (%) reporting sedative-hypnotic drug use among individuals who lived alone and those living in a family

Survey	Gender	Living alone	Living in a family
ICS-MCU (1968)	Male	2.0	3.1
previous 48 hours	Female	7.7	6.6
CHS (1978)	Male	5.4	3.6
previous 48 hours	Female	16.6	7.2
HPS (1985)	Male	14.7	8.1
previous 12 months	Female	24.8	13.6
NADS (1989)	Male	3.3	4.0
previous 30 days	Female	10.6	6.4
HPS (1990)	Male	12.2	8.1
previous 12 months	Female	19.8	11.4

Health Status

Several variables attempting to measure the health of respondents were recorded in the ICS-MCU and the CHS. Three questions asked in both these surveys were whether respondents had consulted a physician within the previous two weeks, whether they had been hospitalized within the previous 12 months, and how many drugs they were currently taking; the latter question was also asked in the NADS. The rates of sedative-hypnotic use for both males and females who had consulted a doctor (Table 6) or had been hospitalized (Table 7) were at least twice the corresponding rates for those who had not seen a doctor or not been hospitalized.

TABLE 6

Proportions (%) reporting sedative-hypnotic drug use among individuals who had consulted a physician within the previous two weeks

Survey	Gender	Consulted a physician within the previous two weeks:	
		Yes	No
ICS-MCU (1968)	Male	7.8	2.1
previous 48 hours	Female	13.7	5.2
CHS (1978)	Male	10.8	2.9
previous 48 hours	Female	16.5	6.4

TABLE 7
Proportions (%) reporting sedative-hypnotic drug use among individuals who were hospitalized within the previous 12 months

Survey	Gender	Hospitalized within the previous twelve months	
		Yes	No
ICS-MCU (1968)	Male	7.8	2.0
previous 48 hours	Female	11.1	5.6
CHS (1978)	Male	12.8	3.1
previous 48 hours	Female	15.9	7.1

Figure 5 shows that the rate of sedative-hypnotic use increased as the number of drugs used, in addition to the sedative or hypnotics, increased.

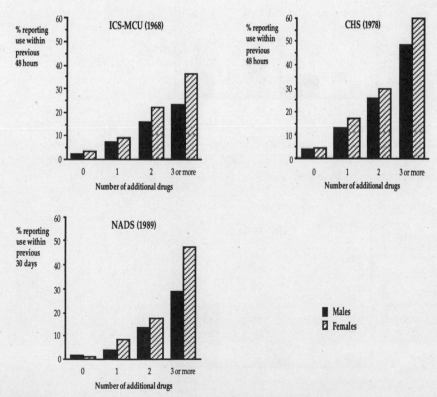

Figure 5
Sedative-hypnotic drug use by number of additional concurrent drugs

A set of questions about anxiety symptoms were asked in the ICS-MCU and these were used to calculate an "anxiety score" which varied between 0 (not anxious at all) to 10 (extremely anxious). Under 7% of the respondents had a score of over three and, therefore, scores of three or more were grouped. The proportion of individuals reporting sedative-hypnotic use increased as the level of anxiety increased (Figure 6).

A version of Bradburn's (1969) Affect Balance Scale (ABS) was used in the CHS as a measure of psychological well-being. The scale consisted of five positively-worded and five negatively-worded descriptions of recent feeling states and respondents were asked to indicate the frequency with which they had experienced these states. The answers were summed for each set of questions giving two separate scores: one for positive effects and one for negative effects. These were combined into a single index, the ABS, which indicated whether positive or negative feelings predominated or were approximately balanced (neutral). The ABS provides a widely accepted measure of psychological well-being (Health and Welfare Canada & Statistics Canada 1981). Rates of sedative-hypnotic use were highest for those in whom negative feelings predominated and lowest for those in whom positive feelings predominated (Figure 7).

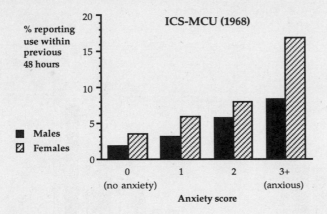

Figure 6
Sedative-hypnotic drug use by anxiety score

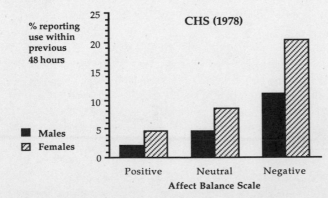

Figure 7
Sedative-hypnotic drug use by Affect Balance Scale

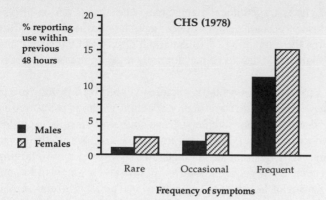

Figure 8
Sedative-hypnotic drug use by frequency of psycho-physiological symptoms (assessed by Health Opinion Survey score)

The ABS was supplemented in the CHS by MacMillan's (1957) Health Opinion Survey (HOS) scale, which has been widely used to assess the extent of anxiety and depression in populations. It does not, in fact, measure opinions but the frequency of occurrence of psycho-physiological symptoms of anxiety and depression and, hence, distress. The HOS score is derived from the responses to 16 questions and ranges from 16 (all symptoms experienced often) to 48 (never experienced). Just over two-thirds of the subjects had experienced symptoms rarely or occasionally (an HOS score of over 40) and less than 3% of this group reported sedative-hypnotic use within the previous 48 hours. However, among those who had experienced symptoms frequently (a score of 40 or less), the use was much higher (11.2% in males and 15.2% in females) (Figure 8).

Discussion

When assessing these results, one should consider the reliability and validity of these studies and their comparability with each other and with other work. All five surveys relied on the memory of individuals to recall the medications that they had taken within the specified time period. The short period of 48 hours used in the ICS-MCU and the CHS was probably selected to minimize the chance that subjects would fail to remember which drugs they had taken. The longer period of 12 months used in the two HPSs (and also in many other studies) is more prone to the potential failure of respondents to recall occasional use leading to under-estimation of utilization.

There are conflicting views concerning the reliability with which individuals can remember medicines that they had taken within the previous 12 months (Anonymous 1974; Balter et al. 1974b; Kelly et al. 1990; Maronde & Silverman 1974; Whitehead & Smart 1972), although few studies have been performed to try to quantify the degree of inaccuracy. In 1968-9, Parry et al. (1970) found that, among a sample of inhabitants of a midwestern United States city, 74% of those who had a sedative, tranquilizer or stimulant dispensed recalled this fact a year later compared with only 64% of those who had an antibiotic dispensed. A long probing interview, with the use of colour photographs of the more commonly used drugs to stimulate the subjects' memories, led to a more reliable recall than that obtained with the "did you take ..." type of question. However, Parry and his colleagues claim that under-reporting of sedative-hypnotic use is probably only of the order of a few percentage points (Balter et al. 1974b; Parry et al.

1970) and this view is supported by Whitehead and Smart (1972), but Smart (1975) thought it might be as high as 20%. In the surveys used here, the questions were of the "did you take ..." type so that the probability of a substantial degree of under-reporting in the two HPS's remains high, but it should be considerably lower in the others due to the shorter recall periods.

The validity of the five surveys as representative pictures of sedative-hypnotic use in Canada is difficult to assess. Although different data collection methods were used in the four national studies, all were random sample surveys so that the results would be representative of the Canadian population. The possibility remains, however, that some groups, e.g. young men, may have been under-sampled, although the use of weighting factors was designed to reduce this problem. The ICS-MCU was not intended to be a representative picture of Canadian health care utilization. Nevertheless, rural, urban and suburban areas were all represented in the survey, although large metropolitan centres were not. In our opinion, the results from the Canadian areas in this study are reasonably representative of non-metropolitan western Canada. Whether these data are generalizable to the whole of Canada is more problematical, especially for women, since the highest rates of use by females in the national studies were consistently reported in Quebec and have been confirmed by the work of Laurier et al. (1992) and Tamblyn et al. (1994). However, the fact that many trends seen in the four Canadian surveys are also found in the ICS-MCU data is encouraging.

If one is trying to assess whether the rate of sedative-hypnotic use in Canada has changed or remained the same between 1968 and 1990, the direct comparison of rates between the five surveys is difficult due to the different time periods used. While we encourage researchers to make greater use of the information in surveys such as the ones considered here, we urge those who plan and perform them to try to achieve some consistency in their work. The overall rate of use in the previous 48 hours was 4.9% (2.9% for males and 6.8% for females) in the ICS-MCU in 1968 and 6.1% (3.8% for males and 8.3% for females) in the CHS in 1978. There are few studies that have used the same recall period and, of these, some have used a broader definition of drug utilization than we have and some a narrower one. As part of their review of drug use in two Ontario communities in 1971 and 1972, Chaiton et al. (1976) found that 8.8% had taken a sedative or a tranquilizer within the previous 48 hours in one community and 10.5% had done so in the other; these are considerably higher than the ICS-MCU rate. In their 1977 study of 429 adult Toronto women, Archer and Benner (1980) found that 14.7% had taken a psychotropic drug within the previous 48 hours, while Cummins et al. (1982) using data from the British Regional Heart Survey, a study of 7,735 middle-aged men carried out in the late 1970s, reported that 8.0% had taken a tranquilizer within the prior 48 hours. These prevalence figures are both higher than the CHS results, even though one recorded all psychotropics and the other only tranquilizers.

In the HPS85 and HPS90, the overall rates of use in the previous 12 months were 11.9% (8.8% for males and 15.0% for females) and 10.7% (8.6% for males and 12.7% for females). Although many studies have used the same recall period, it is again difficult to find directly comparable, contemporary studies in which the same definition of drug utilization was used. Cooperstock (1976, 1978) found that, of 30,353 members of a prescription insurance agency in southern Ontario, 8.0% (6.2% for males and 10.0% for females) had received a sedative-hypnotic prescription during the year 1970-1 and, in 1973-4, the corresponding proportion was 6.0% (4.9% for males and 7.1% for females). More contemporary with the HPS85, Blackburn et al. (1990) reported that the proportion of eligible beneficiaries of the Saskatchewan Prescription Drug Plan receiving sedative-hypnotics during 1985 was 9.5%, having fallen steadily from 12.1% in 1977. In the United States, Cafferata et al. (1983), using data from the 1977 National Medical Care Expenditure Survey, found that, of the 15,504 adult respondents, 12.3% (8.1% for men and 15.9% for women) had obtained at least one psychotropic drug during the year. In both 1971 and 1981, Balter et al. (1974a, 1984) compared the rates of use of anxiolytics and sedatives in several European countries and the United States; the 12-month prevalence rates in each country are shown in Table 8. The rates of 11.9% and 10.7% in the HPS85 and HPS90 are close to the average rate of 12.5% for all countries in the 1981 study. Although not consistent across the country (Figure 2) (Quinn et al. 1992; Tamblyn et al. 1994), Canadian sedative-hypnotic use appears, therefore, to be about average for a westernized society and may even be below it. The recent work of Busto et al. (1989) on benzodiazepine use in Canada between 1978 and 1987 utilizing drug sales data lends support to this conclusion.

Although there are problems of direct comparability between the surveys, they do not rule out all comparisons. For example, sedative-hypnotic use was higher among those with more health problems indicated by more physician contacts, more admissions to hospital, and multiple drugs (Tables 6 and 7; Figure 5). Higher rates were also found among those with anxiety symptoms (Figure 6), those in whom negative feelings predominated (Figure 7), and those who had experienced many psycho-physiological symptoms of anxiety and depression (Figure 8). Therefore, it can be concluded that, in general, throughout the two decades, individuals with psycho-physiological problems were receiving more sedatives and hypnotics than persons without these problems.

TABLE 8

Twelve-month prevalence of use of anxiolytics and/or sedatives for selected countries (as a percentage of the population)

Country	1971[a]	1981[c]	1985	1990
Belgium	16.8	17.6		
Canada	---	---	11.9[d]	10.7[e]
Denmark	15.1	11.9		
France	16.7	15.9		
Germany (West)	14.2	12.0		
Great Britain	14.2	11.2		
Italy	11.2	11.5		
Netherlands	12.7	7.4		
Spain	9.7	14.2		
Sweden	15.8	8.6		
Switzerland	---	14.6		
United States	15.0[b]	12.9		

[a] Balter et al. 1974a
[b] Parry et al. 1973
[c] Balter et al. 1984
[d] Health and Welfare Canada 1987
[e] Stephens & Graham 1993

The two sociodemographic variables most closely associated with sedative-hypnotic use are gender and age (Figure 1). The ratio of the rates of female to male use in all five surveys was approximately 2:1, a ratio that has been found so consistently over time and place that Cooperstock suggested it has "a certain immutability" (1976, 1978). A variety of reasons have been put forward to explain this gender difference. These include differences in the perception of symptoms and the assessment of severity by men and women, a greater willingness to talk about symptoms and disease and a greater readiness to take action among women, and women having more experience with health care, e.g. as a result of reproduction-related morbidity or the role of care-taker of the family's health problems (Cafferata et al. 1983; Cooperstock 1971; Ver-brugge 1985). Since men consume more alcohol than women (Health and Welfare Canada 1990), it is also suggested that, in times of stress and anxiety, women resort to drugs while men resort to alcohol (Neutel 1992). In addition, physicians, who are pre-dominantly male, expect females to be more emotionally expressive than males and, therefore, expect a higher proportion of their female patients to require mood-modify-ing drugs.

In 1986, Bass and Pederson (1986) proposed that there may be a real change in the attitude of Canadian physicians towards prescribing tranquilizers for women. They based this suggestion on a study in which case histories of hypothetical patients, for whom tranquilizers might be recommended, were sent to a random sample of 64 Ontario family physicians who were asked to list the therapies that they would pre-scribe. The study results did not confirm that females would receive more tranquilizer prescriptions than males. Nevertheless, the results of the two HPSs and the NADS, which were contemporary with Bass and Pederson's study, suggest that what physicians say they would do in a hypothetical situation and what they do in practice are not neces-sarily the same.

When considering the difference in the rate of use of sedative-hypnotics between the two sexes, it is important to remember that such results are often reported as "increased use in females." They may also imply *under-use* by males.

A distinct trend of an increasing rate of sedative-hypnotic use with increasing age was found in all five surveys, which also accounts for the high rates among the retired (Figure 3). This result has been reported in most studies of these drugs. In general, as people get older, more health problems are experienced and, as we have shown, poorer health is associated with an increased rate of sedative-hypnotic use. Also, from about the age of 45 onwards, events such as children leaving home, the so-called "mid-life crisis," retirement, widowhood and a greater awareness of one's own mortality begin to occur in the lives of many individuals, all of which may lead to anxiety and sleep dis-turbances that may, subsequently, lead to physician consultation and then to the pre-scription of medication.

Associations between sedative-hypnotic use and other socioeconomic variables have been reported elsewhere but with a lack of consistency. Some have found higher rates of use for those who are separated, divorced or widowed and lower rates for single per-sons (Blennow et al. 1994; Isacson & Haglund 1988; Riska & Klaukka 1984; Swartz et al. 1991). We have confirmed that this difference occurs in Canada, but it rapidly decreases with age so that, among the elderly, there is less difference between the mar-ital groups (Table 2).

The general level of education and income are associated with sedative-hypnotic use in Canada. The four national surveys all indicate that those with a lower level of educa-tion and a low income are more likely to take these drugs (Tables 3 & 4). These two variables are, of course, linked; for example, individuals who achieve a university degree are more likely to obtain a well-paid job, whereas those who do not do well at school and leave early are more likely to end up in a poorly-paid job. We examined sedative-hypnotic use by educational status and income group and the highest rates were found among those aged 45 years or more with both a low educational status and a low income. High rates of use among the lower educated and low income groups have been recorded previously (Allgulander 1989; Isacson & Haglund 1988; Marinier et al. 1985; Riska & Klaukka 1984; Swartz et al. 1991; Vázquez-Barquero et al. 1989). This association may partly explain the higher rates among the unemployed (Figure 3) because the poorly educated are more likely to be unemployed. However, the "unemployed" category also includes those who cannot work due to poor health and a large number of housewives – both groups known to have higher rates of sedative-hypnotic utilization. The results of the surveys (Figure 4) confirm that women who keep house are more likely to use sedatives and hypnotics than women who work outside the home (Cooperstock 1978; Cooperstock & Parnell 1982; Vázquez-Barquero et al. 1989).

Previously we concluded that, between 1968 and 1990, the typical sedative-hypnotic user in Canada was an elderly person, most probably a woman, with a low family income and a less than average education; she did not work outside the home and was afflicted with multiple physical ailments and with related and unrelated emotional problems (Rawson & D'Arcy 1991). There is little to suggest that this portrait has radically changed since then nor that it is likely to do so in the near future.

Since the early 1970s, there has been a concerted effort to reduce the use of sedative-hypnotics, especially benzodiazepines. The results of these surveys suggest that these efforts are having some success in Canada, although perhaps not as great as some would like (Thomson & Smith 1995). In Saskatchewan, overall use of "mood-modifiers" has declined modestly, while the rate of new use of benzodiazepines has fallen steeply from 41.9 per 1,000 in 1978 to 7.8 per 1,000 in 1990 (D'Arcy et al. 1994). However, evidence from the United States and Germany suggests that an enforced reduction in the use of benzodiazepines leads to the increased use of other psychoactive drugs (Linden & Gothe 1993; Reidenberg 1991; Shader et al. 1991; Weintraub et al. 1991), which can have both positive and negative consequences. The question "when will we know that an appropriate level of prescribing of sedative-hypnotic drugs has been achieved?" (assuming it has not already been attained) remains unanswered.

References

Allgulander, C. 1986. History and Current Status of Sedative-Hypnotic Drug Use and Abuse. *Acta Psychiatrica Scandinavica* 73: 465–478.

Allgulander, C. 1989. Psychoactive Drug Use in a General Population Sample, Sweden: Correlates with Perceived Health, Psychiatric Diagnoses, and Mortality in an Automated Record-Linkage Study. *American Journal of Public Health* 79: 1006–1010.

Andersen, R. 1968. *A Behavioral Model of Families' Use of Health Services* (Research Series # 25). Chicago: University of Chicago Center for Health Administration Studies.

Anderson, JE. 1981. Prescribing of Tranquillizers to Women and Men. *Canadian Medical Association Journal* 125: 1229–1232.

Anderson, RM. 1980. The Use of Repeatedly Prescribed Medicines. *Journal of the Royal College of General Practitioners* 30: 609–613.

Anonymous. 1974. International Use of Tranquilizers. *British Medical Journal* 3: 300.

Aoki, FY, VK Hildahl, GW Large, PA Mitenko, and DS Sitar. 1983. Aging and Heavy Drug Use: A Prescription Survey in Manitoba. *Journal of Chronic Diseases* 36: 75–84.

Archer C, and M Benner. 1980. Women's Use of Psychotropic Medication: A Community Survey. *Canadian Family Physician* 26: 867–871.

Balter, MB, J Levine, and DI Manheimer. 1974a. Cross-National Study of the Extent of Anti-Anxiety/Sedative Drug Use. *New England Journal of Medicine* 290: 769–774.

Balter, MB, J Levine, and DI Manheimer. 1974b. Drug Use as Determined by Interviews. *New England Journal of Medicine* 290: 1491.

Balter, MB, DI Manheimer, GD Mellinger, and EH Uhlenhuth. 1984. A Cross-National Comparison of Anti-Anxiety/Sedative Drug Use. *Current Medical Research and Opinion* 8(Suppl 4): 5–18.

Baron, SH, and S Fisher. 1962. Use of Psychotropic Drug Prescriptions in a Prepaid Group Practice Plan. *Public Health Reports* 77: 871–881.

Bass, MJ, and LL Pederson. 1986. Is There a Trend Away from Tranquilizing Women? *Canadian Journal of Public Health* 77: 119–122.

Blackburn, JL, FW Downey, and TJ Quinn. 1990. The Saskatchewan Program for Rational Drug Therapy: Effects on Utilization of Mood-Modifying Drugs. *DICP Annals of Pharmacotherapy* 24: 878–882.

Blennow, G, A Romelsjö, H Leifman, A Leifman, and G Karlsson. 1994. Sedatives and Hypnotics in Stockholm: Social Factors and Kinds of Use. *American Journal of Public Health* 84: 242–246.

Boethius, G, and B Westerholm. 1977. Purchases of Hypnotics, Sedatives and Minor Tranquillizers Among 2,566 Individuals in the County of Jämtland, Sweden: A Six Year Follow-up. *Acta Psychiatrica Scandinavica* 56: 147–159.

Bradburn, NM. 1969. *The Structure of Psychological Well-Being.* Chicago: Aldine Publishing.

Busto, U, KL Lanctôt, P Isaac, and M Adrian. 1989. Benzodiazepine Use and Abuse in Canada. *Canadian Medical Association Journal* 141: 917–921.

Cafferata, GL, J Kasper, and A Bernstein. 1983. Family Roles, Structure, and Stressors in Relation to Sex Differences in Obtaining Psychotropic Drugs. *Journal of Health and Social Behavior* 24: 132–143.

Chaiton, A, WO Spitzer, RS Roberts, and T Delamore. 1976. Patterns of Medical Drug Use: A Community Focus. *Canadian Medical Association Journal* 114: 33–37.

Cooperstock, R. 1971. Sex Differences in the Use of Mood-Modifying Drugs: An Explanatory Model. *Journal of Health and Social Behavior* 12: 238–244.

Cooperstock, R. 1976. Psychotropic Drug Use Among Women. *Canadian Medical Association Journal* 115: 760–763.

Cooperstock, R. 1978. Sex Differences in Psychotropic Drug Use. *Social Science and Medicine* 12B: 179–186.

Cooperstock, R, and J Hill. 1982. *The Effects of Tranquilization: Benzodiazepine Use in Canada.* Ottawa: Health and Welfare Canada.

Cooperstock, R, and HL Lennard. 1979. Some Social Meanings of Tranquilizer Use. *Sociology of Health and Illness* 1: 331–347.

Cooperstock, R, and P Parnell. 1982. Research on Psychotropic Drug Use: A Review of Findings and Methods. *Social Science and Medicine* 16: 1179–1196.

Cooperstock, R, and M Sims. 1971. Mood-Modifying Drugs Prescribed in a Canadian City: Hidden Problems. *American Journal of Public Health* 61: 1007–1016.

Cummins, RO, DG Cook, RC Hume, and AG Shaper. 1982. Tranquillizer Use in Middle-Aged British Men. *Journal of the Royal College of General Practitioners* 32: 745–752.

D'Arcy, C, J Blackburn, and NSB Rawson. 1994. New Use of Benzodiazepines: Trends, Saskatchewan, 1977-90. *Pharmacoepidemiology and Drug Safety* 3(Suppl 1): S49.

Dixon, AS. 1978. Drug Use in Family Practice: A Personal Study. *Canadian Family Physician* 24: 345–353.

Dunbar, GC, MH Perera, and FA Jenner. 1989. Patterns of Benzodiazepine Use in Great Britain as Measured by a General Population Survey. *British Journal of Psychiatry* 155: 836–841.

Fejer, D, and R Smart. 1973. The Use of Psychoactive Drugs by Adults. *Canadian Psychiatric Association Journal* 18: 313–320.

Flight, RJ, NG Davidson, and P Berks. 1983. Self-Reported Use of Alcohol, Cigarettes, Tranquillisers and Sedatives in Patients Admitted to a General Hospital. *New Zealand Medical Journal* 96: 56–58.

Frey, DD, RW Hetherington, and D Glassman. 1978. The Use of Prescription Drugs in Treatment of First-Time Psychiatric Admissions to University Hospital, Saskatoon. *Social Science and Medicine* 12A: 169–174.

George, A. 1972. Survey of Drug Use in a Sydney Suburb. *Medical Journal of Australia* 2: 233–237.

Greenblatt, DJ, RI Shader, and J Koch-Weser. 1975. Psychotropic Drug Use in the Boston Area: A Report from the Boston Collaborative Drug Surveillance Program. *Archives of General Psychiatry* 32: 518–521.

Harris, G, J Latham, B McGuiness, and AH Crisp. 1977. The Relationship Between Psychoneurotic Status and Psychoactive Drug Prescription in General Practice. *Journal of the Royal College of General Practitioners* 27: 173–177.

Health and Welfare Canada. 1987. *The Active Health Report: Perspectives on Canada's Health Promotion Survey 1985.* Ottawa: Minister of Supply and Services Canada.

Health and Welfare Canada. 1990. *National Alcohol and Other Drugs Survey: Highlights Report.* Ottawa: Minister of Supply and Services Canada.

Health and Welfare Canada and Statistics Canada. 1981. *The Health of Canadians: Report of the Canadian Health Survey.* Ottawa: Minister of Supply and Services Canada.

Isacson, D, and B Haglund. 1988. Psychotropic Drug Use in a Swedish Community: The Importance of Demographic and Socioeconomic Factors. *Social Science and Medicine* 26: 477–483.

Johnson, RE, and BH McFarland. 1993. Antipsychotic Drug Exposure in a Health Maintenance Organization. *Medical Care* 31: 432–444.

Josie, GH ed. 1973. *WHO International Collaborative Study of Medical Care Utilization: Report on Basic Canadian Data.* Saskatoon: University of Saskatchewan.

Kelly, JP, L Rosenberg, DW Kaufman, and S Shapiro. 1990. Reliability of Personal Interview data in a Hospital-based Case-control Study. *American Journal of Epidemiology* 131: 79–90.

Kohn, R, and KL White, eds. 1976. *Health Care: An International Study.* Report of the World Health Organization International Collaborative Study of Medical Care Utilization. London: Oxford University Press.

Lapp, JE, R Marinier, and RO Pihl. 1983. Medical Drug Use by Women: Symptoms and Change Attributions. *International Journal of the Addictions* 18: 45–51.

Laurier, C, J Dumas, and J-P Grégoire. 1992. Factors Related to Benzodiazepine Use in Quebec: A Secondary Analysis of Survey Data. *Journal of Pharmacoepidemiology* 2: 73–86.

Linden, M, and H Gothe. 1993. Benzodiazepine Substitution in Medical Practice: Analysis of Pharmacoepidemiologic data based on expert Interviews. *Pharmacopsychiatry* 26: 107–113.

MacMillan, AM. 1957. The Health Opinion Survey: Technique for Estimating Prevalence of Psychoneurotic and Related Types of Disorders in Communities. *Psychological Reports* 3: 325–339.

Marinier, RL, RO Pihl, C Wilford, and JE Lapp. 1985. Psychotropic Drug Use by Women: Demographic, Life-Style, and Personality Correlates. *Drug Intelligence and Clinical Pharmacy* 19: 40–45.

Maronde, RF, and M Silverman. 1974. Drug Use as Determined by Interviews. *New England Journal of Medicine* 290: 1490.

Mellinger, GD, MB Balter, DI Manheimer, IH Cisin, and HJ Parry. 1978. Psychic Distress, Life Crisis, and the Use of Psychotherapeutic Medications. *Archives of General Psychiatry* 35: 1045–1052.

Mellinger, GD, MB Balter, and EH Uhlenhuth. 1984a. Anti-Anxiety Agents: Duration of Use and Characteristics of Users in the USA. *Current Medical Research and Opinion* 8(Suppl 4): 21–36.

Mellinger, GD, MB Balter, and EH Uhlenhuth. 1984b. Prevalence and Correlates of the Long-Term Regular Use of Anxiolytics. *Journal of the American Medical Association* 251: 375–379.

Murray, J, G Dunn, P Williams, and A Tarnopolsky. 1981. Factors Affecting the Consumption of Psychotropic Drugs. *Psychological Medicine* 11: 551–560.

Neutel, CI. 1992. Gender and Family Income in Psychotropic Drug and Alcohol Use. *Chronic Diseases in Canada* 13: 42–46.

O'Reilly, R, and C Rusnak. 1990. The Use of Sedative-Hypnotic Drugs in a University Teaching Hospital. *Canadian Medical Association Journal* 142: 585–589.

Parish, PA. 1971. The Prescribing of Psychotropic Drugs in General practice. *Journal of the Royal College of General Practitioners* 21(Suppl 4): 1–77.

Parry, HJ, MB Balter, and IH Cisin. 1970. Primary Levels of Under-Reporting Psychotropic Drug Use. *Public Opinion Quarterly* 34: 582–592.

Parry, HJ, MB Balter, GD Mellinger, IH Cisin, and DI Manheimer. 1973. National Patterns of Psychotherapeutic Drug Use. *Archives of General Psychiatry* 28: 769–783.

Pflanz, M, HD Basler, and D Schwoon. 1977. Use of Tranquilizing Drugs by a Middle-Aged Population in a West Germany City. *Journal of Health and Social Behavior* 18: 194–205.

Pihl, RO, R Marinier, J Lapp, and H Drake. 1982. Psychotropic Drug Use by Women: Characteristics of High Consumers. *International Journal of the Addictions* 17: 259–269.

Power, B, W Downey, and BR Schnell. 1983. Utilization of Psychotropic Drugs in Saskatchewan, 1977-1980. *Canadian Journal of Psychiatry* 28: 547–551.

Quinn, K, MJ Baker, and B Evans. 1992. A Population-Wide Profile of Prescription Drug Use in Saskatchewan, 1989. *Canadian Medical Association Journal* 146: 2177–2186.

Rawson, NSB, and C D'Arcy. 1991. Sedative-Hypnotic Drug Use in Canada. *Health Reports* 3: 33–57.

Reidenberg, MM. 1991. Effect of the Requirement for Triplicate Prescriptions for Benzodiazepines in New York State. *Clinical Pharmacology and Therapeutics* 50: 129–131.

Riska, E, and T Klaukka. 1984. Use of Psychotropic Drugs in Finland. *Social Science and Medicine* 19: 983–989.

Rosser, WW. 1980. Patterns of Benzodiazepine Usage in a Family Medicine Centre. *Canadian Family Physician* 26: 718–720.

Shader, RI, DJ Greenblatt, and MB Balter. 1991. Appropriate Use and Regulatory Control of Benzodiazepines. *Journal of Clinical Pharmacology* 31: 781–784.

Siciliani, O, C Bellantuono, P Williams, and M Tansella. 1985. Self-Reported Use of Psychotropic Drugs and Alcohol Abuse in South-Verona. *Psychological Medicine* 15: 821–826.

Sketris, IS, ME MacCara, IE Purkis, and L Curry. 1985. Is There a Problem with Benzodiazepine Prescribing in Maritime Canada? *Canadian Family Physician* 31: 1591–1596.

Skoll, SL, RJ August, and GE Johnson. 1979. Drug Prescribing for the Elderly in Saskatchewan During 1976. *Canadian Medical Association Journal* 121: 1074–1081.

Smart, RG. 1975. Recent Studies of the Validity and Reliability of Self-Reported Drug Use, 1970-74. *Canadian Journal of Criminology and Corrections* 17: 326–333.

Smart, RG, and MS Goodstadt. 1977. Alcohol and Drug Use Among Ontario Adults: Report of a Household Survey, 1976. *Canada's Mental Health* 25(3): 2–5.

Stephens, T, and DF Graham eds. 1993. *Canada's Health Promotion Survey 1990: Technical Report.* Ottawa: Minister of Supply and Services Canada.

Swartz, M, R Landerman, LK George, ML Melville, D Blazer, and K Smith. 1991. Benzodiazepine Anti-Anxiety Agents: Prevalence and Correlates of Use in a Southern Community. *American Journal of Public Health* 81: 592–596.

Tamblyn, RM, PJ McLeod, M Abrahamowicz, J Monette, DC Gayton, L Berkson, WD Dauphinee, RM Grad, AR Huang, LM Isaac, BS Schnarch, and LS Snell. 1994. Questionable Prescribing for Elderly Patients in Quebec. *Canadian Medical Association Journal* 150: 1801–1809.

Thomson, M, and WA Smith. 1995. Prescribing Benzodiazepines for Non-Institutionalized Elderly. *Canadian Family Physician* 41: 792–798.

Tuominen, JD. 1988. Prescription Drugs and the Elderly in BC. *Canadian Journal on Aging* 7: 174–182.

Uhlenhuth, EH, MB Balter, and RS Lipman. 1978. Minor Tranquilizers: Clinical Correlates of Use in an Urban Population. *Archives of General Psychiatry* 35: 650–655.

van der Waals, FW, J Mohrs, and M Foets. 1993. Sex Differences Among Recipients of Benzodiazepines in Dutch General Practice. *British Medical Journal* 307: 363–366.

Vázquez-Barquero, JL, JF Diez Manrique, C Peña, A Arenal Gonzalez, MJ Cuesta, and JA Artal. 1989. Patterns of Psychotropic Drug use in a Spanish Rural Community. *British Journal of Psychiatry* 155: 633–641.

Verbrugge, LM. 1985. Gender and Health: An Update on Hypotheses and Evidence. *Journal of Health and Social Behavior* 26: 156–182.

Weintraub, M, S Singh, L Byrne, K Maharaj, and L Guttmacher. 1991. Consequences of the 1989 New York State Triplicate Benzodiazepine Prescription Regulation. *Journal of the American Medical Association* 266: 2392–2397.

Wells, KB, C Kamberg, R Brook, P Camp, and W Rogers. 1985. Health Status, Sociodemographic Factors, and the use of Prescribed Psychotropic Drugs. *Medical Care* 23: 1295–1306.

Weyerer, S, and H Dilling. 1991. Psychiatric and Physical Illness, Sociodemographic Characteristics, and the Use of Psychotropic Drugs in the Community: Results from the Upper Bavarian Field Study. *Journal of Clinical Epidemiology* 44: 303–311.

Whitehead, PC, and RG Smart. 1972. Validity and Reliability of Self-Reported Drug Use. *Canadian Journal of Criminology and Corrections* 14: 83–89.

Wilcox, JB. 1977. Psychotherapeutic Prescribing Patterns in General Practice. *New Zealand Medical Journal* 85: 363–366.

Williams, P, J Murray, and A Clare. 1982. A Longitudinal Study of Psychotropic Drug Prescriptions. *Psychological Medicine* 12: 201–206.

Woods, JH, JL Katz, and G Winger. 1987. Abuse Liability of Benzodiazepines. *Pharmacological Reviews* 39: 251–413.

13

Gender and Depression: Assessing Exposure and Vulnerability to Life Events in a Chronically Strained Population*

R. Jay Turner, Ph.D. and William R. Avison, Ph.D.

Recent studies in psychiatric sociology and epidemiology have focused on identifying the social mechanisms that link one's social environment with risk for psychological distress and disorder. The starting point for much of this work has been the consistently observed associations between distress or disorder and such variables as socioeconomic, marital, and minority status. These relationships have been a major source of compelling hypotheses and, accordingly, have stimulated a significant body of research across a variety of disciplines. One result of these efforts has been the identification of factors thought to be implicated in the stress process.

Over the past decade, another epidemiological observation has generated considerable attention and interest – that of a relationship between gender and psychological distress and disorder. While the pervasiveness of this relationship across diagnostic categories remains a controversial issue (Dohrenwend 1977; Dohrenwend and Dohrenwend 1976; Gove 1978), there is little question that women in Western society experience significantly higher rates of psychological distress in general (Al-Issa 1982) and depression in particular (Nolen-Hoeksema 1987; Weissman and Klerman 1977).

Although some debate on the matter continues (e.g., Newmann 1984), it now seems safe to conclude that the persistently observed gender differences both in level of depressive symptoms and rates of depressive disorder are real rather than artifactual. Considerable evidence has accumulated indicating that these differences are not a function of gender biases in symptom reporting (Clancy and Gove 1974; Gove and Geerkin 1976; Gove et al. 1976; Tousignant et al. 1987), in diagnosis, or in help-seeking behavior (Nolen-Hoeksema 1987; Weissman and Klerman 1977). Moreover, they do not appear to be attributable to genetic factors (Merikangas et al. 1985), and evidence suggests that they cannot wholly, or even largely, be

* Reprinted from *Journal of Nervous and Mental Disease*, Vol. 177, No. 8, R. Jay Turner and William R. Avison, 'Gender and depression: Assessing exposure and vulnerability to life events in a chronically strained population,' pp 443–55, August 1989, with permission from Williams & Wilkins, Baltimore, MD.

explained simply on the basis of gender differences in levels of income, education, or occupation (Ensel 1982; Radloff 1975). Assuming that the tendency for women to experience more depression is not biologically driven, as available evidence clearly allows (Nolen-Hoeksema 1987), the relationship would appear to derive from systematic gender differences in the nature and/or consequences of social experience.

By far the largest body of work inspired by this conclusion has been based on the gender role perspective. This perspective contends that the roles, primarily marital and parenting, normally occupied by men and women are typified by different stresses, rewards, and resources (Gove 1972; Gove and Tudor 1973). Evidence is interpreted as suggesting that the higher rates of distress and disorder observed among women arise directly from greater stress associated with their gender and marital roles (Gove 1978). In our view, the hypothesis that women are exposed to more stress has not yet been effectively tested. Reliable means for estimating the magnitude of role-related stresses and of other enduring strains have so far eluded investigators, and no studies have yet attempted to simultaneously estimate gender differences in the burden of stress imposed by role strains, other chronic stresses, and life events.

An alternative and/or complementary explanation proposes that men and women differ in their capacity to adjust to or resolve stressful circumstances or events, and thus in their vulnerability to such events. A number of different sources of the hypothesized greater vulnerability to stress among women have been suggested, including less access to supportive relationships (Belle 1982), a tendency toward helpless cognitions (Kaplan 1977; LeUnes et al.1980; Radloff and Monroe 1978; Radloff and Rae 1981), and less effective coping strategies (Pearlin and Schooler 1978).

The vulnerability hypothesis has been indirectly supported by findings of no differences or only small differences in the number of stressful life events reported by men and women (Dohrenwend 1973; Radloff and Rae 1981; Uhlenhuth et al. 1974). Direct support has been provided by Kessler (1979) who, nearly a decade ago, reported that the differential impact of stressors was more important than differential exposure in explaining gender differences in psychological distress. Based on this finding, it was suggested that the less adequate coping strategies of women, compared with those of men, are implicated in the greater impact of comparable stress experiences.

In more recent work, Kessler and his colleagues (Kessler and McLeod 1984; Kessler et al. 1985) have taken exception to his earlier conclusion and to similar conclusions by others. They argue that findings from research on specific life crises are inconsistent with the assumption that women are pervasively more vulnerable than men or that they are characterized by a general deficit in coping capacity. They suggest that the different roles occupied by men and women may be associated with variable responsiveness only to particular kinds of events.

Drawing on role theory, Kessler and McLeod (1984) note that women are socialized to be more sensitive to the needs of others and to feel more responsibility for meeting those needs. They hypothesize that "this sense of responsibility for the life events of loved ones could lead women to report more of these events and to experience these events as more distressing" (621). Because such gender differences could not be revealed by aggregate life events scores, their analyses distinguished events that occurred to the respondent from events that happened to others. They found stresses that are centrally associated with womens nurturant roles to be especially significant and concluded that role-related differences in exposure and responsiveness to events occurring to network members represent an important source of the apparent mental health advantage of men.

In providing the first evidence on this important matter, Kessler and McLeod (1984) conducted secondary analyses on data from five separate community surveys, considering that subset of subjects who were white, who were 65 years of age or younger, and who were not students, retired, or disabled. This particular selection of subjects was informed by their interest in considering the significance of labor force participation for understanding gender differences in distress.

This paper builds directly on the work of Kessler and McLeod (1984) and uses similar analytic techniques. Our goal is to assess the "cost of caring" hypothesis within a substantially different population and to further elaborate and specify the significance of "caring" for understanding sex differences in depression. Our data were obtained from a representative sample of community residents who had some form of physical limitation or disability.

Two elaborations are incorporated in our analyses to further specify both the validity and limits of the cost of caring hypothesis. The first of these is a more complete consideration of the relevance of labor force participation for the hypothesis under study. In addition to estimating the impact of women's employment on gender differences in exposure and responsiveness to life stress, we also examine the significance of labor force participation among men as well as the impact of employment on the pattern of stress effects observed for men and for women considered separately.

The second elaboration is to set the question within a life course perspective, recognizing that the kinds of events a person is likely to experience, as well as their meanings and impact with respect to distress, tend to vary depending on one's stage in the life course (Schultz and Rau 1985). Because it is clear that both role demands and prerogatives change over the life course, the impact of undesirable events and gender differences in such impact may also vary with age. To our knowledge the question of whether gender differences in either exposure or vulnerability to stress vary with life stage has never been examined. To address this issue, cross-gender comparisons in both exposure and responsiveness to events occurring to self and events occuring to others are conducted separately among the young, the middle-aged, and the elderly in our sample.

While examination of these issues within a sample of physically disabled subjects raises the question of the extent to which results can be applied with confidence to the general population, there are also several advantages. First, disability, by nature and definition, signifies a reduced capacity to perform one or more roles or activities and thus to meet psychosocial and instrumental needs. This reduced capacity constitutes, we believe, an enduring form of social stress that is generally referred to as chronic strain. Although there is evidence that events with enduring consequences have more compelling effects on psychological distress than do those that are time limited (e.g., Pearlin and Lieberman 1979; Wheaton 1983), the extent to which such distress is attributable to the events involved or to the ensuing strain has been difficult to determine. This confounding of event and strain effects has impeded efforts to assess the role and significance of life strain. Brown and Harris (1978) have argued that preexisting chronic strains may serve to intensify the impact of eventful experiences. This hypothesis, which emphasizes the potential relevance of strain in conditioning individual vulnerability, is consistent with Paykel's (1978) remark that it is not just the event that is significant "but the soil on which it falls" (251).

What is needed to effectively address this hypothesis is a circumstance in which chronic strain is not confounded with the occurrence of recent events. In our view, disabled individuals comprise a population in which this circumstance can be found. The social, occupational, and instrumental difficulties that characterize physical disability are quite distinct from the occurrence of recent life events. Given the assumption that chronic strains and eventful stressors may act synergistically in producing distress, gender differences in vulnerability to life events may be more clearly observable within a population experiencing the strain of physical disability.

A second advantage derives from the relationship between age and the prevalence of physical disability. A representative community sample of physically disabled individuals naturally yields sufficient numbers of older subjects to allow examination of how gender differences in exposure and responsiveness to role-related events may vary at different life stages.

A final advantage is the unique opportunity afforded to examine the relevance of employment. Employment status, of course, has been repeatedly linked with psychological distress or well-being (e.g., Dooley and Catalano 1980; Kasl et al. 1975; Linn et al. 1985; Warr and Parry 1982), but this relationship appears to be substantially stronger among men and its presence among married women has been questioned (Parry 1986). It is not clear whether this apparent gender difference in the mental health significance of employment indicates a greater benefit of working for men or simply reflects the presumably greater stress that men experience when confronted by unemployment. This assumption seems warranted because of gender differences in the stigma attached to unemployment and because of significant differences in the proportions of men and women who need and/or prefer to be working. Our sample of physically disabled individuals includes a substantial number of men, as well as women, who are unemployed and whose unemployment is socially sanctioned and often personally chosen. It thus represents a circumstance in which gender differences in the stress of unemployment are minimized and the significance of the work role for both exposure and vulnerability to stress can be more effectively estimated.

Methods

The results presented in this paper are based on interviews with physically disabled subjects residing in the community. The goal of this longitudinal investigation was to assess social and psychological adjustment among the disabled and to identify factors influencing such adjustment.

Sample

We obtained a representative sample of disabled persons residing in the community through a two-stage clustering technique involving a random selection of enumeration areas as defined by the Canadian Census and the selection of every n^{th} household within each area counting from a random start. Rural households were deliberately oversampled by a factor of three. Screening interviews were conducted at more than 10,000 households in Southwestern Ontario, covering more than 22,000 adults aged 18 and over.

The following question was used to determine eligibility for participation in the study: Do any adults in the household have any physical health condition or physical handicap that has resulted in a change in their daily routine or that limits the kind or amount of activity they can carry out? (For instance: work, housework, school, play/recreation, shopping or participation in social activities or community activities.)

A total of 967 interviews were successfully completed, representing 70% of those who were self-identified as physically disabled. Analyses revealed no differences between lost and completed cases on gender or any differences with respect to type or duration of disability. However, there were significant age differences with the mean age of participants (55.98 years) being somewhat lower than that for lost subjects (61.50 years). This difference appeared to be due primarily to a high percentage of lost subjects among persons 65 and older.

At the time of the initial interview, subjects ranged in age from 19 to 91 years and reported a median duration of eight years of disability. Fifty-four percent of the sample were women, 61% resided in urban areas, and virtually all subjects were white. A wide array of different conditions were reported, with varying degrees of attendant impairment (Turner, et al. 1985). The various heart diseases were the most common, accounting for 16.2% of those categorized as disabled. Arthritis was the second most frequently reported (12.1%), followed by osteoarthritis of the spine (7.9%) and by rheumatoid arthritis and allied conditions (5.4%). The next 12 most frequently reported conditions accounted for between 2 and 5% each and conditions with a frequency of 1% or less made up nearly 24% of the total sample.

Although this is a two-wave panel study, only time 2 data are considered here because the life-stress measure used at time 1 did not distinguish between undesirable events occurring to the respondent and those occurring to significant others. The results to be presented are based upon 731 follow-up interviews completed in 1985-1986, four years after the initial interview. These subjects represent 76% of those studied in the first wave. This number excludes 19 subjects who were successfully interviewed but who no longer met the disability criterion by the time of the second interview. Approximately 13% of the subjects had died during the four-year interval and about 4% were either institutionalized or too ill to be interviewed. Because mortality, institutionalization, and severe illness are analyzable outcomes, our follow-up success rate was nearly 93%. Only 5.6% of the subjects refused to participate in the second wave and only 1.7% could not be located.

For two reasons, in this paper we consider only subjects who were married and living with their spouse at the time of the interview. First, it is well established that gender differences in depression are most pronounced among married subjects (Gove 1972). Second, because we wished to systematically distinguish between events occurring to the respondent and those occurring to significant others, it seemed crucial to assure some consistency in the opportunity for exposure to significant-other events. Because events occurring to one's spouse were expected to represent an important proportion of such events, we chose to exclude cases in which a spouse was not present.

Measurement

Interviews were conducted in the homes of disabled respondents by trained lay interviewers. Depressive symptomatology was assessed by the Center for Epidemiologic Studies Depression Scale (CES-D), which consists of 20 items designed to measure an individual's current level of depressive symptomatology with an emphasis on depressed mood. In four separate field tests of the scale's reliability, Cronbach's (1951) alpha ranged from .84 to .90 (Radloff 1977). In the present study, this coefficient was .88. With respect to validity, the scale has been found to distinguish well between psychiatric inpatient and general population samples and moderately well among levels of severity within patient groups (Husaini et al. 1980; Radloff 1977; Roberts and Vernon 1983; Weissman et al. 1977). The measure also shows good convergent validity, correlating well with other self-report measures of depression (Radloff 1977; Weissman et al. 1977).

The CES-D has also been used to estimate the presence of clinically significant depression. Radloff (1977) suggests that scores of 16 or higher reflect the severity of depressive symptoms that have been found to be characteristic of the levels observed in cases of depressive disorder. However, this cutoff point is intended as a means for identifying high-risk groups rather than for the clinical evaluation of individual cases. We have chosen to focus on depressive symptomatology rather than depressive disorder, which was also measured, because the prevalence of major depression and its dichotomous nature would prohibit the type and range of analyses to be presented.

Life stress was assessed using a 31-item scale of negative events that included items common to many life events indices (Henderson et al. 1981; Holmes and Rahe 1967; Sarason et al. 1978). Because each reported event required a series of additional probe questions, it was necessary to place limits on reporting in order to keep interviews at an acceptable length. For the 12 months preceding the interview, respondents were asked to indicate which of the 31 events they had personally experienced. For 21 of these events, they were also asked whether their spouse had experienced such an event. In a similar manner, for 13 of the 31 they were also asked whether their children had experienced the event and for six events subjects were also questioned with respect to relatives or close friends. This necessary strategy somewhat limits our information on events occurring to relations or close friends. However, when combined with data on children, we believe the information to be sufficient to allow some assessment of gender differences in exposure and vulnerability to events experienced by significant others.

Results

Our presentation of results begins with an examination of gender differences in depression followed by a consideration of variations in exposure and vulnerability to stressful experiences. Because of the possibility of life stage variations in depression and its determinants, our analyses distinguish between young, middle-aged, and elderly subjects. Specifically, separate analyses are conducted on subjects aged 22 to 44 years, 45 to 64 years, and 65 and older. These particular groupings were selected to ensure adequate sample sizes within categories and to be generally consistent with conventional distinctions between young adulthood, middle age, and late adulthood. These three groupings correspond to the adult life stages distinguished by Gordon (1971); Gordon and Gaitz (1976) and by Weissman (1987).

Depression

As noted earlier, the CES-D can be used to roughly distinguish groups who are at elevated risk for clinically significant depression. When the recommended criterion score of 16 or higher was applied to this population, nearly 35% were found to fall into the high-risk category. When this percentage is compared with the average of about 17% that has been observed for general community samples (Boyd and Weissman 1981), our assumption that the disabled represent a chronically strained and high-risk population with respect to depression is clearly supported.

Mean CES-D scores for married men and women both within and across the age categories distinguished are compared in Table 1. Average depression scores for women clearly exceed those for men and the magnitude of the difference is highly consistent across the life course. Although the comparison in the youngest age category does not achieve statistical significance, this inconsistency appears to be an artifact of the smaller sample sizes involved in that comparison. Thus, the widely reported gender difference in depression that we seek to explain is clearly observed in this chronically strained sample and is consistent across the age categories distinguished.

TABLE 1

Mean CES-D scores for married disabled subjects by age and gender

	22-44 yrs		45-64 yrs		65+ yrs		Total	
	M	F	M	F	M	F	M	F
X	12.77	15.05	11.98*	14.24	11.45*	14.62	11.91*	14.56
SD	11.32	11.12	9.29	11.63	8.86	10.01	9.5	11.2
N	44	64	97	109	97	52	238	225

* Difference significant at the .05 level.

The Relevance of Life Stress

As noted earlier, efforts to understand the significance of life stress for gender differences in depression have considered variations in both exposure and vulnerability to such stress. The hypothesis that gender differences in depression may arise, at least in part, from differences in exposure to stressful life events is addressed in Table 2. The mean number of reported life events by gender and age category, distinguishing between events that occurred to the respondent and events reported as having occurred to important others in the respondent's world, is presented. When all events are taken together, a clear difference in exposure is observed. On average, women reported 3.57 events, which exceeds the number reported by men by more than 40%. This elevated exposure to eventful stressors is clearly observed among both young and middle-aged women but cannot be said to apply to those 65 and older.

Examination of the remainder of Table 2 reveals no reliable gender difference in exposure when events occurring to the respondent are considered. However, there are substantial and consistent differences on events occurring to spouse and events occurring to significant others. We conclude from these results that women are exposed to more eventful stressors than are men, that this differential exposure is almost entirely attributable to differences in exposure to events occurring to others, and that the hypothesis that differential exposure to social stress is a factor in gender differences in depression is supported. Identical results were obtained in weighted analyses conducted to ensure that these findings were not materially influenced by the oversampling of rural subjects.

TABLE 2

Mean number of stressful life events for married respondents by age, gender, and to whom the event occurred

	18 - 44 years			45 - 64 years		
	M	F	T	M	F	T
All events	3.82*	5.20	4.64	2.74*	3.41	3.10
	(2.79)	(2.92)	(3.26)	(1.94)	(2.42)	(2.23)[a]
Events to respondent	2.55	2.92	2.77	1.55	1.59	1.57
	(2.67)	(2.36)	(2.32)	(1.56)	(1.50)	(1.53)
Events to spouse	.48*	1.88	.83	.24*	.51	.38
	(1.63)	(1.29)	(1.10)	(.50)	(.83)	(.71)
Events to significant others[b]	.88	1.21	1.84	.96*	1.31	1.15
	(1.11)	(1.11)	(1.12)	(.76)	(1.24)	(1.13)
Sample sizes	44	63	107	97	109	206

	65+ years			All Ages		
	M	F	T	M	F	T
All events	1.72	1.92	1.79	2.53*	3.57	3.03
	(1.47)	(1.88)	(1.62)	(2.10)	(2.89)	(2.57)
Events to respondent	1.81	.96	.99	1.51	1.82	1.66
	(1.15)	(1.24)	(1.18)	(1.66)	(1.88)	(1.77)
Events to spouse	.16*	.35	.23	.25*	.63	.44
	(.43)	(.62)	(.02)	(.51)	(.98)	(.88)
Events to significant others[b]	.55	.62	.57	.76*	1.12	.94
	(.75)	(.82)	(.77)	(.93)	(1.15)	(1.05)
Sample sizes	97	52	149	238	224	462

a   Numbers in parentheses refer to standard deviations.
b   Includes events occurring to children, friends and other relatives.
* $p \leq .05$.

The question of why women report more events occurring to significant others than do men has been addressed by Kessler and his associates (Kessler and McLeod 1984; Kessler et al. 1985). They argue that such differences probably arise from the tendency for women to have a wider field of concern. It is suggested that men and women structure their lives in fundamentally different ways so that women tend to define more people as important. In addition, women are more likely to become aware of undesirable events occurring to others because of a tendency for both men and women to seek out women for support and comfort in times of crisis. It is also possible, however, that at least part of the explanation simply lies in the tendency of women to be more empathic and/or more helpful, which amplifies both the salience and the significance of events occurring to important others.

If events occurring to others are more salient to women than to men, we should observe gender differences in the tendency to forget such events that are not observed for events occurring to oneself. This expectation is based on the assumption that the greater the import of an event, the more reliably it will be recalled. To assess this possibility, we compared the distributions for men and women of events occurring to the respondent and events occurring to significant others during the 12 months preceding the interview. Because stressful life events occur randomly, at least across large samples of individuals, the average number of events reported for each month should be constant across the reporting period if reporting is entirely reliable (Paykel 1983). An observation that fewer events tend to be reported for distant months than for recent months would indicate a tendency to forget more distant events. These comparisons, in terms of both the proportion of all events reported within each month and cumulative proportions across the 12-month period, are presented in Table 3. The results have not been elaborated by life stage because the number of reported events was insufficient to reliably estimate changes in reporting over time within each of the age subgroups.

The left half of Table 3 presents these distributions for events to respondent. For example, during the 11th month before interview males reported 4.7% of the year's events to self while women reported 4.2%. Cumulatively, the proportions reported in each of the first 11 months preceding the interview are quite consistent month to month and quite similar for men and women. However, during the 12th month, 30.6% of all events occurring to male respondents were reported and women reported 32.3% of all events occurring to themselves.

Elsewhere we have shown that these significant departures from expectation during the 12th month do not reflect simple telescoping – the tendency to bring forward in time events that actually occurred before the reporting period. While many of the reported events presumably had an earlier onset, our data suggested that most represented chronic stresses that continued well beyond the 12th month before interview (Avison and Turner 1988, Turner et al. 1986b).

Although the proportion of events to respondent reported by women as occurring in the 12th month exceeds that for men, the difference is not substantial and, overall, there is little evidence of gender differences in the tendency to remember and report events to self. Inspection of cumulative proportions makes a similar point. Comparing the proportion of all events that were recalled as happening in the most distant quarter (months 10, 11, and 12) reveals that both men and women report approximately 40% of all events to respondent as having occurred during that period (1.00 - .600 for men and 1.00 - .609 for women). Computations of the actual numbers of events reported during this period revealed an average of .6 events for men and .7 for women.

TABLE 3
Proportion of life events occurring in each month before interview for married disabled respondents

Month	Events to Respondent					
	N[b]		P		CP	
	M	F	M	F	M	F
1	21	31	.059	.076	.059	.076
2	34	31	.095	.076	.154	.152
3	37	32	.103	.078	.257	.230
4	23	34	.064	.083	.321	.313
5	24	25	.067	.061	.338	.374
6	32	23	.089	.056	.477	.430
7	19	24	.053	.059	.530	.489
8	14	24	.039	.059	.569	.548
9	11	25	.031	.061	.600	.609
10	17	11	.047	.027	.647	.636
11	17	17	.047	.042	.694	.678
12	100	132	.306	.323	1.000	1.000
Total	349	409	1.000	1.000		

Month	Events to All Significant Others[a]					
	N		P		CP	
	M	F	M	F	M	F
1	20	15	.083	.038	.083	.038
2	26	38	.108	.097	.191	.135
3	27	24	.113	.061	.304	.196
4	16	32	.067	.082	.371	.278
5	20	35	.083	.089	.454	.367
6	17	25	.071	.064	.525	.431
7	24	19	.100	.048	.625	.479
8	11	23	.046	.059	.671	.538
9	12	30	.050	.077	.710	.615
10	11	27	.046	.069	.767	.684
11	3	21	.013	.054	.780	.738
12	53	103	.221	.263	1.000	1.000
Total	240	392	1.000	1.000		

[a] Includes events occurring to spouse, children, relatives, and friends.
[b] N, number of stressful events; P, proportion of events occuring in each month; CP, cumulative proportion.

A very different picture emerges when we examine events to all significant others (spouse, children, friends and relatives combined). As with events to respondent, both men and women report a disproportionate number in the 12th month before interview, with women showing a somewhat greater tendency in this regard than men. The most important contrast provided in this data, however, is the clear gender difference in the proportion of all such events reported in the most distant quarter of the year considered. Whereas 39% of all events reported as occurring to significant others by women fell into the 10th, 11th, and 12th months before interview (1.00-.615), only 29% (1.00-.710) of such events reported by men fell into this period. When actual numbers of events rather than proportions are considered, men reported an average of only .28 events during this interval whereas the average for women was .72, or approximately 2.6 times more.

In our view, these differences reflect a greater tendency for married men to forget over time, or to disregard, events occurring to significant others in their social network. Conversely, the fact that women show less "decay of memory" than do men in reporting these events suggests that women are more likely to remember distant events occurring to others, presumably because these events are, for some reason, of greater salience. It is clear that this tendency contributes to the greater number of events to others that were reported by women in this sample. However, it is also clear that something more is involved in the differences in exposure to events to others that we have observed than the relative inability or unwillingness of men to remember such events. A wider domain of concern and greater sensitivity to the needs of others among women appear to be implicated in this exposure difference as Kessler and McLeod (1984) have suggested.

Vulnerability to Stressful Events

To assess the hypothesis of differential vulnerability by sex, we began with an examination of correlations between the number of events reported and depression scores for each of the age categories distinguished. These correlations for total events, as well as separately for events occurring to respondent, events to spouse, and events to significant others, are presented in Table 4. Examination of the results for all events reveals no evidence for a general gender difference in vulnerability. The correlations across age are virtually identical for men and women and what differences are found are both small and inconsistent.

The same can be said when events to respondent are considered. These findings thus contradict the notion that women are generally more vulnerable than men to stressful environmental events. It is worth noting that vulnerability to life events apparently varies somewhat by age, with the youngest group showing the greatest vulnerability, at least when total events and events to respondent are considered.

For events to others a somewhat different pattern is observed. The correlation for women is significantly higher for events to spouse than is found for men, and this difference is rather substantial for both the young and the elderly age groupings. Our findings with respect to vulnerability are thus substantially similar to those observed for exposure. Events occuring to the respondent represent a major portion of total exposure but do not differ markedly by sex. The differences between men and women in exposure to undesirable life events are largely restricted to events occurring to others. Similarly, whereas both men and women appear to be most responsive to events occurring to self, the extent of this responsiveness or vulnerability is quite consistent for both sexes. Evidence for differential vulnerability is found primarily with respect to events occurring to one's spouse. The stronger association observed for women between such events and depression, contrasted with an association similar to that observed for men for events occurring to self, demonstrates this point. Our findings on both exposure and vulnerability to events occurring to others suggests that women may care about more people or care more about the people they know, or both.

TABLE 4

Correlations of CES-D scores with stressful life events for married respondents by age, gender, and to whom the event occurred

To Whom	18 - 44 years			45 - 64 years		
	M	F	T	M	F	T
All events	.31*	.27*	.29*	.08	.23*	.19*
Events to respondent	.45*	.28*	.35*	.19*	.25*	.22*
Events to spouse	-.07[†]	.27*	.20*	.08	.13	.13*
Events to significant others[a]	-.10	-.08	-.07	-.20*[†]	.06	-.01
Sample	44	64	108	97	109	206

To Whom	65+ years			Total		
	M	F	T	M	F	T
All events	.12	.07	.10	.17*	.21*	.21*
Events to respondent	.20*	.10	.15*	.27*	.22*	.25*
Events to spouse	-.07[†]	.22*	.09	.00[†]	.19*	.15*
Events to significant others[a]	-.03	-.15	.07	-.11*	-.01	-.03
Sample	97	52	149	238	225	463

[a]   Includes events occurring to children, friends and other relatives.

*   Indicates that the correlation is statistically significant ($p \leq .05$).

[†]   Indicates a statistically significant difference in correlations ($p \leq .05$).

Less consistent results are observed for events to children, relatives, and close friends. The significant negative correlation observed only for middle-aged men is difficult to interpret with confidence. However, it may reflect a process of social comparison in which the negative experiences to others in one's social network emphasizes one's own good fortune.

As with analyses on exposure, these correlations were also computed with adjustment for the rural oversample. Neither the pattern of results nor the relative magnitude of relationships across gender were materially altered.

Decomposing Exposure and Vulnerability Effects

Results so far presented suggest that both differential exposure and responsiveness to certain kinds of events may be implicated in the observed gender differences in depression. In this section we consider exposure and vulnerability simultaneously in order to estimate the relative contribution of each in explaining this important sex differential.

Following Kessler and McLeod (1984), we use a demographic-mean decomposition procedure suggested by Iams and Thornton (1975) for estimating the proportion of the observed gender difference in depression attributable to differential exposure on the one hand and differential vulnerability on the other. In this procedure we use regression equations to disaggregate mean differences in CES-D scores. Within each gender category, we first regressed our measure of depression on events occurring to the respondent, on events to spouse, and on events to significant others, controlling age variation. Using means and unstandardized coefficients from these analyses, this decomposition technique enables us to estimate the effect of differences in mean number of events (exposure) and in responsiveness (vulnerability) as reflected by different unstandardized regression coefficients.

Specifically, for any age group, we can estimate the proportion of the mean difference in CES-D scores that is due to: a) women's differential exposure to events to self; b) women's differential exposure to events to spouse; c) women's differential exposure to significant other events; d) women's differential vulnerability to events occurring to self; e) women's differential vulnerability to events to spouse; and f) women's differential vulnerability to significant other events. The differential exposure component represents the increase or decrease in the mean difference on the CES-D that would be observed if men were exposed to the same number of events as women, controlling for differences in vulnerability. This component is calculated as $(X_f - X_m)(B_f + b_m)/2$. In an analogous manner, the differential vulnerability component represents the expected change in CES-D mean differences if men and women were equally vulnerable to life events, controlling for differences in exposure. This component is calculated as $(b_f - b_m)(X)_f + (X_m)/2$. In computing effects in this manner we do not estimate exposure-vulnerability interactions, but allocate any such effects equally to the two main components.

The results of these decomposition analyses applied to the total sample are presented in Table 5. For the sake of simplicity and given the consistency of observed gender differences in depression across the life stages, we have chosen to forego separate subgroup analyses. Each entry in Table 5 indicates the amount of change in the mean difference that would be expected if men and women were equivalent on that particular factor. Positive numbers reflect the amount that the mean difference would be reduced in the presence of such equivalence, whereas negative numbers indicate the amount of increase in the difference that could be anticipated. Thus, positive entries indicate that women are more exposed to or more vulnerable than men to a particular kind of event, whereas negative numbers indicate that men are more exposed or vulnerable. These expected changes are expressed as a percentage of the observed mean difference in depression scores.

It can be seen from Table 5 that differential responsiveness or vulnerability accounts for more than 22% of the difference in mean depression scores observed. However, it is clear that the elevated vulnerability to life events on the part of women is specific to events occurring to their spouse and to significant others. Indeed, for events to self, men are clearly more vulnerable than women. The -1.10 shown for events occurring to respondent indicates that, if women were as responsive to such events as are men, the mean difference in depression scores would be increased by over 40%. Thus, with respect to vulnerability generally, we have mixed findings with men being substantially more vulnerable to the events occurring to self and women being substantially more vulnerable to events occurring to others. In contrast, differences in exposure to events appear to contribute relatively little toward our understanding of distress differences, amounting to less than 14%.

Our observation that men are more vulnerable than women to events to self argues against hypotheses that women are more depressed because they tend to be less capable of dealing with stressful circumstances due to less adequate coping ability, social support, or whatever.

TABLE 5

Decompositions of gender differences in CES-D means for married respondents controlling on age

Life Events	Decomposition		
	Vulnerability[a]	Exposure[b]	Total
Events to respondent			
Difference	-1.10	.46	-.64
Percentage	40.89	17.21	-27.79
Events to spouse			
Difference	1.14	.23	1.37
Percentage	42.38	8.55	50.93
Events to significant others			
Difference	.56	-.32	.24
Percentage	20.82	-11.90	8.92
Total			
Difference	.60	.37	.97
Percentage	22.30	13.75	36.06
Mean difference in depression			2.69

[a] Vulnerability = $(b_f - b_m)(\bar{X}_f + \bar{X}_m)/2$

[b] Exposure = $(\bar{X}_f - \bar{X}_m)(b_f + b_m)/2$

The results indicating that women are more responsive or vulnerable to events occurring to others is completely consistent with the hypothesis that gender differences in depression, at least among the married, can be partly attributed to costs associated with caring more about others.

Relevance of Labor Force Participation

To assess the impact of labor force participation, we performed the same exposure and vulnerability decompositions within contrasting categories of labor force participation, both across gender and for men and women separately (Table 6). For these computations, we have restricted our analyses to subjects aged 22 to 64, thus avoiding the confounding of retirement with unemployment. Because our data are derived from individuals with physical disabilities, the possibility must be contemplated that employment differences in depression could arise from the fact that individuals with more severe limitations may be both less likely to be employed and more likely to have higher levels of psychological distress. To eliminate the possible influence of variations in severity of disability, we computed the mean decompositions controlling for level of functional limitation. Functional limitations were assessed with an Activities of Daily Living (ADL) scale, based on the work of Katz (1963) and modified to encompass both the degree of difficulty and the need for assistance in performing 13 specific tasks. Although unemployed subjects were found to be more severely limited based on ADL scores than were the employed, the results displayed in Table 6, which control variations in limitations, match closely results obtained when this control was not applied.

An examination of the mean difference scores displayed in Table 6 emphasizes the apparent significance of paid employment for understanding gender differences in depression. Where labor force participation is held constant, gender differences in depression are minimized relative to that observed for the comparison involving employed men and unemployed women (2.25 and 1.80 vs. 4.44). In fact, the usual pattern of higher levels of depression among women is reversed in the circumstance in which nonworking men are compared with working women, although this difference falls far short of statistical reliability. This pattern of results, of course, is consistent with evidence that lack of employment is a risk factor for depression in women just as it is in men (Aneshenel and Pearlin 1988; Merikangas 1985) and that the role carries with it important mental and physical health advantages for women (Verbrugge 1982; Waldron and Herold 1984) Detailed consideration of the significance of employment for depression among the women in this sample or of the contribution of the quality of labor force participation in understanding gender differences in depression are beyond the scope of this paper. In the present context, our interest is restricted to the consideration of the influence of employment on exposure and vulnerability to eventful stressors in both cross-gender and within-gender comparisons.

In examining this issue, it should be noted that the mean difference in level of depressive symptoms achieves statistical significance for only two of the six contrasts shown. However, results on the amount of change that would occur if the contrast groups were equal on that particular factor are independent of the size of the mean difference and thus remain interpretable. In contrast, the percentage entries are based directly on the mean difference, and thus small absolute differences can translate into large percentage differences. For this reason, percentages have been omitted entirely for the unemployed man-employed woman contrast where the mean difference is only -.34. The reader should bear in mind this connection between the percentage entries and the size of the mean difference in interpreting results presented in the other cells of this Table 6.

Looking first at the bottom third of this table, the mean differences in CES-D scores indicate that the mental health advantage of employment is only slightly greater for men than for women. However, dramatic gender differences are observed in the apparent significance of employment for exposure and vulnerability to various kinds of events. As the "total" entries indicate, variations in exposure and/or vulnerability provide a partial explanation for the difference in mean depression scores observed for employed and unemployed men. By contrast, despite the fact that larger total differences are observed for women, these differences do not assist in explaining employment-related depression differences among women. In fact, if employed and unemployed women were equally exposed and equally responsive to all kinds of events, the depression difference would increase by 2.35 or nearly 110%. This result derives from the fact that employed women are substantially more exposed and more vulnerable to stressful events occurring to themselves and somewhat more exposed to events occurring to their spouses than are unemployed women. On the positive side, working women are substantially less vulnerable to events to significant others than are unemployed women. Thus, although involvement in the paid worker role appears to buffer the impact of events occurring to significant others, the net effect of employment with respect to exposure and vulnerability to stressful life events is, for women, negative rather than positive. The implication of this finding is that the positive corollaries of the paid worker role must be substantial indeed, inasmuch as they must compensate for the clear tendency for working women to be both more exposed to, and more affected by, eventful stressors.

TABLE 6

Decompositions of gender differences in CES-D means by labor force participation for married respondents aged 22 to 64, controlling for age and severity of disability

Decomposition	Men (N = 72) in Labor Force vs Women (N = 66) in Labor Force			Men (N = 69) not in Labor Force vs Women (N = 107) not in Labor Force		
	V^a	E	T	V	E	T
Events to self	1.44 (64.00)[b]	1.35 (60.00)	2.79 (124.00)	-1.43 (-79.44)	-.24 (-13.33)	-1.67 (-92.77)
Events to spouse	.07 (3.11)	.78 (34.67)	.85 (37.98)	.78 (43.33)	.14 (7.78)	.92 (51.11)
Events to significant others	.64 (28.44)	-.24 (-10.67)	.40 (17.78)	1.68 (93.33)	-.43 (-23.89)	1.25 (69.44)
Total	2.15 (95.55)	1.89 (84.00)	4.04 (179.56)	1.03 (57.22)	-.53 (-29.44)	.50 (27.78)
Mean difference in depression		2.25	NS		1.80	NS

Continued on next page

Table 6 - *continued*

Decomposition	Men in Labor Force vs Women not in Labor Force			Men not in Labor Force vs Women in Labor Force		
Events to self	-.21 (-4.73)	-.11 (-2.48)	-.33 (-7.43)	-.07	1.51	1.44
Events to spouse	.01 (.23)	.45 (10.14)	.46 (10.36)	1.02	.28	1.30
Events to significant others	1.74 (39.19)	-.19 (-4.28)	1.55 (34.91)	.68	-.57	-.11
Total	1.54 (34.68)	.15 (3.38)	1.69 (38.06)	1.63	1.22	2.84
Mean difference in depression		4.44	(p < .001)		-.34	NS
Events to self	1.25 (48.45)	.10 (3.88)	1.35 (52.33)	-1.67 (-77.67)	-1.44 (-66.98)	-3.11 (-144.65)
Events to spouse	-.49 (-18.99)	.03 (1.16)	-.46 (-17.83)	-.07 (-3.26)	-.32 (-14.88)	-.39 (-18.14)
Events to significant others	-.11 (4.26)	.38 (14.73)	.27 (10.46)	1.18 (54.88)	-.03 (-1.40)	.15 (53.48)
Total	.65 (25.19)	.51 (19.77)	1.16 (44.96)	-.56 (-26.06)	-1.79 (-83.26)	-2.35 (-109.30)
Mean difference in depression		2.60	p < .10		2.15	NS

[a]   V, vulnerability; E, exposure; T, total.
[b]   Numbers in parentheses, percentage of CES-D mean difference.

Among men, the presence or absence of the paid worker role has relatively little impact upon either exposure or vulnerability to life events, with one significant exception. Directly opposite to the case for women, unemployed men appear to be substantially more vulnerable to stressful events occurring to themselves than are employed men.

In general, the findings presented earlier (Table 5) appear to be confirmed by the gender contrasts shown in the upper two thirds of Table 6 that take account of labor force participation. Thus, the tendency for men to experience more events to significant others is uniformly observed, as is the tendency for women to be more affected by such events. The greater vulnerability of women to events occurring to spouse is found in three of the four contrasts, as is the tendency for women to be exposed to more spouse events. We conclude that the hypothesis that women's greater risk for depression can partially be attributed to the costs of caring more about others continues to be generally supported even when labor force participation is considered.

Table 6 also adds specification to some of the previously reported findings. Although the tendency for men to be more vulnerable than women to events to self is clearly observable in two of the four contrasts, the difference is completely reversed when working women are compared with working men. This reversal derives from the tendency, reported earlier, for employment to reduce vulnerability to such events among men while increasing vulnerability among women. A second specification relates to the observation of women's greater exposure to events to self. Comparison of the relevant entries across the four contrasts reveals that the crucial factor is employment among women. Little difference in exposure is observed in comparisons involving unemployed women while, regardless of the employment status of men, employed women report relatively higher levels of such exposure.

Conclusions

The results presented above have addressed the question of whether the well-established relationship between gender and depression can be at least partially understood as arising from systematic sex differences in exposure and/or vulnerability to stressful life events. Consistent with the findings of Kessler and McLeod (1984), our results point clearly to an affirmative answer. Women in our sample reported significantly more negative events than did men, but this difference did not primarily involve events occurring to the respondent. Rather, the observed differential in exposure derived almost entirely from differences in the number of events reported as happening to important others. Male/female comparisons on the reliability with which events to self and events to others were reported indicated that, over time, men were equally likely to remember events to self but less likely than women to remember temporally distant events occurring to others. This observation suggests that men may reduce their burden of stress by consciously or unconsciously blocking out, or not attending to, some stressful events previously experienced by their significant others. However, differential recall accounts for only part of this gender difference in exposure to events to others. Something akin to a wider domain of interest and concern and/or a greater sensitivity to the well-being of others appears to be implicated in women's greater exposure to stress, as Kessler and McLeod (1984) have suggested.

Taken together, our results with respect to vulnerability to stress allow two significant conclusions. First, women appear to be more affected than men by events occurring to significant others, particularly to their spouse. Stated differently, there is evidence that women are more responsive to the negative experiences of others and this differential responsiveness has significant mental health implications. The cost of caring hypothesis is thus supported by these data.

Second, the hypothesis that women tend to be more depressed because they are less capable than men of dealing with stressful circumstances is clearly refuted. Our finding from the decomposition analyses (Table 5) that men tend to be more vulnerable to events occurring to self indicates that women are at least as capable as are men of adjusting to, or resolving, negative personal experiences. That the reverse is so with respect to events occurring to others is consistent with the argument that the role of married women includes the experience of responsibility for the well-being of family members. Because concern over the happiness of others or over events that emerge on such happiness is clearly limited, the adequacy of personal coping skills may be irrelevant to the impact of such events on mental health.

It is important to emphasize that our conception of vulnerability refers to variations in the rate at which stressors translate into depressive symptoms. Thus, vulnerability is a construct defined by the associations of stress with health. Accordingly, this approach can only estimate vulnerability with respect to the specific outcome being assessed. Our findings concerning differential vulnerability, therefore, do not necessarily apply to other health outcomes thought to be influenced by social stress.

Because depression is a significant public health problem that falls disproportionately on women, the intervention implications of our conclusions require comment. The second conclusion described above discredits the idea that gender differences in depression would be reduced if the capacity of women to resolve difficulties and cope with stress could be enhanced. Clearly, public health programs with such goals would be no less appropriate for men than for women. With respect to the cost of caring, our findings might be taken to suggest that a reduction in concern for, or interest in, others would lead to improved mental health among women. However, abundant evidence for a positive association between social support and psychological well-being suggests that such a change might negatively affect the mental health of women, as well as that of men and children. There are, then, both scientific and moral bases for arguing that programs might better be directed toward making men more like women in this regard than the reverse.

Our findings on the significance of employment for understanding gender differences in depression confirmed certain previous observations and provided important new information. That gender differences are minimized in comparisons where employment status is controlled suggests that the elevated level of depression typically observed among women derives, in part, from the fact that a higher proportion of men tend to be employed.

Employment status and depression are significantly related among both men and women and the mental health advantage of employment appears to be about equal. However, within gender analyses reveal a dramatic gender difference in the apparent significance of employment for exposure and vulnerability to various kinds of stressful events. For men, increased exposure and vulnerability to negative events among the unemployed accounts for almost half of the depression difference observed by employment status. Thus, although differences in the occurrence and impact of eventful stressors account for part of the mental health advantage associated with working, it is clear that the significance of employment for men goes well beyond associated differences in the burden of stress as we have measured it.

By the same reasoning, the mental health significance of employment appears to be even greater for women than for men. For women, observed employment status differences in stress do not contribute toward explaining employment-related depression differences. On the contrary, control of such differences would significantly increase, rather than decrease, the depression difference observed. That employed women tend to be less depressed than unemployed women despite the increased burden of depression-relevant stress associated with employment suggests that, overall, the paid worker role must have especially powerful beneficial effects for women. The effort to understand the determinants of this important association should be high on the research agenda of scientists interested in the health significance of social roles and role requirements.

Two final issues, each bearing upon the generalizability of the results presented, require comment. First, the extent to which these findings, based on a physically disabled and thus chronically strained population, are generalizable to the total population of married adults is uncertain. In those analyses that replicated the work of Kessler and

McLeod (1984), our results correspond completely with their findings, which were based upon a vary large sample achieved by assembling several representative community samples. That the size of the effects we observed tended to be larger than they reported is consistent with the hypothesis that stress effects are amplified in the presence of chronic strain. Our own efforts to replicate these findings within a nondisabled comparison sample revealed no clear sex differences in responsiveness to events occurring to others. However, the magnitudes reported by Kessler and McLeod were rather small and effects of similar size might not be detectable in our substantially smaller comparison sample. Despite this inconsistency, the weight of available evidence suggests that the relevance of gender differences in the cost of caring for understanding depression is not limited to the physically disabled or chronically strained. Second, because our findings are restricted to married subjects, they cannot be assumed to apply to unmarried men and women. Indeed, analyses reported elsewhere (Turner et al. 1986a) suggest a rather different relationship between sex and caring about others among the unmarried.

Acknowledgement

This study was supported by the National Health Research and Development Program of Health and Welfare Canada through a research grant and a National Health Scientist award to R. Jay Turner.

We would like to thank Carl Grindstaff, Ben Singer, and Blake Turner for helpful comments and three anonymous reviewers whose suggestions contributed importantly to the quality of this paper.

References

Al-Issa, I ed. 1982. Gender and Adult Psychopathology. In *Gender and Psychopathology*, 83–101. New York: Academic.

Aneshensel, CS, and LI Pearlin. 1987. Structural Contexts of Sex Differences in Stress. In RC Barnett, L Biener, GK Baruch eds. *Gender and Stress*, 75–95. New York: Free Press.

Avison, WR, and RJ Turner. 1988. Stressful Life Events and Depressive Symptoms: Disaggregating the Effects of Acute Stressors and Chronic Strains. *Journal of Health and Social Behaviour* 29: 253–264.

Belle, D. 1982. The Stress of Caring: Women as Providers of Social Support. In L Goldberger, S Breznitz eds. *Handbook on Stress: Theoretical and Clinical Aspects,* 496–505. New York: Free Press.

Boyd, JH, and MM Weissman. 1981. Epidemiology of Affective Disorders: A Re-examination and Future Directions. *Archives of General Psychiatry* 38: 1039–1046.

Brown, NB, and T Harris. 1978. *Social Origins of Depression: A Study of Psychiatric Disorder in Women.* London: Tavistock.

Clancy, K, and WR Gove. 1974. Sex Differences in Mental Illness: An Analysis of Response Bias in Self-Reports. *American Journal of Sociology* 80: 205–216.

Cronbach, LJ. 1951. Coefficient Alpha and the Internal Structure of Tests. *Principles of Educational Psychology Measurement* 18: 132–165.

Dohrenwend, BS. 1973. Events as Stressors: A Methodological Inquiry. *Journal of Health and Social Behaviour* 14: 167–175.

Dohrenwend, BP. 1977. Reply to Gove and Tudor's Comment on Sex Differences in Psychiatric Disorders. *American Journal of Sociology* 82: 1336–1345.

Dohrenwend, BP, and BS Dohrenwend. 1976. Sex Differences and Psychiatric Disorders. *American Journal of Sociology* 81: 1447–1454.

Dooley D, R Catalano. 1980. Economic Change as a Cause of Behavioral Disorder. *Psychological Bulletin* 87: 450–468.

Ensel, WM. 1982. The Role of Age in Relationship of Gender and Marital Status to Depression. *Journal of Nervous and Mental Disease* 170: 536–543.

Gordon, C. 1971. Role and Value Development Across the Life Cycle. In JW Jackson ed. *Role: Sociological studies IV,* 65–105. London: Cambridge University Press.

Gordon, C, and C Gaitz. 1976. Leisure and Lives: Personal Expressivity Across Life Span. In R Binstock, E Shaws eds. *Handbook of aging and social sciences,* 310–341. New York: Van Nostrand.

Gove, WR. 1972. The Relationship Between Sex Roles, Marital Status and Mental Illness. *Social Forces* 51: 34–44.

Gove, WR. 1978. Sex Differences in Mental Illness Among Adult Men and Women: An Evaluation of Four Questions Raised Regarding the Evidence on the Higher Rates of Women. *Social Science and Medicine* 12: 198.

Gove, WR, and MR Geerkin. 1976. Response Bias in Surveys of Mental Health: An Empirical Investigation. *American Journal of Sociology* 82: 1289–1317.

Gove, WR, J McCorkel, T Fain, and M Hughes. 1976. Response Bias in Community Surveys of Mental Health: Systematic Bias or Random Noise? *Social Science and Medicine* 10: 497–502.

Gove, WR, and JF Tudor. 1973. Adult Sex Roles and Mental Illness. *American Journal of Sociology* 78: 812–835.

Henderson, S, DG Byrne, and P Duncan-Jones. 1981. *Neurosis and the Social Environment.* New York: Academic.

Homes, TH, and RH Rahe. 1967. The Social Readjustment Rating Scale. *Journal of Psychosomatic Research* 11: 213–218.

Husaini, BA, JA Neff, and SB Harrington, et al. 1980. Depression in Rural Communities: Validating the CES-D Scale. *Journal of Community Psychology* 8: 20–27.

Iams, HM, and A Thornton. 1975. Decomposition of Differences: A Cautionary Note. *Sociological Methods and Research* 3: 341–352.

Kaplan, H. 1977. Gender and Depression: A Sociological Analysis of a Conditional Relationship. In WE Fann, I Karacan, AD Pokorny, et al eds. *Phenomenology and Treatment of Depression,* 81–113. New York: Spectrum.

Kasl, SV, S Gore, and S Cobb. 1975. The Experience of Losing a Job: Reported Changes in Health, Symptoms and Illness Behavior. *Psychosomatic Medicine* 37: 106–122.

Katz, A. 1963. Social Adaptation in Chronic Illness: A Study of Hemophilia. *Journal of Public Health* 53: 1666–1675.

Kessler, RC. 1979. Stress, Social Status, and Psychological Distress. *Journal of Health and Social Behaviour* 20: 259–272.

Kessler, RC, and JD McLeod. 1984. Sex Differences in Vulnerability to Life Events. *American Sociological Review* 49: 620–631.

Kessler, RC, JD McLeod, and E Wethington. 1985. Cost of Caring: A Perspective on the Relationship Between Sex and Psychological Distress. In IG Sarason and BR Sarason eds. *Social support: Theory, research and application.* The Hague: Martinus Nijhoff.

LeUnes, AD, JR Nation, and NM Turley. 1980. Male-Female Performance in Learned Helplessness. *Journal of Psychology* 104: 255–258.

Linn, M, R Sandifor, and S Stein. 1985. Effects of Unemployment on Mental and Physical Health. *American Journal of Public Health* 75: 502–506.

Merikangas, KR. 1985. *Sex Differences in Depression.* Paper presented at the Murray Center (Radcliffe College) Conference: Mental Health in Social Context. Cambridge, MA.

Merikangas, KR, MM Weissman, and DL Pauls. 1985. Genetic Factors in the Sex Ratio of Major Depression. *Psychological Medicine* 15: 63–69.

Newmann, JP. 1984. Sex Differences in Symptoms of Depression: Clinical Disorder or Normal Distress? *Journal of Health and Social Behaviour* 25: 136–160.

Nolen-Hoeksema, S. 1987. Sex Differences in Unipolar Depression: Evidence and Theory. *Psychological Bulletin* 2: 259–282.

Parry, G. 1986. Paid Employment, Life Events, Social Support, and Mental Health in Working-Class Mothers. *Journal of Health and Social Behaviour* 27: 193–208.

Paykel, ES. 1978. Contribution of Life Events to Causation of Psychiatric Illness. *Psychological Medicine* 8: 245–253.

Paykel, ES. 1983. Methodological Aspects of Life Events Research. *Journal of Psychosomatic Research* 27: 341–352.

Pearlin, LI, and MA Lieberman. 1979. Social Sources of Emotional Stress. In RG Simmons ed. *Research in community and mental health,* 217–248. Greenwich, CT: JAI Press.

Pearlin, LI, and C Schooler. 1978. The Structure of Coping. *Journal of Health and Social Behaviour* 19: 2–21.

Radloff, LS. 1975. Sex Differences in Depression: The Effects of Occupation and Marital Status. *Sex Roles* 1: 249–265.

Radloff, LS. 1977. The CES-D Scale: A Self-Report Depression Scale for Research in the General Population. *Journal of Applied Psychology Measurement* 1: 385 401.

Radloff, LS, and MK Monroe. 1978. Sex Differences in Helplessness with Implications for Depression. In LS Hansen and ES Rapoza eds. *Career Development and the Counseling of Women,* 199–221. Springfield, IL: Thomas.

Radloff, LS, and DS Rae. 1981. Components of the Sex Difference in Depression. In RG Simmons ed. *Research in community and mental health,* 77–110. Greenwich, CT: JAI Press.

Roberts, RE, and SW Vernon. 1983. The Center for Epidemiological Studies Depression Scale: Its use in a Community Sample. *American Journal of Psychiatry* 140: 41–46.

Sarason, IG, JH Johnson, and JM Seigel. 1978. Assessing the Impact of Life Changes: Development of the Life Experience Survey. *Journal of Consulting and Clinical Psychology* 46: 932–946.

Schultz, R, and MT Rau. 1985. Social Support Through Life Course. In S Cohen and SL Syme eds. *Social Support and Health,* 129–149. New York: Academic.

Tousignant, M, R Brosseau, and L Tremblay. 1987. Sex Biases in Mental Health Scales: Do Women Tend to Report Less Serious Symptoms and Confide More than Men? *Psychological Medicine* 17: 203–217.

Turner, RJ, S Noh, WR Avison, and S Croak-Brossman. 1986a. *Marital Status and Depression: Vulnerability to Stress in Life Course Perspective.* Paper presented at the American Public Health Association Annual Meeting, Las Vegas.

Turner, RJ, S Noh, WR Avison, and S Croak-Brossman. 1986b. *Sources of Attenuation in the Stress-Distress Relationship: An Evaluation of Modest Innovations in the Use of Events Checklists.* Paper presented at the Second National Conference on Social Stress, Durham, NH, 1986.

Turner, RJ, S Noh, and DM Levin. 1985. Depression Across the Life Course: The Significance of Psychosocial Factors Among the Physically Disabled. In A Dean ed. *Depression in Multidisciplinary Perspective,* 32–60. New York: Brunner/Mazel.

Uhlenhuth, EH, ES Lipman, MB Balter, and M Stern. 1974. Symptom Intensity and Life Stress in the City. *Archives of General Psychiatry* 31: 759–764.

Verbrugge, LM. 1982. Women's Social Roles and Health. In P Berman and E Ramey eds. *Women: A Development Perspective,* 49–78. Bethesda, MD: National Institutes of Health. (Publication no. 82-2298).

Waldron, I, and J Herold. 1984. Employment, Attitudes Toward Employment and Women's Health. Paper presented at the meeting of the Society of Behavioral Medicine, Philadelphia.

Warr, P, and G Parry. 1982. Paid Employment and Women's Psychological Well-Being. *Psychological Bulletin* 3: 498–516.

Weissman, MM. 1987. Advances in Psychiatric Epidemiology: Rates and Risks for Major Depression. *American Journal of Public Health* 77: 445–451.

Weissman, MM, and GK Klerman. 1977. Sex Differences and the Epidemiology of Depression. *Archives of General Psychiatry* 34: 98–111.

Weissman, MM, D Sholomskas, M Pottenger, et al. 1977. Assessing Depressive Symptoms in Five Psychiatric Populations: A Validation Study. *American Journal of Epidemiology* 106: 203–214.

Wheaton, B. 1983. Stress, Personal Coping Resources, and Psychiatric Symptoms: An Investigation of Interactive Models. *Journal of Health and Social Behaviour* 24: 208–229.

14

The Impact of Working Conditions, Social Roles, and Personal Characteristics on Gender Differences in Distress[*]

Graham S. Lowe and Herbert C. Northcott

Central to an understanding of the work experiences of employed men and women is the issue of how job conditions influence overall physical and psychological well-being. Most major studies of how working conditions affect employee health and illness focus primarily on males (Caplan et al. 1980: 212; Kasl 1978: 15; Stellman 1978: 286; Haw 1982). Systematic research into job stress among women is thus a prerequisite to developing broader generalizations about the stress process.

Presently, there are two major models of job stress in the literature: the first focuses on job conditions and is used primarily to explain distress among males; the second model looks at the multiple demands of domestic and work roles and typically is used to account for the distress experienced by employed women. Because most of the studies of female job stress examine the relationship between domestic roles and paid employment, the comparisons are usually between employed, married women and housewives (Haw 1982: 135-136). In order to reconcile the two models of job stress, it is necessary to make direct comparisons between men and women who perform similar types of tasks. This facilitates an assessment of the relative impact of working conditions, gender-related social roles, and personal characteristics on employee distress levels. This article provides such an analysis by examining the distress reported by 992 unionized mail processors and letter carriers – about half of whom are women – employed by the Canada Post Corporation in Edmonton, Alberta.

Job stress can be generally defined as the result, typically measured in terms of negative health symptoms, of the imbalance between job demands and an individual's coping resources. Unpleasant working conditions include underload, in which case stress results from the underutilization of a person's capabilities, and alternatively, stress may be a reaction to overload, in which job demands exceed a workers' capabilities (see Kasl 1978: 12; Beehr and Newman 1978: 669–670; Fraser

* Reprinted, abridged and revised, from *Work and Occupations*, Vol. 15, Graham S. Lowe and Herbert C. Northcott, 'The impact of working conditions, social roles, and personal characteristics on gender difference in distress' pp. 55-77, 1988, with permission from Sage Publications, Thousand Oaks, Calif.

1983: 13; Haw 1982: 134). In this study, we measure job stress in terms of self-reported psychological distress, namely depression, irritability, and psychophysiological symptomatology. Studies of male employees amply document the relationships among working conditions, workers' perceptions of these conditions, and resulting psychological distress and poor physical health (see Kasl 1978; Fraser 1983; Beehr and Newman 1978; Cooper 1983, for literature reviews). One of the most comprehensive investigations of job stress, comparing men in 23 occupations, confirmed that certain working conditions produce mental and emotional strains (Caplan et al. 1980). The greatest job stressors are underutilization of skills and abilities, low job complexity, little participation in decision making, work role ambiguity, role conflict, unwanted overtime, heavy workload, and low social support from others at work. These stressors tend to cluster together. In fact, of all 23 occupations examined by Caplan and his colleagues, machine-paced assembly-line workers had the worst job conditions and highest overall distress. In other words, work that is routine, closely supervised, and repetitive leads to depression, anxiety, irritation, and a range of psychophysiological complaints.

While Caplan et al.'s (1980) study demonstrates that working conditions and job stress vary across occupations, and while a number of studies compare distress among males and females generally, there have been few attempts to examine men and women within the same occupation. Consequently, we are unable to generalize much beyond the suggestion that women tend to experience greater psychological and physiological distress than men (Haw 1982). At issue is whether or not men and women performing identical tasks will have similar stress reactions to the same working conditions. On one hand, evidence from epidemiological few surveys suggest that job conditions have little direct impact on sex differences in psychological distress (Kessler 1982). Yet, on the other hand, there is documentation that the psychological functioning of both men and women at work can be largely accounted for by job conditions, especially the degree of initiative, thought, and independent judgement required (Miller et al. 1979). One of the few studies of men and women performing identical tasks provides even stronger support for the argument that working conditions rather than gender determine job stress. A study of U.S. postal workers in machine-paced jobs found that sex per se accounted for less than 1% of the variance in anxiety, depression, and gastrointestinal and musculoskeletal complaints (Hurrell and Smith 1981). Nonetheless, there is a need to further investigate how men and women respond to the same working conditions (Miller 1980: 341; also see Messing and Reveret 1983).

Let us briefly review some of the reasons why males and females in the same job might report different levels of distress. Variations in health problems reported by men and women may reflect differences in reporting due to gender role socialization rather than differences in actual experience. In our culture boys are encouraged to display "manly" stoicism and not to admit to physical "weaknesses," including sickness. Girls, on the other hand, learn that emotional expressiveness is quite appropriate socially. This suggests that males might be less likely to report health problems than females.

Nevertheless, despite the possibility that differences in male and female health problems may be exaggerated, many researchers believe that, on the whole, health reports reflect real gender differences, rather than discrepancies in reporting. There are two major explanations for these "real" differences: the differential exposure (or social role) hypothesis and the differential vulnerability hypothesis. The first explanation argues that men and women are exposed to different work stressors as a consequence of sex segregation in the workplace. Even when men and women are exposed to the same work stressors, their distinctive non-work social roles may contribute to different patterns of distress. Because being a spouse, parent, and homemaker tend to be more demanding social roles for women than men, they produce higher levels of female distress. This argument suggests that role overload (too many demands) and role conflict (competing demands) are mainly experienced by women. For example, some studies suggest that married women continue to do the bulk of domestic work even when employed outside of the home (Meissner et al. 1975). Furthermore, in these non-work roles, it is argued that women look after the needs of other family members often to the neglect of themselves (Gove 1984). Men, on the other hand, are not expected to play a nurturant role and, indeed, are likely to benefit from female nurturance.

The second major explanation for possible real gender differences in distress revolves around the concept of vulnerability. That is, given the same stressor, males may be more or less vulnerable than females. While this may reflect differences in physical constitution, men and women can also be differentially vulnerable to a stressor because of psychological disposition, itself a combined product of physiological make-up and attitudes acquired through sex role socialization. To illustrate this point, suppose both men and women are required to lift heavy mail bags. One would expect that because males tend to be physically stronger than females, they would therefore be less vulnerable to physical strain. But suppose that the job of lifting heavy mail bags paid the same low wages to men and women, creating a potential source of strain. If pay is more important to men than women, then males would be more vulnerable to this particular stressor. In sum, the differential vulnerability hypothesis views men and women in the same job as vulnerable to different physical and psychological sources of distress.

If the vulnerability hypothesis is correct, then we would expect men and women doing the same job in the Post Office to have different work perceptions and stress reactions. On the other hand, if there is little or no truth to the claim that men and women have different vulnerabilities, then all workers in a particular job would have more or less identical job perceptions and job-related distress symptoms. Simply stated, we will examine whether it is primarily job or gender that determines an employee's reactions to workplace stressors (Feldberg and Glenn 1979).

One can find evidence supporting both perspectives. Gore and Mangione (1983) report that employment and marriage have a positive effect on mental health for both sexes. Similarly, other studies show that wives employed outside of the home usually have lower rates of depression than housewives – as do employed men (Rosenfield 1980). Nevertheless, there are few studies examining how employment outside the home actually reduces distress among wives (Haw 1982). It is equally plausible that the double burden of job and family may create additional stresses for wives, stresses from which their husbands are shielded by virtue of the traditional domestic division of labor (see Haynes and Feinlab 1980). Furthermore, one can find evidence supporting the view that different obligations and expectations of societal gender roles underlie sex differences in mental health. For example, married women may develop mental health problems due to the frustrations, low skills levels, and low prestige associated with their traditional homemaking role (Gove 1972; Gove and Tudor 1973), while the roles of household head and paid employee may contribute to the mental health of married men. Further evidence suggests that the interactive effects of family responsibilities and employment may create considerable distress for women but not for men (see Nathanson 1975; Cleary and Mechanic 1983).

In order to determine the extent to which men and women may react differently to working conditions, it is necessary to compare males and females performing similar jobs. The central question guiding our analysis is whether observed male-female differences in distress, operationalized by means of three widely used self-report measures – depression, irritability, and psychophysiological complaints – result from gender-related social demands (spouse, parent, homemaker) or are primarily a reaction to working conditions.

The Study Population

Our data come from a survey of unionized postal workers employed by the Canada Post Corporation in Edmonton, Alberta. The study was conducted in collaboration with two unions[1]: the Letter Carriers Union of Canada (LCUC), which at the time of this study represented 776 letter carriers (including a small group of mail truck drivers), and the Canadian Union of Postal Workers (CUPW), which represented 753 primarily manual employees inside the city's main postal plant, where mail is processed for delivery. Broadly speaking, the two union groups represent polar opposites in blue-collar work. The letter carriers, being relatively free from supervision, enjoy a fairly high level of job autonomy. In contrast, CUPW members encounter factory-like conditions in the main postal plant, where tasks are routinized, closely supervised, and often automated. The fact that almost half of the total population studied was female provides a unique opportunity to investigate whether gender-specific characteristics do indeed make a difference in how employees respond to stressful work situations. Respondents belong to strong unions, thereby ensuring that job requirements and conditions are standard for everyone in a job classification. Moreover, both "inside" (CUPW) and "outside" (LCUC) workers are subjected to the same employee relations policies and bureaucratic organization. This all but eliminates the confounding effects of studying workers who have similar job titles but work in different organizations. In short, our study population is especially suited to an investigation of the relationships among job characteristics, gender, and employee stress symptomatology.

The two unions cooperated with the researchers throughout the study, advising on research design, commenting on questionnaire drafts, and providing mailing lists of their memberships. A pretested questionnaire containing items tapping a variety of work- and stress-related variables was mailed to all union members early in 1983. A total of 992 completed questionnaires were returned, for a response rate of 65% (68% for CUPW, 62% for LCUC). Following Heberlein and Baumgartner (1978), we used a five-stage mailing procedure: letters from both researchers and union officials, a questionnaire with a postcard for keeping track of respondents without violating confidentiality, a follow-up letter, a duplicate questionnaire sent to nonrespondents, and a final follow-up letter.

Lacking complete demographic data on the membership of the unions either in the Edmonton area or nationally, we are unable to claim that our results are fully representative at either level. However, we did ascertain that the sex structures of our respondent groups and of the larger populations were comparable and can therefore draw some tentative conclusions about the Edmonton membership. Furthermore, the fairly uniform working conditions for Canadian postal employees in large urban centers also permit some generalizations. More tentatively, our findings may be viewed as indicative of broad trends in gender differences in stress reactions to working conditions.

In most respects, respondents from LCUC and CUPW had similar personal characteristics. For both groups, the mean age was 34, the average years of education was 12, about 60% were married, and over one-third had at least one dependent child. There were, however, some notable differences: mean length of employment with Canada Post was seven years for CUPW members, compared to nine for LCUC; 31% in CUPW worked part-time (averaging 24 hours weekly), compared to only 9% in LCUC; only 6% of LCUC members worked afternoon or evening shifts, whereas 59% of CUPW members were on these shifts; and, finally, CUPW had a higher percentage of women in its membership – 57% versus 36% for LCUC. The proportion of women in these two unions was relatively high, considering that only 30% of all union members in Canada at that time were women (Statistics Canada 1982: 623).

Measures

Perceived Job Characteristics

Because perceived stressors in the work environment are typically used to explain employee distress, it is essential to know if women provide the same job evaluations as men for identical tasks. We address this question by examining six job dimensions obtained by a factor analysis of 29 description items, each scored on a seven-point Likert scale (adapted from the 1977 U.S. Quality of Employment Survey; see Quinn and Staines 1979). A varimax rotation was used and only those items with factor loadings of .40 or above were included. The following six factors emerged: (1) supervision (discipline handled fairly, supervisor gets people to work together, supervisor concerned about employee welfare, supervisor is friendly, supervisor is competent, supervisor is helpful to me, supervisor treats some employees better than others; alpha = .90); (2) variety/challenge (use my skills and abilities, can be creative, work is meaningful, work is interesting; alpha = .78); (3) work intensity (work very hard, work very fast; alpha = .72); (4) autonomy (can decide what I do, decide when to take breaks, determine work speed, decide how job gets done; alpha = .65); (5) financial rewards (good pay, good job security, good fringe benefits; alpha = .53); and (6) coworkers (coworkers take a personal interest in me, coworkers are helpful; alpha = .68).

Factor loadings for the remaining seven items did not produce discrete task dimensions. However, because the literature places importance on role conflict and time pressure as potential strains (see, for example, House et al. 1979; Caplan et al. 1980), we also included time pressure as tapped by a single item (never enough time) and two items measuring competing demands, or work role conflict (can't satisfy everybody, no conflicting demands; alpha = .46). A test for a possible gender effect in how workers perceive these eight job characteristics yielded no significant differences for men and women performing identical tasks (see Northcott and Lowe 1987). Furthermore, factor analysis performed separately for males and females (results not reported) yielded similar factor structures. We are thus fairly confident that these key job characteristics are perceived in similar ways by workers of either sex.

Finally, we measured work place social support, given its potential moderating effect on stress. A summary score was created from responses to the question, "How much can each of the following people be relied on when things get tough at work? Immediate supervisor, shop steward or union representative, other people at work," each answered on a four-point scale ranging from "very much" to "not at all."

Working Conditions

We also included five "objective" measures of the work environment: (1) union membership (CUPW/LCUC) to tap in a general sense the objective differences between the work done by the letter carriers and letter processors; (2) part-time status, because part-time employees may be exposed to proportionately less job stress; (3) working afternoon or evening shifts, a factor that has been identified in previous studies as a major stressor; (4) average hours of weekly overtime, which is also a principal source of stress; and (5) seniority, residualized on age to tap the effects of time on the job independent of age.

Personal Characteristics

The key personal characteristic we examined is respondent's sex. We also measured respondent's age and education (in years), as well as family income.

Social Roles

The following social roles directly linked to gender are included in our analysis: marital status (measured by three categories: married or living common-law; never-married; and divorced, separated, or widowed); having an employed spouse; the number of children aged 6 to 17 living at home; the number of children under the age of 6 living at home; and nonwork social support (measured with the same question as for workplace social support, but with reference to the respondent's spouse, friends, and relatives). Further, in order to assess the degree to which home life and work activities are compatible for postal employees, we asked the two-thirds of our respondents who were either married, living with someone, or were single parents, "How much do your job and your family life interfere with each other?" (1 = a lot, 7 = not at all).

Stress Outcomes

We utilized three dependent variables that document the self-reported health effects of stressful working conditions: depression, irritability, and psychophysiological complaints. The complexity of the stress process requires the use of multiple outcome measures (Gore and Mangione 1983: 311). To measure depression, we used a summary score of the 20-item CES-D scale (Markush and Favero 1974). Irritability is measured by a summary score for a seven-item anger/aggression scale developed by Petersen and Kellam (1977). Both scales have good inter-item reliability (alphas of .92 for depression and .89 for irritability). All items use a five-point response scale with 1 meaning that the symptom is never experienced and 5 indicating that it is always present. Finally, we used a summary score for six psychophysiological complaints (general tiredness, loss of appetite, irritability, sleeplessness, dizziness, and headaches). Symptoms are assessed with reference to the previous three months and are measured on a five point scale in which 1 is "never" and 5 is "always." This scale has a reliability alpha of .81.

Our analysis proceeds as follows: first, we compare the reported incidence of depression, irritability, and psychophysiological symptoms among males and females in each of the two unions (CUPW and LCUC). Second, we attempt to explain distress by regressing five blocks of variables – gender, personal characteristics, social roles, working conditions, and perceived job characteristics – on the three stress outcomes. Lastly, we perform regression analysis separately for males and females to determine if our independent variables influence distress differently for women than for men.

Results

With respect to family versus work demands, letter sorters were far more likely than letter carriers to experience tension between job demands and home life. Females, especially in the letter sorter group, were more likely than their male co-workers to report conflict between work and home. This greater conflict between work and non-work roles experienced by our female respondents supports the argument that home and family obligations fall disproportionately on women. Our data also show, however, that the nature of one's job affects these links between work and family. As shown in the following, letter sorting is more stressful than letter carrying. Consequently, letter sorters of both sexes are more likely than letter carriers to report that their job interferes with their family life. Shifts, weekend work, and changing schedules are all sources of interference. Furthermore, stress that arises on the job does not stay at work but gets carried home. People in stressful jobs come home with less energy and with a "shorter fuse" than do those who work at more rewarding tasks in a pleasant environment. It also takes the distressed employee longer to unwind. In other words, both work scheduling and work-generated distress interfere with family life. By contrast, letter carriers, who work weekdays in a less stressful environment, are far less likely than letter sorters to report that their work interferes with their family life.

Table 1 shows the percent distributions for males and females on our three measures of distress. Respondents are categorized as letter carriers (LCUC members) and letter sorters (CUPW members). Comparing male letter carriers with male letter sorters, and female letter carriers with female letter sorters, we see that the letter sorters regardless of sex are more likely to report depression, irritability, and psychophysiological complaints than the letter carriers. Further, comparing men and women doing the same work, we see that women tend to experience higher levels of distress than men regardless of their general work situation, and that this gender difference tends to be more pronounced for the letter sorters than for the letter carriers.

To summarize, there are variations in stress between the two work groups that we hypothesize are due to the effects of different working conditions. Further, with respect to gender, we detect a tendency for women to experience a somewhat greater frequency of distress in each of the work groups. Thus working conditions seem to induce similar stress symptoms in men and women, with the important caveat that women report somewhat higher levels of symptomatology than men.

We will now investigate the relative importance of gender in explaining variations in stress outcomes. In our regression procedure, we sequentially enter five blocks of predictor variables: gender, personal characteristics, social roles, working conditions, and perceived job characteristics. We estimate three separate equations, one for each distress measure. The regression analyses are summarized in Table 2.

TABLE 1
Perceived job characteristics and self-reported distress, for letter carriers and letter processors, by gender

	Percent Giving Negative Response			
	Letter Carriers (LCUC)		Letter Sorters (CUPW)	
	Males	Females	Males	Females
Perceived Job Characteristics[1]				
Supervision	33	33	59	56
Variety and Challenge	36 *	52	60 *	70
Autonomy	18	20	50	53
Financial Rewards	9	6	12	13
Co-workers	30	26	25	26
Intensity	55 *	67	59	64
Competing Demands	40	37	54	54
Time Pressure	30	27	41 *	31
Social Support at Work	58 *	45	64 *	55
Self-Reported Distress[2]				
Percent Irritable:				
Often or Always	2	4	8	10
Sometimes	31	30	30 *	39
Percent Depressed:				
Often or Always	1	2	3	5
Sometimes	33	35	41 *	53
Percent Reporting Psycho-physiological Symptoms:				
Often or Always	2	7	9	13
Sometimes	43 *	54	51 *	59
(n)	(304)	(173)	(221)	(290)

* The difference between males and females is significant at $p \leq .05$.

1 The job characteristics variables are each composites of several items (except Time Pressure). The items are rated on a 7-point scale and scale values 1 to 3, or 4 to 7 (depending on the item), indicate a negative perception of working conditions. "Social support at work" is also a composite, but is rated on a 4-point scale, where 1 and 2 indicated little or no support. The figures reported in this table are the percentages of respondents indicating a negative perception of work characteristics (less than a value of 3.5 or more than a value of 4.5, as appropriate, on the summary scales) or indicating a lack of social support at work (less than 2.5 on the social support summary scale).

2 The irritability, depression and psychophysiological distress measures are composites of 7, 20, and 6 items respectively. Frequency of recent occurrence is assessed on a 5-point scale (1. never, 2. rarely, 3. sometimes, 4. often, 5. always). In this table "often" or "always" is a summary scale value greater than 3.5, while "sometimes" is scale values 2.5 to 3.5.

Regression of gender, personal characteristics, social roles, working conditions, and perceived job characteristics on depression, irritability, and psychophysiological symptoms

	Depression			Irritability			Psychophysiological Symptoms		
	b	B	ΔR²	b	B	ΔR²	b	B	ΔR²
I. Gender (female)	.13 *	.11	.02	.11 *	.08	.01	.21 *	.15	.03
II. Personal Characteristics									
Age	-.00 *	-.07		-.00	-.06		-.00	-.04	
Education	-.00	-.02		.01	.02		.00	.00	
Income (family)	-.00 *	-.11	.04	-.00	-.07	.03	-.00	-.08	.02
III. Social Roles									
Marital Status (married)	.00	.00		-.03	-.02		.05	.03	
Marital Status (widowed, divorced, separated)	.02	.01		.01	.00		-.12	-.04	
Working Spouse	.04	.04		.08	.06		.02	.02	
No. of Children 6-17	-.01	-.01		.01	.01		.01	.01	
No. of Children under 6	-.01	-.01		.01	.01		-.02	-.02	
Non-Work Social Support	-.01	-.06	.03	.01	.04	.01	.01	.03	.00
IV. Working Conditions									
Union (CUPW/LCUC)	.07	.06		.01	.01		.04	.03	
Part-time	-.08	-.06		-.10	-.06		-.03	-.02	
Shift (non day)	.05	.04		.13 *	.09		.19 *	.13	
Overtime	.00	.02		-.00	-.00		.01	.06	
Seniority (residualized on age)	-.00	-.01	.04	.00	.06	.04	.00	.04	.06
V. Perceived Job Characteristics									
Supervision	.02	.04		-.04 *	-.09		-.00	-.01	
Variety/Challenge	-.07 *	-.17		-.06 *	-.13		-.06 *	-.13	
Intensity	.01	.03		.01 *	.03		.03 *	.07	
Autonomy	-.03	-.07		-.03	-.06		-.00	-.01	
Financial Rewards	-.04 *	-.08		-.04 *	-.07		-.06 *	-.10	
Co-workers	-.04 *	-.11		-.02	-.04		-.03	-.07	
Time Pressure	.01	.03		.00	.00		.01	.04	
Competing Demands	.09 *	.25		.12 *	.26		.12 *	.26	
Social Support at Work	.02	-.06	.18	-.02	-.05	.18	-.03 *	-.09	.18
CONSTANT	2.85			2.60			2.61		
R²	.31			.27			.29		
(n)	(819)			(819)			(819)		

ΔR² = change in R2 from one block of explanatory variables to another

*p ≤ .05

Scanning the first columns in Table 2, our initial observation is that gender has a small but significant impact on self-reported depression. Specifically, after controlling for all other work and nonwork variables, women still experience slightly higher levels of depressive symptomatology than men. Gender alone, however, accounts for only 2% of the variation in depression scores.

The most impressive change in the R2 comes when the nine perceived job characteristics are entered into the regression equation. The proportion of explained variance rises from 13% to 31%. The prior addition of personal characteristics and social roles produced an R2 of only .09, suggesting that these factors are far less important in explaining depression than the subjective perceptions of the work performed. Similarly, objective working conditions account for little of the variance in depression. Among the perceived job characteristics, four exert a significant impact on depression in the regression analysis: variety/challenge, financial rewards, coworkers, and competing demands. We should point out that two other variables – family income and age – do have weak yet significant negative influences on depression scores.

Examining the relative importance of job characteristics more closely, we see that competing demands, or work role conflict, is the major predictor of depression, followed by the degree of variety and challenge provided by the job. The influence of friendly and helpful coworkers, good financial rewards, gender, family income, and age is modest, although statistically significant. In sum, job characteristics, especially competing demands and having little variety and challenge, contribute more to depression than do gender, other personal characteristics, or social roles.

Table 2 also reports a similar regression analysis, this time using irritability as the dependent variable. Once again, the initial observation is that gender exerts a small but significant impact on irritability even after controlling for the effects of all other independent variables. Another parallel with the analysis of depression is that while the amount of variance explained in steps I through IV is quite low, the introduction of the nine job characteristics in step V boosts the R2 substantially (from .09 to .27). None of the personal characteristics or social role measures entered into the equation at steps II and III have significant bearing on irritability scores.

Another strong similarity with the depression analysis is that perceived job characteristics are the best predictors of irritability. Thus irritability is a likely distress symptom in jobs perceived by incumbents to have competing demands, little variety or challenge, inadequate supervision, and relatively poor financial rewards. Recall that competing demands and variety/challenge were also the strongest predictors of depression. Nonetheless, it generally seems that depression and irritability are distinct manifestations of distress. Specifically, supervision affects only irritability, whereas coworker relations are significant only for depression.

In the analysis of the irritability data, we find one other significant predictor variable. Working afternoon or evening shifts contributes in a minor way to irritability, and is a marginally more important predictor than gender. In sum, 27% of the variation in irritability can be accounted for in our regression equation by four specific job characteristics, and by work shift and gender.

The last of the three distress measures we study is a summary score for psychophysiological symptoms. These results are also reported in Table 2. Our first observation is consistent with the previous regression results: gender exerts a minor but significant influence on distress while personal characteristics and social roles have very little explanatory power. Of the working conditions variables in the equation, shift work contributes significantly to psychophysiological symptoms, as was also true for irritability.

Once again, perceived job characteristics are the strongest predictors of distress. A total of five of these characteristics, even more than for depression and irritability, are statistically significant. As in the case of depression, financial rewards exert a weak negative influence on the dependent variable. And for the first time in the three regression equations, social support at work (from coworkers, supervisors, or union officials) and work intensity have a significant impact. Once again, competing demands emerges as the single most important explanatory variable, with variety/challenge also having an important impact.

Finally, as in the two previous analyses, there is a substantial jump in the R2 between steps IV and V, when perceived job characteristics are entered into the equation. In comparison with general working conditions, social roles, personal characteristics, and gender, workers' perceptions of specific task characteristics are the most important determinants of all three manifestations of distress.

A consistent finding is that gender has a weak yet significant relationship with the three types of distress – depression, irritability, and psychophysiological symptoms – independent of all other work and nonwork variables. Our data do not permit further exploration of why there is a small gender effect. We did, however, explore whether or not work and gender interact to produce different stress reactions for men and women. To test possible interaction effects, we added interaction terms (gender X each independent variable, all entered as a block) to the regression equations in Table 2. The results (not reported) fail to add significantly to the R2s in these tables. In other words, men and women tend to experience the same problems when in the same situation. However, women tend to report higher levels of distress than men.

Table 3 disaggregates our data by sex, presenting separate regression equations for males and females. This allows us to further examine whether each predictor variable in the equation has the same impact on both sexes, or whether women respond to potential stressors differently than men. We have included all of the independent variables in the regression equations (except gender, which is now the control variable). Table 3 shows that a few variables do appear to affect women differently than men. For example, shift work may be more of a problem for men, contributing to higher irritability and psychophysiological symptoms scores. While shift work has a similar effect for women, this effect is not statistically significant. Financial rewards are negatively related to all three distress measures for men, but are less important in explaining female distress. Similarly, family income is a significant predictor of psychophysiological symptoms among men but not women. In addition, there are some variables uniquely influencing female distress. Specifically, work intensity and being widowed, divorced, or separated are significantly related to the level of psychophysiological symptoms among females, but not among males. Having helpful and friendly coworkers seems to alleviate this type of distress for women. Finally, competing demands (role conflict) is the only variable significantly related to all three forms of distress among workers of either sex. In short, the previous influence of role conflict in occupational stress is confirmed by our data. Furthermore, it is important to note that despite the differential impact of several variables on male and female distress Table 3 suggests that there are far more similarities than dissimilarities regarding the impact of personal characteristics, social roles, and working conditions on the distress experienced by men and women.

TABLE 3
Regression of personal characteristics, social roles, working conditions, and perceived job characteristics, on three measures of distress, controlling for gender

	Depression				Irritability				Psychophysiological Symptoms			
	Males		Females		Males		Females		Males		Females	
	b	B	b	B	b	B	b	B	b	B	b	B
Personal Characteristics												
Age	-.00	-.06	-.01	-.10	-.01	-.09	-.00	-.04	-.00	-.07	.00	.06
Education	.01	.03	.00	.00	.01	.02	.00	.01	.01	.02	-.01	-.04
Income (family)	-.00	-.10	-.00	-.11	-.00	-.09	-.00	-.02	-.00	-.12*	-.00	-.06
Social Roles												
Marital Status (married)	.00	.00	-.02	-.02	.10	.07	-.18	-.13	.08	.06	-.01	-.01
Marital Status (widowed, divorced, separated)	.09	.03	-.03	-.01	-.03	-.01	.00	.00	-.02	-.01	-.28	-.12*
Working Spouse	.04	.03	.05	.04	.03	.02	.11	.09	.05	.03	-.02	-.02
No. of Children 6-17	.00	.00	-.02	-.02	.00	.01	-.01	-.01	-.00	-.00	.03	.04
No. of Children under 6	-.02	-.02	-.01	-.01	-.08	-.07	.07	.06	-.08	-.07	.06	.05
Non-Work Social Support	-.02	-.08	-.01	-.03	.01	.04	.01	.03	.01	.05	.00	.01
Working Conditions												
Union (CUPW/LCUC)	.03	.02	.11	.09	-.06	.04	.07	.05	.06	.04	-.01	-.01
Part-time	-.17	-.08	-.04	-.03	-.28	-.11*	-.02	-.01	-.21	-.08	.08	.06
Shift (not day)	.09	.07	.00	.00	.19	.12*	.08	.06	.27	.18†	.11	.08
Overtime	.00	.03	-.00	-.02	.00	.01	-.01	-.04	.01	.04	.02	.07
Seniority (residualized on age)	-.00	-.03	-.00	-.03	.00	.04	.00	.08	.00	.02	.00	.09
Perceived Job Characteristics												
Supervision	.01	.02	.02	.06	-.05	-.11*	-.04	-.08	.00	.01	-.02	-.04
Variety/Challenge	-.06	-.17†	-.08	-.19f	-.04	-.10	-.10	-.19f	-.04	-.09	-.10	-.21f
Intensity	.00	.01	.02	.05	.00	.01	.03	.06	.01	.01	.07	.16†
Autonomy	-.03	-.08	-.02	-.04	-.04	-.10	-.01	-.01	-.03	-.07	.03	.06
Financial Rewards	-.05	-.12†	-.02	-.03	-.08	-.15†	.02	.03	-.09	-.16f	-.01	-.02
Co-workers	-.04	-.10*	-.05	-.13*	-.01	-.02	-.02	-.04	-.01	-.01	-.06	-.14†
Time Pressure	.02	.06	-.00	-.00	.01	-.02	-.01	-.02	.03	.07	.00	.01
Competing Demands	.08	.21f	.11	.30f	.12	.25f	.12	.27f	.12	.27f	.10	.22f
Social Support at Work	-.02	-.06	-.02	-.06	-.02	-.05	-.01	-.04	-.03	-.08	-.03	-.10
CONSTANT	3.01		2.84		2.97		2.31		2.77		2.71	
R²	.32		.28		.31		.25		.32		.27	
(n)	(437)		(382)		(437)		(382)		(437)		(382)	

NOTE: *p < .05; †p < .01; fp < .001.

With two exceptions, none of the personal characteristics or gender-related social roles we measure have statistically significant effects in Table 3. The two exceptions both pertain to psychophysiological symptoms: family income is negatively associated with this form of distress for men (the association for women is also negative although not statistically significant), while being widowed, separated, or divorced has a negative impact among females (the effect for males is similarly negative although not statistically significant). A final general comment on Table 3 is that R2s are typically higher for men than women. Indeed, the R2s for all three distress measures for men are either .31 or .32, while female R2s range from .25 to .28. This suggests that the model tested in this study to explain male and female distress may be somewhat more complete for men than for women.

Let us now briefly examine each of the distress measures individually. Looking first at depression, competing demands is undeniably the crucial variable, more so for women than men. Variety/challenge is also central. Less important, yet still significant for both sexes, is relations with coworkers. Financial rewards affect depression among men, but this variable is less influential for women. None of the other variables make a significant contribution.

Regarding irritability, we find two similarities with the results for depression. First, receiving competing demands is the major contributor to distress for all workers. Second, financial rewards are linked to irritability symptoms, although for men only, while women are more strongly influenced by the variety/challenge variable. Males also respond more to poor supervision and performing part-time or shift work. In short, work variables, not social roles or personal characteristics, are the principal factors explaining irritability.

Lastly, for psychophysiological symptoms, competing demands again emerges as the strongest predictor of this form of distress for all respondents. The variety/challenge job characteristic is almost as important as competing demands for women but is less significant for men. Work intensity (working hard and fast) contributes significantly to psychophysiological symptoms among female employees only. Relations with coworkers also influences women but not men, while the reverse is true of financial rewards. Furthermore, males react more stressfully to two factors than do women: shift work and a relatively low family income.

Discussion

Let us now return to the two models of job stress outlined at the beginning of the article. The first model examines working conditions and typically is applied to male employees. The second model focuses on the multiple demands of domestic and work roles, usually as they influence stress levels among employed married women. Both models are structural, being primarily concerned with how work and nonwork roles contribute to distress. We examine both work and nonwork variables and find that work variables are the most important predictors of distress. While gender alone has a weak, significant impact on all three distress measures, its explanatory power is greatly overshadowed by the strong, pervasive influence of job conditions.

Some qualifications are in order, however. At a general level, we have compared the relative influences of two different categories of variables, one representing objective characteristics, the other encompassing individual perceptions. While perceptions do vary according to objective job conditions, it is perhaps understandable that perceptions of one's objective world are better predictors of distress than are objective indicators. Furthermore, there are some gender differences. For example, we find that women do tend to experience somewhat greater distress than men. Even though none of our nonwork social role variables (with the one exception of marital status noted above in Table 3) had significant net effects in the regression analyses, it is possible that the observed gender effect may be due to factors that we have not measured.

The main thrust of this article was to explain male and female variation, if any, in job-related distress. In this one respect, our regression analyses contain some findings of general relevance to the study of occupational stress. The fact that each of the three outcomes (depression, irritability, and psychophysiological complaints) were affected somewhat differently by the predictor variables, despite their moderately strong inter-correlations (not shown), suggests that we need to know more about the precise etiology of these different forms of distress. More important for our understanding of occupational stress, however, is the fact that two job characteristics exerted a significant influence on all three types of distress. For males and females combined, the extent to which one experienced competing job demands and the degree of variety and challenge perceived in one's tasks were key predictors of distress. The same can be said for competing demands based on the regression equations disaggregated by sex. Interestingly, however, while variety/challenge affects both sexes in terms of depression, it is somewhat more influential for females than males with respect to irritability and psychophysiological symptoms.

The central importance of competing demands is consistent with findings from the University of Michigan studies on occupational sources of distress (see Kahn 1980; Caplan et al. 1980: 85). Subordinate employees who receive conflicting or ambiguous demands on the job are clearly in a stressful situation. This is not confined to blue-collar jobs, as Sutton's (1984) research on teachers demonstrates. The distressfulness of competing demands for workers in our study may involve indirect or interactive effects not captured in our model, such as possible interactions with the type of supervision received. However, competing demands are only a partial explanation for the psychological and psychophysiological distress experienced by our respondents. As Karasek (1979) convincingly argues, a worker's decision-making discretion to meet job demands is a fundamental ingredient of the stress process. Many of the postal employees we surveyed, especially those working in the confines of the main postal terminal, performed routine tasks with little scope for decision making. We find that variety and challenge in a job is moderately associated with autonomy (r = .44) and supervision (r = .37). Clearly, more thorough research into the relationships among the various aspects of task structure is needed, especially in more heterogeneous samples than ours. However, the evidence we have presented suggests that a cluster of characteristics focused around job demands, routinization, and decision-making discretion are crucial for explaining levels of employee distress.

Finally, it is especially noteworthy that the social role variables had a virtually negligible impact on distress. We thus take issue with Cleary and Mechanic (1983) when they argue that being a working parent contributes to depression for women but not for men. More broadly, our data are consonant with other evidence suggesting that, among married persons who have children, working wives are no more depressed than husbands (see Gore and Mangione 1983). As for the absence of significant effects in terms of personal characteristics, we must caution against drawing any firm conclusions. This is mainly because of the relatively homogenous character of our sample; a more diverse group of employees may, for instance, show distress differences along education and income lines.

We have gone beyond previous stress research in attempting to identify which specific job characteristics and working conditions induce stress among male and female workers. Our analyses show that certain aspects of both the specific tasks performed and the larger working environment influence women somewhat differently than men. For example, doing shift work is a more stressful experience for men than women, and low family income tends to have a stronger stress effect on men. Furthermore, for females but not for males, having friendly and helpful coworkers contributes somewhat to lower depression levels, while increased work intensity tends to exacerbate psychophysiological symptoms. Also remarkable about our regression results (in Table 3) is that social support on or off the job has virtually no net direct effect on distress for either men or women, as some previous research might lead us to predict (see House 1981; Caplan et al. 1980). The links between social support on the job and the supervision and coworker variables ($r = .34$ and $.37$, respectively) require further exploration in this regard. A far more adequate test of the effects of social support would incorporate direct, indirect, and interactive effects into a model of distress (Wheaton 1985). Our basic point, though, concerns the rather direct and pervasive influence of job characteristics on self-reported distress among both males and females. That is, we find that distress experienced by postal workers is more a function of working conditions than a function of gender differentials in vulnerability or of gender-related non-work social roles. Nevertheless, there do appear to be some gender differences particularly in the amount of distress experienced. Only by extending this research to men and women performing similar tasks in a diversity of work settings will we more fully comprehend the sources of gender variation in job stress.

Notes

1   These two unions have since merged into one union (CUPW).

References for Further Reading

Cooper, CL and R Payne eds. 1988. *Causes, Coping and Consequences of Stress at Work.* New York: Wiley.

Karasek, R, and T Theorell. 1990. *Healthy Work: Stress, Productivity, and the Reconstruction of Working Life.* New York: Basic Books.

Mirowsky, J, and CE Ross. 1989. *Social Causes of Psychological Distress.* New York: Aldine de Gruyter.

Sauter, SL, JJ Hurrell, and CL Cooper eds. 1989. *Job Control and Worker Health.* Chichester: Wiley.

White, J. 1990. *Mail and Female: Women and the Canadian Union of Postal Workers.* Toronto: Thompson Educational Publishing.

References

Beehr, TA, and JE Newman. 1978. Job Stress, Employee Health, and Organizational Effectiveness: A Facet Analysis, Model, and Literature Review. *Personnel Psychology* 31: 665–699.

Canadian Labour Congress, Labor Education and Studies Center. 1982. *Towards a More Humanized Technology: Exploring the Impact of Video Display Terminals on the Health and Working Conditions of Canadian Office Workers.* Ottawa: Canadian Labor Congress.

Caplan, RD, S Cobb, JRP French, Jr., R van Harrison, and SR Pinneau, Jr. 1980. *Job Demands and Worker Health: Main Effects and Occupational Differences.* Ann Arbor: University of Michigan, Institute for Social Research, Survey Research Center. First published in April 1975 by NIOSH, HEW pub. no. H1OSH 75–160.

Cleary, PD, and D Mechanic. 1983. Sex Differences in Psychological Distress Among Married People. *Journal of Health and Social Behavior* 24: 111–121.

Cooper, CL. 1983. Identifying Stressors at Work: Recent Research Developments. *Journal of Psychosomatic Research* 27: 369–376.

Feldberg, RL and EN Glenn. 1979. Male and Female: Job Versus Gender Models in the Sociology of Work. *Social Problems* 26: 524–538.

Fraser, TM. 1983. *Human Stress, Work and Job Satisfaction: A Critical Approach.* Occupational Safety and Health Series 50. Geneva: International Labor Office.

Gore, S, and TW Mangione. 1983. Social Roles, Sex Roles and Psychological Stress: Additive and Interactive Models of Sex Differences. *Journal of Health and Social Behavior* 24: 300–312.

Gove, WR. 1972. The Relationship Between Sex Roles, Marital Status, and Mental Illness. *Social Forces* 51: 34–44.

Gove, WR. 1984. Gender Differences in Mental and Physical Illness: The Effects of Fixed Roles and Nurturant Roles. *Social Science and Medicine* 19: 77–91.

Gove, WR, and JF Tudor. 1973. Adult Sex Roles and Mental Illness, 1. *Amerrican Journal of Sociology* 78: 812–835.

Haw, MA. 1982. Women, Work and Stress: A Review and Agenda for the Future. *Journal of Health and Social Behavior* 23: 132–144.

Haynes, SG, and M Feinlab. 1980. Women, Work and Coronary Heart Disease: Prospective Findings From the Framingham Heart Study. *American Journal of Public Health* 70: 133–144.

Heberlein, TA, and R Baumgartner. 1978. Factors Affecting Response Rates to Mailed Questionnaires: A Quantitative Analysis of the Published Literature. *American Sociological Review* 43: 447–462.

House, JS. 1981. *Work Stress and Social Support.* Reading, MA: Addison-Wesley.

House, JS, AJ McMichael, JA Wells, BH Kaplan, and LR Landerman. 1979. Occupational Stress and Health Among Factory Workers. *Journal of Health and Social Behavior* 20: 139–160.

Hurrell, JJ, and MJ Smith. 1981. Sources of Stress Among Machine-Paced Letter-Sorting-Machine Operators. In G Salvendy and MJ Smith eds. *Machine Pacing and Occupational Stress,* 253-259. London: Taylor & Francis.

Kahn, RL. 1980. Conflict, Ambiguity, and Overload: Three Elements of Job Stress. In D Katz et al. eds. *The Study of Organizations,* 419-428. San Francisco: Jossey-Bass.

Karasek, RA. 1979. Job Demands, Job Decision Latitude and Mental Health: Implications for Job Redesign. *Administrative Science Quarterly* 24: 285–308.

Kasl, SV. 1978. Epidemiological Contributions to the Study of Work Stress. In CL Cooper and R Payne eds. *Stress and Work,* 3-48. New York: John Wiley.

Kessler, RC. 1982. A Disaggregation of the Relationship Between Socioeconomic Status and Psychological Distress. *American Sociological Review* 47: 752–764.

Markush, RE, and RV Favero. 1974. Epidemiological Assessment of Stressful Life Events, Depressed Mood and Psychophysiological Symptoms: A Preliminary Report. In BS Dohrenwend and BP Dohrenwend eds. *Stressful Life Events: Their Nature and Effects,* 171-190. New York: John Wiley.

Meissner, M, EW Humphreys, SM Meis, and WJ Scheu. 1975. No Exit for Wives: Sexual Division of Labour and the Cumulation of Household Demands. *Canadian Review of Sociology and Anthropology* 12: 424–439.

Messing, K, and J-P Reveret. 1983. Are Women in Female Jobs for Their Health? A Study of Working Conditions and Health Effects in the Fish-Processing Industry in Quebec. *International Journal of Health Services* 13: 635–648.

Miller, J. 1980. Individual and Occupational Determinants of Job Satisfaction: A Focus on Gender Differences. *Sociology of Work and Occupations* 7: 337–366.

Miller, J, C Schooler, ML Kohn and KA Miller. 1979.Women and Work: The Psychological Effects of Occupational Conditions. *American Journal of Sociology* 85: 66–94.

Nathanson, CA. 1975. Illness and the Feminine Role: A Theoretical Review. *Social Science and Medicine* 9: 57–62.

Northcott, HC, and GS Lowe. 1987. Job and Gender Influences in the Subjective Experience of Work. *Canadian Review of Sociology and Anthropology* 24: 117–131.

Petersen, AC, and SG Kellam. 1977. Measurement of the Psychological Well-Being of Adolescents. *Journal of Youth and Adolescence* 6: 229–246.

Quinn, RP, and GL Staines. 1979. *The 1977 Quality of Employment Survey.* Ann Arbor: University of Michigan, Institute for Social Research, Survey Research Center.

Rosenfield, S. 1980. Sex Differences in Depression: Do Women Always Have Higher Rates? *Journal of Health and Social Behavior* 21: 33–42.

Statistics Canada. 1982. *Annual Report of the Minister of Supply and Services Canada Under the Corporations and Labor Unions Return Act, Part II: Labor Unions, 1980.*

Stellman, JM. 1978. Occupational Health Hazards of Women: An Overview. *Preventative Medicine* 7: 281–293.

Sutton, RI. 1984. Job Stress Among Primary and Secondary School Teachers: Its Relationships To Ill-Being. *Work and Occupation* 11: 7–28.

Wheaton, B. 1985. Models for the Stress-Buffering Functions of Coping Resources. *Journal of Health and Social Behavior* 26: 352–364.

15

Exploring the Correlates of Self-Provided Health Care Behaviour*

Alexander Segall and Jay Goldstein

Introduction

The expanding body of self-care literature is currently characterized more by debate than by data. Ongoing arguments centre on: the nature of the linkage between self-care and professional medical care; whether or not self-care is a social movement; and whether self-control and personal autonomy will ultimately result in the deprofessionalization of health care and the decline of medical dominance. In addition, one of the most frequently encountered unresolved disputes concerns the potential consequences of increased lay responsibility for health-related matters.

One point on which there is agreement, however, is the fact that our present knowledge of self-care is fragmentary and a great deal of further investigation is required. Indeed, 10 years ago Levin, Katz and Holst stated that there is a "... need to give high priority to systematic study of self-care" (Levin et al. 1976: 49). They felt the first step should be general population surveys designed to describe the nature and variety of self-care behaviours. More recently, Dean (1981) has restated the importance of descriptive baseline studies of the current extent of self-care practices. Yet despite the fact that self-care is typically described as the basic or primary level of care in all societies, we know very little about lay health care beliefs and behaviour. There is still a need for studies of non-patient populations to identify the dimensions of self-care behaviour and to determine the factors which shape this behaviour. There is a continuing need for more self-care research including: retrospective surveys, prospective health diary studies, and socio-historical analyses. Once this descriptive data base has been established it will be possible to adopt a more analytical approach to the study of self-care. Without these behavioural data the controversies will likely continue unabated, and self-care will remain "... a much discussed but little analyzed – or understood – phenomenon" (Shiller and Levine 1983: 1351).

* Reprinted from *Social Science and Medicine*, Vol. 29, Alexander Segall and Jay Goldstein, 'Exploring the correlates of self-provided health care behaviour', pp. 153–61, 1989, with permission from Elsevier Science Ltd., Oxford, England.

Self-Care: The Lack of Conceptual Clarity

Conceptual clarification is vital to future self-care research. Williamson and Danaher contend that self-care has been "ineptly conceptualized" and consequently "inadequately researched" (Williamson and Danaher 1978: 107). What is the meaning of the concept? In an early discussion of lay initiatives in health, Levin, Katz and Holst (1976) defined self-care as a process by which the layperson functions on his/her own behalf to promote health, to prevent illness, and to detect and treat disease when it occurs. According to this definition, self-care is a lay phenomenon, and the layperson is a self-provider who can function effectively as the primary resource in the health care system. This conceptualization has been quite influential and has been accepted as the working definition by many subsequent studies of self-care (Schiller and Levin 1983; Linn and Lewis 1979; Fleming et al. 1984; Green 1985).

Dean (1981) offered a slightly different conception of self-care. She suggested that self-care includes not only health maintenance/lifestyle behaviour, utilization of preventive services, symptom evaluation, and various self-treatment activities, but also interaction with the professional sector. Both of these definitions illustrate that the concept of self-care focuses on aspects of health/illness management which are believed to be subject to individual control and involve some type of lay initiated deliberate action.

The concept of self-care thus includes a range of potential behaviours such as: health maintenance, illness prevention, symptom evaluation and self-diagnosis, self-treatment (both non-medication practices and self-medication), self-referral (use of lay social network as a health resource), consultation with a variety of non-medical (alternative) health care practitioners, and the use of professional medical care services. In each case, the critical factor is that these self-care practices are lay initiated and are undertaken as a result of a self-determined decision making process. In other words, the essence of self-care is self-control. However, it is important to note that this conceptualization does not present self-care and professional care as mutually exclusive, but rather as integral and inter-related components of the health care system. Self-care is a factor "... in nearly all illness episodes, including those that ultimately receive professional care" (Levin and Idler 1983: 184).

Barofsky (1978) in a discussion of the functions of self-care, suggests a typology for differentiating between various forms of self-care behaviour. The four types of self-care he identifies are: (1) regulatory self-care (routine health maintenance activities such as eating, sleeping and personal hygiene); (2) preventive self-care (adherence to self-selected practices such as exercise, dieting or self-examination); (3) reactive self-care (self-initiated responses to symptoms which have not yet been labeled by a physician as illness or disease); and (4) restorative self-care (compliance with a professionally prescribed treatment regimen of medication and behavioural change). Although this categorization scheme is potentially useful for organizing discussions of self-care and for guiding research, it does, however, raise an important definitional problem. While the first three types of lay care are always self-initiated, the fourth type involves complying with professionally initiated care. Consequently, it is important to question the inclusion of compliance behaviour within the conceptual framework of self-care.

This lack of conceptual clarity is not limited to Barofsky's writing. For example, Dean, Holst and Wagner contend that since compliance with professional directives may be based on lay decision making, it is therefore also a form of self-care (Dean et al. 1983: 1012). In contrast, Levin and Idler begin their recent review paper on self-care in health by asserting that "these activities are undertaken without professional assistance, although individuals are informed by technical knowledge and skills derived from the pool of both professional and lay experience" (Levin and Idler 1983: 181). Just what, then, are the limits of self-care? How can these divergent viewpoints be integrated into a coherent conception of self-care? It is apparent that self-care is not limited exclusively to care provided by the lay community. The use of professional health care services can also be included within the rubric of self-care if indeed it stems from lay decision making. The critical issue is not whether the care is self or other provided, but whether the care is self-managed (i.e., ultimately within the control of the individual). However, it does not seem legitimate to treat compliance behaviour, which may be an expression of coerced conformity, as a form of self-care.

Additional conceptual clarification is obviously required. Perhaps the distinction between primary self-care (actions based on the individual's knowledge and experience) and secondary self-care (actions based on information obtained in consultation with lay and professional others) may be helpful in this endeavor (Dean 1986). In any case, the components of self-care behaviour must be more precisely identified, and the boundaries of self-care more clearly established. Theoretical refinement, definitional consensus and a better specification of the behavioural referents of this construct must accompany a call for more self-care research.

Issues in Self-Care Research

"Self-care in its various forms, preventive, curative and rehabilitative, is neither contemporary nor reactionary. It is the basic health behavior in all societies past and present" (Dean 1981: 673). Indeed, contemporary self-care behaviour must be placed in a sociohistorical context to be properly understood. Self-provided health care is firmly rooted in the traditional values of individualism, self-reliance and popular democracy. While the current research interest in self-care may be a new development, personal responsibility for health and active public participation in self-care practices certainly are not new. Green (1985) suggests that in recent years there has been an increase in the visibility of self-care, rather than an increase in the prevalence of self-managed health. It is difficult to determine whether this is a cause or a consequence of expanding research interests in self-care.

Various factors have been cited to explain the present renewed (if not new) interest in self-care among both the general population and health care professionals. Precipitating factors include: the epidemiological shift in disease patterns from acute to chronic morbidity and the accompanying need to shift medical intervention from cure to care; growing public dissatisfaction with the fragmented and depersonalized nature of medical care and a recognition of the limits of modern medicine; the increasing number of alternative health workers and access to nonallopathic therapies; and heightened consciousness of the effects of lifestyle on health and a desire to exercise personal responsibility in health-related matters. The recent 'rediscovery' of self-care and the prevalent tendency to characterize lay initiatives in health as a social movement have contributed to the false impression that this is a new form of behaviour.

Self-care has been variously described as a lay movement in its 'infancy' (Levin 1976a), and as an 'emerging' or 'nascent' social movement (Levin et al. 1976). This so-called social movement is viewed as a further collective outcome of the 'rising tide of populism' (Levin 1977: 117) which seeks greater personal control in many aspects of life and has spawned the civil rights movement, the feminist movement and consumerism. Kronenfeld (1979), proceeding on the assumption that self-care is a social movement, argues that the activists involved in this movement are essentially young people with high levels of education and income.

Is self-care really a social movement? According to Fleming et al. (1984) some aspects of self-care (e.g., consumerism) may represent a 'recent social movement' but others (e.g., home remedies) are really a part of traditional health behaviour and folk healing practices. The most complete answer to this question is provided by Schiller and Levin (1983). They review and then apply the formal characteristics of a social movement to self-care behaviour and conclude that self-care is not presently a social movement because there is no clearly articulated ideological base, common purpose, coherent organizational structure, or strategy for concerted action. Levin and Idler agree with this conclusion and state that "self-care is not a movement in the classical use of the term" (Levin and Idler 1983: 193). However, the pre-conditions for a self-care movement seem to exist, and to argue that self-care is not presently a social movement does not deny the possibility that it may become one in the future.

"If self-care has always existed along-side expert care, then, what is self-care – a movement either for or against" (Schiller and Levin 1983: 1349). Fleming et al. (1984) examined the impact of self-care practices on health services utilization but failed to provide conclusive evidence as to whether self-care is a substitute for or a supplement to professional medical care. There is reason to believe that this study failed to produce a decisive answer because the basic research question was not correctly formulated. If self-care existed prior to the emergence of health specialists and the professionalization of medical care, and if the overwhelming proportion of everyday care is self-provided, then it is professional health care which is supplementary to self-care! In Dean's words "lay care continues to be viewed as residual and supplemental to professional care in spite of the well documented fact that professional care is the supplemental form of health care (Dean 1986: 275). Indeed, it has been argued that public health policy needs to be modified to reflect the fact that professional care, while vital, is supplementary to lay self-care (Levin 1982). This suggests that in addition to clarifying the concept of self-care, the central research questions about the nature of self-provided health care need to be reformulated.

Studying Self-Care Behaviour

To date, self-care research has focused almost exclusively on actions undertaken in response to illness, including self-diagnosis and treatment (e.g., Schiller and Levin 1983; Fleming et al. 1984; Dean et al. 1983; Freer 1980). Among the range of possible self-treatments available, self-medication has been most frequently studied. Furthermore, the health maintenance components of self-care have typically been excluded. In addition, since this limited body of research has been preoccupied with self-care practices, the fundamental assumptions about the underlying beliefs which shape this behaviour have gone untested.

It is time to take a more comprehensive approach to the study of self-care. Consequently, in this research, lay health beliefs and self-initiated/provided health care were investigated since "existing levels of self-care are part of social life and constitute a fabric of beliefs and practices more profoundly cultural than medical" (Levin and Idler 1983: 193). More specifically, the objectives of the present study were: (1) to describe the nature and extent of self-care behaviour found among a sample of Canadians; and (2) to explore some of the correlates of self-provided health care. The data used in this analysis were derived from a broader study of the relative influence of folk and professional medical systems on lay health beliefs and healing practices.[1]

Research Design

Information on lay health beliefs and self-care behaviour was collected as part of the 1983 Winnipeg Area Study, which is an annual survey of the residents of Winnipeg, Canada. A random cross-sectional sample of 701 addresses was selected from all dwelling units listed in the 1982 property tax assessment file for the City of Winnipeg. Nursing homes and temporary residences were excluded from the sample. The household was the primary sampling unit and one adult per household was selected for a 1-hr interview. The eligibility criteria were that the dwelling was the individual's usual place of residence and the person was between 18 and 80 years of age. All of the interviews were conducted in the respondents' home during February and March, 1983. A total of 524 respondents were interviewed for a response rate of 75%. The sample was compared to the adult population of Winnipeg (using 1981 Census of Canada statistics) and was found to be quite representative of the city on a number of characteristics such as age, sex and household size.

Self-Care Measures

The self-care practices considered in this study were: self-treatment responses to symptoms of illness, self-medication activities, and the use of home remedies. The measure of self-treated symptomatic response involved presenting the respondents with a list of 10 conditions and asking 'What type of treatment would you use if you experienced this condition?' The symptomatic conditions were: feeling of dizziness; bowel irregularity; constant tiredness; frequent headaches; rash or itch; shortness of breath; unexplained loss of weight; difficulty sleeping at night; loss of appetite; and stomach upset/indigestion. The response categories provided were: 'A person shouldn't bother much about this because it is not usually important'; 'A person should try to take care of it him/herself'; and 'A person should see a doctor about it right away'. Each respondent was assigned a scale score on the basis of the number of these symptomatic conditions that he/she would manage with self-provided care.[2] In other words, this is not a direct measure of self-care behaviour, but rather a measure of the respondents' behavioural intention or tendency toward self-treatment.

Respondents were asked a series of questions about their recent self-medication activities. First, they were asked about the types of medication they had used during the past 2 weeks. Then for each medication identified, they were asked several follow-up questions such as: was the medication prescribed or recommended by a doctor?; was it already available in the home?; for what health problem was it used?; and was it effective? For the purposes of the present analysis, scores on the self-medication measure were simply dichotomized on the basis of whether or not the respondents had taken or used a non-prescription medication during the 2-week period prior to the interview.[3]

Finally, the respondents were asked about their familiarity with home remedies. To explore this aspect of self-care behaviour, respondents were asked to indicate if they knew any home remedies that they believed were effective and would recommend others use. If the response was positive, they were then given an opportunity to explain each home remedy in an open-ended format. This question yielded a wealth of information about the nature and types of home remedies used. However, it is not possible to incorporate all of this information into the present paper. Scores on the home remedies measure were assigned on the basis of the number of home remedies cited.[4]

Correlates of Self-Care

A number of studies have addressed the question – Who uses self-care? (Fleming et al. 1984; Green 1985; Levin and Idler 1983; Dean et al. 1983). Unfortunately, no clear answer emerges from their findings. According to Green (1985), self-care has been found to be related to socio-economic status and education, but not to sex or marital status. Fleming et al. (1984) report rather weak relationships between age and sex and the self-care measures investigated (i.e., non-prescribed home treatment and the use of lay consultation). Dean, Holst and Wagner (1983) surveyed self-care behaviour in Denmark and concluded that independent of age and sex, the social variables included in the analysis (e.g., marital status, education, income) 'exerted surprisingly little influence' on self-care responses to common illnesses. Levin and Idler (1983), in a recent review paper, contend that the available data on the relationship between self-care and demographic factors such as age, sex, marital status, and social class are contradictory and lead to no clear conclusions.

The sociodemographic attributes measured in the present study include: the respondent's sex, age (actual age in years), marital status (married, common-law, single, divorced, widowed or separated), education (elementary or less, junior high school, some high school or graduated, post-secondary, some university or graduated), income (total annual family income), religion (Catholic, Anglican, Protestant, Evangelical and no preference), ethnic self-identity (simply Ethnic, e.g., Ukrainian; Ethnic-Canadian, e.g., French-Canadian; and simply Canadian), and generation (first, second, third).

In addition to sociodemographic factors, the potential correlates of self-care explored in this study were: perceived health status, level of understanding of medical knowledge, attitude toward medical care (i.e., skepticism), and lay health beliefs (i.e., health maintenance and locus of control beliefs). Perceived health status has been identified as a potential correlate of self-care by a number of investigators (Green 1985; Dean et al. 1983), and was measured by four questions: (1) 'Generally speaking, how would you describe your present health?' The response categories were excellent, good, fair and poor. (2) 'In the past 12 months how healthy have you felt physically?' Responses were arranged on a 7-point scale ranging from very healthy to very unhealthy. (3) 'During the past 12 months, how many days did you stay at home in bed for all or most of the day because of an illness?' (Actual number of days were coded.) (4) 'During the past 12 months, how many days did you cut down on the things you usually do because of an illness?' (Actual number of days were coded.) Each question was treated as a separate indicator of health status in the analysis of self-provided health care.[5]

Level of lay knowledge about medical conditions was gauged by asking the respondents a series of questions about the symptomatology and treatment of stomach ulcers, diabetes, leukaemia, coronary thrombosis and hypertension. This measure is based upon a previous study designed to compare the level of medical knowledge among patients with physician estimates of patient comprehension of medical information (Segall and Roberts 1980). The measure was included to test level of medical knowledge in a non-patient population and to evaluate whether this factor is related to self-care. Two questions about each medical condition were presented to the respondents in a forced choice format with three specific responses and a 'don't know' category. Each answer was then categorized as: correct understanding; misunderstanding (incorrect response); or lack of understanding (no response or don't know). Scores on this measure of lay understanding of medical knowledge were calculated by summing the number of correct responses.[6]

A measure of the respondents' attitude toward physicians was included in the study to explore the relationship between medical skepticism and self-care. A series of Likert-type attitudinal statements was presented to the respondents who were asked to indicate their level of agreement (ranging from strongly agree to strongly disagree on a 5-point scale). Responses were subjected to a varimax rotation factor analysis and two dimensions of medical skepticism were identified: (1) a skeptical attitude about the things that doctors say; and (2) a skeptical attitude about the things that doctors do.[7] Both of these subscales of medical skepticism were included in the analysis of self-care behaviour.

Finally, two lay health beliefs were investigated. First, health maintenance beliefs were measured by presenting the respondents with a list of everyday activities in which an individual can engage and asking 'How important do you believe the following things are to your overall health?' Response categories were: very important, of some importance, and of no/little importance. Each respondent was assigned a scale score on the basis of the number of these activities identified as very important for health maintenance.[8] The types of regulatory and preventive self-care health beliefs examined were: adequate rest and sleep, a good diet, low calorie snacks, maintenance of proper weight, participation in social and cultural activities, having close friends, prayer or faith, control of stress, regular physical activity such as exercise, being a non-smoker, being a non-drinker, seat belt use, and self-examination.

Beliefs about the individual's ability to control health/illness were also investigated. A number of researchers have suggested that the locus of control concept may be related to self-care and should be incorporated in future studies (Levin et al. 1976; Levin 1982; Freer 1980). Consequently, the Multidimensional Health Locus of Control Scales were used to measure these beliefs (Wallston et al. 1978; Lau 1982; Lefcourt 1984). The respondents were asked to indicate their level of agreement with a series of Likert-type items designed to measure both internal and external locus of control beliefs. Response categories were: strongly agree, agree, undecided, disagree and strongly disagree. Responses were subjected to a varimax rotation factor analysis and three dimensions of control were identified: (1) internal preventive control beliefs, (2) external provider control beliefs (doctors and medical care), and (3) external chance outcome beliefs (health is a matter of good fortune and beyond everyone's control).

While the Multidimensional Health Locus of Control Scales measured both internal and external dimensions, only the data on internal preventive control beliefs were included in this analysis of self-care behaviour. This is based upon the finding reported by Wallston et al. (1983) that people who expect their own behaviour will affect their health (i.e., those with internal locus of control health beliefs) are more positive toward self-treatment and more actively involved in their own care. The internal preventive control belief subscale consists of four items with fairly high factor loadings: 'People's ill health results from their own carelessness' (0.61); 'Whenever I get sick it is because of something I've done or not done' (0.72); 'When I feel ill, I know it is because I have not been getting the proper exercise or eating right' (0.68); and 'If I take care of myself, I can avoid illness' (0.67).[9]

Data Analysis

The first step in the statistical analysis of the data was to assess the nature of the relationship between each of the variables: sociodemographics, perceived health status, level of medical knowledge, attitude toward medical care, health maintenance beliefs, preventive control beliefs, self-treated symptoms, self-medication, and home remedies. Correlation coefficients (r) were calculated to determine the significance and strength of the relationships between these variables. Next a stepwise multiple regression analysis was performed. For this procedure the three self-care practices measured were treated as dependent variables and all other factors as independent variables. The independent variables were allowed to 'compete' with each other as they were entered into the regression equation in order to identify the best set of predictors of each of the self-care behaviours measured. Finally, a hierarchical regression analysis was performed based on the results of the stepwise regression. Only those variables which had met the minimum significance level for entry into the models were used in the hierarchical regression. The purpose of this last stage of the data analysis was to evaluate the relative explanatory power of each of the subsets of independent variables (sociodemographics, health status, knowledge, attitudes, beliefs) in accounting for variance in self-provided health care.[10]

Health Beliefs and Self-Care Practices: Some Descriptive Evidence

What types of regulatory and preventive self-care health beliefs are prevalent in this population? Responses to the items in the health maintenance beliefs scale varied considerably. The majority of the respondents (i.e., 70% or more) attached a great deal of importance to lifestyle activities such as: getting adequate rest or sleep, having a good diet, as well as being a non-smoker. Many respondents (i.e., between 50 and 69%) also felt that activities such as: maintaining proper weight, having close friends, getting regular exercise (younger people), and self-examination (females) were very important to a person's overall health. The other items in the scale were dismissed as of little or no importance to health maintenance, although there was some variation by subgroup. For example while only 42% of the sample said that prayer and faith were important, this increased for older respondents. Finally, it is worth noting that despite the existence of mandatory seat belt legislation, only about one third of the respondents felt the use of seat belts was an important health maintenance factor.

Responses to the items in the preventive control beliefs scale also varied. Respondents were almost equally divided in their beliefs about whether or not ill health results from personal carelessness (42% agree vs. 40% disagree); and whether getting proper exercise and proper eating can prevent illness (45% agree vs. 46% disagree). Fifty-seven percent of the respondents believe that illness can be avoided if an individual takes care of him/herself.

What types of reactive self-care practices are prevalent in this population? The vast majority of the participants in the study disagreed with statements such as: 'I can't do much for myself when I'm sick' (80%); and 'When a person is sick, there is very little he/she can do to get well' (86%). Obviously, the population surveyed firmly believes in the appropriateness of self-provided care in response to illness. Is this reflected in their self-care behaviour? Data on the self-treatment of symptomatic conditions indicate that few respondents would define these conditions as unimportant and simply ignore them. The typical response was either to consult a physician right away or to engage in some form of self-treatment (both medication and non-medication). Apparently, these types of symptomatic conditions seldom go untreated. The majority of respondents would see a doctor without delay if they experienced a loss of weight (93%), shortness of breath (84%), or frequent headaches (80%). The conditions which were most likely to be self-treated were stomach upset (61%), bowel irregularity (52%), and difficulty sleeping at night (52%). It seems that the interpretation and evaluation of the meaning of various bodily conditions (self-diagnosis), and the decision to engage in some form of self-treatment is symptom-specific.

Turning to self-medication activities it was found that 63% of the sample had taken or used at least one non-prescribed medication in the 2-week period before they were interviewed. The medications cited (in order of frequency) were pain relievers, vitamins, skin ointments, and cold remedies. In about 75% of these cases, the respondents already had the medication in their home and overwhelmingly (90% plus) felt it was an effective treatment for their health problem.

Finally, 41% of the sample indicated that they were familiar with home remedies, believed them to be effective, and would recommend that others use them. Of those respondents who described their home remedies, the majority cited only one or two at the most. These home remedies were generally used for colds, gastro-intestinal problems, skin irritation and burns.

Assessing the Correlates of Self-Care

What factors are related to self-care behaviour? Do these factors correlate with all of the aspects of self-provided health care investigated in this study? To try to answer these questions, a correlational analysis was performed (Table 1).

Starting with the sociodemographic attributes of the respondents, sex was significantly associated with the use of home remedies. Female respondents were more likely than males to provide information about home remedies. A somewhat surprising finding, in view of the well documented gender differences in illness behaviour, is the fact that sex was not related to either self-treated symptoms or self-medication activities. However, this finding may be a result of the specific self-care measures used in this study.

Age was significantly related to the number of self-treated symptomatic conditions and to the recent use of non-prescribed self-medication. In both cases there was an inverse relationship, indicating that younger respondents were the ones who were more likely to engage in these self-care behaviours. Furthermore, being unmarried was also associated with the tendency to try to achieve symptomatic relief with some form of self-provided treatment.

Social class factors such as education and income were not correlated very highly with self-care behaviour. Only the respondents' level of formal education was directly related to the tendency to self-treat symptoms.

Turning to the sociocultural variables, the relationship between religion and the use of home remedies was statistically significant. More specifically, having no stated religious preference was associated with the use of home remedies. Finally, ethnic identity and generation did not correlate with any of the self-care measures. What then can be concluded about the pattern of self-care among different social groups? It appears that no one sociodemographic attribute is systematically related to all of the self-care behaviours investigated, and that no single dimension of self-care is associated with all of these social, cultural and economic characteristics.

TABLE 1

Zero order correlation coefficients for the relationship between sociodemographics, health status, medical knowledge, medical care attitudes, health beliefs and self-care behaviour

	Self-care behaviour		
	Self-treated symptoms	Self-medication	Home remedies
Sociodemographics			
Sex	-0.07	-0.01	0.15***
Age	-0.24***	-0.27***	-0.07
Marital status	-0.12**	-0.09	0.03
Education	0.19***	0.06	0.03
Income	0.06	0.04	-0.09
Religion	-0.07	-0.02	0.11*
Ethnic identity	0.08	-0.01	0.06
Generation	0.07	0.06	-0.09
Health Status			
Present health	0.12**	0.21***	0.05
Past health	0.05	0.15***	-0.02
Cut down days	-0.08	-0.19***	0.03
Bed days	-0.01	-0.18***	0.01
Medical knowledge	0.08	0.10*	0.13**
Medical care attitudes			
Skepticism about what doctors say	0.06	0.06	0.12**
Skepticism about what doctors do	0.17***	0.05	0.21***
Health beliefs			
Health maintenance	-0.22***	-0.13**	0.08
Preventive control	0.09	0.03	0.03

* $p \leq 0.05$.

** $p \leq 0.01$.

*** $p \leq 0.001$.

Several indicators of health status were included in the present analysis of self-care. The correlation coefficients reported in Table 1 indicate that the only clear and consistent relationship was between the four measures of health status and self-medication activities (although perceived present health was also positively associated with self-treated symptoms). Those individuals who reported that both their present health and their health over the past 12 months was either good or excellent were the ones who had self-medicated. In addition, the disability days measures were negatively associated with self-medication. The causal connection between these variables is an intriguing one. Does this relationship reflect the efficacy of self-care practices?

Next, level of lay medical knowledge and attitudes toward medical care (skepticism) were examined to see if they were correlates of self-care. The relationship between medical knowledge and the measures of self-care used in this study appears to be somewhat difficult to interpret. It seems that respondents who have a better understanding of medically diagnosed conditions are more likely to use non-prescribed medication and home remedies for the self-management of ill health. However, while a higher level of medical knowledge was positively associated with self-medication and the use of home remedies it was not significantly related to self-treated symptoms. Skeptical attitudes about the things that doctors say and do were found to be correlated with some of the self-care measures. For example, skepticism focused on the doctor's ability to cure sickness was significantly correlated with two of the three aspects of self-care considered in this study.

Finally, no statistically significant associations were found between internal preventive control health beliefs and the self-care behaviours investigated. In contrast, health maintenance beliefs were significantly related to self-treated symptoms and self-medication. However, in both cases the relationship was inverse, suggesting that those individuals who believe in the importance of self-initiated activities to maintain good health may not be the ones who actively engage in self-care responses to ill health. This finding indicates the importance of more clearly differentiating between preventive and curative self-care beliefs and behaviour.

In order to explore these relationships further, two forms of multiple regression analysis were performed: stepwise multiple regression to identify the best set of predictors of each of the self-care practices; and hierarchical multiple regression to assess the ability of the different types of independent variables to explain the variance in the three measures of self-care behaviour. Table 2 summarizes the results of the stepwise multiple regression analysis.

TABLE 2

Stepwise multiple regression analysis of the relationship between sociodemographics, health status, medical knowledge, medical care attitudes, health beliefs and self-care behaviour

Independent variables in model	Standardized regression coefficient
Self-care behaviour = self-treated symptoms	
Sex	-0.06
Age	-0.19
University education	0.11
No religious preference	0.07
Present health	0.12
Medical knowledge	0.08
Skepticism: what doctors do	0.16
Preventive control beliefs	0.09
Health maintenance beliefs	-0.21
$R^2 = 0.16$, adjusted $R^2 = 0.14$, F = 10.90, P ≤ 0.0001	
Self-care behaviour = self-medication	
Age	-0.27
Junior high education	0.10
Anglican	-0.12
Catholic	-0.15
Present health	0.15
Cut down days	-0.09

Continued on next page

Table 2 - *Continued*

Independent variables in model	Standardized regression coefficient
Bed days	-0.09
Medical knowledge	0.05
Skepticism: what doctors say	0.13
Health maintenance beliefs	-0.13
$R^2 = 0.15$, adjusted $R^2 = 0.13$, $F = 7.67$, $P \leq 0.0001$	
Self-care behaviour = home remedies	
Sex	0.15
Age	-0.11
Senior high education	-0.07
Income	-0.08
Generation	-0.11
Medical knowledge	0.10
Skepticism: what doctors say	0.07
Skepticism: what doctors do	0.19
Health maintenance beliefs	0.08
$R^2 = 0.12$, adjusted $R^2 = 0.10$, $F = 7.18$, $P \leq 0.0001$	

Starting with the sociodemographic variables, the results reveal that sex is an important predictor of self-treated symptoms and the use of home remedies, but not self-medication activities as measured. Age and education are important in explaining all three types of self-care behaviour. While a university education is associated with the self-treatment of symptoms, lower levels of formal education are associated with the other two types of self-care. Income is included in only one of the predictive models (home remedies). Two of the sociodemographic variables (marital status and ethnic identity) did not meet the minimum significance level for inclusion in any of the models.

Turning to perceived health status, once again the clearest relationship seems to be between the various indicators of self-reported health and self-medication. In contrast, none of the health status measures were included in the set of best predictors of the use of home remedies. Medical knowledge and at least one of the two measures of medical skepticism appear in all of the models. Finally, health maintenance beliefs were associated, more clearly than preventive control beliefs, with the measures of self-care behaviour.

The total explained variance (adjusted R^2) in the dimensions of self-care ranged from 10% (home remedies) to 14% (self-treated symptoms). How much of this variance can be accounted for by health beliefs, or skeptical attitudes compared to other factors such as perceived health status or sociodemographic attributes? In an effort to answer this question, hierarchical regression was performed using the variables identified by the stepwise regression. This procedure reveals the amount of variance in the dependent variables explained by each of the subsets of independent variables (Table 3).

TABLE 3

Hierarchical regression analysis of the relationship between socio-demographics, health status, medical knowledge, medical care attitudes, health beliefs and self-care behaviour

Subsets of independent variables	Variance in self-care behaviour explained (adjusted R^2)		
	Self-treated symptoms	Self medication	Home remedies
Sociodemographics	0.07 (F = 9.79, $P \leq 0.001$)	0.09 (F = 10.82, $P \leq 0.001$)	0.04 (F = 5.58, $P \leq 0.001$)
Health status	0.00 (F = 1.24, NS)	0.03 (F = 5.06, $P \leq 0.01$)	*
Medical knowledge	-0.00 (F = 0.89, NS)	-0.00 (F = 0.83, NS)	0.02 (F = 9.71, $P \leq 0.001$)
Medical care attitudes	0.02 (F = 3.50, $P \leq 0.01$)	0.01 (F = 2.18, $P \leq 0.05$)	0.04 (F = 7.19, $P \leq 0.001$)
Health beliefs	0.03 (F = 8.04, $P \leq 0.001$)	-0.00 (F = 0.79, NS)	0.00 (F = 1.98, NS)

*   None of the four health status measures met the significance level (0.15) for entry into the model for 'home remedies'.

Sociodemographics accounted for one-half of the explained variance in self-treated symptoms. Social attributes of the individual also explained over one-half of the total variance in self-medication and slightly less than one-half of the total variance in home remedies. As might have been expected from the results of the stepwise analysis, health status explained some of the variance in self-medication activities but not in the other two self-care behaviours. Similarly, medical knowledge and health beliefs each contributed to the explanation of only one dimension of self-care behaviour. Medical care attitudes (along with sociodemographics) were the only variables significantly related to self-treated symptoms, self-medication and home remedies. These findings suggest that different explanatory factors will have to be identified to account for the diverse activities encompassed by the concept of self-care. Furthermore, the inconclusiveness of the findings illustrates the need to clarify the conceptual distinction between preventive/regulatory and curative/reactive self-care and to operationalize more precisely the behavioural dimensions of each of these types of self-provided care. It is rather self-evident to conclude that this study leaves a good deal of the variance in self-care behaviour unexplained and awaiting further research.

Personal and Professional Responsibility for Health: Implications for Self-Care Research

While a better empirical understanding of self-care beliefs and behaviour is beginning to emerge, there is still a long way to go. In the meantime, it is likely that the controversies surrounding self-care will persist and the debate will continue regarding the implications of promoting individual responsibility for health. Self-care has become a popular topic since Illich (1975) issued his call for action and challenged the public to demystify and overcome professional dependency and re-establish personal autonomy and control of their health. Proponents of self-care have extolled its virtues. For example, Levin (1976b) portrays self-care as a force for helping people: to make decisions for themselves, to take initiative in dealing with their health and responding to their illness, and to use professional resources in a 'self-protecting' manner. In his view, self-care will ultimately contribute to an "improvement of the efficiency of the overall health care system" (Levin 1976a). In reviewing the advantages of self-care, Green adds that "self-care brings with it the possibilities of reducing chronic illness, promoting wellness, and raising the level of well-being" (Green 1985: 326).

However, self-care also has its critics (Crawford 1977; Crawford 1986; Knowles 1977). The gist of the argument against self-care is that increased personal responsibility for health brings with it the potential for 'victim blaming.' In other words, self-care is based on the assumption that the individual has the power to control conditions which give rise to ill health. The critics argue that this is more apparent than real. In reality, a consequence of self-care is that the individual is made responsible for things which may not be preventable at the personal level (e.g., environmentally and occupationally induced sickness). Thus illness may become equated with personal failure, and the sick person may be blamed and in this way victimized. Critics further argue that self-care may be used as a justification for decreasing the level of formal health services provided, and most importantly that this emphasis on individual responsibility distracts attention from a structural analysis of the social, political and economic aspects of ill health.

Bolaria (1979) has echoed this sentiment in the Canadian context. In his words, self-care "... obscures the extent to which health and illness depend upon socially determined ways of life, obfuscates the social causes of disease, shifts responsibility for health and illness back onto the individual, individualizes what is essentially a social problem, and promotes a course of action oriented toward changing individual behaviour and lifestyles rather than the existing social, economic, and political institutions and the health sector" (Bolaria 1979: 351). Katz and Levin (1980) acknowledge that there are dangers associated with self-care, but respond to the criticism by maintaining that the public will derive benefits from self-care such as decreased dependency and a heightened individual and socio-political awareness of the hazards to health. In their opinion, self-care cannot be understood within the ideological framework of 'victim blaming.'

One issue on which both the proponents and opponents of self-care seem to agree is that self-care is being medicalized. At various points in his writing, Levin has acknowledged that self-care faces the "threat of professional cooptation" and "may be subject to medicalization and the hegemony of the health professions." In concluding a 1976 paper on the layperson as primary health practitioner, Levin expressed concern about the ways in which the professionalization of this lay health resource could be avoided (Levin 1976a). Crawford (1980) characterizes self-care as the transfer of medical competence to the individual and contends that medicalization has already occurred. This assertion is supported by the fact that the content of self-care educational programs often reflects medical norms and values, and medical technology explicitly designed for lay use is now available. Furthermore, both self-care and medical care situate the problem of ill health and its solution at the individual level. Thus Crawford concludes that self-provided health care represents a further extension of medical jurisdiction because professional, scientific biomedical ways of understanding the aetiology, symptomatology and treatment of illness/disease are reflected in the conceptions and practices of self-care. It seems then that "self-care practices probably are medicalized to a certain extent, but with the current lack of descriptive research no one can really say" (Idler 1979: 730). This could be a good starting point for future self-care research.

Acknowledgements

The research reported in this paper was supported by grants from the Social Sciences and Humanities Research Council of Canada, the University of Manitoba Institute for Social and Economic Research, and, in part, by a National Health Research Scholar Award to the first author.

Notes

1   The health beliefs and behaviour investigated included: lay conceptions of health, illness explanations, health maintenance beliefs, health locus of control beliefs, popular health beliefs, belief in the efficacy of medical care, willingness to adopt the sick role, symptom evaluation and response, self-treatment and medication activities, use of the informal social network as a health resource, and utilization of health services. Only selected findings are presented in this paper.

2   The minimum value was 0 and the maximum was 10 on this scale of self-treated symptoms (mean = 3.10, SD = 2.02).

3   This is admittedly a limited measure of self-medication activity and does not take into account the volume of non-prescribed drugs consumed or the specific illness episodes managed with this type of self-care. A fuller discussion of these aspects of self-provided care is included in a paper currently being prepared which is entitled: A Community Survey of Self-Care Medication Behaviour.

4   The minimum value was 0 and the maximum was 4 on this measure of home remedy use (mean = 0.72, SD = 1.05).

5   The last three measures of perceived health status raise the issue of the accuracy of respondent recall over a 12-month period. The literature generally suggests that physician and self-assessed health status are highly correlated and essentially stable over time. Thus self-report provides a valid and apparently reliable measure of health.

6   The minimum value was 0 and the maximum was 10 on this measure of lay medical knowledge (mean = 5.3, SD = 2.4).

7   Factor one (skepticism about the things that doctors say) has an eigenvalue of 1.92 and consists of three items with fairly high factor loadings: 'I have my doubts about some things doctors say they can do for you' (0.58); 'Doctors often tell you there's nothing wrong with you, when you know there is' (0.70); and 'I believe in trying out different doctors to find out which one I think will give me the best care' (0.75). The minimum value was 3 and the maximum was 9 on this subscale (mean = 5.99, SD = 1.95). Factor two (skepticism about the things that doctors do) has an eigenvalue of 1.09 and consists of three items with equally high factor loadings; 'If you wait long enough, you can get over most sicknesses without going to the doctor' (0.77): 'Some home remedies are still better than prescribed drugs for

curing sickness' (0.70); and 'A person understands his/her own state of health better than most doctors' (0.52). The minimum and maximum values were the same on this subscale (mean = 5.58, SD = 1.88).

8   The minimum value was 0 and the maximum was 13 on this scale of health maintenance beliefs (mean = 7.20, SD = 2.85).

9   This factor has an eigenvalue of 1.87.

10   For the correlational and regression analyses, dummy variable recodes were used when required.

References

Barofsky, I. 1978. Compliance, Adherence and the Therapeutic Alliance: Steps in the Development of Self-Care. *Social Science and Medicine* 12: 369.

Bolaria, BS. 1979. Self-Care and Lifestyles; Ideological and Policy Implications. In JA Fry ed. *Economy, Class and Social Reality,* 350–363. Butterworths: Toronto.

Crawford, R. 1986. Individual Responsibility and Health Politics. In P Conrad and R Kern eds. *The Sociology of Health and Illness: Critical Perspectives,* 369–377. St Martin's Press: New York.

Crawford, R. 1980. Healthism and the Medicalization of Everyday Life. *International Journal of Health Services* 10: 365.

Crawford, R. 1977. You are Dangerous to Your Health: The Ideology and Politics of Victim Blaming. *International Journal of Health Services* 7: 663.

Dean, K. 1986. Lay Care in Illness. *Social Science and Medicine* 22: 275.

Dean, K, E Holst, and M Wagner. 1983. Self-Care of Common Illnesses in Denmark. *Medical Care* 21: 1012.

Dean, K. 1981. Self-Care Responses to Illness: A Selected Review. *Social Science and Medicine* 15A: 673.

Fleming, GV, et al. 1984. Self-Care: Substitute, Supplement or Stimulus for Formal Medical Care Services. *Medical Care* 22: 950.

Freer, CB. 1980. Self-Care: A Healthy Diary Study. *Medical Care* 18: 853.

Green, KE. 1985. Identification of the Facets of Self-Health Management. *Evaluation and the Health Professions* 8: 323.

Idler, E. 1979. Definitions of Health and Illness and Medical Sociology. *Social Science and Medicine* 13A: 723.

Illich, I. 1975. *Medical Nemesis.* London: Calder & Boyars.

Katz, A, and L Levin. 1980. Self-Care is Not a Solipsistic Trap: A Reply to Critics. *International Journal of Health Services* 10: 329.

Knowles, JH. 1977. The Responsibility of the Individual. In JH Knowles ed. *Doing Better and Feeling Worse,* 57–80. New York: Norton.

Kronenfeld, J. 1979. Self-Care as a Panacea for the Ills of the Health Care System: An Assessment. *Social Science and Medicine* 13A: 263.

Lau, RR. 1982. Origins of Health Locus of Control Beliefs. *Journal of Personality and Social Psychology* 42: 322.

Lefcourt, H ed. 1984. *Research With the Locus of Control Construct.* Orlando, Fla: Academic Press.

Levin, LS, and E Idler. 1983. Self-Care in Health. *Annual Review of Public Health* 4: 181.

Levin, LS. 1982. Health Service Via Self-Service. *Social Policy* 13: 44.

Levin, LS. 1977. Forces and Issues in the Revival of Interest in Self-Care: Impetus for Redirection in Health. *Health Education Monographs* 5: 115.

Levin, LS. 1976a. The Layperson as the Primary Health Care Practitioner. *Public Health Reports* 91: 206.

Levin, LS. 1976b. Self-Care: An International Perspective. *Social Policy* 7: 70.

Levin, LS, AH Katz, and E Holst. 1976. *Self-Care: Lay Initiatives in Health*. New York: Prodist.

Linn, L, and C Lewis. 1979. Attitudes Toward Self-Care Among Practicing Physicians. *Medical Care* 17: 183.

Schiller, PL, and JS Levin. 1983. Is Self-Care a Social Movement? *Social Science and Medicine* 17: 1343.

Segall, A, and LW Roberts. 1980. A Comparative Analysis of Physician Estimates and Levels of Medical Knowledge Among Patients. *Sociology of Health and Illness* 2: 317.

Wallston KA et al. 1983. Expectancies about Control Over Health; Relationship to Desire for Control of Health Care. Person. *Personality and Social Psychology Bulletin* 9: 377.

Wallston, KA et al. 1978. Development of the Multi-Dimensional Health Locus of Control (MHLC) Scales. *Health Education Monographs* 6: 160.

Williamson, JD, and K Danaher. 1978. *Self-Care in Health*. London: Croom Helm.

16

Predictors of Successful Aging: A Twelve-Year Study of Manitoba Elderly[*]

Noralou P. Roos and Betty Havens

The elderly are not a homogeneous group. Some are beset by multiple chronic and/or acute conditions and spend considerable time in hospital. Still others, especially women, live a very long life but are afflicted by increasing frailty or declining mental status, passing their last years in nursing homes. Some elderly manage to avoid all of these scenarios, maintain themselves independently in the community and are described as "aging successfully" (Rowe 1987; Stallones 1987).

While other investigators have attempted to study successful aging, our analysis is unusual in its longitudinal design, its large representative sample, and in focusing on successful aging of an already elderly cohort. It addresses three questions:
1. What proportion of an elderly cohort will age successfully?
2. What are the health care expenditure patterns associated with successful aging?
3. Which characteristics of individuals predict successful aging? (From among all those interviewed in 1971, who will successfully age? And among those who survive to 1983, what are the factors which predict successful aging?)

Methods

In 1971 a large (N = 3,573) representative sample of individuals ages 65-84 living in the community was interviewed as part of the Manitoba Longitudinal Study on Aging (Manitoba Department of Health and Social Development 1973; Mossey et al. 1981). In 1983 and 1984 survivors of this cohort were reinterviewed. In addition, the health care expenditures of this cohort over the period 1970 through 1983 were available from administrative records of the universally insured provincial health care program.

The sample was selected as follows: 2.5 percent of the residents of urban areas and 5 percent of the residents of non-urban areas. Analyses were reweighted by the sampling proportions within strata to reflect population figures. A place of residence variable (urban/not) was included in each multivariate model to control for sampling fraction.

* Reprinted with permission from *American Journal of Public Health,* Vol. 81, No. 1, Naralou P. Roos and Betty Havens, 'Predictors of successful aging: A twelve-year study of Manitoba elderly', pp. 63–68, 1991. Copyright 1991 by the American Public Health Association.

Individuals were excluded from the analysis if they were not resident in the province (as judged by coverage in the health care system) for the period of the study, 1970 through 1983 or until death (310); if they were alive and resident in the province in 1983 but not reinterviewed (147); or if the 1971 or 1983 interview was conducted entirely through a proxy (101). (Proxy interviews were used primarily where individuals were too ill or confused to respond.) Native Manitobans (90) were also excluded from the analysis. The final sample for this analysis included 2,943 elderly. A comparison of baseline characteristics of those included and excluded in the study found no difference in age and sex or self-reported health status. However, the interviewer was significantly more likely to rate the respondent's mind as steady or strong in general for those retained in the study.

Successful aging was defined using the 1983 reinterview as follows:
• Alive in 1983.
• Not resident of a nursing home in 1983.
• Did not receive more than 59 days of home care services in 1983.
• In the 1983 interview:
Rated health excellent to fair.
Not dependent in any activities of daily living (getting in and out of bed,
    dressing, bathing, eating, using stairs).
Did not use a wheelchair.
Did not need help in going outdoors.
Able to walk outdoors.
Scored seven or more correct answers on Mental Status Test.
Interviewer judged respondent's state of mind to be steady and strong or a bit weak only after some interview time had elapsed.

Cause of death was taken from death certificates. Less than 1 percent of the individuals (N = 26) died of accidents, poisonings or violence and therefore lost the chance to age successfully.

Claims data have been shown to provide a highly accurate, reliable, and valid representation of health care use (Roos et al. 1982; Roos et al. 1989). Claims were used to estimate health care expenditure patterns associated with healthy aging over the 14-year period 1970-83 (or until death). The following types of utilization were tracked: days spent in hospital (with days spent in intensive care treated separately); days spent in nursing home; days enrolled in the home care program; all physician visits and surgical fees (for both inpatient and outpatient procedures).

Since nursing home services in Manitoba have been universally insured only since 1973, costs incurred by nursing home residents prior to July 1973 were estimated as described elsewhere (Roos et al. 1989). Since September 1974, home care services in the province have also been universally provided at no charge to consumer.

Manitoba hospitals and nursing homes are funded on the basis of global budgets. (Detsky et al. 1983) An estimate of mean costs per day in hospital ($322) and nursing home ($49) was calculated by dividing total Manitoba Health Services Commission payments (including capital repayment) to hospitals and to nursing homes in fiscal 1984 by the number of days of care produced that year by these institutions. The cost of a day in intensive care was estimated to be $1,610, five times the cost of a hospital day. Although per diem costs escalated markedly in both the hospital and nursing home sectors over the time period studied, constant dollar costs were used. The estimate of home care costs per day ($4) were derived by dividing service costs per user over a six-month period by the 182 days in that period (Chappell and Horne 1987). Total payments for physician visits and consultations were divided by the total numbers of visits to obtain an average cost per visit ($17). All costs are in constant 1984 Canadian dollars.

Variables available from the 1971 interview represent potential predictors of successful aging, while diagnoses made during physician visits over the period 1970 through 1982 and variables constructed from administrative records recording events occurring to spouse (death or admission to nursing home) during this same period are potential factors associated with successful aging. Thus predictors of successful aging may include characteristics of the individual's demographic, ethnic and cultural background, socioeconomic characteristics, and characteristics of the support network. The individual's mental status was also assessed in 1971, as well as satisfaction with life, and several characteristics of health status. Factors studied for association with successful aging include changes in the individual's support network over time (whether the individual's spouse predeceased him or her and whether the spouse entered a nursing home prior to the interviewee's death or 1983).

The extent to which specific diseases pose threats to successful aging was examined using both self-reports in 1971 and claims-derived measures of physician contact for five conditions judged to place an elderly individual at "risk for recovery" (Jones 1974). The Manitoba Cancer Registry was used to determine whether the individual had been diagnosed as having cancer (other than skin). Whether individuals had regular contacts with physicians (and therefore would be available for the early detection and treatment of disease) was measured by the percent of years the individual was alive between 1970 and 1982 during which one or more (or two or more) visits were made to physicians. (See Appendix for a complete listing of predictor variables.)

Two dependent variables were examined: successful aging (yes-no); and successful aging versus survival to 1983 in a dependent state.

In the analyses, using the first dependent variable, all individuals sampled were used to determine which variables were predictive of successful aging. The second analysis examined the association between all dependent variables and successful aging among those who survived to 1983.

Because of the large number of independent variables, a two-step process was followed for each group of variables (see Appendix for grouping). First, the relation of each variable to each dependent variable was tested by univariate analyses. A forward step-wise fitting algorithm for the multiple logistic regression model was used to determine which variables among each group of predictor variables made a contribution to each model at a p value level of 0.05. Age and sex were included in every model. From among those variables within a set which were substantially correlated with one another (i.e., absolute value of Pearson correlation coefficient .5 or greater) only one was selected for modeling. The variables which made the most contribution to model fit, or, where there was little difference, the variables most commonly used in previous studies were selected.

A final multiple logistic regression model was fit including the variables from each set selected as described above. Contributions to the model of the combined effect of 1) sex and income, 2) sex and spousal death/nursing home entry, 3) income and spousal death/nursing home, were assessed by including interaction terms in the model.

The data were randomly split with one-half of the records used to develop the models and to estimate the coefficients of the logistic regression models (Mosteller and Tukey 1977). The final model was tested on the other half of the records to see if the same variables entered the model and whether the coefficients were estimated in similar magnitude. All data have been pooled for presentation since the larger sample provides more stable estimates of the coefficients.

Results

By our definition, 20 percent of those individuals ages 65 to 84 interviewed in 1971 were judged to have successfully aged in 1983, 22.6 percent were alive but dependent, and 57.5 percent were deceased (Table 1). Males were more likely to be deceased by 1983 than females. Although females ages 65 to 74 were somewhat more likely to have aged successfully than males, there was little difference in successful aging by sex in the older age group (p = .466). Recalculating the percentages in Table 1 (not shown) and focusing upon those who survived to 1983 shows no difference in the percentage of females versus males in the youngest group who successfully aged (p = 0.172). However, among survivors in the oldest age group, males were more likely to successfully age than were females (32.7 percent versus 18.0 percent, p = 0.006).

Remaining independent (the definition of successful aging) is associated with a higher level of satisfaction with life in older age (see Table 2). Separate comparisons by age confirmed this relationship (data available on request to author). However, maintaining functional independence is not a guarantee for being satisfied with one's life in advanced old age. Moreover, losing one's independence is not necessarily judged a disaster. Among those reporting their satisfaction with life to be excellent, 30.4 percent were classified as "alive but dependent" in 1983.

Individuals who remained independent made markedly fewer demands on the health care system (Table 3). About two-thirds (67.7 percent) of those aging successfully used less than $10,000 worth of health care resources over the 14-year period 1970 through 1983, averaging $736 per year. In contrast, those who lived to 1983 in a more dependent state averaged $3,850 per year over the 14-year period. Those who died before 1983 had the highest resource use, averaging $5,955 per year lived. Further analyses (not presented in Table 3) demonstrated that the low resource utilization patterns of those aging successfully were observed both for males ($768 per year lived) and females ($710) and were independent of age ($744 per year for those aged 65-74 in 1971 and $671 for those aged 75-84).

TABLE 1

Characteristics of individuals in 1983 by age in 1971

| Characteristics of Individuals in 1983 | Age in 1971 | | | | All % |
| | 65-74 | | 75-84 | | |
	Male %	Female %	Male %	Female %	
Has successfully aged	24.0	31.5	7.0	5.9	20.0
Alive but dependent	19.9	29.8	12.3	24.4	22.6
Deceased	56.1	38.7	80.7	69.8	57.5
Number (N)	908	930	521	584	2943

TABLE 2
Satisfaction with life in 1983 in those defined as successfully aged versus those alive but dependent

Satisfaction	Characteristics of Individuals in 1983		
	Aged Successfully	Alive but Dependent	N
In 1983, how would you describe your satisfaction with life in general at present?			
Excellent	69.6	30.4	182
Good	60.5	39.5	556
Fair	46.9	53.1	193
Poor-Bad	18.1	81.9*	40

*Mantel Haenszel Trend Test: $p < .001$

TABLE 3
Total health care expenditures over period 1970-83 by individuals' differing 1983 health status

	Characteristics of Individuals in 1983			
	Aged Successfully	Alive but Dependent	Deceased	All
Total Health Resource Use[a] 1970-83 or to Time of Death (%)				
0-$10,000	67.7	30.5	23.5	33.9
10-25,000	20.7	18.4	22.1	21.0
25-50,000	9.5	19.6	21.8	18.8
50-100,000	2.0	14.0	17.0	13.3
$100,000 or more	0.1	17.5	15.7	13.0
Mean Resource Use per Individual (In $ over Period 1970-83 or to Time of Death)				
Total use ($)	10304	53906	50643	43354
Use per year lived ($)	736	3850	5955	4441
Number	583	666	1694	2943

[a]   Resource use is estimated in 1984-85 Canadian dollars as follows: $1,610 per day in intensive care, $322 per hospital day, $49 per nursing home day, $17 per physician visit, $4 per day on home care, and actual $ amount for surgical procedures.

Table 4, using multivariate analysis, suggests that the most important factors distinguishing those who successfully aged from all others interviewed in 1971, apart from age, were: bad outcomes occurring to a spouse, self-reported health in 1971, retirement because of poor health, not developing cancer or diabetes, and not having good mental status. Females were no more likely to age successfully than were males.

TABLE 4
Adjusted relative odds of successful aging as estimated by the multiple logistic regression model. I. Comparing those who age successfully with those who died or became functionally dependent by 1983

	Relative Odds Estimate	95% Confidence Interval
Age of Individual in 1971		
65-69 / 80-84	28.8	(13.9, 59.7)
70-74 / 80-84	12.7	(6.1, 26.3)
75-79 / 80-84	4.5	(2.1, 9.7)
Sex		
female / male	1.2	(1.0, 1.5)
Spouse Assessed/Placed in Nursing Home (1971-82)		
yes / others	0.2	(0.1, 0.5)
Spouse Died 1971-82		
yes / others	0.4	(0.2, 0.6)
Self-Rated Health 1971		
excellent / poor bad	7.0	(4.0, 12.4)
good / poor bad	4.0	(2.4, 6.8)
fair / poor bad	2.4	(1.4, 4.2)
Reason for Retiring (1971)		
poor health, compulsory / others	0.6	(0.5, 0.8)
Cancer (1970-82)		
no / yes	3.5	(2.4, 5.1)
Had Physician Visit(s) for Diabetes (1970-82)		
no / yes	1.7	(1.3, 2.5)
Interviewer Assessed State of Mind (1971)		
steady and strong / else	2.5	(1.4, 4.6)
Score on Mental Status Index (1971)		
High score (9 or 10) / Lower score (0-8)	1.6	(1.1, 2.4)

Model Chi-Square = 514 with 15df. Region of residence included in the model to control for sampling fraction. Logistic regression results were based on comparing 583 individuals who aged successfully with 2,350 individuals who died or became functionally dependent by 1983. The score on the mental status index, not having diabetes, and rating one's health as fair, reached the 0.05 level of significance in only one of the split half models and the final model.

Factors which distinguish those who successfully aged from those who survived to 1983 but were functionally dependent are shown in Table 5. After controlling for age, self-rated health was again a strong predictor of successful aging. Individuals who did not have diabetes were also more likely to age successfully, although cancer had no similar impact. The odds of successful aging were decreased if one's spouse died or was assessed for or placed in a nursing home.

TABLE 5
Adjusted relative odds of successful aging as estimated by the multiple logistic regression model. II. Comparing those who age successfully with those who were alive in 1983 but dependent

Specification of Variable	Relative Odds Estimate	95% Confidence Interval
Age of Individual in 1971		
65-69 / 80-84	11.5	(5.3, 25.0)
70-74 / 80-84	5.6	(2.6, 12.3)
75-79 / 80-84	2.7	(1.2, 6.2)
Sex		
female / male	0.8	(0.6, 1.0)
Spouse Assessed/Placed in Nursing Home (1971-82)		
yes / others	0.1	(0, 0.4)
Spouse Died 1971-82		
yes / others	0.4	(0.3, 0.8)
Self-Rated Health 1971		
excellent / poor bad	5.5	(2.9, 10.6)
good / poor bad	3.0	(1.7, 5.5)
fair / poor bad	2.2	(1.2, 4.0)
Reason for retiring (1971)		
poor health, compulsory / others	0.7	(0.5, 0.9)
Cancer (1970-82)		
no / yes	1.0	(0.6, 1.7)
Had Physician Visit(s) for Diabetes (1970-82)		
no / yes	1.5	(1.0, 2.2)
Interviewer Assessed State of Mind (1971)		
steady and strong / else	1.9	(1.0, 3.9)
Score on Mental Status Index (1971)		
High score (9 or 10) / Lower score (0-8)	1.9	(1.2, 2.8)

Model Chi-Square = 208 with 15df. Included in the model was region of residence to control for sampling fraction. Logistic regression results based on comparing 583 individuals who aged successfully with 662 individuals who were alive in 1983 but dependent. Age 75-79, having a spouse who died, retiring because of poor health, having a visit for diabetes, reporting fair health and having a high score on the mental status index, reached the 0.05 level of significance in only one of the split half models and the final model.

Discussion

Successful aging has been defined in terms of an individual retaining the ability to function independently (Rowe 1987; Stallones 1987). Those who age successfully remain out of institutions and do not have continuing input from a home health agency. They remain mobile and competent in all the activities of daily living. While these individuals defined their health status in 1983 as fair or better, we deliberately did not label these individuals the "healthy aged." Healthy implies the absence of disease and further, individuals with the "same disease" may have a different sense of well-being and ability to function (Guralnik and Kaplan 1989).

Our results are interesting not only because of the variables they include, but also for the variables which they do not include. None of the measures of socioeconomic status were significant in the final models, even though the measures available in 1971 were extensive. Also, an index combining high scores on the education, occupation and income variables was constructed but did not prove significant.

Two recent studies (Wigle and Mao 1980; Wilkins and Adams 1983) have reported that low incomes are associated with poor health outcomes for Canadians despite universally insured medical and hospital care. Guralnik and Kaplan (1989) also found income predictive of a high level of functioning in the 19-year follow-up of Alameda County residents. Two factors may help to account for our contradictory findings compared to these earlier studies. The income effect may decrease with age because: not as many poor people as others survive long enough to be classified as "old"; the income gradient among the elderly may narrow with government transfer payments improving the lot of the poor, while advancing age is depleting the resources of the wealthy. Haan, et al. (1987) compared age-specific mortality rates among White Alameda County residents of poverty and non-poverty areas. While in the younger age groups the mortality rates in poverty areas were much higher, among those ages 65 and older, there was essentially no difference. Finally, the one group in Canadian society which is most economically disadvantaged, Native Canadians, were excluded from the analysis.

This study presents strong evidence that regular contact with physicians, even among elderly individuals (one of the highest risk groups in the population), is not related to successful aging. Regular contact with the health care system was measured with a high degree of accuracy. Neither the percentage of years in which individuals made one or more visits, nor the percentage of years in which two or more visits were made, was associated with successful aging.

Many measures of disease and functional status were not useful predictors of successful aging. None of the measures of poor functional status in 1971, including indicators that an individual needed help in the activities of daily living or in instrumental activities, none of the self-reported health conditions (including stroke, arthritis, etc.) and only one of the conditions for which physician visit data were available (diabetes) was negatively associated with successful aging.

These findings are contrary to most preconceptions and to some literature. The National Institute of Mental Health's Human Aging II Study (Granick and Patterson 1976) a longitudinal follow-up of a small number of very healthy males, found even asymptomatic disease was negatively predictive of longevity. However, that study focused on longevity alone and longevity is only one (albeit an important) aspect of successful aging.

Having cancer was negatively associated with successful aging but primarily influenced longevity; people with cancer were less likely to live long enough to age successfully by our criteria. However, if such individuals did survive to 1983 (6.7 percent of those surviving to 1983 had cancer), they were just as likely to have aged successfully as those without cancer.

Since age is strongly related to mortality, odds ratios for categories associated with successful aging are greater for the model whose comparison group included decedents (Table 4). The magnitude of the odds ratio for the female sex decreased somewhat from model one to model two (Table 5) reflecting the fact that, although more females may survive, their chance of aging successfully appears to be lower than that for males who survive (Jette and Branch, 1981). A comparison of self-rated health in the two models suggests the distribution of self-rated health in 1971 among those who subsequently died was similar to that among those who remained alive but dependent.

Previous work in Manitoba demonstrated that self-rated health was a predictor of mortality over a six-year period independent of objective health status (Mossey and Shapiro 1982) and this relationship has been confirmed by others (Idler et al. 1990). The present study extends these findings by demonstrating that self-rated health is not only an important predictor of mortality over the longer 12-year period, but is also one of the few factors associated with successful aging among those who survive. Muller (1982) suggested that the predictive contribution of self-rated health could be partly due to Mossey and Shapiro's including indicators developed from utilization data in their measure of objective health status. She suggested pessimism and depression might be the actual causal factors. Although measures of life satisfaction in 1971 were predictive of successful aging in early models, they made no contribution here to the final models which included the self-rated health measure.

There were measures unavailable to this project which might have made useful contributions. The most obvious limitation of the data was the lack of biological measures of function (blood pressure, etc.) and the lack of measures of health practices (smoking history, alcohol consumption, regular physical activity, etc. although the latter could be approximated by the questions pertaining to leisure time activities). The Alameda County study found individuals with more low risk practices to have lower mortality rates (Wingard et al. 1982). The Framingham Study, after 21 years of biennial observations, also reported that alcohol intake, smoking, ventricular rate, and education were related to good functioning status for men although, for women, the only significant predictor other than age was education (Pinski et al. 1987).

In conclusion, a significant group of elderly do age successfully. These individuals express more satisfaction with their lives and incur substantially fewer health expenditures than other elderly. Individuals at particular risk of not aging successfully include those with poor self-assessed health, whose spouse has died, whose mental status is somewhat compromised, who developed cancer, and those who are forced to retire or retire because of poor health.

Acknowledgements

This research was supported by a grant (6607-1440-57) from the National Health Research and Development Program (NHRDP). The 1971 interview was funded by the Government of Manitoba, Department of Health, with the 1983 interview funded by NHRDP grant (6607-1302-06) and the Government of Manitoba, Department of Health. The assistance of Robert Tate, Carmen Steinbach, Bogdan Bogdanovic, Betje Jacobs, and Debbie Molina is acknowledged with thanks. The authors are indebted to the Manitoba Health Services Commission, the Manitoba Cancer Treatment and Research Foundation, and the Manitoba Department of Vital Statistics which helped make this research possible. Interpretations of the data are the authors' own.

Dr Roos holds a Career Scientist Award from the National Health Research and Development Program of Health Canada and is an Associate of the Canadian Institute for Advanced Research. Ms. Havens is also a Provincial Gerontologist and Acting Assistant Deputy Minister of Community Health Services, Manitoba Department of Health.

Appendix

Variables Available to the Analysis (All Items from 1971 Interview Except as Indicated)

- **Ethnicity and Cultural Characteristics of Individual**
  National descent
  Language spoken
  Date of arrival in Canada
  Language of interview
- **Socioeconomic Characteristics of Individual**
  Level of education attainment (number of years or grades completed in school)
  Major occupation when employed
  Current employment in major or other occupation
  Major reason for continuing working (if applicable)
  Total monthly income (a total of income reported from three sources:
      own resources – wage, rents, interest, etc.; pensions or allowances;
      other sources – children, etc.)
  Disposable income (calculated by subtracting monthly expenses from monthly
      income)
  Percent of income from private sources
  Whether income satisfied current needs
  Whether income would satisfy future needs
  Would extra income be spent on food, medical needs, etc.
  Ownership of current residence
  Characteristics of residence
      Heating satisfactory, lighting satisfactory, complete bathroom available,
          bathroom sharing, a room of one's own?
      Residence in a senior citizen's housing unit
- **Characteristics of Individual's Social Network**
  Marital status
  Living arrangements (with spouse, with spouse and others, other)
  Number of relatives, amount of contact with them and "nearness"
  Frequency of contact with neighbors, friends
  Death of spouse between 1971 interview or person's death or December 31, 1982*
  Spouse assessed for or entered nursing home during same period*
- **Individual's Mental Status**
  Score on 10 question mental status test (Kahn et al. 1960)
  Frequency of forgetting names of friends or relatives, time of day.
      How quickly recalled?
  Interviewer's assessment of respondent's:
  -state of mind (steady and strong to weak or unsteady)
  -attitude (friendly to hostile)
  -comprehension of questions (satisfactory to unsatisfactory)

- **Satisfaction with Life**
  In general
  Score on 20 questions Life Satisfaction Index "A" (Neugarten et al. 1961)
- **Individual's Health Status**
  Self-reported health: "For your age, would you say your health is excellent, good, fair, poor or bad?"
  Reporting any of 15 health problems including diabetes, chest problems such as asthma or emphysema
  Under treatment for any of these conditions
  Amount of time in bed at home because of illness in last year: none, less than one week, one week to a month, more than a month
  Help required in basic activities of daily living (getting in and out of bed, dressing, bathing, eating, using stairs)
  Number of activities requiring help from someone outside the house (light house work, making tea, preparing a hot meal, shopping, laundry, heavy housework, financial affairs)
  Number of activities requiring help from someone inside or outside the house (nursing care, cutting toenails, going out of doors, watching TV or reading)
  Required attention of physician or nurse when last sick
  Moved because of ill health
  Retired because of poor health
  Living in a senior citizen housing unit (individuals tend to move to these rental units when they have difficulty maintaining themselves at home usually for health and/or economic reasons)
  Unmet health care needs for eyeglasses, hearing aid, false teeth, cane, special shoes, wheelchair or medicine
  Mean number of physical visits (per year alive) for conditions identified as increasing an individual's "risk of not recovering from an illness" (Jones 1974) e.g., angina, arthritis, arrhythmia, diabetes, hypertension over period 1970-82*
  Number of above listed conditions for which made one or more physical visits (per year alive); for which made two or more physician visits (per year alive)*
  Cancer (excluding skin cancer) diagnosed 1970-82**
- **Participation in Leisure Time Activities**
  21 alternatives including visiting, telephoning, listening to radio or TV, work, etc.
  Which activities are most important
- **Access to Care**
  Difficulty getting to see a doctor/dentist because of transportation, language problems or distance
  Percentage of years alive in which one or more visits to physicians were made; in which made two or more visits, 1970-82*

*   Indicator derived from claims files of Manitoba Health Services Commission.
**   Indicator derived from files of the Manitoba Cancer Registry.

References

Chappell, N, and J Horne. 1987. *Housing and Support of Services for Elderly Persons in Manitoba*. Ottawa: Canada Mortgage and Housing Corporation.

Detsky, AS, SR Stacey, and C Bombardier. 1983. The Effectiveness of a Regulatory Strategy in Containing Hospital Costs: The Ontario Experience, 1967-1981. *New England Journal of Medicine* 309: 151–159.

Granick, S, and RD Patterson eds. 1976. *Human Aging II. An Eleven-Year Follow-up Biomedical and Behavioral Study*. Washington, DC: Government Printing Office. Department of Health, Education and Welfare.

Guralnik, JM, and GA Kaplan. 1989. Predictors of Healthy Aging: Prospective Evidence from the Alameda County Study. *American Journal of Public Health* 79: 703–708.

Haan, M. GA Kaplan, and T Camacho. 1987. Poverty and Health. Prospective Evidence From the Alameda County Study. *American Journal of Epidemiology* 125: 989–998.

Idler, EL, SV Kasl, and JH Lemke. 1990. Self-Evaluated Health and Mortality Among the Elderly in New Haven, Connecticut, and Iowa and Washington Counties. Iowa, 1982-1986. *American Journal of Epidemiology* 131: 91–103.

Jette, AM, and LG Branch. 1981. The Framingham Disability Study: II. Physical Disability Among the Aging. *American Journal of Public Health* 71: 1211–1216.

Jones, EW. 1974. *Patient Classification for Longterm Care: User's Manual*. Washington, DC: Government Print Office. Department of Health, Education and Welfare.

Kahn, RL, AI Goldfarb, ME Pollack, and A Peck. 1960. Brief Objective Measures for the Determination of Mental Status in the Aged. *American Journal of Psychiatry* 117: 326–328.

Manitoba Department of Health and Social Development. 1973. *Aging in Manitoba*. Winnipeg: Queen's Printer.

Mossey, JM, B Havens, NP Roos, E Shapiro. 1981. The Manitoba Longitudinal Study on Aging: Description and Methods. *Gerontologist* 21: 551–558.

Mossey, JM, and E Shapiro. 1982. Self-Rated Health: A Predictor of Mortality Among the Elderly. *American Journal of Public Health* 72: 800-808.

Mosteller, F, and JW Tukey. 1977. *Data Analysis and Regression*. Reading, MA: Addison-Wesley.

Muller, C. 1982. Health Status and Survival Needs of the Elderly (Editorial). *American Journal of Public Health* 72: 789–790.

Neugarten, BL, RJ Havighurst, and SS Toblin. 1961. The Measurement of Life Satisfaction. *Journal of Gerontology* 16: 134–143.

Pinsky, JL, PE Leaverton, and J Stokes. 1987. Predictors of Good Function: The Farmingham Study. *Journal of Chronic Diseases* 40(Suppl 1): 159S–167S.

Roos, LL, NP Roos, SM Cageorge, and JP Nicol. 1982. How Good are the Data? Reliability of One Health Care Data Bank. *Medical Care* 20: 266–276.

Roos, LL, SM Sharp, and A Wajda. 1989. Assessing Data Quality: A Computerized Approach. *Social Science and Medicine* 28: 175–182.

Roos, NP, F Shapiro, and R Tate. 1989. Does a Small Minority of Elderly Account for a Majority of Health Care Expenditures: A Sixteen Year Perspective. *Milbank Memorial Fund Quarterly* 67(3-4): 347–369.

Rowe, JW. 1987. Seeking the Keys to Successful Aging. *Geriatrics* 42: 99–100.

Stallones, RA. 1987. Epidemiological Studies of Health: A Commentary on the Framingham Studies. *Journal of Chronic Diseases* 40(Suppl 1): 177S–180S.

Wigle, DG, and Y Mao. 1980. *Mortality By Income Level in Urban Canada.* Ottawa: Health and Welfare Canada, Health Protection Branch,.

Wilkins, R, and OB Adams. 1983. Health Expectancy in Canada, Late 1970s: Demographic, Regional, and Social Dimensions. *American Journal of Public Health* 73: 1073–1080.

Wingard, DL, LF Berkman, and RJ Brand. 1982. A Multivariate Analysis of Health-Related Practices. A Nine-Year Mortality Follow-up of the Alameda County Study. *American Journal of Epidemiology* 116: 765–774.

Part IV
Health Care Providers (Or Caring)

Introduction - Empty Spaces

Health care providers and the "system of health professions" have received more research attention than any other area in the health field, perhaps because the area is closely tied to the more general sociological literature on occupations and professions. Before moving to a brief overview of recent trends in the sociology of providers, a note on "empty spaces."

Because most higher status health professionals were male and because the gendering of occupations and women's work in health care has been attributed to women's "natural" caring role, examination of female health care occupations is relatively new. Women's caring occupations and the impact of women's life situation on them, for example, the interaction between domestic and public or paid work, also has only recently claimed attention. Not only have women informal caregivers been ignored, but theories of the professions have tended towards general androcentric explanations, which ignored gender (and race) issues and structures as an explanation of the dynamics of health professions. Although these issues were neglected in the past, the number of articles on women or on women's health issues is now burgeoning, as this volume and this section, attest.

More generally, lower status health care workers have been almost totally ignored. The orderlies, paramedicals, and service personnel who keep hospitals functioning are almost invisible and occupy a different world than do the higher status healing or caring occupations.

Until the advent of feminist writers, almost all research was confined to research on workers in the public realm. Just as health matters had been overidentified with the health care system, so health care work had been viewed as referring to those in health care who were paid for such services. The caring for the ill which takes place within families, almost entirely carried out by women, has been out of sight and out of mind. In that sense sociologists have been captured by the visibility of the public realm at the expense of the "private." This situation is also beginning to be rectified.

The context within which health occupations and professions function is often mentioned, but contextual factors are seldom explicitly included in theories in the area. The exception to this generality is neo-marxian theories, which, because of their emphasis on the operation of modes of production or social formations as a whole, are more prone to view health professions and health systems within their broader social context. Contextual factors are not, of course, only the province of marxists; neo-institutionalists, some Weberian closure theorists, and even some pluralist interest group theorists, note that contextual factors are important although these are seldom integrated into the explanations provided.

Finally, although there is much in the general sociological literature on postmodernism and, most relevant to the professions, the knowledge/power approach of Foucault, there is as yet little readily available Canadian literature using these concepts. Much of what is written about the professions, then, still remains clearly within the "modernist" fold.

Theorizing in the Provider/Professions Area

Most analysts agree that theorizing in the professions area moved from "trait" through "functional" to more power oriented theories – the latter derived from Marx or Weber. There has been an historical sequence of viewing the professions from their own perspective – as displaying particular characteristics (such as esoteric knowledge, codes of ethics emphasizing the rights of patients, etc.) to taking a much more cynical view. Recently, from both the political right and the left, medicine, as well as other high status professions, are viewed as groups seeking monopoly powers through state legitimation, and the power, prestige and income that go along with this status.

The dominant perspectives currently are those based on a notion of "closure" theory derived from Weber's emphasis on groups seeking to control a market. Neo-marxists, by comparison, look for the linkages between class and professions or ground the analysis of professions in the context of the class struggle, a class coalitional perspective, and/or situate the health professions as part of the "rise and decline" of the welfare state.

Much of the literature on the health occupations and professions arises from a Freidsonian tradition based on the notion of the dominance of the medical profession in health care. Freidson asserted that medicine controls not only the content of health care but also clients, other health care occupations, and the context within which health care is given (health policy). The historical trajectory whereby medicine came to be all-powerful has received considerable analysis. In the recent literature there are now numerous critiques of the dominant role of medicine and arguments about whether or not medicine is as powerful as it once was. Even those who contend that medicine is still dominant feel that medical control over health and health care is at least being challenged. But, while some claim medicine retains the essential elements of its dominance, others feel that the profession is being de-professionalized or proletarianized.

More recently, of course, greater attention has been paid to alternative or previously excluded health occupations such as chiropractic, naturopathy, and accupuncture, and to occupations subordinate to medicine; nursing has been particularly well treated. All of these tend to be viewed as part of a system of health care occupations and professions still at least partially controlled by medicine. Other healers were excluded by medicine from the formal health care division of labour (e.g., chiropractic or naturopathy) or accepted within it only in a subordinated (nursing or physiotherapy) or limited (dentistry or pharmacy) role (Willis 1989).

The conclusions to recent Canadian analyses are that medicine, while undoubtedly declining in dominance, is still the single most powerful health occupation, but is now surrounded by many other providers, all with increasing degrees of legitimation or state recognition and all eager to escape from under medicine's thumb. The rise of these "other" occupations was aided by strategies, seemingly drawn from sociological accounts of the rise of professions, emphasizing credentialism, new and different (from medicine) theories of health, caring, or rehabilitation, and/or promising greater efficiencies and effectiveness. From a situation of almost total medical control, the hierarchical system of health care professions and occupations now is somewhat flatter than it was. But the explanation for these changes must be sought, not only in the internal dynamics of the system, but in those external factors which influence or determine inter-professional relationships.

There is a change towards a post-Freidsonian perspective which seeks to escape from the inconsistencies within previous medical dominance theory, to contextualize trends in professional power, and to remedy the lack of attention paid to the gender aspects of the professions. In fact, ever since Freidson's original formulations there have been critics pointing to the lack of connections of medical dominance theory to its social context. Given developments regarding constraints on state actions by the globalization of capital and by perceived fiscal constraints, the context of health care, and in particular the roles of the state and of broader structural class groupings are now seen to be crucial to any explanation of fluctuations of power amongst providers and between providers and patients. For example, a powerful, but still far from fully substantiated approach takes medicine's congruence with powerful class forces as major determinants both of its rise to power in the late nineteenth and early twentieth centuries and of present challenges to its power. One explanation for the changing power structure within health care is that medical and upper class or bourgeoise/state interests and/or ideology no longer coincide.

As noted, the theoretical tools to carry out these connections are still somewhat underdeveloped. Although neo-marxian theory re-emphasizes the contextual conditions under which medicine or other health care professions rise and fall, the theoretical and empirical linkages tying social structural factors with the historical trajectory of the professions is still inadequate. Conversely, the major alternative, or supplement, to neo-marxist theory can seemingly deal with interprofessional rivalries through the Weberian concept of market closure, yet such theories often degenerate into simple, pluralist interest group analyses with all of the problems attendant on this approach, or, if developed on a more macro level, closely approximate neo-marxist theory. Perhaps there is a convergence, and certainly it is difficult to know whether some writers are Weberian or Marxist. Both of these approaches, of course, have been severely criticized for not adequately noticing, or accounting for, the high degree of gender segregation within health care occupations and for their inability to explain gender related factors, although closure theory has somewhat better credentials in this respect than does marxist theory. In fact, there is a rapidly changing gender composition for some of the professions (but not others), at the same time as state policy seems oriented to shuffling off some of its current health care responsibilities onto the private (family) sphere in which women are the main unpaid "carers" and workers.

All of this is occurring at a time when welfare states generally are under attack from the right and from the neo-conservative movement. There has been a decrease in power or of the "relative autonomy" of national states as a result of economic depression and to the internationalization of capital. State-run or financed health care systems are under fiscal pressures at the same time as more market oriented ones are also open to criticism because of the obvious inefficiencies in a health care system left to the mercy of private insurance markets.

The overall trends seem to be a decrease in medical dominance, an increase in the power of other providers, and an incipient move to more patient power, at the same time that health care is attacked as being ineffective in improving the health status of the population or at least as reducing inequalities in health status. This is accompanied by a managerial demiurge within health care systems. In Alford's term, the corporate rationalizers are in the ascendance (Alford 1975). In Canada this managerialism is reinforced by an implicit business/state coalition aiming to rationalize health care as part of the project to reduce government expenditures.

In This Part

The chapters in this part point to some of the issues mentioned above as well as exemplifying the new wave of research with women as the major focus. The part begins, not with a provider, but with a first person description of an encounter with providers and the health care system. Sharon Batt documents her own story of breast cancer and the problems and issues of diagnosing and attempting to cure this disease. Major issues emerge, not only of the ambiguities of diagnosis and treatment and the stresses produced by these, but also of the difficulties of obtaining humane treatment and care in a highly technically oriented health care system. Patient needs are often lost sight of in the complexities of the health care system or are slighted by providers used to assuming a controlling role.

Next, examining medicine, nursing, and chiropractic, Coburn reveals that these occupations showed somewhat different historical trajectories. Medicine in Canada shows a pattern of "rise and fall," although as yet the fall is not great nor equivalent to a full process of proletarianization. Nursing exemplifies the forces implicit in a gendered division of labour and presents a complex picture of professionalization and proletarianization (although not necessarily deskilling). Throughout its history nursing has struggled against the dominance of medicine – as has chiropractic. The latter occupation, although early on excluded from the health care division of labour, has managed to gain legitimation, if at the cost of a narrowing of its aims and scope of practice. The boundaries between medicine, the dominant profession, and the state are permeable rather than impassible. Medicine early on infiltrated state organizations, while the state now seeks to control practitioners, partly through controlling, or at least constraining, medical organizations themselves. Although the state implicitly used medicine to control the health care division of labour, the state is now directly involved in managing the health care system rather than simply acting as paymaster. There is emerging a form of state-constrained meso-corporatist control of the professions.

Williams, Domnick-Pierre and Vayda note that in 1959 women constituted only 6 percent of medical school graduates, whereas by 1989 the total was 44 percent. By 1990 women were 50 percent of medical students (not reported are large differences amongst medical schools in the percentage of women students – women form a much larger percentage of medical classes in Quebec than elsewhere). The increasing percentage of women may prove one impetus for changes in medicine. Women physicians practice somewhat fewer hours than do men, but also, their practices might be qualitatively different. Are these differences the result of the "double role" of women or of different attitudes and values? Surveys analyzed by these authors indicate that there are few differences between men and women physicians on economic and medico-political issues, partly, the authors believe, because of the socializing influences of medical school. But, from focus group research with small numbers of women practitioners, there does seem to be a possible difference in orientations to practice in which women doctors are more "whole patient" oriented than are men physicians. Although increasing percentages of women physicians may lead to differences in practice, actual political change may be muted by common socialization and the fact that women (now but not necessarily in the future) are relatively marginalized within the medical political power structure.

One important indication of the possible decline of medical dominance and the impact of feminism on health care is the revival of midwifery. Across Canada midwifery is much in the news as it becomes, more or less, an accepted part of health care. Cecilia Benoit reports on the role of midwifery in Britain and the United States as well as in Canada. She notes that, despite many cultural similarities, midwifery has emerged in somewhat different form in these three countries. Midwifery thus has to be understood as responsive to particular social structures. Midwifery has long been a part of the British health care system, but Benoit notes that it is a bureaucratized and medically dominated midwifery. Midwifery in the United States has been forced in the direction of a focus on costs and fees rather than patients needs. Although Canada is moving in the direction of making midwifery a legitimate part of health care the question arises – what kind of midwifery? Benoit's own research in Newfoundland and British Columbia indicates that the increasing acceptance of midwifery into the formal health care system in Canada is a two-edged sword. Midwifery may be seduced by a "professionalism" which would lead them to separation from their clients and exclusion of those with "inadequate credentials." Thus there is the danger that midwifery will become more like the orthodox medical model it was originally set up to oppose.

Television advertisements now continually ask us to use pharmacists as our "patient advisors." Muzzin, Brown, and Hornosty characterize pharmacy as a profession with a somewhat beleagured jurisdiction. Over the years pharmacy has used various ideologies to justify its role and to emphasize its uniqueness. In particular, in response to changing markets and inter-professional challenges pharmacy is now trying to justify a new and somewhat expanded role as patient counsellors (as opposed to earlier ideologies which emphasized the pharmacist either as expert or as an advisor to physicians). The authors use Becker's notion of "situational development" to explain divergent enactments of these ideologies by pharmacists in hospitals or elsewhere. They also examine the possible role of gender regarding the enactment of these ideologies in practice. They conclude that adherence to the new "patient counselling" ideology is most strongly effected by work setting (in which community pharmacists are most supportive and hospital pharmacists the least). Gender is not as important as structural location. Pharmacy thus faces its future somewhat divided over its proper role, a division leading to a disjunction between pharmacy education and pharmacy practice.

We are used to thinking of health care as taking place in hospitals or doctors offices, yet Aronson notes that it is estimated that 90 percent of care for the elderly is given in the "private sphere" and only 10 percent by the formal health care system and by social services. The main caregivers in the family are female. Studying the intersection of "biography" and "structure" Aronson analyzes interview data from 32 teachers – either elderly or middle-aged women with elderly mothers for whom they felt responsible, that is, both caregivers and carereceivers. Her analysis indicates the contradictions between the wish to support relatives versus the stress and resentment at having to do so, and the needs of elderly women versus the culturally expressed and structurally determined barriers to the expression of these. Violation of what is viewed as appropriate women's roles produces feelings of guilt and stress. Aronson shows how structurally produced expectations interact with and constrain individual needs or wants. What is needed to adequately cope with the problems of women as caregivers and as receivers is broader cultural change along with the provision of better alternatives for care of elderly women in the public realm. Yet, the general trend for neo-conservative governments is precisely the opposite, to put more pressure on families as caregivers at the same time as cost-cutting eliminates public services.

All of the above confirms the notion of a changing health care division of labour. There is a decline in medical dominance and an increasing appreciation of the role of women caregivers inside and outside of the health care system. Analysts are now more aware of the degree to which health care dynamics reflect, and reinforce, broader social structural factors such as class dynamics, gender relations, and the role of the state.

References

Alford, RR. 1975. *Health Care Politics*. Chicago: University of Chicago Press.
Willis, E. 1989. *Medical Dominance: The Division of Labour in Australian Health Care.* 2nd ed. Sydney: George Allen and Unwin.

17

Thrown* (an encounter with the health care system)

Sharon Batt

> Down, Down, Down.
> Would the fall never come to an end.
> Lewis Carroll, *Alice in Wonderland*
> "What a queer planet" he thought. "It is altogether dry,
> and altogether pointed, and altogether harsh and forbidding."
> - Antoine de Saint-Exupery, *The Little Prince*

Until I got breast cancer, I had thought about it on only three occasions.

When I was a university student in Vancouver in the '60s, my mother wrote to tell me that her sister had breast cancer and was moving from Detroit to live with my family in Ottawa. Mom was upset because Helen had known of the diagnosis for some years but had refused breast surgery. Helen was stubborn so her decision would have seemed merely in character – except that she was a nurse. "Maybe she knows something we don't," I said to my mother. My mother had a different interpretation – that Helen wanted to die.

In fact, my aunt did die a few years later. Around that time I went to a clinic for a routine checkup and an intern examined my breasts.

His eyebrows shot up in alarm. "Very lumpy!" he said.

He told me to go for another opinion which, after two sleepless nights, I did. The doctor was a tall woman with greying hair. After she examined me, she asked, "How old was the doctor who sent you here?"

"Maybe 25."

"I don't think he's felt many breasts in his life," she said dryly. "This is perfectly normal tissue. He's given you a needless scare."

After that, I had a marked bias towards women physicians. I didn't think about breast cancer again for 20 years.

By then I was living in Montréal. I attended an international feminist book fair, and a highlight on the program was an address by the black American poet Audre Lorde. She gave an uncompromising talk which set off a turmoil of debates about race. Afterwards, I headed for the bookstalls. All her books were sold out except for a slim volume called *The Cancer Journals*, based on Lorde's experience with breast

* Excerpted from *Patient No More: The Politics of Breast Cancer,* by Sharon Batt, Gynergy books, 1994, Charlottetown, PEI; with permission of the publisher.

cancer. I didn't want to read about cancer. But I wanted to read Audre Lorde. Reluctantly, I bought the book.

Four months later I, too, was diagnosed with breast cancer.

ii

It happened this way. In September I took a cycling vacation in France. Late one afternoon, while showering off the day's hard-won sweat, I ran a soapy hand over my left breast and froze. There, in the lower crescent of flesh, I felt a small, hard lump. I continued to shower, focussing on the evening ahead, the delectable dinner I knew awaited me; but some magnetic force kept drawing my hand to the spot. Sometimes the lump was gone. Then it wasn't. Over the next few days, the reluctant search became a nightly ritual.

By day, I didn't think about it. I felt well, ergo I was well. This straightforward philosophy of health had served me well until now. Indeed, at 43, I felt superb. The lump was an incongruous presence in my vibrant body.

Back in Montreal, I confronted the mammogram machine. The technician scrunched my breast between two horizontal plates then tightened the clamp. "Don't breathe," she said, and vanished.

"OK, breathe," she said, coming out, and squashed my breast vertically.

Downstairs at the breast clinic I gave the X-rays to the surgeon on duty, a taciturn man who seemed to know what he was about. He snapped the X-rays onto a lighted surface, he palpated my breast, he pulled out a long needle. "Mosquito bite," he said. The needle pierced the lump and he twisted it around. I winced.

"Sorry," he said. Then, "Ninety-nine percent sure it's nothing."

I believed him. Despite my unease about the lump, despite my aunt and *The Cancer Journals*, breast cancer seemed a distant menace. I held onto the reassuring slogans I'd heard for years: get a mammogram, see your doctor, breast cancer can be cured. As for those 99 percent odds – most breast lumps are benign.

When I came back for the results of the needle biopsy, things turned ominous. Some cells were irregular.

"I can take another needle sample, or remove the whole lump. I'd prefer to take it out. Then we can be sure."

I must have looked doubtful. The surgeon flipped the report around so I could see it. "Ambiguous cells, insufficient sample."

"What does that mean?" I demanded, suddenly aggressive. It seemed to me he'd messed up the test. And what about the 99 percent odds? Or the mammogram, which showed nothing unusual? I was sinking in quicksand.

My antagonism was not going over well. In fact, the whole encounter had tilted, had spun us both out of control. Now the surgeon was protesting vehemently, "I do not cut off women's breasts, I do not cut off women's breasts!"

I hadn't even considered that possibility. And why was he so defensive? Terrified, I fled.

That night, my friend Jeannie came over to visit. I could think of nothing but the lump and when I told her about it, she asked to feel it. By now I'd decided to have it out. Jeannie has strong opinions and she thought I was capitulating to the medical system.

"If I had all my lumps out, my breasts would look like a moonscape," she said.

"The cells were irregular. I want it out."

She insisted on a mutual breast feel, the kind of ritual we had in high school.

"It's really hard," she said, surprised. Then, soberly, "I'd get it out."

To get my bearings before the operation, I read about breast cancer. Already, I'd skimmed the section in *The New Our Bodies Ourselves* trying to absorb medical jargon: *estrogen receptor assays, permanent section, two-step biopsy*. Everything the surgeon had done checked out, which reassured me, but the book began to undermine my comforting assumptions. For example, it said, "breast cancer mortality rates have not declined significantly in the past half-century despite progressively earlier detection and treatment" (Boston Women's Health Collective 1984: 531). And, "mammograms use radiation and radiation can cause cancer" (p. 495). The more I read, the more astonished I was. Breast cancer, I learned, kills thousands of North American women every year, second only to heart disease. In women 35 to 55, it's the number one killer. I was 43.

As a feminist and a journalist, I fancied myself well informed, especially about women's issues. Yet I knew next to nothing about breast cancer. Now, it seemed that the little I thought I knew was wrong. I was puzzled and vaguely irritated with myself.

My life split onto two tracks. One was life-as-usual: my work as a magazine editor, evenings with friends, a screenwriting workshop, swimming at the gym. The summer of regular cycling had given me a taste for rigorous training and I felt in peak condition. I wanted to try triathlon competition. A fitness test at the Y confirmed my sense of well-being. "Remarkable!" said the women who tested me. "Only professional athletes score higher than this." I could hardly have cancer and feel this well.

Between routines, my thoughts were scattered. I sent postcards to friends in other cities and slipped in an anxious phrase or two: "by the way ... it seems I may have cancer." Mentally, I sketched out a will. I drew back from long-term projects and thought morbidly about winding up unfinished business: my last to-do list and will.

iii

The morning of the biopsy, Jeannie takes me to the day surgery. She will come back and get me, then stay overnight at my place. After a general anaesthetic, you aren't supposed to spend that night alone.

I lie ready in my hospital gown. A nurse slips on a pair of white cotton boots that go over my knees. "It's cold in the operating room," she says. My surgery boots reassure me; I'm no longer naked. The nurse sticks a needle in my behind and the drug rolls through me in waves.

Only moments later, it seems, I'm back in the recovery room. I feel fine. Just a slight ache in my left breast, which is bandaged. The surgeon has kept his promise. So far, so good. I fade back into the anaesthetic.

I'm awake again and the surgeon is standing by the bed, looking serious. He begins pacing up and down.

"I don't like having to tell you this..." he begins.

Malignant. I can't believe it.

"How big was it?" My last refuge. Small is better.

"A centimetre. Not very big."

Still, he's ordered scans and X-rays. Bone. Liver. Lungs. All the places breast cancer goes, I recall from my crash reading. *Metastasize*, a Greek word, means "to change place." When breast cancer changes place it usually kills you. And he's lined up another operation, to remove lymph nodes. I'm to stay in the hospital.

I don't want these tests, this operation. I haven't told my family yet. I don't know what lymph nodes are but I think maybe I want to keep mine. I drift back into the anaesthetic. When I surface again, he's gone. I ask the nurse about the lymph node operation.

"The doctor should have explained it." She's annoyed.

"I think he did." My memory of the surgeon's visit flickers and fades, a lost dream.

"It's the anaesthetic," she says, concerned. Now she's on the phone to the doctor, cancelling the operation. A reprieve.

Jeannie comes back. "It's cancer," I tell her. The word doesn't seem real. It catches on the way out. She hugs me and I feel tears on my cheeks. I don't know if they're hers or mine.

iv

Well. Sick. Well. Sick. I can't hold the two ideas in my head at the same time. And all week, I don't. I keep switching tracks. At work at my desk, then to the hospital for a test. Finally, the terrible hours at night when I'm in bed but awake, soaked in sweat.

Sometimes I switch from the normal track onto the cancer track, like the morning I stop at a red light on the way to work and notice the woman in the next car staring at me. I am talking feverishly to myself, gesturing wildly at an invisible other who is listening patiently to my discourse about cancer.

I step up my research. For most of my reading I rely on the library at McGill but find only one book in the catalogue under breast cancer: a battered copy more than 10 years old of *Breast Cancer: A Personal History and Investigative Report* by Rose Kushner. I also find a sociology doctoral thesis called *Decision Difficult: Physician Behaviour in the Diagnosis and Treatment of Breast Cancer.*

Kushner's book, I sense, is outdated; otherwise, it's a godsend. A Washington journalist who had a mastectomy in the 1970s, Kushner was so outraged by physicians she talked to at some of America's leading hospitals that she carried out an intensive investigation to learn the facts for herself. Then she wrote a book to tell other women what she'd learned.

She also began a personal crusade to change breast surgery practices. She argued that surgeons should separate the diagnostic biopsy, which determines whether a breast lump is malignant, from the mastectomy that was standard treatment for breast cancer in the 1970s. No woman, Kushner reasoned, should come out of the anaesthetic to be hit with the double whammy of cancer *and* a lost breast. She also knew, from her experience as a former med student, that the operating-room test for malignancy could be wrong. A quick-frozen section might look malignant, but the more reliable lab test, done later, could show it was not. If the surgeon acted on the first analysis, he would inevitably remove a certain number of healthy breasts (Kushner 1986a).

Kusher tells her own story with disarming wit, and I feel I'm listening to a big sister who's been there. Her investigation reads like a detective novel – mystery: breast cancer. Her questions are so much like my own, I stop feeling foolish for being confused. And her discussion of diagnostic errors gives me hope. Maybe, just maybe, my lump isn't really malignant.

The sociology doctoral dissertation has a different tone – the dispassionate language of social science. The writer, Kathryn Taylor, spent three years following physicians as they treated women in a Montreal breast cancer clinic. She wanted to understand how doctors stayed motivated "in the face of high degrees of uncertainty and failure in their endeavour to cure." Uncertainty ... failure? I'm not sure I'm ready for this. And it gets worse: "... no overall improvement in breast cancer survival since statistics were first collected in the 1930s. Early detection is not leading to improved mortality rates ..." Breast cancer patients underwent "painful, uncertain and often unsuccessful treatment plans ..." (Taylor 1984: 2).

At some point as I read, the book falls to the floor. I wander in a daze around my apartment. I can't take this in, I don't want to. Until now, breast cancer has meant having an operation, no big deal. I've had the surgery and I don't feel very different. Now I am truly frightened. *Pain, Uncertainty. Death. No progress.*

Monday, a week after my biopsy, I go back to see the surgeon. When the doctor is impatient he says things twice. "You have an interductal carcinoma," he tells me. "You have an interductal carcinoma." He's telling me the diagnosis was not a mistake. What's worse, the bone scan has a "hot spot." The cancer could be in my bones. He orders an X-ray of my upper spine. He's obviously miffed about the cancelled operation. He wants to get on with it, but I have some questions.

"Is the operation risky?"

He says it could leave my arm paralyzed.

I'm incredulous. "Permanently?"

"Perhaps permanently."

I imagine a gimpy arm, cancer everywhere. Pains shoot through my neck where the bone scan was positive.

"Will I be able to work? Do sports?"

I've said something wrong. The doctor stands up and calls the nurse into the office.

"I need a witness," he declares. "Doctors have rights too."

The room tilts into the vortex again. It's spinning faster than before. I blurt out questions while he takes notes and answers methodically. "The operation won't affect the cancer," I say accusingly. "It won't stop it." I've read this. A lymph node operation will only show how far the disease has spread.

"No. It doesn't stop the cancer."

"And my arm could be permanently paralyzed?"

"Perhaps. We have to cut nerves."

"I don't see the point."

"To complete the staging!" He's exasperated. "We need the operation to complete the staging!"

I stare, blankly. Staging is something they do in the theatre. I'm sitting in a surgeon's office with a diagnosis of cancer and he's talking props and lighting.

"I need to talk to another doctor," I shout "I want another opinion."

"I *insist* you have another opinion," he throws back, seizing the upper hand. "There's no point treating a patient who doesn't believe in the doctor!"

I glance sideways at the nurse. What is she thinking? She's watching the doctor; when he signals that the discussion is over; she leaves.

"What about this bandage," I demand. In the turmoil, we've both forgotten that the bandage is to come off my breast today. "Am I supposed to remove it myself?"

"You could." He's staring down at his desk.

"Are there stitches in there for me to take out?" I know this is ludicrous, but I'm so mad I can't stop.

"No stitches," he says with a sigh. He gestures to the open door of the examining room. "Why don't you let me take it off."

I hesitate a minute, than capitulate. After he removes the bandage, he nods to a small mirror on the wall. "You can look at it if you like." He sounds conciliatory. Awkward emotions hang in the air; like the aftermath of a lovers' quarrel.

I can hardly see my reflection through the tears. I blink. My breast looks the same as before except for some swelling and a bright red line, like a deep scratch, that follows the curve underneath. I try to take in this line – so long; this red – so vivid. I can feel the surgeon watching, I sense he wants me to be pleased. I'm not. I'm still livid from our interview. I reach for my clothes.

In the reception room, I hurtle past the nurse towards my coat. She calls me over and gives me the name of another doctor who works in the same office.

"A different type altogether," she says. "You'll see. Try him, and if you want to change, no problem." She continues talking me down. "Dr T was tired. I could see that. But even when he's not tired," – a long pause – "you take people as they come. He can be ... difficult." She lowers her voice and leans forward. "But Sharon, he's one helluva surgeon."

She arranges an appointment with the other doctor and persuades me to return to Dr T one more time, to discuss the X-rays of my neck.

"Now Doctor G," she confides, "he's a different type. I always say, when you go to see Dr G, bring a book. A thick one."

vi

Added to the enigma of cancer is the enigma of doctors. Not only have I never been seriously ill, I've had scant contact with people who work in medicine. Jeannie's father was a doctor but mine was a lawyer, my mother a psychologist. It strikes me now that my whole family and virtually all my friends are journalists, lawyers, writers, therapists. They live by words and concepts. Aunt Helen was a nurse, yes, but she lived in Detroit and visited. Before I talk to another doctor, I want to understand what motivates them.

Perhaps Kathryn Taylor's dissertation will throw some light on this question, I think. Taylor analyzes the way doctors go about telling women they have breast cancer. Typically, she says, they use one of two strategies. One type – she calls them "experimenters" – take a scientific approach. They emphasize rational thinking and technical skills. Their colleagues, whom Taylor classes as "therapists," rely on clinical experience more than on science for their expertise, and view clinical skill as an almost mystical talent (Taylor 1988: 33–34).

The two types of doctors have very different ways of talking to patients. Experimenters are explicit. They use medical jargon and statistics; they cite published studies to back up their recommendations. One, for example, announced to his patient, "Your lesion is in the inner upper quadrant, so it may have infiltrated the internal mammary chain of the lymph node system making reliance on the results of an axillary dissection only tentative. The protocol for your stage of disease suggests radiating the internal chain, prophylactically of course ..." (Taylor 1984: 37).

These doctors know the patient has no idea what they are saying and wouldn't remember it anyway, but they reason that full disclosure of a breast cancer diagnosis will protect them against malpractice suits. By talking up scientific research, they hope to discourage the patient from seeking alternative treatments they consider quackery. Finally, the experimenters feel it is useless to evade the hard facts about breast cancer because patients will ultimately get them from the media.

The therapists use a different language. They speak in euphemisms and describe cases from their clinical experience to explain the diagnosis. They meet direct questions with evasion. One begins the interview by saying, "There was something we didn't like about your [pathology] report ..." The patient, shaking and crying, sobs that when she was 16, her mother died of cancer. She asks if she too has cancer. "Well, it's sort of a tumour," the doctor responds, "but mind you ... probably not like [your mother] had ... we call it infiltrating ductal carcinoma, just your everyday garden variety type ..." To which the patient replies, "Oh, thank God! ... I thought I had cancer ... thank you doctor ... I'm sorry I got this upset ..." (Taylor 1984: 43).

These physicians invoke tradition to justify their evasiveness: things have always been done this way. They don't believe patients really want to know the diagnosis and assume a frank disclosure will trigger depression and grief. They take it on themselves to shield the women from such traumatic emotions.

Dr T is an experimenter type I muse, as I sit with my thick book in Dr G's office. The reason for the book is becoming obvious. I've already waited several hours and notice that women who disappear into Dr G's office seem to be there an awfully long time. When my turn finally comes, everyone, including the nurse, has gone home.

Dr G is a tall, thin man with blond hair and an angular face. As he examines my breast, he seems to take an especially long time palpating under my arm, all the while staring thoughtfully at the ceiling.

"What is it?" I ask nervously. "Did you find something?"

"Oh, no no no," he protests, as if I were trying to corner him. "A manual exam is never certain. You need a lab report to be sure."

So why all this *feeling*, I wonder, as I pull on my clothes. I sit down in his office for the interview. In the window behind his head the October sky is black but I hold firm when he ventures that I am probably in a hurry to get home. I haven't waited hours in his office to be rushed out the door. I tell him I'm not sure I want to have my lymph nodes removed, especially if it might leave my arm paralyzed. "If it doesn't stop the cancer, why risk it?" I want to know. And don't the lymph nodes have something to do with the immune system?

"Well, you're quite right, the operation won't change your diagnosis," he agrees. He trips along rapidly, hurling out information as he goes. The nurse is right. He is totally different from Dr T – Taciturn vs Garrulous. Whether he's an experimenter or a therapist I'm not sure; maybe he's a mixed type. The odds of a paralyzed arm are very small, he assures me. "I'd say one percent. In all likelihood, you'd be in the 99 percent that has no problem."

I've lost this gamble before, I think. And don't I need my lymph nodes to fight the cancer?

"Now you may just have something there," he begins. "As a matter of fact, we'll be starting a protocol in January to look at that very thing." This digression disorients me and I recall something Kathryn Taylor says in her dissertation: *The experimenters often volunteered information that their patients had not requested* (Taylor 1984: 38).

"We'll be looking at whether it's better to go right into radiation and chemotherapy without surgery" he finishes.

I'm stuck on the word protocol. Whatever it is, it sounds hopeful, an escape from the operation. "Then maybe I should wait until January ..." I begin.

"Oh, no no no!" he cries. "I wouldn't advise that!"

"Why not?"

"You might get in the wrong group."

Another stumper. They have wrong groups? I go back to the immune system. I am almost never sick and have no allergies, so I think mine must be working pretty well. I don't feel comfortable about having it tampered with.

"If the lymph nodes are part of the immune system and you take out the lymph nodes …."

"Look," he says, "you have cancer. Your immune system let you down."

Low blow. He's hit the button that crashes my logical defenses: so what if I feel healthy? I have cancer.

Now on the offensive, Dr G launches into his wind-up.

"I recommend that you have this operation. If you want, I can do it for you. I've done lots of breast surgery, though lately I've been moving into neck and throat …"

Another spanner. What's wrong with breast cancer, I wonder. Aren't there enough of us packing the waiting rooms?

In the end, both doctors are saying the same thing: have the operation. I thank him and leave.

I could go to yet another surgeon, but see little point. I'm veering back towards Dr T The incision on my breast scarcely hurts at all and looks like it will heal without a trace. The nurse's words echo, "One helluva surgeon." Dr G's career shift to neck and throat makes me nervous. What still worries me about Dr T is that we can't talk to one another.

vii

"No one can talk to surgeons," declares my friend Eleanor, on the phone from Toronto. "They're the engineers of the medical profession."

The postcards worked. My friends are kicking in, in unexpected ways. One night Eleanor phones and announces that she has an in-law who is an oncologist in Montreal. She sounds pleased, as if offering something useful.

"What's an oncologist?" I want to know.

A suppressed giggle, then, "A cancer specialist."

After a late-night consultation about my mishaps in doctorland, she called the family oncologist for inside advice. Doctors, he said, could be placed on a continuum of communicative skills, with surgeons weighing in rock bottom. "Medical students who are totally inarticulate go into surgery," was how he put it. The ones who like to talk become psychiatrists. Everyone else falls in between.

This makes a certain sense and is curiously comforting. The disastrous dramas aren't all my fault. And I can stop looking for a surgeon-confessor because I probably won't find one. The in-law also endorsed the hospital where I was being treated. "It seems you've fallen into a nest of good guys," says Eleanor.

viii

"Have you had an accident lately where you could have hurt your neck?" Dr T begins.

"Yes, in September. A bicycle accident."

Three days before I was to leave for my cycling vacation, a parked motorist flung his door open in my path and threw me to the pavement. Tests showed nothing broken and I opted to take my long-awaited trip despite a doctor's sensible counsel that I spend my three-week vacation in bed.

Now the X-rays show a cracked vertebra in my neck. The hot spot on the scan isn't cancer after all.

The terror that has gripped me for a week melts into ecstasy. A cracked vertebra! I had assumed the bone scan, an intimidating affair, was a definitive test. Down in the sub-basement of the hospital, I'd passed through metal doors marked Nuclear Medicine and was injected with something radioactive. Two hours later, I returned and stretched out, fully clothed, under a large metal disk. To the left, a tiny TV screen sent pulsating signals as the disk passed over my body. The machine looked impressive, but evidently it couldn't tell the difference between cancer and a cracked bone on the mend. Someone might have told me, I think. Still, I am elated and agree to the lymph node operation.

It's Dr T's turn to look relieved.

ix

Breaking the news of my diagnosis is a complicated affair. I have hardly told anyone. My mother, for example. She'll worry, and I'll have to deal with that. Besides, I can still hardly say the word cancer to myself, let alone lob it, grenade-like, into a conversation.

At work, my imminent lymph node operation prods me to tell my boss, the magazine's editor-in-chief. I'll be taking a week off and some explanation is called for. I know I can allude to some vague medical problem and he won't probe, but I decide to say I have breast cancer. His concern doesn't surprise me, but I'm not prepared for his stricken look. Only later, when he tells me his girlfriend's mother died of breast cancer, do I understand the intensity of his response.

I've become so self-absorbed, I am blind to the needs of others. A few days before I go into the hospital, my neighbour Stuart invites me out for supper. Stuart and I have lived in the same walk-up apartment block for years. When he is between girlfriends we hang out together, two singles at ease with each other. As the dinner progresses, the time seems right to explain why I'm not my usual self. Stuart's shock seems to evolve naturally into sympathy; as we part in the hallway late that evening, I feel I've added a plank to my expanding scaffold of support. I learn later that his brother has just died of a drug overdose. The added burden of my news sends him into a serious depression.

My mother is a worrier of the first rank and I put off telling her as long as I can. When I do, she is much calmer than I expect her to be and we have one of our best conversations in years.

"I thought you would freak out," I confess.

"At times like this, I think it's more helpful to be supportive," she says quietly. She offers to send some relaxation tapes that helped her sleep after dad died.

Aside from Jeannie and Stuart, my other close friend in Montreal is Mary Meigs, a writer my mother's age. The previous summer, Mary was one of eight women chosen for the cast of *The Company of Strangers*, a film about older women. Mary calls me a few days after I tell her I have cancer.

"The most terrible thing has happened," she says. "Gloria has cancer too."

Gloria is Gloria Demers, a woman of about my own age who wrote the script for the film. She has lung cancer. Soon afterwards Mary introduces us and Gloria becomes my first cancer buddy: we compare notes about treatments, doctors and our fear of dying.

x

The operation is slated for Tuesday morning, two weeks after the biopsy. On Monday night an intern comes in to have me sign a consent form for the operation. He's tow-headed and freckle-faced, a 30-year-old Dennis the Menace.

"Is the operation difficult?" I ask, fishing for reassurance.

"Well, more difficult than an appendectomy," he offers. "But nothing like a heart bypass."

I picture him late at night, hunched over a textbook at a page headed "Axillary Dissection for Breast Cancer." He's going to assist Dr T.

"Let's just say I'm glad he's doing it and not me," he jokes.

With the operation over, the orderly wheels me back to my room. We pass a group of interns and I spot my towheaded visitor of the night before. He sees me too and peels free of the ambulatory pack.

"An incredibly clean dissection!" he declares, beaming down as I roll by. Before I can say anything, he's reabsorbed by the multilegged clump which glides into a waiting elevator. Lymph nodes, I imagine, are strung together like Christmas-tree lights. I picture mine slipping free of my armpit, unencumbered by nerves and other vital parts. I sink back on the pillow. I won't have a gimpy arm after all.

I share my hospital room with a woman I'll call Mrs. Salisbury. She's in her 70s and has a colostomy bag strapped around her waist. She used to be a nurse, has raised two children and had a difficult marriage. Most of the day she sits unsmiling in a chair against the wall, reading, her white hair pulled back in a pony tail. Her reading alternates between the *Consumers Distributing* catalogue and the *National Enquirer*. She will probably outlive me, I think.

"You got flowers," she says, glumly, as the orderly helps me into my bed. "And phone calls."

The flowers are from Stuart. One night he comes to visit me, another night Jeannie, then Mary arrives with Gloria. With the operation over, the week goes by quickly. Friday I'll be discharged.

But first there's a tumour conference, a sort of show-and-tell with me, Exhibit A, lying on a bed. My friend Louise Dulude and my sister Sylvia have driven down from Ottawa and are sitting in the shadows, against one wall. A dozen or so doctors circle the bed as the surgeon presents my case.

"A tumour of one centimetre was removed from the six o'clock position of the left breast," he announces, lifting off my gown. A dozen pairs of eyes close in on the red slit at the bottom of my breast. I shut my eyes. When I open them, the doctors are filing out of the room.

Later the surgeon comes upstairs to tell me the results of the dissection and explain the treatment. The news isn't good. One of the lymph nodes had cancer cells in it, meaning that the cancer has spread beyond the breast area and is circulating through my system. Millions of maurauding cells are busy dividing, looking for a place to settle. The team recommends six months of chemotherapy, then six weeks of radiotherapy to the spot where the tumour was removed, then a drug called tamoxifen for the rest of my life. Sylvia and Louise hold me up.

xi

Chemotherapy terrifies me. Poisons sent into the bloodstream are supposed to kill the cancer cells when they're dividing. They also kill healthy cells that are dividing. Cancer patients often lose their hair during chemotherapy because cells in the hair follicles divide rapidly, like cancer cells.

The surgeon had said the group recommended CMF, a relatively mild drug mix that usually doesn't cause hair loss. Now the oncologist is suggesting I take part in a trial, a study designed to test three levels of a different combination, CAF, with no tamoxifen. The A stands for Adriamycin, one of the most toxic chemotherapy drugs known. I had thought it was used only for advanced cases.

"What about the tumour conference?" I ask, stunned, "Were you there?"

"If it was Friday, I must have been there," he says enigmatically.

I'm back in the baffling world of medi-speak, complicated this time by the issue of research trials. In her thesis, Taylor says that patients in these studies are followed more closely than those who don't take part. They may benefit from a newer treatment. She also points out that experimenter-physicians face a conflict of interest when it comes time to recruit a patient. The physician is obliged to help the patient make a fully informed choice; the researcher wants to place eligible patients in the trial.

In the larger picture, knowledge about which treatments work best won't advance if women don't take part in studies. Sylvia, Louise and I had discussed this after the tumour conference. Louise was especially sold on the concept of collective responsibility. In theory, I agree. Now, faced with donating my body to this particular experiment, I'm not so sure.

The consent form makes the decision exquisitely concrete. Before I take Adriamycin, I have to sign a paper. It's the kind of release form you sign if you decide to go rafting on the Nahanni. If you crack your head open on a rock, you can't sue the rafting company, because you chose to spend your vacation shooting the rapids. The Adriamycin form releases the drug company from liability if my heart suffers permanent damage – one of the risks of a trip with Adriamycin.

I feel I'm not understanding something.

"Heart damage is a possibility," says the oncologist. "However, with the dosage we'll be giving you, and the duration, and your age, it's not likely."

We're back to probabilities. I try to weigh the unspecified high probability of dying of breast cancer with this unspecified low probability of a permanently damaged heart. Fine for the oncologist to say heart damage is unlikely; the drug company obviously isn't taking any chances.

The oncologist is a stocky man of about my own age with a beard and limpid brown eyes. "You just have to trust me," he says, his eyes underlining the plea. "I wouldn't recommend it if I didn't think it was the best choice."

Taking a deep breath, I sign.

I need to talk to someone. A friend recommends her GP, a woman. I like her. She laughs a lot and talks with an earthy casualness, much different from the reserve of the male cancer specialists.

"I don't think there's anything you could have done to prevent it," she says, "except to have had a baby at 15. That seems to help." She grins.

I ask her about Adriamycin. This brings a merry cry. "The red killer!" she exclaims. Her mother, still alive in her 70s, had it. "Mind you, mother's heart is terrible," she adds. She puts the treatments in this perspective. "With chemotherapy and cancer, we're at about the same place we were when we used to treat syphilis with arsenic. If it doesn't kill you, it can help you."

I expected something more precise from medicine, but nothing about cancer seems precise. The bone scan, the survival odds, now the chemo.

Rose Kushner's book explains that cancer's chemotherapy era is a by-product of war weaponry. The discovery during World War II that mustard gas kills by poisoning cells led research chemists to reason that liquified mustards could be used to combat cancer. The catch-22 was that lethal chemicals are indiscriminate; years of tests ensued before relatively safe chemotherapy combinations were developed. In the testing process, many cancer patients were "lost," not to cancer but to toxic chemicals (Kushner 1986).

Chemotherapy's great successes, with childhood leukemia and early adult Hodgkins disease, came in the '50s. With breast cancer, the results were more modest, explained *Our Bodies, Ourselves*. "Currently, only premenopausal women have shown much improved survival with chemotherapy and the gain is small – about 15 percent."

I face my first chemo session with trepidation. The drugs are administered intravenously at the hospital's oncology ward in a room with several beds and large leather-covered chairs. I sit on one of the beds, waiting for the nurse to hook me up to the IV drip. Wearing protective gloves, she readies the thick plastic bags of fluid to hang from the metal rack next to my bed. The fluids are yellowish or clear except for the bright red one: Adriamycin.

"How do you feel?" asks the nurse.

"Scared." My hands are clammy.

"I'd say that's normal."

She pokes the needle into a large vein in the back of my hand; the fluid starts to flow, and I feel a cold sensation as it begins to course through my veins. One, two, three, four, five packs of fluid. Three are chemotherapy drugs, two are to reduce nausea from the drugs. The whole procedure takes about two hours.

Afterwards I'm drowsy. At home I sleep a few hours, passing in and out of a drugged haze. A neighbour, Mimi, knocks on the door and asks if I want to go out for supper. I hesitate – I'm a little unsteady on my feet; I also think I might throw up in the restaurant. I decide to chance it. I'm fine through the meal, but walking home I feel woozy and sit down on a step with my head between my knees until the feeling passes. Later that night I'm jolted awake by the sudden rush of saliva to my mouth and I hurry to the bathroom. In the morning I'm a bit dazed but otherwise I feel my usual self.

The day of my first chemotherapy treatment I am menstruating. Ten days later, at the office, I realize I've begun bleeding again. In a panic, I call the oncology nurse. "The chemo's affecting your ovaries," she says. That night, Stuart and I go to Jeannie's for dinner but I'm in a terrible mood. I sense that my body will never be the same again.

Just before Christmas my hair starts to come out. For the most part this happens in the shower, when I'm rinsing it. The wet strands cover my hand like seaweed. I pull them from one hand; they stick to the other. In two weeks, except for some fuzz, my hair is all gone.

I've already bought a wig. Cancer Society pamphlets advise buying a wig before hair loss, so I go to a discreet salon. Inside, the owner's assistant has bright pink hair while Pierre himself wears a toupee which he lifts off and wiggles, like a magician doing a trick for a child. I choose a dark, curly wig that costs far more than I planned to spend. Pierre gives me separate bangs which, he explains, I can sew to the inside of a scarf to wear on days when I don't want to wear the wig.

xii

During the next six months, my sense of crisis subsides and I gradually reshape my life. After my week in hospital, my boss asks if I want to take a leave of absence or to work part-time. The thought of either frightens me – stay home all day thinking about cancer? My job is my occupational therapy. Except for doctors appointments and the two days a month I have chemotherapy, I don't miss a minute at the office.

After a few months I reconsider and decide to work three days a week. For three years I've been in a job that doesn't challenge me. It pays better than any job I've ever had, it's moderately interesting and my co-workers are congenial, but a sense of urgency sets in now that my future looks like a finite set of months or years rather than a hazy forever-and-ever. The part-time arrangement will give me enough to live on and I can initiate freelance projects of my own choosing. Heading into my third chemo session, I work up a proposal for a radio documentary on a question that's plagued me since my diagnosis: cancer and its relationship to thoughts and emotions. To my delight, it's accepted!

After the surgery I force myself to swim regularly. When I try to reach out with my left arm, a sharp pain runs through my armpit, as if a tough thread that's too short is holding me together. My arm splashes awkwardly into the water an inch or two above my head. I gain gradually, by centimetres, until one day the thread snaps. For a terrified moment I think my arm is going to drop to the bottom of the pool but instead it curves gracefully over my head.

In the communal shower; the fading incision in my breast causes me no embarrassment but my baldness does. I keep my bathing cap on. Out on the street, the wig is another story and feels like part of a costume. I continually worry that it's crooked.

"What does it look like?" asks a friend, calling from Alberta.

"I'm not sure," I tell her. "Sometimes I think I look cute, but most of the time I think I look like a middle-aged lady in a wig."

A few people, like Jeannie's adolescent son Frank, demand to see my head. A pregnant pause ensues as Jeannie and her partner Henri wait for my reaction. We've just finished supper and are relaxing around the table. I pull off the wig. Another silent moment. Then Frank cries out, "baby hair!" and we all laugh.

Usually I'm more comfortable in public wearing a colourful scarf wrapped around my head, with the fringe of hair sewn underneath. No one seems to guess this is a ruse; in fact the scarf so often draws compliments from people who don't know I have cancer, I begin to think it may actually look stylish. In private, though, the sight of my baldness in a mirror unsettles me. The reflected image recalls the haunted faces of prisoners in death camps ... and photos I've seen of cancer patients.

Strange bodily symptoms also trigger panic. One evening Mary and I go to see *Bagdad Cafe*. Halfway through the film, my concentration goes. I see the images flickering on the screen but I'm not listening, I'm thinking about the pains shooting up and down my neck. *The cancer is in my bones.* Just then Mary leans over and whispers, "My neck hurts! We're sitting too close." I'm so relieved I almost laugh out loud.

Other symptoms are real. For several days after each chemo treatment, breathing is an effort. My chest feels heavy yet not congested. Before going to sleep, I wonder if I'll be able to keep breathing the whole night. "It could just be stress," suggests the oncologist. Later he retracts this. "It is the treatments," he concedes. In February, I begin having mild hot flashes. Within a week they're intense and frequent. During the day this is merely disconcerting; I halt in mid-sentence to mop my face. At night I snatch what sleep I can between sweats that leave the bedclothes drenched and clammy.

I spend hours in the waiting room at the hospital. Chemotherapy lowers your resistance to infections so that something as minor as a hangnail can have fatal complications. Before the nurses can give a chemo treatment, the oncologist has to check the results of a blood test to make sure I can withstand another onslaught. While I'm waiting, I often talk to other patients. I want to know their stories. One day a pretty blond woman, younger than I am, comes into the waiting room wearing sunglasses. It's not that sunny, I think, as we tentatively exchange bits of our histories. She has breast cancer too. "I was fine for two years, she says. "Now," she pauses and removes the glasses to dab her eyes, puffy from crying, "it's come back."

Another day I'm next to a Japanese woman. Her lovely face is tense with strain. She tells me she's 40, married, with a young child. She had a two-centimetre lump in her breast which the doctor thought was a cyst, but it turned out to be cancer. "All removed," she says, her hand circling where her breast once was. At first her husband refused to believe it. "So few Japanese women get breast cancer. But we've had to accept it, it's true."

By all indications, I'm "tolerating the treatments well," as the medical jargon puts it. My blood count varies within the normal range and, though I get noticeably more tired as the months wear on, I'm able to swim, ski, and keep up a moderately active schedule. I still vomit the night after my monthly dose of CAF, but the next morning I'm back to normal.

Gloria Demers is not so fortunate. Her blood count is so low she has to have blood transfusions. One night we go out with Mary to a Chinese restaurant. I'm ravenous, as I have been ever since the chemo started, but Gloria won't touch even her soup. When she and Mary drop me off, Gloria gets out of the car; hugs me tightly and says, "I know we're both going to make it." I hug her back, but I don't know what to say. I think she may be dying.

I've asked Kersti Biro, a friend and amateur photographer, if she'll take some photos of me before my hair grows in. Much as I hate being bald, my months on chemo mark an important transition in my life. I need to understand it. Kersti sets up her tripod in my apartment while I make lunch and we spend a long afternoon together, talking and laughing. She shoots four rolls.

xiii

"Is there any chance I will be cured," I ask the oncologist, "or are we just trying to postpone the inevitable?"

I'm about to have my last chemotherapy treatment and I still can't figure out whether this regimen of poison was the right choice.

"There is a chance you might be completely cured," he answers. "You may never have cancer again."

"How good a chance?"

"What odds could you live with?"

"Ninety-five percent," I say. If I had 95 percent odds of surviving breast cancer, I would truly feel cured. I could throw off the burden of worry that has weighed on me since the diagnosis.

The big brown eyes turn doleful and he shakes his head sadly.

Six weeks of radiation mark the last stage of treatment. First, I have to be measured. I'm prone once more, breast bared, while two cheerful young men mark me up as if they are surveyors charting a field. Their gung-ho mood upsets me; I feel vulnerable and exposed. As the chief marker blocks out an area around my breast with a grease pencil, I break into a dramatic sweat. This bewilders him and he asks, "Were you running or something?" I don't feel like explaining the intricacies of the female body and its response to chemotherapy, so I give a helpless shrug. By the time he reaches the final step, in which he tattoos five pinpricks to permanently delineate the section to be radiated, I am completely undone. Back home, I burst into tears.

The radiation is scheduled every weekday for six weeks. I insist on an early time slot so I won't miss too much of my three days per week at the office. I sense this demand is interpreted as "patient being difficult." When someone calls to say a cancellation has freed up the eight AM slot, I feel I've gained a tiny measure of control. While the sessions themselves only last about 15 minutes, the whole procedure bites several hours out of my day, including travel time to and from the hospital, waiting for treatment, and more waiting to see the doctor; who has to decide each week if I'm strong enough to continue the invisible bombardment.

I find radiation sessions more impersonal than chemotherapy. The technician positions me carefully on a narrow bed between two fat metal wings, with my marked-up breast poking through the white gown. Then she exits and closes the door. The bed and wings begin moving through a series of positions, each stop punctuated by a harsh buzzing. Someone, apparently hoping to make this experience sublime, has pasted California feel-good posters in strategic spots on the ceiling and on the massive arms of the machine. One shows two cuddly raccoons and the caption, "A friend is someone who gives you a nice warm feeling." The message misses the mark. As the bed glides silently backwards, I imagine I'm on a mortuary slab, moving by remote control into a crypt.

Still, I do have a warm feeling because the end of treatments is in sight and the spring weather is glorious. One night I have a vivid dream in which my hair grows back, thick and long. About the same time, a man I met at a fall playwriting workshop phones and we splurge on tickets to an international theatre festival: 10 plays in two weeks. He seems curious about the cancer rather than frightened by it. "What's that red line?" he asks one night, as we lean over coffee discussing the merits of the play we've just seen. I look down to see a boundary mark poking above the neck of my tank-top. Another evening, we have to park blocks from the performance venue; the play is an experimental piece from Spain that I don't want to miss. As we tear across a parking lot, he begins lagging behind. "Are you sure you have *cancer*?" he puffs. "I think they got the diagnosis wrong."

It's clear that my friends are no more savvy about breast cancer than I was before I got it.

"What's chemotherapy?" asks the one from Alberta, calling for a health bulletin and a chat. "Is that where they zap you with a big machine?" Others ask, "Did they get it all out?" Or they nod reassuringly and say, "At least they can cure it."

When I try to convey the uncertainty of my prognosis, they are puzzled or incredulous. Everyone wants closure, but I'm getting stubborn. I'd like closure too, but the doctors won't give it to me. And if I can't have it, I'm not about to let my friends have it either.

I'm most baffled by my own misconceptions about breast cancer and those of a close circle of women friends. In the '70s we worked together on a feminist magazine in

Edmonton, of which I was the editor. At one time or another, Karen, Louise, Linda and Eleanor all wrote for the magazine or edited sections of it. If we don't know anything about breast cancer, who does? I wonder. I want to understand the reasons for our collective ignorance which, I am now convinced, must be a characteristic of our generation – the very women who are now turning 40, when breast cancer begins to strike. We should all have read Rose Kushner and Audre Lorde when their books appeared, but we didn't.

At the end of April, one of the hospitals sponsors a cancer information symposium and Rose Kushner is the invited speaker. My admiration for Kushner has grown in the months since I discovered that worn volume in the library. I sent for an updated version of the book and was delighted when it arrived, complete with an autographed inscription: "For Sharon Batt, Good luck, Rose Kushner, January 1989." That Kushner is alive so many years after her diagnosis gives me courage. I wait expectantly for her to appear before the packed auditorium.

She's in her 50s now, rather heavy-set with a broad, open face. She shows slides and tells wry jokes with the ease of a practised public speaker. But her voice is hoarse and she sounds weary.

"What causes breast cancer?" she asks, rhetorically. "Well, the latest theory is ..."

She dies the following February, 16 years after her diagnosis in 1974.

I hate the mysteriousness of my disease and desperately want to know what causes it. One of the astonishing things I learned from Kushner's book is that breast cancer was known in ancient Egypt, as far back as 3500 B.C. The Greeks knew about it too and it was the crab-like appearance of advanced breast tumours that inspired the Roman physician Galen to give cancer the name it has today ("cancer" is Latin for "crab"). What have researchers been doing all these centuries, I wonder.

Many of the books I've read say that environmental carcinogens don't cause breast cancer, but they never explain what *does* cause it. When the cancer centre at McGill advertises a talk on the environment and cancer, Mary and I attend. The lecturer, an epidemiologist, explains the difficulties of epidemiological research, in which patterns of illness in the population are used to suggest disease causation. "Epidemiologists study useful relationships but we can't say anything definite about them," he quips. "Laboratory scientists establish causal relationships, but they don't study anything useful."

One thing he is willing to say is that the effect of environmental carcinogens in causing cancer is cumulative. He illustrates this point with two slides of a camel. In the first, the camel stands tall, proudly bearing its multilayered pack. In the second, an extra item has been added to the pack and the camel, spindly legs splayed, is about to collapse. People worry that a whiff of exhaust from a passing truck will give them cancer, he says, but apparently it takes many whiffs – an unspecified number. Those elusive cancer probabilities.

He goes on to talk about specific environmental causes of cancer. It turns out that he has just completed a large study that examined every recorded case of cancer in Montreal during a certain period of time. He then traced the employment history of each person in the study. When he finishes analyzing the data, he tells us, he will be able to suggest which occupations pose hazards for specific kinds of cancer. There's only one catch: he excluded women from his study. He mentions this casually, in passing. So much for finding out if breast cancer has occupational causes.

After the lecture, Mary and I exchange impressions. We are both distressed that the epidemiologist omitted women from his study – all the more so because his manner was sympathetic. He simply spoke as though a study without women was perfectly normal. Even worse, neither of us was brave enough to stand up and challenge his assumption.

By June, I'm midway through my radiation treatments. The Montreal papers are filled with news of the Fifth International AIDS conference, which has drawn thousands of medical researchers to the city – and thousands of AIDS activists too. I'm impressed by the AIDS activists, even envious. They seem to know so much about the disease and they have such nerve. They are out on the streets staging angry demonstrations; they are in the meeting rooms, telling the scientists to hurry up with their research; they are in the media, talking about AIDS and wearing buttons that say Silence=Death. The AIDS quilt is on display at the Olympic Stadium and I go to see it. Stretched out the length of a football field are hundreds upon hundreds of squares, lovingly made by friends and relatives in memory of their dead.

After seeing the quilt, I go to Jeannie's to watch a TV program about breast cancer. It's an NBC special called *Destined to Live* and it features about 20 women; some famous, some not, speaking of their experience with the disease. They tell moving anecdotes about their terror upon diagnosis, but the overall tone of the program is upbeat. Everyone feels and looks great. They talk about the wonderful changes that have taken place in their lives since having cancer: a baby, a new job, marriage. "Cancer is the best thing that ever happened to me," beams one woman. Watching this show, you would think no one ever died of breast cancer. The long list of sponsors names every cancer agency and medical organization imaginable.

Something inside me snaps. The documentary captures one side of breast cancer – the need for hope – but so much is missing.

I remember an essay in Audre Lorde's *The Cancer Journals,* called "The Transformation of Silence into Language and Action." In it, she talks about her need to overcome her fear of speaking out. When she learned that she might have cancer, she became aware that her greatest regrets were her silences, those occasions when she lacked the courage to put her beliefs into words. She urges women to confront their fears, especially the fear of being visible. "For those of us who write," she says, "it is necessary to scrutinize not only the truth of what we speak, but the truth of that language by which we speak it" (Lorde 1980: 22).

The feeling I have to put into words is obvious: it's my fear of death from breast cancer. I sit down and write an article in which I reject the chipper, optimistic attitude that seems so prevalent. We have much to learn from AIDS activists, I argue. We must educate ourselves about the disease, about the amount of money that is spent on it, and about the policies that govern where that money goes. We must ask why the cause of breast cancer is still not known after all these years. We must also voice our anger about the thousands of women who die each year of breast cancer.

I send the article to the local newspaper and enclose one of Kersti's photos showing my bare, bald head. When the article appears, the photo enlarged to twice the original size, the effect is shocking, even to me. I am more than out of the closet, I have thrown myself into a public arena where the rules are as mysterious as the disease itself. One thing I do understand: there's no going back.

References

Boston Women's Health Collective. 1984. *The New Our Bodies Ourselves.* New York: Simon and
    Schuster.

Kushner, R. 1986. *Alternatives: New Developments in the War on Breast Cancer.* A revised version of her original book. New York: Warner.

Lorde, A. 1980. *The Cancer Journals.* San Francisco: Spinsters Ink.

Taylor, K. 1984. Decision Difficult: Physician Behaviour in the Diagnosis and Treatment of Breast Cancer. McGill University Doctoral Dissertation (Sociology), Montreal.

Taylor, K. 1988. Physicians and the Disclosure of Undesirable Information. In Margaret Lock and Deborah Gordon eds. *Biomedicine Examined.* Dordrech,: The Netherlands: Kluwer Academic Publications.

18

State Authority, Medical Dominance, and Trends in the Regulation of the Health Professions: The Ontario Case*

David Coburn

Introduction

The focus of this paper is on the relationships between the state and the professions. It is commonly assumed that public powers were devolved onto professional organizations by the state. There is little argument that the state did provide legislation which gave professions considerable scope and that the professions made full use of the degrees of freedom provided. At the height of its power, organized medicine, the 'dominant' health care profession, showed many of the attributes of a 'private government' (Friedson 1970; Taylor 1960). The provision of a public framework for private power has most often been seen as the appropriation of public authority by a private body rather than as the extension of the domain of the state.

Many writers insist that the professions have used their extra-ordinary powers partially or mainly to protect or enhance their own self-interests rather than the interests they are presumed to serve, i.e., those of the general public. Again, medicine is the most often used example (Friedson 1970). However, analysts of contemporary developments regarding medicine now claim that the state, corporations, health institutions, other health occupations, and even patients are infringing on medical privilege. Medicine, it is said, is declining in power (although the issue is contentious, see refs: Coburn 1988a; Friedson 1985; Larkin 1983; McKinlay and Arches 1985; Navarro 1989; Willis 1983)).

The idea that medicine is (or was) dominant in the health care division of labour suggests that in analyzing health care occupations what we are talking about is not simply *an* occupation or profession in relationship to the state but a whole series of interacting occupations and professions. In this 'system of professions' (see e.g., refs. Larkin 1983; Willis 1983; Abbott 1988), medicine is at the apex. Given medical dominance, it is argued here that many (but not all) state-health occupation relationships were mediated or shaped by the relationship of medicine with the

* Reprinted from *Social Science and Medicine*, Vol. 37, David Coburn, 'State authority, medical dominance, and trends in the regulation of the health professions: the Ontario case', pp. 841–50, 1993, with permission from Elsevier Science Ltd., Kidlington, UK.

state. A decline in the power of organized medicine has brought more direct state-health occupation interaction.

Apart from the changing role of medicine, an additional cue for this paper was Terrence Johnson's (1982) point that the professions and the state are not 'external' to one another but intermingle and interpenetrate, i.e. their boundaries are permeable. For example, state health bureaucracies were once largely staffed by medical men and medical power was partly constituted within the state. Conversely, the decline of medical dominance has brought with it an infiltration of 'public' or 'state' power into what once were purely professional organizations. This latter point highlights the fact that professional organizations are one means of controlling an occupation. The origin of this control may be either internal or external to the occupation itself.

Much of the political science literature in the area of the relationships between organizations in civil society and the state echo these concerns (Coleman and Skogstad 1990; Atkinson and Coleman 1989). Organization-state relationships tend to be viewed in terms of combinations of weak-strong organizations interacting with weak-strong states. Some analysts focus on 'meso-corporatism' – the notion that incorporation into policy-making by organizations is given in exchange for (elite) control or professional control of its membership (Cawson 1985).

This paper examines changing state-profession relationships focusing on the points mentioned: medicine as a dominant occupation mediating between the state and other health occupations; the permeability of state-profession boundaries; and the dual nature of occupational organizations. The examples used are from historical and recent events concerning the health professions in Ontario.

Since state-profession relationships encompass most of the field in the literature on the professions, we can only touch on this area. What follows is a partial rather than a complete analysis of state-profession interaction (which would take a monograph to cover).

I have argued previously that medicine rose to a position of dominance in health and health care in Canada in the late 19th and early 20th centuries. Today, however, there is an increasing state 'rationalization' of resources and personnel in the health field arising from the industrialization of health care and from government fiscal responsibility for health insurance. Whereas previously medicine had direct or indirect control over the context of care and over other health occupations, state rationalization involves the reduction of medical control over the health care division of labour and the re-structuring of state-profession and interprofessional relationships. Examples of this changing situation given here focus on recent health professions legislation in Ontario, the Health Professions Act. Increasing (but still partial) state control of medicine has brought a more direct relationship between the various other health occupations and the state. Medical infiltration of state agencies has been succeeded by state and public involvement in professional organizations.[1]

Health Professions and the State in Ontario

There is even more uncertainty about the role of the state and its internal dynamics than there is dispute over the nature and fate of the professions. The major focus here, however, is on the professions rather than on the state.

Canada is a federal state with ten provinces and two territories in which professional regulations and relationships with state authority are somewhat different in each jurisdiction. I am therefore limiting this discussion of health professions and the state to

Ontario, the most populous province in Canada with nearly 40% of Canada's total population of about 27 million. However, I believe that the general trends in Ontario are, *at a very general level* and to a greater or lesser extent, also true for most of the other provinces. Its proponents claim that recent health professions legislation in Ontario (which we will describe later) is amongst the most advanced in the world (certainly, other provinces have shown an interest in the Ontario legislation. (See for example, the recent Royal Commission on Health Care in British Columbia 1991.) Whether or not this is the case (Quebec carried out 10 years ago at least some of the changes proposed in Ontario, see ref. Contandriopoulos et al. 1986), the Ontario experience shows a new stage of state-profession relationships. But these relationships may be profoundly influenced by broader economic, political and social developments. The changing nature of federal-provincial ties, the role of Quebec and constitutional change, could have a major impact on state-profession interaction.

Medicine and the State

Given a system of health occupations in which medicine was predominant, analysis of the linkages between the health professions and 'public authority' must necessarily focus on the notion of medical dominance. The historical evidence suggests that there have been in Ontario three 'phases' of state-medicine-health profession relationships. Early on, i.e. in the 19th century, there was state regulation in the creation of a monopoly 'for medicine'; later, with the increasing devolution of state powers onto medicine and medicine's control over the emerging complex division of labour in health care there was state control over health care 'by medicine'; since the Second World War, with the rise of a complex health division of labour and the involvement of the state in the rationalization of health care, there is the regulation of state-health occupation interactions 'through professional organizations.' We are at the beginning of the end of medically mediated state-health occupation relationships. The 'other' health occupations are in (partial) alliance with the state in seeking to escape medical aegis, but the powers sought are much less than those previously enjoyed by medicine.

The state has never been 'neutral' *vis-à-vis* the health professions. The state accorded medicine a monopoly on the 'free' market in health care in the 19th century and later reinforced that monopoly through restricting the activities of other occupations and of the public (for example, through an all-inclusive definition of medicine in the Medical Act, through making certain drugs only available through prescription by a physician, through restricting the role of public health institutions etc.).

Medicine succeeded in obtaining Legislative sanction for a medical monopoly (in the 1860s in Ontario, earlier in Quebec). Medicine then organized, establishing internal control before either incorporating dissenters and competitors or excluding them from the health care system (Willis 1983; Torrance 1987). As the complex health care division of labour grew, mainly in the hospital, many health occupations were 'born' under medical control (Torrance 1987). Throughout most of the 20th century medicine largely controlled the Canadian health division of labour (Coburn et al. 1983).

I have argued that medicine-state relationships were those first of externality, then of the penetration of medicine into the state, and then of creeping state infusion into medicine. What are examples of these relationships? In the 19th century the state left the medical 'market' to itself. In the last decade of the century state financing of medical schools in Ontario was rejected because state aid would then be used by physicians to make money in the private market. A variety of healers existed, there was a pluralistic medical system. But, through appeals to a political and social elite, medicine did gain a monopoly, though this monopoly was opposed by other types of healers as well as by many politicians and was not at first supported by either the courts or the public. For example, the courts were reluctant to prosecute or to penalize 'illegal' midwives. However, through their legal monopoly, physicians eventually did come to exert *de facto* control over the emerging complex system of health occupations.

Preceding and concomitant with the attainment of a legal and later actual monopoly over care came numerous conflicts *within* medicine over control of the occupation. In the 19th century a medical elite sought to control the occupation in its own image and to 'raise-up' the country healers within orthodox medicine or to exclude those beyond the pale. The College of Physicians of Ontario (separate from the Ontario Medical Association), the body which embodied medicine's legal monopoly and self-governing powers over education, admittance or registration of physicians, prosecution of the unorthodox etc., was the site of struggles amongst various medical factions. Throughout the late 19th century and particularly in the early 20th century, there was opposition by ordinary medical practitioners to the schoolmen (academic physicians) and to the elite of the profession whom practitioners saw as dominating the College in their own interests.

Practitioners accused medical schools of encouraging greater numbers of medical students in order to enhance their incomes or prestige whereas practitioners saw increasing numbers as leading only to greater competition. Ordinary physicians were incensed by increased College fees and the control over the profession, through the College, by what they saw as an urban medical elite with little understanding of medical practice outside of the big cities. Manifestations of these struggles included the formation of practitioner organizations (The Medical Defence Association) and attempts to gain control over the College Council by rural practitioners through election of their own candidates (McCaughey 1984; Naylor 1986).

During much of the 20th century, up to about the date of the Saskatchewan doctors' strike in 1962, medical men came to rule their own occupation and to exclude, limit or subordinate, competitor occupations such as chiropractic and midwifery, dentistry and pharmacy, and nursing (for the use of these terms see Willis 1983). There were (partially) successful attempts to reduce competition within the occupation, to reduce external competition from other healers, and, somewhat later, to control self-care within the family. Health care bureaucracies were staffed by doctors from the top down, i.e. Ministers of Health and their Deputies were invariably doctors, and physicians occupied key Ministry posts. Medical leaders heavily influenced if not directly wrote state policy (Coburn 1990, McGinnis 1980). Many state functions, such as the administration of a state-funded system to provide health care to the indigent in Ontario, were devolved onto medical organizations (Taylor 1960). Medicine became a 'private government' (Taylor 1960).

Physician state bureaucrats, government politicians, and medical leaders had a common frame of reference: 'what was good for medicine was good for Canadians as a whole.' According to the constitution of the Canadian Medical Association, two officials from the Federal Department of Pensions and National Health, one of whom was the Deputy Minister, were members of the CMA Council. A medical official of the federal Department of Health asserted: "We do our utmost to maintain at every turn the interests of the practitioners of Canada as well as organized medicine" (McGinnis 1980). So close were the relationships between physicians in the public service and medical organizations that it is difficult to say who precisely wrote federal policy regarding health insurance during World War II, physician-bureaucrats or such groups as the 'Group of Seven,' a Canadian Medical Association medical elite advising federal committees. The CMA came to feel that: "The Minister is endeavouring to carry out the recommendations that the Executive, representing the medical men of Canada, made to the Royal Commission [World War II Royal Commission on Health Insurance]" (Canadian Medical Association Archives 1943). Furthermore, as McGinnis (1980) notes, the federal government used the medical profession as a 'source of objective opinion' regarding the role of paramedical and alternative healers.

Medicine directly or indirectly controlled the 'paramedical' health workers such as laboratory technicians either through their direct control over the education and professional organizations of these occupations or through their control over the labour process, i.e. patient care. The state was involved, but only indirectly through state control over educational institutions or hospitals and through enacting legislation in conformity with medical wishes.

The real change began when the 'free-market' for health care failed most dramatically during the Depression. At that time various regions, municipalities or provinces began to introduce doctor or hospital insurance schemes. After World War II, organized medicine tried to forestall government action by extending a burgeoning and largely doctor-sponsored private insurance system. But Saskatchewan's example, in the 1950s and 1960s, first of provincial hospital and then of provincial medical insurance, was followed in subsequent decades by government policy on the federal level which enabled the development of nation-wide provincial health plans. And, though some physicians are fond of focusing on state intervention in medical care as the source of friction between governments and medicine, even in the doctor-sponsored medical plans there were conflicts which remarkably presaged later government-medicine showdowns.

Beginning in the early 1960's provincial and federal government involvement in the health insurance area led to efforts to restructure the health care system. Thus began a period of decline in medical control over health and health care, one which is still continuing. This decline is evident in many aspects of state-medicine relationships including the failure of doctors' strikes, in Saskatchewan in 1962, in Quebec in 1970, and, most recently, in Ontario in 1986 (not necessarily complete failures, doctors often gained a good many concessions – and there is currently [1992] a partial doctors' strike in British Columbia). The decline of medical power is also evident in an increased public regulation of the professions, and in a sequence of rising state control starting with control over fees but eventually manifest in global payments for physicians' care, and attempts to control the numbers of physicians produced and where they practice (Coburn 1988a; Barer and Evans 1986; Barer et al. 1988).

During much of the 20th century too, the increasing complexity of medicine and medical care, and the fragmentation of medicine into various organizations, groups and specialties, led to a diminishing of the powers of the Ontario College of Physicians and Surgeons. For example, more and more the Universities and the Medical Schools rather than the College came to control medical education. The state is now highly involved in medical education because of its control over university and hospital funding and because it directly funds hospital internship and residency places.

With the advent of government sponsored health insurance physician control over provincial and federal health organizations declined. Physicians were replaced in positions of authority by health bureaucrats, planners, managers and accountants. This was true at all levels. In Ontario, for example, all health ministers until 1968 had been physicians, after that time (apart from a brief period in 1971-72) all health ministers have been laypersons (the first lay deputy-minister of health was appointed in 1975).

These events had a major impact on the medical profession and on the health occupations generally. Two aspects of this relationship were crucial: first, state-doctor relationships more and more came to resemble those of employer-employee; second, medical dominance and the sometimes convoluted divisions of tasks amongst health occupations was viewed by the new breed of state and academic health technocrats as a hindrance to efficiency and effectiveness. The centrality of medicine forced the state to begin to structure its own relationship with medicine and to 'rationalize' state-medicine-health occupation relationships.

At the same time as the state had an interest in reducing costs (or at least slowing the rate of increase), health ministries had to respond to social movements pushing for different forms of care. For example, the women's movement was instrumental in increased lay control over reproduction and childbirth. The women's movement had additional indirect effects in stimulating the actions of the largely female health 'semi-professions' such as nursing in their attempts to escape from medical control. For example, as a result of pressure from nursing, with the support of women's movements, the Ontario Ministry of Health explicitly directed that hospital committees should include more nurses. The largely female para-medical health occupations had powerful organizational support and could appeal to the general feminist drive for equality in their own power struggles.

Midwifery is another illustrative instance. By the early 20th century medicine had succeeded in largely eliminating midwives as (legal) competitors. Throughout the 1970s and 1980s, however, the growth of lay midwifery, catering to a largely middle-class clientelle, led to a push to legalize midwifery practice. Lay midwifery received legal recognition in Ontario in 1991 despite the fact that there were certainly less than 100 lay midwives in the entire province.

In the meantime professional organizations proliferated. And, amidst this proliferation came a separation of those organizations which claimed to represent the interests of the occupation from those whose sole, major, or partial function was protection of the 'public interest.' In most provinces, the Provincial Colleges of Physicians separated out from provincial associations (although in Ontario these had always been separate). In nursing, nurses unions were forced to organize as separate entities from provincial associations because of court decisions which declared that the latter were dominated by 'managerial' nurses.

While the various provincial associations were yet controlled by the profession they were increasingly 'unionate' (in Quebec even more explicitly so). The provincial Colleges more and more came to be constrained by legislation and to have lay or public representation (even though still only a small minority). The Colleges were now viewed by the state, and even by many practitioners, as an arm of government (though the extent to which this is the case is vastly exaggerated by practitioners).

The state sought to control health and health care, to regularize the relationships amongst the health occupations (which were in increasing rivalry), as well as to protect 'the public interest' in the sense of physician-public relationships. These pressures led to increasing government regulation of the health occupations and professions, first, in Quebec in the 1970's (see refs Contandriopoulos, et al. 1986; Renaud 1984; Renaud 1987) then in Ontario (in 1974) and other provinces. The most recent move has been in Ontario (in 1991) with new legislation governing 24 health occupations.

Medicine itself was becoming more diverse. Though the separation between researchers, medical educators, administrators, and practitioners is not necessarily reflected in organizational conflict, these groups have divergent interests (Freidson 1986; Marsden 1977). Certainly, there are at times vicious internal struggles over control of the provincial and federal medical associations between various 'political' factions within the profession. In Ontario sub-groups on the left (the Medical Reform Group), or on the right (the Association of Independent Practitioners) arose. In other provinces conflict was more muted, or, as in British Columbia, more or less open warfare between highly conservative groups and those slightly more liberal. Control over provincial and federal medical organizations was seen as the means to push the occupation in the desired directions.

At the same time as medicine experienced internal divisions (although these should not be exaggerated), more and more health occupations sought to escape medical domination. Examples of these, and their changing relationships with state authority and with medicine, are nursing and chiropractic.

Nursing

One source of pressure for increasing 'regularization' of the professions and of interprofessional relationships came from occupations which sought to escape their subordination to medicine. However, these 'rising' occupations were ultimately willing to accept much lesser degrees of self-regulation than medicine felt its natural right. Nursing is an example. Nursing in Canada has always been under medical control, but also under the control of hospitals and state authorities (Coburn 1988a). Even the numbers of nurses for most of the 20th century was largely determined by the need by hospitals for (unpaid) student nurses to staff these institutions. This control was cemented through the co-optation of major segments of the nursing elite by hospitals and by medicine. Nursing dissent was suppressed, not only by external forces but also by the nursing elite itself.

Nursing was originally granted the right of registration (which included protection of title) only in the 1920's. This minimal right lasted until contemporary developments in which, in some provinces, Alberta for instance, nurses have been granted a monopoly over nursing services. Nursing has been the health occupation most recently in the news with nursing strikes in Alberta, British Columbia, Quebec, Saskatchewan and Manitoba (many of these illegal). There is much concern about an alleged nursing shortage, about the poor working conditions of nurses and about their lack of power. Nursing-state relationships have thus been characterized by the role of buffer organizations such as the hospital and by nursings' subordinate status (on both the occupational level and on the labour process level) to medicine.

Nursing experienced a market crisis during the Depression at the same time as nurses moved into the hospital in large numbers (this movement partially a consequence of the spread of private hospital insurance schemes). After World War II, nursing was soon characterized by the twin thrusts of professionalization by an elite and unionization by the rank and file (Coburn 1988b). But nursing also became even more internally fragmented between nurse managers, an educational and professionalizing elite (most of these with the BScN), and rank and file (diploma) nurses.

The history of nursing largely consists of attempts to escape these various forms of subordination. The task for nursing in pre-war Canada, however, was difficult. The role of nursing as 'doctors hand maidens' was freely accepted even by many within nursing.

The change today is startling. Though nursing is divided, at least one segment of the nursing elite is actively seeking to promote and channel nursing discontent. Nursing militancy is being used as part of nursing's efforts to crawl out from under the thumb of hospital and medical dominance. On many issues nursing has publicly opposed the avowed goals and aims of organized medicine.

Insofar as nursing organizations are concerned, developments in nursing parallel those in medicine. There have been struggles for control over the occupation by those with differing visions of the future of nursing. Even within different organizations, such as the Registered Nurses Association of Ontario (RNAO), there have been internecine battles. In Ontario (unlike in most other provinces), nursing has three organizations: a College, a federation of unions (the Ontario Nurses Association – 80% of working nurses are unionized in Canada), and a 'professional,' and presently somewhat fragile, organization, the RNAO. The RNAO now mainly represents a managerial, educational, and professionalizing elite. Furthermore, there is the real possibility of existing divisions within nursing leading to separation of 'professional' (B.Sc.N.) from more 'practical' (diploma) nursing.

Within nursing, as in medicine, there are struggles over alternative visions of nursing's future. Nursing is deeply divided by interests and ideologies. Control over nursing organizations was the key to steering nursing in the direction various interest groups wanted nursing to go.

Current health professions legislation in Ontario gives nursing *occupational* autonomy *vis-à-vis* medicine while the nursing labour process is still controlled by medicine and by hospitals. This occupational self-regulation is, however, not the dominance which medicine once possessed. The state now has a new form of control over nursing through public representation on College councils and committees and through public regulation of the Colleges. And there is a powerful and continuing state influence over nursing practice and education through state financing of hospitals, nursing colleges, and universities.

Chiropractic

The fate of chiropractic and its relationships with the state and with medicine in Canada, as in some other countries (see refs Willis 1983; Baer 1984), can be described as one of "increasing legitimation at the cost of narrowing of scope of practice" (Biggs 1989; Coburn and Biggs 1986). Chiropractic in Canada has moved from being a competitor of medicine, one which medicine succeeded in excluding from the official health care system, to becoming, in its official rhetoric if not in the day-to-day practice of chiropractors, 'part of the health care team' – specialists on the spine. Much of the early exclusion was due to the power of medicine. At that time most people in positions of authority in the various Ministries of Health were physicians and medicine could appeal to its relationship with science to justify its role as the judge of what was acceptable. According to medicine, chiropractic had no basis in research and theory.

Chiropractic survived because people used it – in that sense we should distinguish, as Starr 1982 has done, between 'cultural authority' and state sanction (although these two are no doubt related). State sanction is itself limited and constrained – particularly because of the division between politicians and bureaucrats. The latter *may* have been controlled by the professions and the former partially influenced, but medicine could never completely manage political party policy.

Chiropractic, however, from being a complete alternative to medicine, has been partly tamed and 'medicalized.' Its education now consists to a great deal of traditional 'medical' basic science. In order to be able to deal with patients directly rather than having to have a medical referral chiropractic has had to teach 'general diagnosis' in a manner little different from medical schools. Many of the original claims to being a complete alternative to medicine have been downplayed as chiropractic has sought to distance itself from anything faintly disreputable. An example is the changing relationships between chiropractic and naturopathy (Gort and Coburn 1988). Chiropractors early on used joint registration as chiropractic-naturopaths to try to expand their scope of practice. But, attempting to gain state recognition, chiropractic leaders later disavowed naturopathic treatments as 'non-scientific' and cut all ties with naturopathy. Thus, the relationships of various health occupations with medicine, though central, are not the only ones of importance – Abbott (1988) does have a point when he talks about the 'system' of professions.

Organizations within chiropractic now include a Board of Regents of Chiropractic (developed out of a more heterogeneous Board of Regents of Drugless Practitioners), an Ontario Association of Chiropractors, and a group governing the Canadian Memorial Chiropractic College, the Board of Governors of the CMCC. Amongst these, and between these and practicing chiropractors, there has been a great deal of friction. This conflict has largely revolved around the degree to which the occupation would try to become more 'legitimate' through rejection of many of its earlier broad claims and beliefs, and about the scope of practice to which chiropractic should aspire. There have been furious battles between 'straights' and 'mixers' the former focusing their treatments on spinal manipulation only, the latter focusing on other bodily functions and other treatment modalities. Many of these conflicts have taken the form of attempts to gain control over key organizations, committees, and the educational process.

Chiropractic has eagerly sought state legislation though its relationships with the state have been essentially as 'outsiders.' Chiropractic has been much more successful in lobbying politicians than they have been with the physician dominated bureaucracy (although, as noted, this situation has now changed). Under the new Ontario health professions legislation, chiropractic also will have a College, in nearly all respects similar to that of medicine, nursing and numerous other health occupations. Chiropractic, like nursing, is quite willing to pay the price of (somewhat) increased state regulation through a redefined College, in return for greater (implied) official recognition.

The Health Professions Legislation Review

All of these developments have culminated in Ontario in recent health profession legislation. I have noted that the state has always been involved in regulation of the health professions but that for most of this century medicine had been a major vehicle through which the health occupations were controlled. That is, state power was mediated through medical dominance.

After the implementation of medical insurance in 1967-71 major federal and provincial health commissions proliferated. These were mainly concerned with attempts to reorganize health care services. An important commission in Ontario was the Committee on the Healing Arts in 1970 (Ontario Committee on the Healing Arts 1970). This commission's major conclusion was that the health care system had to be rationalized for greater efficiency and reduced costs. Medical power had distorted the system. The Committee's recommendations eventually led to a proposal to give twenty separate health occupations common legislation. However, medicine and dentistry raised so much opposition that the proposed legislation was dropped and the revised regulations governed only medicine, dentistry, nursing, pharmacy and optometry. The Health Disciplines Act (1974) granted the Colleges self-regulation, but a self-regulation within more restricted boundaries than previously.

There were additional reforms. Not only were College powers restricted but for the first time, the Colleges were forced to include lay representatives on their governing councils and on their patient complaints and disciplinary committees. Furthermore, patients dissatisfied with the decisions of the Colleges' complaints committees (or practitioners not satisfied with the outcomes of their application for registration) could appeal these decisions to a Health Disciplines Board consisting entirely of laypersons Still, lay members constituted only about 25% of Council members and one of three persons in Complaints and Disciplinary hearings, and were often easily co-opted.

Since the time of the introduction of the Health Disciplines Act many occupations have been lobbying government for similar legislation. There have also been a number of highly publicized court cases relating to stillbirths at (lay) midwife attended births or concerning harm suffered by some patients as a result of particular naturopathic treatments. These practical difficulties, combined with increasing health costs and the drive to 'rationalize' the confusing and overlapping jurisdictions of various health professions, produced mounting pressure for reform of professional legislation. The Health Professions Legislation Review, inaugurated in 1982 and reporting in 1989, noted that:

The Review was created at a time when much pressure for change to the existing regulatory legislation was being exerted. Members of the public were expressing doubts about the thoroughness of governing bodies' investigations of complaints against their members, and demanding more open and responsive complaints and discipline processes. A large number of unregulated health care groups were pressing the Ministry to become regulated. Health professions currently regulated by a number of outdated statutes were seeking to be regulated under the Health Disciplines Act. Hospital administrators were expressing frustration with the rigidity that the existing regulatory system imposed on their ability to employ the most efficient and cost-effective mix of health care providers. Finally it was recognized with the Government that the existing patchwork of legislation made coordinated policy direction of the health professions impossible to achieve (Health Professions Legislation Review 1989).

The commission consisted of a committee of legal experts to review all of the health occupations and to propose a new system based on 'the public interest' and on review of the system of inter-professional relationships which were viewed as anachronistic and hindering 'rationalization.' From the start, however, the Review accepted the assumption of professional 'self-regulation' even if 'in the public interest' (rather than partial or complete regulation by government or lay boards).

After much consultation with hundreds of professional and a very few public interest groups, taking a total of eight years, the committee finally made its complete proposals known in January of 1990. Nearly 75 health occupations had originally sought incorporation in the legislation (including such diverse 'health professions' as the Canadian Prescription Footwear Association, Clinical Biomedical Engineers, Colon Therapy Association of Canada and the Toronto Society for Bioenergetic Analysis). Many of them undoubtedly thought that incorporation under new legislation meant either immediate or later inclusion under fee-for-service health insurance. It did not. Those who did not have such illusions saw the Review as a first step towards public payment, as a means of gaining a monopoly over a particular area of practice, as granting them a form of public recognition as a health 'profession,' or possibly as leading to primary contact with the public.

Eventually 24 of the original 75 'professions' were included in omnibus legislation (including midwifery as an occupation separate from medicine and from nursing; chiropractic; massage therapy; dietetics; etc.). The two major innovations of the legislation are the distinction between scopes of practice and 'licensed acts' and further restriction over professional self-government. Concerned with a more 'rational' division of labour in the health field the review narrowed the areas over which an occupation had exclusive jurisdiction. The health professions now do not have a monopoly over whole areas of endeavour (as defined in scopes of practice) but instead have the authority to perform specific 'licensed acts.' There are thirteen licensed acts in all, e.g.: "(1)... diagnosis... (2) Performing a procedure on tissue beyond the dermis, below the surface of a mucous membrane, in or below the surface of the cornea, or in or below the surfaces of the teeth, including the scaling of teeth... (12) Managing labour or conducting the delivery of a baby ..." (Ontario Regulated Health Professions Act 1991). Medicine has the authority to perform twelve of these (all but "(11) fitting or dispensing a dental prosthesis..."), Occupational Therapy has none. Medicine, physiotherapy and chiropractic all have the licensed act of, for example: "Moving the joints of the spine beyond a person's usual physiological range of motion using a fast, low-amplitude thrust." This legislation would thus loosen the boundaries amongst the professions because some acts may be performed by more than one health profession, and any act not specifically mentioned may be performed by any regulated health profession.

Inter-professional relations concerning changes in functions, scopes of practice, the regulation of new professions or the deregulation of existing professions were to be governed by another board composed entirely of laypersons, The Health Professions Regulatory Advisory Council. This Council is advisory to the government of the day on such matters as which professions should be regulated and which should no longer be regulated.

The second thrust of the legislation is to increase public participation in the chief 'self-governing' professional organization, namely the Colleges. All of the occupations included are to have their own governing bodies or Colleges (in addition to their professional associations), these Colleges all with similar forms and functions. Medicine is now not alone but part of a large group of regulated health professions.

The Colleges will have increased lay representation on their governing councils, as well as on their registration committees and complaints and disciplinary committees. Lay members would now constitute over 40% of the Governing Councils of the Colleges (up from approximately 25% mandated by the Health Disciplines Act and compared to no lay representation before that). As at present patients could appeal the decisions of the Colleges' Complaints Committee to a totally lay board, the Health Disciplines Board. But now both College Council meetings and the proceedings of Disciplinary Committees are to be open to the public.

Finally, and after much argumentation over wording, the relationship between the Minister of Health and the Colleges was changed to a more directive one. That is, under the previous Health Disciplines Act the Minister had the power to request the Colleges' to take action, under the new Act the Minister may require the Colleges to take action.

The Review argues that:

The new scope of practice system will provide better public protection while permitting more efficient and cost-effective delivery of health care services. A larger number of regulated health professions – new as well as traditional professions; predominantly female as well as predominantly male professions – will be given equal status and a public policy forum in which to express their views. Colleges will have the powers necessary to regulate health professionals effectively, and will be more accountable to the public for how they exercise their powers (Health Professions Legislation Review 1989).

In sum, the Colleges have become not simply professional organizations designed to self-regulate the profession by members of the profession itself, but, with reduced powers, part of a system of organizations, all with lay input and responsive to quasi-state influence if not direct control. The Colleges, the central vehicles for professional self-regulation, thus have much narrowed powers from that earlier in the century, have much more rigorous and detailed duties, are directly answerable to state authority, and have much greater public representation.

Politically, the more 'established' occupations (particularly dentistry) have tended, to one degree or another, to resist this new legislation whilst the currently unregulated or partially regulated 'rising' occupations were much more favourable, or at least amenable, to increased lay input and more state regulation of the professions through the new proposed system (Rappolt 1990). The governments of the day thus had a great deal of support, both from public interest groups and from many of the occupations seeking regulation, for reform (hence why these reforms were not even more fundamental than those proposed is another question – for example, there were suggestions from patients' rights groups that patient complaints should be heard by a completely independent commission rather than by a professional body). Certainly medicine, dentistry and other professions had their influence diluted as meetings regarding the proposed legislation were crowded with dozens of representatives of occupations all desiring legislation giving them at least some elements of state sanction. Medicine was numerically if not politically swamped by numerous other occupations who saw in regulation a chance to escape from medical dominance as well as a means of gaining official recognition.

The contemporary situation is thus a far cry from the days when the state abdicated control over what happened in the health care system to medicine. Not only is the state now directly involved in controlling and re-organizing the health care system, but it has moved to 'rationalize' inter-professional, state-profession, and public-profession relationships. The gaining of power by numerous health occupations has, however, resulted in these occupations being partially and more directly controlled by the state through their own 'self-governing' organizations.

The crucial nature of self-regulation regarding professional autonomy is emphasized by many, e.g. Coburn 1988a; Friedson 1986. In fact, Freidson equates self-regulation with professional autonomy. Yet, greater power for some occupations has meant lesser power for medicine and greater state and lay input into professional regulation in general. Medical mediation has been transformed into direct state-health occupation links.

Conclusions

Historically, state regulation of health occupations in Ontario was mediated through medical control over the health care division of labour. The state structured control over health care through medical dominance. The state and medicine have permeable boundaries which initially permitted medicine to control health care bureaucracies or departments, if not provincial legislatures. But medical organizations, and those of other health professions, have been the sites of conflict in which factions or groups within the occupation sought to gain control over the occupation itself. Occupational elites attempted to 'construct' their occupations in their own image.

With the creation of a mass market for care, and as the state became involved in health care through its financing of health insurance plans, the relationships amongst the state, medicine, and other health occupations changed. The state came to directly affect medical dominance through its attempts to rationalize health care. At the same time this rationalization involved and supported the efforts of other health occupations to escape from medical control. Partly through its financial control over the health care system and over education (which areas we could not treat here), but also partly through a re-structuring of professional organizations, governments now shape professional 'self-government.' The latter changes, as exemplified in the Health Professions Legislation Review and the subsequent Regulated Health Professions Act in Ontario, point to the dual role of key professional organizations as means to control the occupation from the inside but also as vehicles to control the occupation from 'outside' (Coleman and Skogstad 1990; Cawson 1985[1]). This interpretation of occupational organizations parallels the somewhat contradictory interpretations of the role of, e.g. labour organizations or of political parties, as, on the one hand, vehicles for the expression of particular views, and, on the other, as methods of organizing and possibly co-opting those they supposedly represent. Medical self-governing organizations are increasingly most often neither one or the other but some combination of both.

Medical organizations, namely, the Colleges, have been forced to take into account 'the public interest' even if their actions do not necessarily reflect this public mandate (on the latter point the College of Physicians and Surgeons of Ontario recently came under severe criticism for ignoring the sexual abuse of patients by physicians). Professional organizations, even those whose goals were to directly represent professional self-interest, have become much more complex.

As medicine has moved from 'dominance' more towards 'autonomy' so the paramedical or 'other' health professions have moved towards autonomy and somewhat away from subordination to medical authority. The spread of direct state authority through the reforms of the College system was fully supported by the rising para-medical professions because it was accompanied by a limited state mandate which meant an increased autonomy from direct medical control. In essence the College system serves to give the numerous new set of professions as occupations (not as individual practitioners) 'relative autonomy' yet also clearly indicates that what the state mandates it can also take away.

Acknowledgement

The historical material on which this paper is based was gathered as part of a larger project on 'The Rise and Fall of Medicine in Canada' funded by the Social Science and Humanities Research Council of Canada Grant No. 410-85-0539.

Notes

1   There are conflicting views about whether or not certain 'mediating elites' in medicine are being co-opted for state purposes, or are simply making a strategic concession to government in order to preserve their fundamental clinical autonomy. See Tuohy and O'Reilly 1992.

References

Abbott, A. 1988. *The System of Professions.* Chicago: University of Chicago Press.

Atkinson, M, and W Coleman. 1989. Strong States and Weak States: Sectoral Policy Networks in Advanced Capitalist Economies. *British Journal of Political Science* 19: 47–67.

Baer, HA. 1984. A Comparative View of a Heterodox Health System: Chiropractic in America and Britain. *Medical Anthropology* 8: 151–168.

Barer, ML, and RG Evans. 1986. Riding North on a South-Bound Horse? Expenditures, Prices, Utilization and Incomes in the Canadian Health Care System. In RG Evans and GL Stoddart eds. *Medicare at Maturity.* Banff, Alberta: Banff Centre School of Management.

Barer, ML, RG Evans, and RJ Labelle. 1988. Fee Controls as Cost Controls: Tales from the Frozen North. *Milbank Quarterly* 66: 1–64.

Biggs, CL. 1989. *No Bones about Chiropractic? The Quest for Legitimacy by the Ontario Chiropractic Profession, 1895 to 1985.* Ph.D. Dissertation, University of Toronto.

British Columbia Royal Commission on Health Care and Costs. 1991. Published by the Commission, Victoria: British Columbia.

Canadian Medical Association Archives. 1943. Minutes of the Executive Committee, 7: 24 October.

Cawson, A. ed. 1985. *Organized Interests and the State: Studies in Meso-Corporatism.* Beverly Hills: Sage.

Coburn, D. 1988a. Canadian Medicine: Dominance or Proletarianization? *Milbank Quarterly* 66(Suppl 2): 92–116.

Coburn, D. 1988b. The Development of Canadian Nursing: Professionalization and Proletarianization. *International Journal of Health Services* 18: 437–456.

Coburn, D. 1990. Medicine-Nursing and Chiropractic: The Rise and Fall of a Profession (Manuscript). Department of Behavioural Science, University of Toronto.

Coburn, D, and CL Biggs. 1986. Limits to Medical Dominance: The Case of Chiropractic. *Social Science and Medicine* 22: 1035–1046.

Coburn, D, G Torrance, and J Kaufert. 1983. Medical Dominance in Canada in Historical Perspective: The Rise and Fall of Medicine. *International Journal of Health Services* 13: 407–432.

Coleman, WD, and G Skogstad eds. 1990. *Policy Communities and Public Policy in Canada.* Toronto: Copp Clark Pitman.

Contandriopoulos, A-P, C Laurier, and C-H Trottier. 1986. Towards an Improved Work Organization in the Health Care Sector. In RG Evans and GL Stoddart eds. *Medicare at Maturity: Achievements, Lessons and Challenges.* Banff, Alberta: Banff Centre School of Management.

Freidson, E. 1986. *Professional Powers: A Study of the Institutionalization of Formal Knowledge.* Chicago: University of Chicago Press.

Freidson, E. 1985. The Reorganization of the Medical Profession. *Medical Care Review* 42: 11–35.

Freidson, E. 1970. *Profession of Medicine.* New York: Dodd, Mead and Company.

Gort, EH, and D Coburn. 1988. Naturopathy in Canada: Changing Relationships to Medicine, Chiropractic and the State. *Social Science and Medicine* 26: 1061–1072.

Health Professions Legislation Review. 1989. *Striking a New Balance: A Blueprint for the Regulation of Ontario's Health Professions.* Toronto: Queens Printer.

Johnson, T. 1982. The State and the Professions: Peculiarities of the British. In A Giddens and G Mackenzie eds. *Social Class and the Division of Labour.* Cambridge: Cambridge University Press.

Larkin, G. 1983. *Occupational Monopoly and Modern Medicine.* London: Tavistock.

Marsden, L. 1977. Power Within a Profession: Medicine in Ontario. *Sociology of Work and Occupations* 4: 3–26.

McCaughey, D. 1984. Professional Militancy: The Medical Defence Association vs the College of Physicians and Surgeons of Ontario, 1891-1902. In CC Roland ed. *Health Disease and Medicine: Essays in Canadian History.* Toronto: The Hannah Institute for the History of Medicine.

McGinnis, JPD. 1980. *From Health to Welfare: Federal Government Policies Regarding Standards of Public Health for Canadians.* Ph.D. dissertation, University of Alberta, Edmonton.

McKinlay, JB, and J Arches. 1985. Towards the Proletarianization of Physicians. *International Journal of Health Services* 15: 161–195.

Navarro, V. 1989. Professional Dominance or Proletarianization?: Neither. *Milbank Quarterly* 66 (Suppl 2): 57–75.

Naylor, CD. 1986. Rural Protest and Medical Professionalism in Turn-of-the-Century Ontario. *Journal of Canadian Studies* 21: 5–20.

Ontario Committee on the Healing Arts. 1970. *Report*, Vols 1-3. Toronto: Queen's Printer.

Ontario Regulated Health Professions Act. 1991. Bill 43 and Bills 44 to 64. Toronto: Queen's Printer.

Rappolt, S. 1990. *The Orientation of Ontario's Health Professions.* M.Sc. Thesis, University of Toronto.

Renaud, M. 1987. Reform or Illusion: An Analysis of the Quebec State Intervention in Health. In D Coburn, C D'Arcy, G Torrance and P New eds. *Health and Canadian Society: Sociological Perspectives.* 2nd ed. Toronto: Fitzhenry and Whiteside.

Renaud, M. 1984. Quebec: The Adventures of a Narcissistic State. In J Kervesdorie et al. eds. *The End of an Illusion.* Berkeley: University of California Press.

Starr, P. 1982. *The Social Transformation of American Medicine.* New York: Basic Books.

Taylor, MG. 1960. The Role of the Medical Profession in the Formulation and Execution of Public Policy. *Canadian Journal of Economic and Political Science* 25: 108–127.

Torrance, G. 1987. Historical Introduction. In D Coburn, C D'Arcy, G Torrance and P New eds. *Health and Canadian Society, 2nd ed.* Toronto: Fitzhenry and Whiteside.

Tuohy C, and P O'Reilly. 1992. Professionalism and the welfare state. *Journal of Canadian Studies* 27: 73–92.

Willis, E. 1983. *Medical Dominance: The Division of Labour in Australian Health Care.* Sydney: George Allen and Unwin.

19

Women in Medicine: Toward a Conceptual Understanding of the Potential for Change*

A. Paul Williams, Karin Domnick, Eugene Vayda

In 1959 only 6% of Canadian medical school graduates were women, but by 1989 they accounted for 44% (Ryten 1989) and in 1990, women accounted for almost half of Canadian medical students (Sullivan 1990). The rapid increase in the number of women entering medicine in Canada and the United States poses important questions about the potential for change, whether more women in medicine will transform not just the demographic face of the profession, but also the way in which medicine is practiced. In contrast to Eisenberg's 1985 (Eisenberg 1985) caveat that "physician's gender has not been shown to have a measurable effect on practice styles," evidence now suggests that women do practice differently from their male colleagues. Recent U.S. data indicate that women are more likely than men to work as general practitioners, in groups, in urban settings, and in salaried positions (Barondess 1981; Bobula 1980; Weisman et al. 1980; Adams and Bazzoli 1986; Bowman and Gross 1986). Data from Canada (Contandriopoulos and Fournier 1987; Woodward et al. 1990; Bryant et al. 1991), Australia, (Fett 1976; Dennerstein et al. 1989), Great Britain (Elston 1980; Wakeford and Warren 1989), and Sweden (Frey 1980) suggest that women physicians also work fewer hours than their male colleagues, see fewer patients, and are more likely to take time away from professional activities. Two national surveys of Canadian physicians conducted by the authors confirm these findings and suggest that women physicians also tend to be less involved in their professional associations (Stevenson and Williams 1985; Williams et al. 1990b).

This growing research evidence focuses attention on two key issues concerning the potential for change as more women enter medicine. On a quantitative level, it has been suggested that because of shorter working weeks, lighter patient loads, and higher numbers of career interruptions, women physicians will produce fewer medical services than men. The logic is that because of the persistence of an historical division of labor in the family, women still hold primary responsibility for child rearing and this inevitably conflicts with professional activities, limiting "out-

* Reprinted from the *Journal of the American Medical Women's Association*, Vol. 48, No. 4, A. Paul Williams, Karen Domnick Pierre, and Eugene Vayda, 'Women in Medicine: Towards a Conceptual Understanding', pp. 115–21, 1993, with permission of the publisher.

put" (Wheeler 1990). While such arguments generally fail to comment on the quality or appropriateness of the medical services provided (Lomas et al. 1986) differences in service volume are seen to have important implications for physician workforce planning: if observed gender differences in practice persist and women continue to enter medicine in increasing numbers, more physicians may have to be trained to maintain the current profile of service provision (Contandriopoulos and Fournier 1990; Wakeford and Warren 1989; Mickelburgh 1992) assuming, of course, that profile continues to be accepted.

The second, more important issue, concerns fundamental qualitative change in medicine and the role of the physician. Either by nature or by nurture, it has been suggested that women have a more humanistic and patient-centered approach to medical practice. Women physicians have been described as less oriented to "high tech" medicine, more sensitive and responsive to the psychosocial needs of their patients, and more appreciative of the role of the family in health and illness (Eisenberg 1983; Levinson et al. 1987; Hayes 1981). Burkett and Kurz (1981) found that women are more likely than men to cite "the desire to help people" as their primary motivation for entering medical school and less likely to cite "the desire for financial rewards" in the same context. However, the evidence on this issue is less clear cut. Recent studies of both medical students and practicing physicians have failed to find persistent gender differences in attitudes toward the role of the physician (Maheux et al. 1988) various sociopolitical questions (Dornbush et al. 1991) and the operation of the health care system (Williams et al. 1990b) suggesting a levelling effect of medical school socialization (Leserman 1981).

The question remains whether observed gender differences in the organization and conduct of medical practice are primarily a function of women's double role as professionals and family care givers and the pragmatic workload management this double role entails, or, alternatively, whether such differences also reflect the fact that women bring with them distinctive attitudes and values that shape the way they practice. The former possibility has implications for physician workforce planning, but the latter suggests a more profound change in the nature of medicine and the role of the physician.

This paper addresses the ongoing discussion of the impact of women's progressive entry into medicine and suggests that a shortcoming of the discussion has been its preoccupation with the descriptive examination of women physicians' professional characteristics and practices. While rightly drawing attention to the ongoing demographic transformation of the profession and generating valuable data about the current practice patterns of women and men, sufficient attention has yet to be paid to the development of a clearer conceptual understanding of the nature of gender differences and the implications for change. Using data from a national study of Canadian physicians, this paper reexamines the nature of the relationship between gender differences in practice and underlying attitudes and values. The aim is to emphasize the complexity of this relationship and to identify alternative hypotheses about the potential for change as more women enter medicine. We suggest that this potential will be mediated by the socializing impact of medical school and the extent to which women physicians are included in or excluded from positions of power within the organized profession. We suggest also that to understand and document change, consideration must be given to arguments that women and men view the world in qualitatively different ways (Gilligan 1982).

The first section of the paper is a brief summary of our national study of Canadian physicians presented here as a focus for discussion. The second section presents data that describe similarities and differences in the practice patterns and attitudes of women and men physicians. In the third section, key hypotheses suggesting alternative scenarios for change are identified. In the final section we discuss our findings in light of the hypotheses and consider factors influencing the prospects for change.

Method

In a previous paper, we reported quantitative data from a 1986-1987 national survey of 2,400 Canadian physicians documenting gender differences in practice patterns and attitudes (Williams et al. 1990a). In this paper we briefly review those differences in light of the qualitative results of a follow-up focus group and open-ended discussions with women physicians, as well as the results of recent studies of gender differences in physicians' attitudes. These research results are not offered as proof of underlying relationships, but as a means of drawing attention to important conceptual issues. Central among these is the question of reconciling research findings, including our own, that show both differences and similarities in the attitudes of women and men physicians. A failure to demonstrate gender differences in attitudes suggests that observed differences in practice are primarily pragmatic in nature, not a function of more fundamental differences in gender orientation. This in turn suggests that the potential for change is primarily a matter of change in demographics and workloads rather than in medicine and the role of the physician.

As reported elsewhere (Williams et al. 1990a; Stevenson et al. 1988; Williams et al. 1990b) a representative national survey of Canadian physicians was conducted at the Institute for Social Research, York University, Toronto, between November 1986 and May 1987. The survey was a follow-up to an earlier one conducted in 1982. Questionnaires were mailed to 3,529 eligible physicians including all respondents to the 1982 survey who could be located, plus an additional sample selected randomly from the 1986 *Canadian Medical Directory.* An extensive follow-up regime yielded 2,378 completed questionnaires, 297 (12.4%) from women and 2,101 (87.6%) from men, and an effective response rate of 68% (Northrup 1988). Analysis of patterns of response/non-response and comparisons to the results of a 1987 Canadian Medical Association survey of 41,000 physicians (Adams 1989) failed to identify any systematic bias in the results (Williams et al. 1990).

To assist in interpreting the results, a number of follow-up discussions were conducted with women physicians. The most important of these was a focus group convened in June 1988. A random sample of 25 of the 49 women physicians living in the Toronto area who had participated in the survey were sent a summary description of gender differences observed in the national survey and invited to attend. Budgetary restrictions precluded a larger, more geographically diverse sample. Thirteen women participated in a three-hour discussion of their practices, the influence of childbearing and rearing on practice, and gender differences in attitudes toward patient care and professional issues. The group included general practitioners and specialists and women with families of different sizes and ages. The discussion, facilitated by the female member of the research team (KDP), was tape recorded and transcribed. Although this focus group included only a small number of women physicians living in a major metropolitan area in central Canada, we present the results because they raise important issues of interpretation and suggest a number of important hypotheses about the potential for change in medicine.

Results

Physician Survey

The results of our national survey confirmed a number of previously reported gender differences in professional workloads and practice organization (Williams et al. 1990a). More women than men preferred alternative practice types: 18% of women compared to 29% of men worked as solo practitioners while 23% of women but only 17% of men were in private (fee-for-service) group practice. Women were also more likely than men to practice general rather than specialty medicine (67% vs 49% respectively) and to work in urban areas (69% vs 60%). Even when year of graduation, specialty, and practice type were controlled in multiple regressions, women worked significantly fewer hours during typical weeks than men (38 hours vs 45 hours) and conducted fewer patient visits (90 vs 113). Similarly, even when age, specialty, practice type, hours worked, and patient visits were statistically controlled, the estimated net, before-tax income (1985) of women physicians was significantly lower than that of men ($77,000 vs $103,000).

The survey failed to find significant gender differences in physicians' attitudes, however. For instance, on a multiple-item scale measuring "approval of medicare," women and men had mean scores of 2.8, just below the scale midpoint of 3, indicating a lukewarm response to universal government health insurance. Similarly, both groups had mean scores of 3.1 on a scale measuring "satisfaction with medicare," reflecting a slightly more positive assessment of practice under the federal-provincial health insurance system. Both women and men supported the principles that physicians should control their own incomes (3.5) and that patients should pay hospital user fees (3.3), but neither supported a return to private and commercial control of health insurance (2.8 vs 2.9). Women were slightly more approving than men of community-based health strategies and incentives to establish group practice, but these differences lost statistical significance when other factors were controlled.

Focus Group

A key issue for the focus group was the extent to which the progressive entry of women into medicine implied a process of "feminization" beyond changes in professional demographics and workloads. In spite of our survey results and the equivocal evidence reported in the literature, the focus group participants held that such a process was proceeding.

The women confirmed the gender differences in practice organization and workloads and agreed that they worked fewer hours and conducted fewer patient visits per week than their male colleagues. They felt, nevertheless, that they "worked quite enough," as much as or more than the 35 to 40 hours typical in most professions. In part, shorter working weeks were seen to be a function of the need to manage time, since they felt that they were bearing most of the burden for child raising and family care. Said one participant, "Even though my husband helps me a lot, I'm still the one who has all the responsibility."

The balance of career and family was a major concern summed up in the phrase, "Women leave work too early and get home too late." The women physicians felt that their family reality influenced choices among alternative working arrangements. Group practice was viewed as offering advantages for workload management, including the ability to schedule on-call periods and time off by having other group doctors cover. Salaried group and hospital practice were seen by some group members as freeing physicians from financial and administrative responsibilities. By providing predictable hours, incomes, and benefits, physicians in collaborative practice could be less concerned about juggling large numbers of patients during long hours to maintain or increase fee-for-service incomes. Similarly, health care teams including other physicians, nurses, and ancillary personnel could bring a broader base of knowledge to patient care. Said one woman physician, "There is a lot medicine does not know. I'm glad there will be other health care givers to share the load."

Similar pragmatic considerations were seen to influence incomes. A number of focus group members said that women physicians will often opt for reduced hours and lower incomes in order to devote more time to their families. Particularly in two-income families, women physicians often felt less pressure to maintain or increase high levels of "production" to generate fees. However, the women physicians stressed that such decisions were not simply pragmatic; they also reflect important differences in how women and men approach medicine. Compared to men, they felt that they were more "patient centred" and placed greater emphasis on the "art" of medicine.

This emphasis on relations with patients and on human contact was also seen to motivate women's choices of specialty. Whereas higher incomes might attract men to specialties such as surgery, the group participants felt women would tend to be drawn to specialties that are more "caring" and less technical; "less lucrative" was seen to be of secondary importance. One group member suggested that women are less likely to enter surgery because there is little interaction with patients, "The surgeon goes in, does his thing ... [and] the patient usually gets better." In contrast, "women physicians were seen to prefer fields like family medicine, geriatrics, and obstetrics, which focus more on nurturing relationships than on technological "cures.""

The women physicians pointed to additional differences between women and men that influenced how they practiced. One said, "Women are more process oriented and men more task oriented." These women also considered themselves to be better listeners and communicators than their male colleagues. One woman contrasted her style to that of her husband with whom she shared a practice:

He might see a hypertensive [patient] and manage his blood pressure. He would see the hypertension and I would see a whole person with a family and problems and stress. I'd ask, "How are things going?" [This] inevitably leads to a more time-consuming consultation. He would see ten patients an hour, while I might see only four.

Women physicians' lower incomes may also reflect a tendency to spend more time with each patient and to bill for fewer, less technical, and less expensive procedures. One woman observed that men are "driven to earn $200,000 a year, and it's the 'macho' expectation that a doctor has to work X hours per day." She added, "I don't want to be a money-making machine."

The women in the group conceded, nevertheless, that on political issues they often shared male positions. Like many of their male colleagues, they defended their right as physicians to control their incomes. They also supported the autonomy of the medical profession against what was perceived as a trend toward increasing government regulation. They unanimously agreed that they were "physicians first and women second" and

criticized the 1984 Canada Health Act, which had led to a provincial ban on extra billing – the practice of charging patients fees in excess of those covered under universal
government health insurance – and had precipitated a 25-day physicians' strike in
Ontario in l986 (Stevenson and Williams 1985). One group member who had trained
and practiced in Eastern Europe before immigrating to Canada pointed to a decline in
the quality of care and to a rise in corruption under government controlled health services; another suggested that government attempts to control physicians would only
discourage personal initiative. Although not advocating a return to private health care,
there was a tendency to see physicians as scapegoats for government inefficiency and
underfunding.

The government will not call the public to task for overusing the system. It's easy to knock
hospitals for not meeting their budgets and accuse doctors of being greedy. It's politically unwise
to tell the public not to run [to the doctor] for every sniffle or every hang-nail . . . (but) the system
can't afford it.

There was, however, a strong feeling among the group members that political issues
were less important and central to their experiences as women physicians; they placed
greater importance on the human dimension of their work. Although they might agree
with the positions of the organized profession toward government, the whole area of
medical politics was secondary to their relations with patients and families. The women
also judged themselves to be less active than men in their professional organizations;
only a minority regularly attended medical association meetings. In part, this lack of
political involvement was related to family responsibilities; one woman physician
observed that association meetings were often scheduled in the evenings and conflicted
with family time. However, the primary reason given was their greater interest in issues
of patient care.

On the question of gender bias in medical school, the group members suggested that
instead of being discriminated against, they felt that male professors and students had
generally been supportive and that women had been encouraged to pursue their own
interests, to "come and do our thing." These women did not feel that they had been
"streamed" or "channelled" into traditional female specialties such as family medicine
and obstetrics or excluded from male fields such as surgery; choices among specialties
had been primarily their own decisions, made in keeping with their inclinations toward
greater patient contact and involvement. They felt that gender had not impeded their
careers. Most of the group members felt that they had enjoyed a *greater* degree of
autonomy and choice than their male colleagues who, by contrast, had been under constant pressure to conform to professional conventions and to adopt the traditional male
physician's role. According to one woman, men are "driven to have careers and be
high-income earners," while "women can afford to bring a different orientation to medicine because they have other socially acceptable choices available to them."

Hypotheses

Our research results pose a number of important questions about the potential for
change associated with the progressive entry of women into medicine. While confirming significant gender differences in professional practice, our data provide a more tentative indication that such differences may be rooted in underlying orientations toward
medicine. Our evidence for distinctive orientations can be questioned as being unrepre-

sentative. Nevertheless, like other studies cited earlier, our focus group suggested that the experiences of women physicians are qualitatively different from those of men and constitute a potential for change that goes beyond workload management to the heart of the doctor-patient relationship. We found this prospect sufficiently compelling to examine theoretical hypotheses offering alternative interpretations of our results and, more generally, of the potential for change.

Professional Socialization

The first hypothesis is that any initial gender differences among medical students are progressively diminished by the intense and homogenizing effects of professional socialization and that remaining differences are not meaningful. In Mastering Medicine, Coombes (1978) describes how medical students are conditioned to suppress their personal inclinations and to adopt the appearance and persona of the "physician." Haas and Shaffir (1981) relate how students initially react with distaste, albeit suppressed, to some of the attitudes of their mentors toward patients, but gradually find it necessary to behave in a similar fashion to accomplish their immediate tasks and eventually consider such behavior acceptable. Recent work by Maheux et al. (1988) suggests that initial attitudinal differences among freshman medical students tend to decline and that "conservatism" increases as students progress through medical school. Women who choose a historically male-dominated profession may, by virtue of this very decision, be similar to their male peers (Eisenberg 1983). And the predilections of medical school admissions officers may produce a further narrowing of demographic and attitudinal differences among medical students of both genders (Coombes 1978).

Professional Marginalization

The second hypothesis states that even if women bring distinctive values and orientations to medicine, the potential for change is limited by the extent to which they are isolated from the mainstream of the profession. Although women make up an increasingly large proportion of physicians, they still tend to be concentrated in less prestigious and less lucrative specialties including family practice, pediatrics, and psychiatry (Adams 1989). Women also tend to be underrepresented and lack female role models in positions of authority and power within the organized profession (Stevenson and Williams 1985; Levinson et al. 1991). To the extent that women are "streamed" into professional niches seen to be more compatible with traditional female roles (Woodward et al. 1990) gender equality is diminished and the significance of women's increasing access to medicine is minimized. Alternatively, women physicians may themselves seek work settings that provide both greater flexibility of hours and a more humanistic style of medicine. While still posing the risk of a segregated job market and raising questions about the way medicine is practised in traditionally male specialties, the possibility of choice would suggest change over time as more women become physicians. A key issue, therefore, is the extent to which women control their own career choices within medicine.

Overcoming the Numbers Threshold

A third hypothesis suggests not only that women bring different values and orientations to medicine, but also that their increasing entry into medicine establishes an important potential for change. In her benchmark study of women's entry into male-dominated corporations, Kanter (1977) described a threshold effect that occurs when women move numerically beyond minority. According to Kanter, as a minority, women will tend to conform to and express the norms and behaviors of the male majority in order to be accepted and to succeed. However, as their numbers grow and they become a more visible and cohesive group comprising about a third of the population, they may begin to act more freely, to develop female role models, to express their own identifiable interests as women, and, eventually, to change male values and behavior. In spite of the increasing numbers of women entering medicine during the past 20 years, in Canada women still account for less than a fifth of all physicians (Adams 1989). In principle, therefore, even if women hold values and orientations different from those of male physicians, the expression of such differences will be restricted by women's minority status as well as by their relative youth and lack of experience within the profession. A failure to find systematic evidence of gender differences in medical practice could mean simply that the articulation of underlying differences will be more evident once women push past their minority status.

Discussion

These hypotheses suggest alternative explanations for our research results with important implications for understanding change. A central issue is the apparent inconsistency in results like our own, which document gender differences in practice, but provide equivocal evidence of parallel differences in physicians' underlying orientations.

Our survey findings appear to support the professional socialization thesis, that, to the extent there are gender differences in physicians' orientations, they are limited. Like other surveys, ours failed to demonstrate significant gender differences in physicians' attitudes. Even the focus group participants affirmed that there are important similarities between women and men on issues of medical economics and politics.

However, the focus group results suggest a more expansive interpretation of the survey findings. They hint that the career choices of women in medicine, while linked to caregiving responsibilities, are also rooted in distinctively female orientations. At the heart of these orientations is the focus on the patient: when women look at medicine they tend to see human needs first while men may see the elevated social status and income associated with a prestigious profession. This predisposition toward the "art" of medicine is perceived by women to motivate their choices of specialty, practice setting, and workload. It can also account for the lower professional incomes of women physicians who may spend more time with individual patients (Ohlsfeldt and Culler 1986).

A key to reconciling these findings and moving toward a more meaningful understanding of the potential for change in medicine lies in research indicating that women and men have qualitatively different ways of viewing their world. An important statement of this argument is found in the work of Gilligan (1982) who observes that female and male children develop along different psychological "trajectories" with distinctive gender-based conceptions of the moral domain. While male thinking is characterized by impersonal logic and law, women are more attuned to the web of social relationships that surrounds them and is sustained by interpersonal communication and mutual responsibilities. Because this fundamental distinction has often not been recognized, important gender differences may have been ignored. With respect to medicine, Gilligan's work suggests that research focused on the personal relationships between doctors and patients, what women in our focus group called the "art" of medicine, will reveal important gender differences. Conversely, research focused too narrowly on more impersonal issues of medical workloads and economics may either fail to find differences or, alternatively, suggest that women physicians do not meet the same norms as their male colleagues.

This distinction between the *realms* of values and of orientations is thus an important consideration in understanding the potential for change. Recent research indicates that while a principal effect of medical school socialization is to change attitudes toward social issues, attitudes toward human relations are not changed. Dornbush et al. (1991) found that the attitudes expressed by third year medical students were more politically conservative than they had been when the students first applied to medical school; however, there was no corresponding change in attitudes toward the doctor-patient relationship. The effects of professional socialization are not monolithic and they may not obliterate all attitudinal differences; socialization to a historically male-dominated profession may be more marked in areas of traditional male concern including the defense of professional freedom against external intrusion (Stevenson et al. 1988).

Particularly intriguing is the suggestion by women physicians in our focus group that male physicians may be more constrained than women by medical socialization. If women in medical schools are streamed *away* from the more prestigious and lucrative specialties like surgery (Dickstein 1990), another important effect of medical education may be to stream men *toward* these specialties and infuse in them the belief that success is measured primarily in terms of mastery of complex medical technology, high levels of productivity, and high incomes.

There are two further considerations suggested by our hypotheses. First, change may not be a linear function of the number of women entering the profession. Following the logic of Kanter's threshold hypothesis (Kanter 1977) change should become increasingly apparent as women reduce and finally overcome their minority status in the profession. An important effect of the increasing number of women physicians may be to establish alternative norms focused less on quantitative production than on the quality of patient care. If men, in addition to women, choose to follow these norms, it seems possible, for instance, that the documented trend in Canada and the United States for *male* physicians to take on lighter workloads (Woodward et al. 1990; Wheeler et al. 1990) could be reinforced, or that men, like women, will begin to provide a different mix of services involving more counseling but fewer surgical services (Cohen et al. 1991).

Second, women physicians' apparent reluctance to engage in political/professional activities may reduce the potential for change or at least slow its pace. While again emphasizing a humanistic orientation, this reluctance could mean that women continue to play a relatively marginal role in the organized profession. Although in Canada women have served as medical association leaders at both the national and provincial levels, these have tended to be the exception rather than the rule.

In summary, our research suggests prospects for change and for understanding its potential. It points to the complexity of professional values and orientations that span more than one field or realm. This complexity suggests the need to devise research strategies that look beyond the quantitative issues of volume and productivity to the qualitative experience of patient care. Women physicians suggest that they practice a distinctive style of medicine that benefits their patients; more needs to be known about the nature and extent of such differences and the implications for costs and quality.

The effects of the growing number of women in medicine are likely to be complex. If differences in women physicians' practice patterns and choices of specialty persist over time in Canada, as they apparently have in other Western industrialized countries (Uhlenberg and Cooney 1990) they will produce further changes in patterns of medical service delivery as more women enter medicine. However, if men also adopt the alternative role models and the practice norms established by women, change will be compounded. Only longitudinal research that combines qualitative and quantitative methodologies will be able to monitor and assess such changes.

Although women constitute an important potential for change in medicine, it would be misleading and unfair to imply that the prospect for change rests solely on their shoulders. The fact that so many women are now entering what was until recently a male-dominated profession is itself evidence of the effect of social forces that are reshaping conceptions of health and illness and the role of the physician.

References

Adams, O. 1989. Canada's Doctors – Who They Are and What They Do: Lessons from the CMA's 1986 Manpower Survey. *Canadian Medical Association Journal* 140: 212–221.

Adams, EK, and GJ Bazzoli. 1986. Career Plans of Women and Minority Physicians: Implications for Health Manpower Policy. *Journal of the American Medical Women's Association* 41: 17–20.

Barondess, A. 1981. Are Women Different? Some Trends in the Assimilation of Women in Medicine. *Journal of the American Medical Women's Association* 36: 95–104.

Bobula, JD. 1980. Work Patterns, Practice Characteristics and Incomes of Male and Female Physicians. *Journal of Medical Education* 55: 826–833.

Bowman, M, and ML Gross. 1986. Overview of Research on Women in Medicine–Issues for Public Policy Makers. *Public Health Reports* 5: 513–521.

Bryant, HE, PA Jennett, and M Kishnevsky. 1991. Gender, Family Status, and Career Patterns of Graduates of the University of Calgary Faculty of Medicine. *Academic Medicine* 66: 483–485.

Burkett, GL, and DEA Kurz. 1981. A Comparison of the Professional Values and Career Orientations of Male and Female Medical Students: Some Unintended Consequences of US public policy. *Health Policy Education* 2: 33–45.

Cohen, M, BM Ferrier, and CA Woodward. 1991. Gender Differences in Practice Patterns of Ontario Family Physicians (McMaster Medical Graduates). *Journal of the American Medical Women's Association* 46: 49–54.

Contandriopoulos, AP, and MA Fournier. 1987. *Les Effectifs Medicaux au Quebec. Situation de 1972 a 1986 et Projection pour 1990.* Montreal: Corporation Professionelle des Medecins do Quebec.

Coombes, RH. 1978. *Mastering Medicine: Professional Socialization in Medical School.* New York: Free Press.

Dennerstein, L, P Lehert, R Orams, et al. 1989. Practice Patterns and Family Life – A Survey of Melbourne Medical Graduates. *Medical Journal of Australia* 151: 386–390.

Dickstein, LJ. 1990. Female Physicians in the 1980s: Personal and Family Attitudes and Values. *Journal of the American Medical Women's Association* 45: 122–126.

Dornbush, RL, S Richman, P Singer, and EJ Brownstein. 1991. Medical School, Psychosocial Attitudes, and Gender. *Journal of the American Women's Association* 46: 150–152.

Eisenberg, JM. 1985. Physician Utilization: The State of Research About Physician's Practice Patterns. *Medical Care* 23: 461–483.

Eisenberg, C. 1983. Women as Physicians. *Journal of Medical Education* 58: 534–541.

Elston, MA. 1980. Medicine: Half our Future Doctors? In R Silverstone and A Ward eds. *Careers of Professional Women,* 93-139. London: Croom-Helm.

Fett, I. 1976. The Future of Women in Australian Medicine. *Medical Journal of Australia,* Supplement 2: 33–39.

Frey, H. 1980. Swedish Men and Women Doctors Compared. *Medical Education* 14: 143–153.

Gilligan, C. 1982. *In A Different Voice.* Cambridge, Mass.: Harvard University Press.

Haas, J, and W Shaffir. 1981. The Professionalization of Medical Students: Developing Competence and a Cloak of Competence. In D Coburn, C D'Arcy, G Torrance, and P New eds. *Health and Canadian Society: Sociological Perspectives.* Toronto: Fitzhenry and Whiteside.

Hayes, MD. 1981. The Impact of Women Physicians on Social Change in Medicine: The Evolution of Humane Health Care Delivery Systems. *Journal of the American Women's Association* 36: 82–83.

Kanter, RM. 1977. *Men and Women of the Corporation.* New York: Basic Books.

Leserman, J. 1981. *Men and Women in Medical School: How They Change and How They Compare.* New York: Praeger.

Levinson, W, K Kaufman, B Clark, and SW Tolle. 1991. Mentors and Role Models for Women in Academic Medicine. *Western Journal of Medicine* 154: 423–426.

Levinson, W, SW Tolle, and C Lewis. 1987. Women in Academic Medicine: Combining Career and Family. *New England Journal of Medicine* 321: 1511–1517.

Lomas, J, M Barer, and G Stoddart. 1986. *Physician Manpower Planning: Lessons from the MacDonald Report.* Toronto: Ontario Economic Council, Discussion Paper Series.

Maheux, B, F Dufort, and F Beland. 1988. Professional and Sociopolitical Attitudes of Medical Students: Gender Differences Reconsidered. *Journal of the American Women's Association* 43: 73–76.

Mickelburgh, R. 1992. Provinces Agree to Reduce Medical School Enrollments. *Toronto Globe and Mail,* January 29, Al.

Northrup, D. 1988. *Sample and Field Report: 1986 National Survey of Canadian Physicians.* Toronto: Institute for Social Research, York University.

Ohlsfeldt, RJ, and SD Culler. 1986. Differences in Income Between Male and Female Physicians. *Journal of Health Economics* 5: 335–346.

Ryten, E. 1989. The Output of Canadian Medical Schools in 1989. *Forum* 22: 7–9.

Stevenson, HM, AP Williams, and E Vayda. 1988. Medical Politics and Canadian Medicare: Professional Response to the Canada Health Act. *Milbank Quarterly* 66: 65–104.

Stevenson, HM, and AP Williams. 1985. Physicians and Medicare: Professional Ideology and Canadian Health Care Policy. *Canadian Public Policy* 11: 504–521.

Sullivan, P. 1990. Women close in on 50% share of places in Canada's medical schools. *Canadian Medical Association Journal* 143: 781.

Uhlenberg, P, and TM Cooney. 1990. Male and Female Physicians: Family and Career Comparisons. *Social Science and Medicine* 30: 373–378.

Wakeford, RE, and VJ Warren. 1989. Women Doctors' Career Choice and Commitment to Medicine: Implications for General Practice. *Journal of the Royal College of General Practice* 39: 91–95.

Weisman, CS, DM Levine, DM Steinwachs, et al. 1980. Male and Female Physician Career Patterns: Specialty Choices and Graduate Yraining. *Journal of Medical Education* 55: 813–825.

Wheeler, R, L Candib, and M Martin. 1990. Part-Time Doctors: Reduced Working Hours for Primary Care Physicians. *Journal of the American Women's Association* 45: 47–54.

Williams, AP, KD Pierre, and E Vayda, et al. 1990. Women in Medicine: Practice Patterns and Attitudes. *Canadian Medical Association Journal* 143: 194–201.

Williams, AP, E Vayda, HM Stevenson, et al. 1990. A Typology of Medical Practice Organization in Canada: Data From a National Survey of Physicians. *Medical Care* 28: 995–1003.

Woodward, C, ML Cohen, and BM Ferrier. 1990. Career Interruptions and Hours Practised: Comparisons Between Young Men and Women Physicians. *Canadian Journal of Public Health* 81: 16–20.

20

Rediscovering Appropriate Care: Maternity Traditions and Contemporary Issues in Canada

Cecilia Benoit

Introduction

Scrutiny of health services in industrial democracies indicates that appropriate care for citizens means different things in different places (Roemer 1991). This is the case even in culturally similar territories, including in Britain and its North American frontier societies, the United States and Canada. In each of these countries over the last century, divergences have developed concerning the range and availability of services provided by health professionals.

Great Britain at mid-century established a National Health Service (NHS) administered under the direct tutelage of the central government and financed through country wide taxes. Yet the proportion of the Gross Domestic Product (GDP) allotted to pay for the NHS is substantially lower than in most other industrial democracies, leading to a shortage of medical specialists, waiting lists for certain surgical procedures, and the unavailability of some vital health services for disadvantaged citizens without the means to pay for private professional care (Stacey 1988).[1]

By contrast, the multi-tier government structure of the United States has worked against central planning of health care services; rather, a weakly integrated, pluralistic health care system holds firm (Field 1980). Health care in the U.S., notwithstanding some laudable governmental programs (Ruggie 1992), is essentially a consumer good or item. Ironically, the comparatively large proportion of the GDP required to finance the U.S. health care system does not lead to greater public access or quality care. In fact, current figures indicate that more than thirty-five million Americans possess no health insurance, and sixty million more are underinsured. In addition, the U.S. has a comparatively low rating regarding mortality and morbidity internationally (Light 1986).

Canada's health care system is an amalgam of the British and U.S. models. On the one hand, like its British counterpart, the Canadian federal government takes an active role in financing organized health and other social services. National legislation, including the Canadian Health Act of 1984, provides the general framework for the country's health system, which is based on the principles of comprehensiveness, universality, portability, accessibility and public administration. However, unlike the NHS, and more closely paralleling the U.S. federal-state model, economic management of the Canadian system, as well as the day-to-day administration of services, are largely provincial affairs. Another shared feature concerns mode of payment for medical services: physicians in most areas of Canada closely resemble their American counterparts in working as medical entrepreneurs reimbursed on a fee-for-service basis. The result is a comparatively attractive medicare package freely available to Canadian citizens, accompanied by notable gaps in the areas of primary care, preventive health and health promotion (Sutherland and Fulton 1988).

It is obvious, then, that health care systems are not rational and predictable realizations of science nor, indeed, direct reflections of citizens' health needs. Sociologists are far from certain as to why this is the case, however. An examination of the full range of the debate is beyond the scope of this inquiry (Benoit forthcoming). A brief sketch of some of the concepts central to the rich literature on the health professions and health care systems can highlight the main lines of argumentation.[2]

Many scholars contend that the root cause of inappropriate health care on both sides of the Atlantic is medical dominance. Medical dominance, on the one hand, involves demarcationary strategies employed by physicians to gain occupational monopoly over the provision of crucial health services. Demarcationary strategies are typically accompanied by exclusionary strategies – what G.V. Larkin (1983) has referred to as occupational imperialism – whereby physicians simultaneously exercise power in a downward fashion by subordinating and even eliminating less-powerful occupational groups. The ultimate result of these two forms of medical dominance is that physicians are able to maintain and/or enhance their favoured access to rewards and opportunities, without concern for accountability to those they serve. Eliot Freidson (1970) describes the medical profession as Janus-faced – that physicians not only enjoy work autonomy but also an authoritative position over both non-medical health practitioners and clients. A third source of medical dominance, perhaps the most fundamental of all, is found at the cultural level. It involves deference of the citizenry to a medical profession which orchestrates public opinion for its own self-interest (Light and Levine 1988; Wolinsky 1988).

Not all sociologists place the blame for inadequate health care on the shoulders of Anglo-American physicians. Many scholars highlight macro level social and economic causes, not least of all the corporatization of the social service sector, which has significant negative outcome for both citizens and health professionals, including physicians themselves (Starr 1982; Weller 1977; Light and Levine 1988). Some writers even suggest that medical dominance, including physicians' cherished clinical autonomy – that is, professional control over the content and organization of day-to-day activities – is on the wane. Among other things, this is the outcome of a shift of medical practice to large bureaucracies (Larson 1977; Derber 1982) – what George Torrance (1987) calls "health factories." Physicians employed in the emerging "medical-industrial complex" (Relman 1980), which in the U.S. is comprised largely of for-profit health chains, are subordinated to a new breed of corporate managers more concerned with organizational efficiency and profits than with workers' well-being and appropriate client care. The ultimate result for the medical and complementary health professions is a downward move towards proletarianization (McKinlay and Arches 1985; McKinlay and Stoeckle 1988). In countries with state-financed or organized health systems, such as Canada and Britain, a parallel process of proletarianization is occurring, with the result that physicians and allied health workers are suffering a loss of autonomy to organize the care of clients. In these countries, the motor of change concerns the rationalization of health and other social services by the state in an attempt to resolve the fiscal crisis of the welfare state (Coburn et al. 1983; Weller and Manga 1983; Blishen 1991).

Most recently, feminist scholars, many of them active members of the intertwined health care and women's movements on both sides of the Atlantic, have added further complexity to this debate by singling out gender as a pivotal variable influencing the care of citizens in general and women clients in particular (Stacey 1988; Crompton 1987; Butter et al. 1987). Feminist writers have found a close link between patriarchal control and the health service structure. Women practitioners, assumed to be society's natural "emotional experts," are assigned to primary care specialties or low-ranking positions, typically in bureaucratic settings as salaried employees (Riska 1988; Riska and Wegar 1993). There is a hidden gatekeeping system or a "glass ceiling" in operation which keeps women practitioners at or near the bottom of the health division of labour (Lorber 1984), without the resources and power to substantially improve their own subordinate situation nor that of their clientele (Pizurki et al. 1987; Altecruse and McDermott 1987). In alternative health occupations where women are located, such as midwifery, patriarchal controls have been so influential that female midwives have not only been subordinated but, in Canada and many of the American states, banned from legal practice entirely (Biggs 1983; Burtch 1988; Sullivan and Weitz 1988). Such exclusionary gender tactics not only have consequences for female healers (Witz 1990); birthing women too lose out because they are deprived of appropriate care under the guidance of female midwives. Some writers believe that this situation is now changing as a result of the new "feminist vision of health" taking hold among women physicians, nurses, midwives, other female-based occupations and consumers, joined together to create a less-stratified and more caring health service (Ruzek 1986).

Rather than attempting to evaluate these various perspectives in term of relative analytical usefulness, this chapter advocates a multi-paradigmatic approach in order to ascertain which societal conditions detract from or enhance the appropriate care of birthing families. In addition to notions of medical dominance, corporatism and patriarchy touched on above, it is worthwhile to employ two other concepts found in the sociological literature. The first, "system of professions," is a concept central to the work of Andrew Abbott (1988) and others (Halpern 1992) drawing on the interactionist tradition (Hughes 1958; Bucher and Strauss 1961; Strauss 1978). These writers argue that sociological understanding of health professions necessarily involves scrutiny of the content, organization and control of their caring work – caring work which varies depending upon relations among practitioners within and across professions, as well as due to wider economic, legal and political forces. The health division of labour, in this view, is interactional, arbitrated by segments of, or entire professions, in the task or jurisdictional area, and further patterned by changes in the external environment. When applied to maternity care, the system of professions allows for a more complex understanding of the work of midwives – as more or less autonomous/subservient, depending upon intra- and inter-professional relations and societal conditions.

Second, it is paramount to consider the role of the state in a more multifarious manner than has usually been the case. An adequate conceptualization of the state understands it as more than the silent and supportive partner of medical-corporate-male elites. States in most industrial democracies are complex bureaucracies assigned the difficult task of organizing efficient and appropriate health care systems. In regard to the health professions, states serve as instruments of professional (and not merely male medical) advancement, direct professional education, establish legal limits on the work mandates of health workers, and coordinate administration and funding of the services provided to citizens (Freddi and Bjoerkman 1989; Burrage and Torstendahl 1990; Wilsford 1991; Naylor 1992). In brief, states and health professions "intermingle and interpenetrate each other" (Coburn 1993: 129); at certain times and in certain places, states are weak and dependent, while at other times and in other places states are strong and relatively autonomous from allopathic medicine, private interest groups and patriarchal controls (Swartz 1987). As Elliott Krause (1988: 49) states: "[t]he rise or fall of professional group political/economic or guild power is a complex topic, demanding respect for historical and political processes, profession by profession and nation by nation."

The first section of this chapter draws upon the concepts mentioned above and historical data to outline the social transformation of maternity in Anglo-America, with a particular emphasis on Canada. The second section highlights some of the lingering issues, beyond legalization and legitimation of midwifery, which will likely complicate appropriate care for less advantaged Canadian birthing families. Two primary sources are drawn upon to lend support to this section of the chapter: 1) the author's findings on midwifery and maternity care in Newfoundland and Labrador (Benoit 1991; 1992); and 2) the author's current research project in British Columbia, which seeks to understand the diverse visions and strategies held by provincial midwives and complementary health professionals about quality maternity care.

Maternity Care in Historical and Comparative Perspective

It was natural that a mother who had given birth should offer her advice and assistance to inexperienced women. Once this help had been repeated several times, it was also natural that people had faith in her and called upon her. That is how the first midwife came into being.

The practice of attending birthing families during parturition was, in virtually all preindustrial societies, awarded to women healers, usually referred to as traditional midwives, wisewomen or grannies. Midwifery is one of the oldest specialized social services, demonstrating the willingness of a particular group of female caregivers to respond to calls for help from those in need. The midwife's care of birthing families was already recognized in the earliest books of the Old Testament, and it was an established occupation in ancient Greece and Rome (Lefkowitz and Fant 1982: 162-164). Despite the tainting of this age-old form of midwifery with witchcraft during the European medieval and late agrarian periods,[3] birthing families from humble to aristocratic standing continued to seek out the local female midwife to guide them through their confinements.

Yet the midwife – indeed, any health worker, including the academically-educated physician – during this long stretch of history predating industrialization, was limited in her capacity to provide a safe and happy birth experience. While many practised proper hygiene and provided skilled care, other traditional midwives were poor candidates on both counts. Even for parturient women who managed to secure and pay the services of a competent local midwife, there was no guarantee that her birthing process would unfold in a straight-forward manner. The advantage of labour and delivery in her own home surrounded by those that she had called together – of being "brought to bed" (Leavitt 1986) – was all too frequently accompanied by anxiety, fear, and even death. Thus Katharine Park (1992: 62) notes, "[t]he dangers of pregnancy and childbirth seem to have accounted for the shorter life expectancy of medieval women." At risk above all were infants; from 15 to 30 per cent – even higher in some centuries and particular geographical regions of preindustrial Europe – are reported to have died before reaching their first birthday (Stone 1977). Of course, the shortcomings of the traditional maternity system were not solely the responsibility of midwives. Additional factors include the frequency of pregnancies, arduous work roles during and after the reproductive period and, perhaps most important of all, the diets of the average household, which were deficient in both quality and quantity, and worsened by periodic famines.

In the late 18th century Continental governments, as part of a broad strategy to reduce maternal and infant morbidity and mortality, initiated a variety of pronatalist policies to create a healthy population. In pursuance of this plan, steps were taken to improve the quality of care of birthing families by upgrading the standards of midwifery and other health professions, including obstetrics. In Denmark a national midwifery school was founded in 1787, and legislation passed to regulate the occupation. Similar schools and state-operated systems for the examination and control of midwives appeared around this time in Moscow, St. Petersburg and Austria (Donnison 1981). In many German states a local "Hebammenmeister" was selected to organize midwifery training and to regulate the practice of graduates. In France, following an official inquiry into midwifery practice in 1728, lying-in hospitals were built in strategic locations across the country and staffed by salaried midwives who had received formal training in the newly established state midwifery schools (Ackernecht 1967). In brief, as Deborah Sullivan and Anne Weitz note (1988: 206):

The history of midwifery on the European continent reveals that independent midwifery can flourish under physician supervision and legal limitation as long as it does not compete directly with medicine. While licensure restricted independent European midwives to normal childbirth and prohibited them from using instruments, it left them with considerable functional autonomy...

Space limits do not allow for a thorough examination of the current situation of midwives as professional workers in Continental Europe and the Nordic Countries. It seems that, in at least some areas of the European continent, childbirth has become "medicalized" and the midwife's work "bureaucratized," lending support for the medical dominance perspective mentioned in the introduction (Oakley and Houd 1990). Yet there are divergent cases, including the Netherlands, where independent midwifery practice in the home setting survives the test of time (Van Teiglingen 1992), as well as in the Nordic Countries where autonomous midwifery care in state-supported community clinics is popular. As explored elsewhere (Benoit 1992), the Swedish example of "mothercare centres" is a viable example of this option (Seward et al. 1984). Workable alternatives can also be found today in Finland (Valvanne 1988) and Denmark (Houd 1988). What these different countries share are: 1) extensive state support for birthing families, which go a long way to reduce, although not completely eliminate, health problems associated with social and economic marginality; 2) midwives who are relatively autonomous from medicine and part of a "health team" oriented towards placing the care of birthing families first. These cornerstones of appropriate care of birthing families have been much more difficult to achieve in Anglo-America.

Britain

Like its Continental European neighbours, premodern Britain depended upon the ancient institution of lay midwifery to carry birthing families through the reproductive process. Originally midwifery was practised as a form of mutual support among women in village communities (Donnison 1977). Wise women, chosen mainly on the basis of high moral character and practical knowledge of pregnancy and childbirth, were informally elected to the office of midwife by local inhabitants (Boehme 1984: 371).

As early as the Tudor period, the English monarchy began to take a more active role in the regulation of health services, including those offered by midwives. King Henry VIII initiated the systematic organization of the healing professions, beginning with the incorporation of the Royal College of Physicians in 1512. The original attempt by the English Crown to certify midwives was started around the mid-16th century, at which time the local parish bishop and a trustworthy "doctor of physicke" were appointed to examine hopeful midwives. Yet the British state avoided the path subsequently taken by Continental governments, choosing instead to establish neither national midwifery training nor licensure for British midwives.

Not surprisingly, within a hundred years men were specializing in midwifery – initially calling themselves "male-midwife," "midman," "man midwife," "endroboethogynist" or "accoucheur" and finally "obstetrician" – and taking a place at the birth chamber. Their position was abetted when the British surgeon, Peter Chamberlen the Elder, modified the levers used by medieval barber-surgeons and invented the forceps, which emerged as the "secret instrument" of the new male obstetrics to which midwives were denied access. The forceps made it possible for doctors to intervene in the birth process and to offer women the promise of shorter labours. This development was a direct challenge to the role of the female midwife, traditionally the senior attendant at all normal deliveries (Wertz and Wertz 1977).

It was only at the turn of the twentieth century that the tide began to slowly turn in the favour of the female midwife in Britain. The concerted efforts of various groups calling for maternity reform ultimately proved successful, resulting in the Midwives' Act of 1902. According to Ann Oakley (1976: 51), "the passing of the 1902 Midwives' Act in Britain ensured a future for the female midwife;" Jean Donnison (1977: 174-75) concurs, noting that without the Midwives' Act the British midwife "would probably have vanished from the scene within the next fifty years, squeezed out by her medical competitors."

Yet, compared to its Continental and Nordic neighbours, the British state continue to take a "weak" role in the NHS (Wilsford 1991), reluctant to allot necessary funds to support crucial social services for disadvantaged birthing families and unwilling to stand above sectarian interests of powerful medical and nursing lobbies vying for a stake in the delivery of maternity services. This conservative/partisan stance of the British state resulted in the virtual elimination of the homebirth option, as well as state-funding for maternity care in small hospitals. The majority of British midwives by the 1970s were delegated the position of "assembly-line workers, while [family physicians] and obstetrical consultants control the line" (Sullivan and Weitz 1988: 175). The outcome for birthing women has been fragmented care by "strangers": "The midwives who work in the antenatal clinic and the midwife she [the pregnant woman] may meet at her GP's surgery are different from the midwives who work in the labour ward ... after she has her baby she goes to the postnatal ward, where she is attended by yet more midwives, and then home again to the care of several community midwives, most of whom she has never met before" (Flint 1988).

A small yet vocal segment of British midwives believe that positive change for birthing families is now underway, however. The central government has recently adopted a stronger position in the NHS and moved to decentralize health care services, apparently in order to create a system claimed to be simultaneously more efficient and client-centred (Alaszewiski and Manthrope 1992). The Report on Maternity Services made by the Health Committee of the House of Commons[4] is an outcome of this new governmental approach recommending, among other things, an end to territorial disputes among health professionals concerned with control over parturition and the establishment of genuine continuity of client care by midwives working in the home or small maternity units. Yet obstetricians, family physicians and nurses across the country are not rushing to lay down their battle armour. Nor is the British state reaching into its coffers to provide the essential funds for the called-for restructuring process. As disquieting is the lack of firm agreement among British midwives themselves concerning how best to implement their "visionary principles" underlying quality care for birthing families, which seems to run counter to the professionalization trend observable among the midwifery leadership.[5] Without such an alternative occupational image, British midwives "may become more like doctors instead of more like midwives" (Oakley and Houd 1990: 164), and disadvantaged birthing families are likely to experience little or no improvement in their health status. As shown below, North American midwives today are grappling with similar professional concerns within their own ranks, while economically and culturally marginalized birthing families are deprived of adequate maternity care.

The United States

The earliest style of maternity care in the United States is in many ways analogous to the occupation's origins in Britain, Continental Europe and the Nordic Countries (Wertz and Wertz 1977). One well-known colonial midwife, Ann Hutchinson, was "very helpful in the times of childbirth, and other occasions of bodily infirmities and well furnished with means for those purposes" (quoted in Litoff 1978: 4). The traditional American midwife was required to 'be diligent and ready to help any woman in labour, whether poor or rich.' But this tended to be the extent of the restrictions on her. As Sullivan and Weitz (1988: 2) explain:

Colonial American midwives worked under an incomplete system of municipal licensure. Where licensure existed, unlike on the European continent, it was not accompanied by training programs. As in Britain, American midwives were considered moral guardians rather than health care providers.

Analogous to developments in the Mother Country mentioned above, in a relatively short period of time "male midwifery" had blossomed in the New Colonies. Yet by the turn of the twentieth century the two countries diverged: British midwives gaining official status while their American counterparts facing subordination and, in some states, virtual elimination. The reasons for this divergence are many (Benoit 1991; Sullivan and Weitz 1988). Space concerns allows only mention of the most salient.

As noted above, the British state eventually passed the appropriate legislation that allowed for midwives survival, albeit subordinate to physicians. In the U.S., a democratic ideology discouraged state legislatures from passing statutory requirements for the training and practice of midwives (Starr 1982). Moreover, unlike in the Mother Country, there existed no landed aristocracy in the American Colonies to lobby for the midwife's cause. Equally important, the average American medical practitioner of the time was recruited from the working classes and lacked the protection and support of a

Royal College that physicians on the European continent and in Britain enjoyed (Wertz and Wertz 1990).

Midwifery in the new colony did not decline overnight, however. The open market in health services characteristic of the nineteenth century left all American health workers, including physicians, vulnerable. Physicians were only one among a number of practitioners American families might select. In fact, female midwives often topped the list (Wertz and Wertz 1990: 151-152). Not surprisingly, as late as 1910 approximately fifty percent of all births in New England were still attended by midwives in clients' homes (Kobrin 1966).

Yet most American midwives of the period were poor immigrant women and black grannies who lacked formal credentials, organizational backing, and aristocratic patronage crucial for gaining access to the political machinery then taking shape in urbanizing America (Donegan 1978; Litoff 1986). Furthermore, American midwives were excluded from the educational reforms aiding the cause of the new male obstetrics. The influential Flexner Report of 1910 highlighted the abysmal situation of American medical education, reporting that ninety percent of all physicians received their training from profit-making schools that offered little or no resources for authentic clinical training. Abraham Flexner recommended the elimination of all "diploma mills," and the tightening of education and licensure standards for American physicians. The female midwife, among other lay healers, became an easy target for the reformed medical profession, although even at this late date the high maternal and infant death rates among midwifery attended cases were closely matched by their physician counterparts (Arney 1982). A counterpart to the British nurse-midwife eventually emerged in pockets of the U.S. in the early 1930s. Yet American nurse-midwives remained small in number and their mandate narrowed to serve those urban and rural poor without economic means to pay for obstetrical care (Campbell 1946). The result is that even today the majority of American nurse-midwives, especially in urban areas where the competition from obstetrics remains intense, practice as "obstetrical nurses" who are expected to move to the side lines as soon as the obstetrician appears (Eakins 1986).

The futile effort by American midwives to gain a legitimate footing in the maternity system is complicated by macro social, economic, and political issues. Corporatization of health and other crucial services, usually in large chains owned and operated by private business and/or medical groups, remains characteristic of the U.S. (Light and Levine 1988). The human costs, health-wise, are hardly surprising. Compared to other industrial democracies, the U.S. scores poorly on both infant mortality and maternal morbidity, and is characterized by the over-use of such obstetrical procedures as episiotomies, inductions of labour, fetal monitoring, and forceps and cesarean deliveries (Jordan 1983).

These unanticipated side-effects of medical/corporate dominance in the United States has fostered a variety of critical responses from the American public. It has become widely publicized that "in the bureaucratic setting of the hospital women could no longer receive the individualized, personal care that had accompanied homebirth among family and friends" (Sullivan and Weitz 1988: 24). Yet debureaucratization alone will not likely realize either midwives' autonomy or appropriate care for birthing families. U.S. midwives working in free-standing birthing centres, for example, the majority of which are for-profit enterprises, are forced, as Georg Simmel (1908) stated in a different context, to react with their heads rather than their hearts, calculating the value of their exchange with clients first. At the same time, the needs of indigent birthing families, many who are from culturally disadvantaged groups and without access to familial support systems, remain unaddressed.

As disturbing as the emphasis on fees is the simmering conflict among U.S. midwives themselves concerning the path forward. As observed above in the British case, disquiet among midwives regarding "sisterhood or professionalization" (Reid 1989) suggests that caution is in order concerning accepting midwives claims to provide more appropriate care for birthing families at face value. As observed below, a similar prudence is advised when analyzing the recent declarations of Canadian midwives as the fiduciary agents of birthing families.

Canada

Although no longer the case, Canada throughout the 20th century was unique among industrial democracies for having no legal provision for midwives (Phaff 1986). This negative climate regarding midwifery seems puzzling since Canada is generally held in high esteem world-wide for its comprehensive and equitable medical and hospital service plan. Unlike other industrial democracies with analogous state-supported systems, however, Canada shows poor rates of maternal morbidity. A brief glance at the country's historical roots may shed light on this seeming incongruity.

As observed above regarding the U.S., most families in frontier Canada had little contact with "learned physicians." Instead they tended to rely upon their own healing cures or those of their close kin. In times of special concern, one of the many lay healers – bone setters, homeopaths, eclectics, apothecaries among them – were secured. Parturient women, depending upon their economic standing and cultural background, would call upon one of a variety of kinds of midwives.

Although little is known about the midwives who attended Inuit and Indian birthing women prior to settler contact, evidence can be gleaned from the few native midwives still active today who operate their practices using an unofficial communication link – the "moccasin telegraph" – sending whispers that a birth is imminent (Barrington 1985: 31). The first reference to midwifery among non-native women in the country appears in a deed in the archives of Montreal published by a Mr. Massicotte, "which reveals that the women of Ville-Marie, in solemn concave assembled, on February 12th, 1713, elected a midwife Catherine Guertin for the community" (Abbott 1931: 28). Mention is also made in government documents of the time of Madame Bouchette, a midwife trained in France, who was sent out to the French colony of Quebec in 1722 on an annual salary from the King of 400 livres, and of Mlle. Bery who travelled from France in 1930 to serve the women of St. Foye in the capacity of their community midwife. Due to frail health, she was eventually replaced by a younger colleague, whose government wages were raised from 400 to 600 livres (Abbott 1931: 28). In addition, in the British settlement of Lunenburg, Nova Scotia, it is written that in 1755 the Commander, Colonel Sutherland, requested from the British Crown four pounds per annum for the salaries of two practising midwives. As late as the 1930s, local granny midwives and formally-trained foreign midwives could also be found practising in the 5000 or so coastal communities dotting the Newfoundland and Labrador coastlines (Benoit 1989).

Pressure to transform the original maternity system in the young country began in the late 18th-century. The first Medical Act attempted to regulate the practices of "physic and surgery" in Upper Canada in 1795 by making it illegal to practice midwifery without a license, exempting only those with a university degree. The impracticality of such a ruling soon became apparent, and the small degree-holding segment of the medical profession was left vulnerable to public criticism (Canniff 1894: 22). The original Medical Act was repealed in 1806 and traditional midwifery remained immune from the licensing laws of the Ontario Medical Board for the next half century. In 1866, however, the permission awarded by the provincial government to unlicensed female midwives to practice their art was withdrawn; thereafter midwifery was to be the legal mandate only of those holding medical degrees. Given that no female physicians were licensed in Ontario until the 1880's – and few females occupied this capacity for many decades to come – male counterparts in the province enjoyed a legal monopoly over the birthing chamber by the time of Confederation in 1867 (Biggs 1983).

The growing number of physicians trying to make a living in Toronto and other provincial urban areas could now look to accouchement as a feasible entré to family practice. Although some physicians (known as the "traditionalists") opposed this turn of events embraced by their colleagues (the "radicals"), and called instead for formal training and legalization of midwifery, their efforts proved unsuccessful. The medical majority won the day by convincing governmental authorities that "women don't want midwives about them [for] as a rule they have no confidence in them" (Canada Lancet 1875, 8:60).

Yet traditional midwifery persisted in outlying regions of Ontario where medical practitioners were in short supply well into the twentieth century. Even in the urban areas, competition between physicians and midwives persisted on the home birth front for several decades after Confederation. But "doctor-births" were eventually to become the norm. In fact, only one-sixth of recorded births in Ontario were not attended by physicians by 1897, and only a few of those "medically unattended" births were recorded to have been attended by midwives (Oppenheimer 1983: 40-44; Task Force on the Implementation of Midwifery in Ontario 1987).

Midwives in other parts of the country remained active long after their Ontario counterparts had lost their place in the birth chamber. Although as early as 1788 the colonial government enacted licensing requirements on health practitioners in Quebec, female midwives with a certificate, and duly examined by a health board to determined their proficiency, were granted the right to practice alongside of male physicians operating in Montreal and its surrounding environs. In the countryside, meanwhile, sage-femmes continued to remain unregulated, controlled by the local clergy and by birthing women themselves (Ordinances of the Province of Quebec 1763-91. Ottawa: King's Printer 1971). In 1879, however, the Quebec College of Physicians and Surgeons, following events in Ontario, extended control over female midwifery (Laforce 1990). Quebec midwives in the countryside were permitted to practice for the next half century, provided that a physician certified their competence. Such was also the case in New Brunswick and Saskatchewan where as late as 1924 it is reported that fifty percent of births were medically unattended (Biggs 1983). In the long run, nevertheless, midwifery in most areas of the country was undermined and childbirth attendance emerged as the mandate of the medical profession.

Medical dominance over birthing arrangements in Canada did not easily result in more appropriate care than that previously provided by traditional midwives. This was especially the case for poor and destitute pregnant women who were often left with neither physician nor midwife during their confinement. Some of these forsaken women were given physical aid by philanthropic institutions, including the Society for the Relief of Women during their Confinement, established in 1820 in Ontario (Oppenheimer 1983). Yet such voluntary organizations did not provide accommodation, which left the few hospitals with the task of providing shelter to homeless parturient women.

The result was that as late the 1920s (when the first national statistics became available) the Canadian infant mortality rate was very high by international standards at 92 per 1,000 live births and the maternal mortality rate was 5.6 maternal deaths per 1,000 birthing women (Buckley 1979: 134-5). As one commentator pointed out at the time: "more babies die in Canada yearly, under one year old, from preventive causes than soldiers have been killed during the war" (quoted in Buckley 1979: 133).

Although health teams comprising midwives, physicians and public health nurses working out of community clinics were advocated by some prominent Canadian health reformers, the opposing medical and nursing lobby groups eventually won the day. By 1930, the present-day structure of the country's maternity care system was all but in place. The midwife's modern substitute, the obstetrical nurse, was awarded the less than prestigious position of "doctor's handmaiden" and expected to show "wifely obedience to the doctor, motherly self-devotion to the patient and a form of mistress/servant discipline to those below" (Buckley 1979: 134). The medical profession's perspective on human reproduction, as a potentially abnormal event needing close monitoring and frequent obstetrical intervention, surfaced as the dominant view endorsed by all care givers on the maternity ward, including the new obstetrical nurse. Provinces situated both west and east of Ontario and Quebec eventually followed the same modernization path, suppressing midwifery and promoting the medically dependent obstetrical nursing specialty. The common view was expressed by a physician: "the art of midwifery belongs to prehistoric times; the science of obstetrics is the latest recognition of all ancient sciences" (quoted in Biggs 1983: 32). The question of "lady nurses or midwives" was ultimately decided in favour of the former. Such a maternity care arrangement was not only detrimental to autonomous Canadian midwifery – as Buckley (1979: 149) notes, pregnant women, too, were disadvantaged since "the exclusion of trained midwives ensured that future generations of women would be denied an alternative to the gynaecological and obstetrical monopoly held by the predominantly male profession."

As observed in Britain and the U.S., the maternity care system across Canada is now in transition. Like their counterparts in other industrial democracies, health officials in Canada presently face two major pressures: 1) demand by citizens for more appropriate care; 2) state financial crisis. Health authorities across the country are searching for a new course that is responsive to the citizenry and at the same time more cost-effective. Concerning Canadian birthing families, provincial health authorities are looking to the "new midwifery" to realize their aims of a more equitable and efficient public health service. Legal midwifery is already a reality in Ontario, and will likely be so in Alberta and B.C. in the not too distant future. It also seems likely that midwifery services will be financed, analogous to medical services, via general taxes.

Although a signal of decline in male-medical dominance over normal pregnancy and childbirth, legalized midwifery in Canada does not necessarily signal improved care for birthing families. Space concerns allow only brief mention of some of the most pressing problems that create an uneasy relationship between the new professional/legal midwife and birthing families.

Contemporary Issues Inhibiting Appropriate Maternity Care

As suggested above, the new midwifery in Canada is under trial on many fronts, not least of all in respect to neighbouring occupations competing for control of the maternity mandate. Perhaps the most fundamental challenge Canadian midwives face, however, concerns their work relationship with birthing families. Midwifery advocates and feminists scholars have often asserted that lay midwives of the past and independent midwives today share a unique relationship with birthing families. The result is that pregnant women in particular and their significant others in general have greater voice and control over the reproductive process than is typically the case in client encounters with the formal health care system. Assuming that this claim is indeed the case, then trends now underway across the country may render the idealized midwife-client relationship problematic. A segment of the literature on midwifery and other service occupations indicates that there lies a potential danger in the "professionalization project" officially endorsed by the midwifery leadership in Ontario, Alberta and, most recently, British Columbia. Rather than equal partners in the reproductive process, midwives claiming esoteric knowledge and superior technique may become strangers holding authoritative positions vis-à-vis birthing families.

In brief, Canadian midwifery today faces a difficult dilemma: while providing attractive work benefits and economic security, professionalization may exert a severe price. What may be at stake is precisely the aspect of maternity care midwives claim to be their unique contribution – bonding with clients. The current potential in Ontario for the emergence of two types of midwives themselves are divided about the necessity of academic training and the other trappings of professionalization endorsed by career-oriented counterparts. Is midwifery then another case of the "tyranny of experts," whereby those claiming privileged knowledge gain power over "unenlightened" colleagues as well as the citizens they serve? In an attempt to shed light on this pivotal question, I draw upon primary data on the social transformation of Newfoundland and Labrador midwifery.[6]

Canadian midwives are apt to point out that a woman's passage through pregnancy and childbirth is a relatively straightforward process involving physical and psychological changes during a momentary interlude in her life. Yet such a biopsychological construction of pregnant women creates a false picture of homogeneity. Broad social factors – economic, religious, cultural, educational, and legal -- can significantly affect a pregnant woman's personal experience, greatly complicating the situation for the attending practitioner, including the midwife.

As mentioned above, prior to the emergence of government sponsored health care in most Western countries, impoverished pregnant women often found that even if they could pay the midwife's fees, they could not afford to follow her recommendations. As a case in point, a granny respondent noted that one of her clients went into labour while gathering dried cod from the family's fishflakes but was told by her fisher husband to "wait until all the fish are in before you call the midwife." While today in Canada birthing families of all social classes enjoy universal access to organized medical (and perhaps soon midwifery) care, economic considerations still make many Canadians far from the ideal candidates for the new midwifery. This is especially the case for clients of disadvantaged, ethnic, and rural background and those in single-headed households. Newfoundland and Labrador women falling into one of these categories often view their passage through pregnancy and childbirth "as something to get over with." In fact, "delivering" themselves up to physicians and hospital maternity workers and being drugged during the entire birth process is valued by some women as a rare opportunity to temporarily escape from the heavy social demands normally placed upon them. If the new Canadian midwife is to successfully reach out to these disadvantaged clients, she will need unique social-economic understanding of their families and communities. Will the new midwife's knowledge base bring about such a crucial awareness? How will such knowledge be transmitted in the midwifery schools of the coming decades, most of which are designated to be located in academic institutions worlds apart from that of disadvantaged birthing families? Will midwifery graduates be willing to relocate to distressed rural and urban communities in order to witness first-hand the hardships daily experienced by many families during the childbearing cycle?

Birthing families' religious and cultural backgrounds may likewise problematize the new Canadian midwife's promised partnership. Sociological writings provide numerous illustrations of restrictive definitions of women's reproductive role imposed by religious and patriarchal considerations (Okely 1975; Shorter 1982). In Newfoundland and Labrador society pregnancy was traditionally known as "Eve's curse" and women's labour pains were seen as penance for the "glory of God the Father." My granny respondents recollected, for example, that it was common for unwed mothers to be publicly ridiculed. Granny midwives were expected to pressure such "fallen" women into confessing the name of their child's father. Those granny midwives who possessed intimate knowledge of the birthing woman and open communication with female relatives in attendance, however, managed to side-step such onerous customs. An active midwife practising in one of the province's urban hospitals, where such an opportunity to form alliances with birthing women and female kin is not available, reports a contemporary religious-patriarchal problem blocking easy partnership with her birthing client:

There was very heavy influence from the partner. He was very back-to-the-land. They belonged to the Rastafarian group and were very much into homebirth. They finally went [into the hospital] and it was awful. Even after the birth, the wretched man was refusing to let her have pain medication. This was after major surgery, after a cesarean and an episiotomy to boot.

The new Canadian midwife tends to envision her task of primary caretaker of birthing families as involving a relatively unproblematic information sharing with a receptive clientele, both united in the goal of assuring a natural and rewarding passage through pregnancy and childbirth. Client's educational backgrounds, however, may thwart such expectations. During the Victorian era, for example, pregnant women of the middle and upper classes often adopted a "sick role," regarding themselves as ill throughout the entire reproductive cycle. Obsessed with discovering minor "complaints and disorders," they dutifully reported these to their family doctor (Ehrenreich and English 1973: 26-36). Newfoundland and Labrador midwives working in urban areas complain that a similar obsession frequently prevails among many of the middle-class women they attend, who fervently listen to their prenatal instructors, read all the medical literature on reproductive care and believe that every one of their thoughts and actions have fundamental bearing on fetal development. Such women tend to harbour deep fears of their passage through labour and delivery, inevitably creating problems for the new midwife who views maternity as a non-medical, stress-free event.

If, as some of my Newfoundland and Labrador respondents indicate, birthing clients can be overly obsessed with medical information, they can also possess too little of it. Much to the chagrin of Newfoundland and Labrador midwives, economically-disadvantaged and Aboriginal women tend to ignore or refuse to accept scientific evidence that heavy cigarette smoking, high alcohol consumption, and poor diet may negatively affect their own health and that of their newborn. Perhaps worse off are teenage mothers, who, often still children themselves, tend to have little knowledge of either pregnancy or childbirth. Such naiveté is not a new phenomenon. A granny midwife recalled one young girl sitting at the foot of her bed prior to the onset of her labour pains with her "hair all curled and putting lipstick on. Looked like she was going to a party, like a little doll." A Labrador midwife practising in a regional hospital spoke of an Inuit teenager who avoided help throughout her entire pregnancy cycle, showing up on the maternity ward only when she was seven centimetres dilated. Another Labrador midwife mentioned a young birthing woman who fearfully wanted to know at what point in the birthing process "hot irons" would be placed on her feet. How will the new Canadian midwife solve such client problems surrounding inappropriate education about reproduction? What will be her novel educational tools that overcome the shortcomings of the existing maternity system which fails to adequately address these concerns?

Finally, the envisioned partnership between the new midwife and birthing families does not coincide well with the litigation trend in Canadian society. Newfoundland and Labrador granny midwives and those located in community cottage hospitals, due to their long-term ties with local birthing families, had no fear of malpractice suits. Such suits are increasingly common today, however, particularly in urban centres where the "informed" clientele tends to concentrate. The financial implications of litigation can be every bit as daunting for midwives as for physicians. As one midwife put it: "litigation is a problem now. That's what has spoiled the job for many midwives. They feel that everything must be written down, but all the time you're thinking will this stand up in court?"

Such problems hindering easy partnership with clients are reduced, although not eliminated, when maternity care is organized at the community level and midwives negotiate with allied health professionals regarding the appropriate care of local families. There is an example of such an alternative maternity care arrangement in the lived memory of Newfoundland and Labrador midwives: the cottage hospital. These were small health institutions operated by a health team of physicians, nurses, midwives and allied workers, all of whom were salaried employees working together to provide home and hospital care to several thousand people residing in the immediate and adjacent geographical area. These comparatively small 30-50 bed institutions operated, employing five to ten midwives on their modest maternity wards, never grew large enough to generate the tight medical and managerial authority structures characteristic of bureaucratic hospitals. One cottage hospital midwife described some of the advantages for birthing families:

The women really got good care in the cottage hospital. It was unreal, the care they got there. If there wasn't any complications, they had a midwife and you really got to know them 'cause we stayed working at the hospital for awhile. So we got to know the women personally, a close relationship. We sat with them and held their hands all the way through it. They felt relaxed and at home with us. We had time for them. I believe they really liked the old cottage hospital style ... A small place, with warmth.

Another describes how a non-compartmentalized environment also enhanced rapport between attendant and client:

Coming to the cottage hospital to have a baby was like nothing, really. They came in, had their baby, and you'd try to give it to the mother right away to feed, just to stimulate sucking. You didn't take the baby away to a so-called nursery. The baby was no distance from the mother; she could hear it cry. It was just because the cottage hospital was so small. The mothers stayed three days or so and then packed and went home with their little ones in tow. We looked out to them in the community for fourteen days after that.

By the 1980s, however, the Newfoundland and Labrador government followed the bureaucratization trend in organizing health services found in other areas of Canada. The result was a gradual demise of the cottage hospitals across the province. Due to under-funding, medical and support staff left and were not replaced. Eventually even normal deliveries could no longer be safely performed on maternity wards. Unable to cope with the larger forces deciding their fate, unemployed cottage hospital midwives, along with their kin, packed their belongings and travelled in search of more promising habitats. The transplanted midwives had little choice but to seek employment in the new large hospitals, by then defined by health authorities as the only safe places for deliveries, with physicians, not midwives as the major attendants. Only in hinterland regions of Newfoundland and Labrador was midwifery allowed to survive the test of time and even today midwives attend most normal deliveries (Benoit 1991). Elsewhere, however, an era of midwifery practice in small organizations had drawn to a close.

As noted above, this situation of male-medical dominance and bureaucratic organization of maternity services is in flux across Canada. My ongoing research project, which seeks to develop a sociological understanding of the caring ideologies and practices of B.C. midwives and complementary health professionals indicates that the community health centre option is viewed as a viable alternative by some of my midwifery respondents. Yet it is disconcerting to find that other candidates of the new midwifery in my study would choose to follow their medical counterparts working in private group practice. This latter model of maternity care will likely aid midwives in their struggle to gain professional status and attractive incomes. Appropriate care of disadvantaged birthing families, however, may not be so easily accomplished. Left unresolved are the issues that trouble North American physicians in private group practice: geographic distribution of midwives in rural communities and among marginalized urban groups; health promotion, counselling and home visits, which tend to be bypassed in fee-for-service arrangements; accessibility to midwifery services outside of clinic office hours; consumer voice regarding the maternity services available; and negotiation with other health professionals serving birthing families.

In brief, it seems that Canadian midwives today like their U.S. and British sisters alluded to above, are split into two camps: 1) those who identify with the professional model characteristic of their medical and nursing counterparts; 2) those who affiliate themselves with birthing families and allied health workers and work to create a decentralized, state-supported health service that balances the concerns of the public with that of the professionals themselves.

Summary and Conclusion

The historical and primary date reported in this chapter present a mixed assessment of the concepts of medical dominance, corporatization and patriarchy for understanding the complex social forces hindering appropriate maternity care in present-day Anglo-America. While crucial for analyzing the changing position of the medical profession on both sides of the Atlantic, a legitimate topic of sociological concern in its own right, these umbrella terms fall short of explaining significant variation in both the organization of maternity services and infant and maternal outcomes in the culturally-similar countries of Britain, the U.S. and Canada. Examination of the historical records of these three countries reveals that male-medical dominance and bureaucratic organization of maternity care have been commonplace but not all-encompassing. While all show improvement in public access to maternity services in the twentieth century, of the three countries examined, Canada offers birthing families the most comprehensive medical package, while the British are more progressive in regard to the midwifery option. A unique amalgam of economic, racial, and ethnic problems in the U.S., exacerbated by powerful business and medical interest groups, results in the most inadequate maternity service of the three countries, as indicated by comparatively poor infant mortality rates and maternal morbidity outcomes.

Sociological interpretation of these findings requires additional tools of analysis: 1) the system of professions to capture the assorted historical and cross-national articulation of health professions competing/negotiating over the maternity mandate; and 2) theories of the state to conceptualize the indeterminate role of Anglo-American governments elected by the citizenry to provide appropriate health services yet at the same time to resolve fiscal crisis.

A sociological understanding of the shifting professional and political forces shaping the maternity services on both sides of the Atlantic indicates a more complicated reality behind the assumed natural partnership between the new Canadian midwives and pregnant women by virtue of their gender. Broad structural forces – economic, religious-cultural, educational, legal – place significant constraints on the new midwife-client relationship. Canadian midwives, moreover, like their medical counterparts, can be seduced by the trappings of professionalization, moving to exclude lay and nursing (henceforth, non-legitimate) members from the new midwifery, embracing scientific over practical ways of knowing, developing professional associations that veto public input, and favouring private group practice rather than the community/health centre alternative. Sociologists attempting to understand the fit between patriarchal/medical subordination of female health occupations such as midwifery, and the social forces which enhance the quality of care for birthing families, should be attentive to the possibility that the new Canadian midwife may unwittingly become more like a traditional physician than a twentieth century midwife.

Notes

1   The proportion of the GNP which the British government allocated for the NHS in 1987 was 6 percent. This was considerably lower than, during the same time period, in Canada (8.8 percent), the U.S. (11.2 percent), and in most countries of Western Europe (e.g., 8.1 percent for former West Germany; 8.6 percent for France; 7.2 percent for Italy). In fact, only Spain, Portugal and Greece spend less per capita on health care services than Britain. Data source: D Wilsford 1991, pp. 21 and 279.

2   The concept of "deprofessionalization," which Marie Haug (1973: 197) defines as the professions losing "their monopoly over knowledge, public belief in their service ethos, and expectations of work autonomy and authority over clients," will not be mentioned here. Little solid data are presented to support this claim and/or the concept is used simultaneously with the concept of "proletarianization," both of which are often assumed to follow from the increasing "corporatization" of the health division of labour (Hafferty 1988). This latter concept will therefore be highlighted in this chapter.

3   According to Achterberg (1990: 122), this was not least because "midwives had access to fetal tissue, which – while forbidden by the Church – was in great demand as a magical charm by healers and practitioners of the magical arts."

4 House of Commons, Session 1991-92, Health Committee (Chair Nicholas Winterton), Second Report, Maternity Services, Volume I, March 4, 1992. HMSO, London.
5 I am referring here to the political process by which occupational groups attempt to uplift their economic standing and prestige within the division of labour by adopting the university as the site of training forming professional associations that exclude outsiders, including clients, and obtaining from the state exclusive power or licensing and disciplining members on the basis of embracing ethical codes.
6 For a detailed analysis of the contemporary issues causing an uneasy partnership between Canadian midwives and birthing families, see Benoit (1989) and Benoit (1991).

References

Abbott, A. 1988. *The System of Professions.* Chicago: University of Chicago Press.

Abbott, M. 1931. *History of Medicine in the Province of Quebec.* Toronto: Macmillan.

Ackerknecht, E. 1967. *Medicine at the Paris Hospital 1794-1848.* Baltimore: Johns Hopkins Press.

Achterberg, J. 1990. *Woman as Healer.* Boston and Shafesbury: Shambhala.

Alaszewiski, A, and J Manthrope. 1992. Restructuring the Professions in the U.K. Paper presented at the International Sociological Association Conference, "Professions in Transition," Leicester University, Leicester, England.

Altecruse, J, and S McDermott. 1987. Contemporary Concerns of Women in Medicine, In S Rossner ed. *Feminism within Science and Health Professions,* 65-88. Oxford: Pergamon Press.

Arney, W. 1982. *Power and the Profession of Obstetrics.* Chicago: University of Chicago Press.

Barrington, E. 1985. *Midwifery is Catching.* Toronto: NC Press.

Benoit, C. 1989. Traditional Midwifery Practice: The Limits of Occupational Autonomy. *Canadian Review of Sociology and Anthropology* 26 (4): 633–649.

Benoit, C. 1991. *Midwives in Passage: The Modernization of Maternity Care.* Memorial University of Newfoundland: ISER Press.

Benoit, C. 1992. Midwives in Comparative Perspective: Professionalism in Small Organizations. *Current Research on Occupations and Professions* 6: 199–216.

Benoit, C. 1994. Paradigm Conflict in the Sociology of the Professions. *Canadian Journal of Sociology* 19(3): 303-329.

Biggs, L. 1983. The Case of the Missing Midwives: A History of Midwifery in Ontario from 1795-1900. *Ontario History* 65 (1): 21–35.

Blishen, B. 1991. *Doctors in Canada.* Toronto: University of Toronto Press.

Boehme, G. 1984. Midwifery as Science: An Essay on the Relationship Between Scientific and Everyday Knowledge. In N Stehr and V Meja ed. *Society and Knowledge,* 365-385. New Brunswick, NJ: Transaction Books.

Buckley, S. 1979. Ladies or Midwives. In L Kealey ed. *A Not Unreasonable Claim,* 131-149. Toronto: The Women's Press.

Bucher, R, and A Strauss. 1961. Professions in Process. *American Journal of Sociology* 66: 325–334.

Burrage, M, and R Torstendahl eds. 1990. *Professions in Theory and History.* London: Sage.

Burtch, B. 1988. Midwifery and the State. In A McLaren, ed. *Gender and Society,* 349-371. Toronto: Pitman Ltd.

Butter, I, E Carpenter, B Kay, and R Simmons. 1987. Gender Hierarchies in the Health Labor Force. *International Journal of Health Services* 17(1): 133–149.

Campbell, M. 1946. *Folks Do Get Born.* New York: Rinehart.

Canada Lancet. 1875. Editorial 8: 60.

Canniff, W. 1894. *History of the Medical Profession in Upper Canada, 1783-1850.* Toronto: W. Biggs.

Coburn, D, G Torrance, and J Kaufert. 1983. Medical Dominance in Canada in Historical Perspective: The Rise and Fall of Medicine. *International Journal of Health Services* 13: 407–432.

Coburn, D. 1993. State Authority, Medical Dominance, and Trends in the Regulation of the Health Professions: The Ontario Case. *Social Science and Medicine* 37(2): 129–138.

Crompton, R. 1987. Gender, Status and Professionalism. *Sociology* 21: 413–428.

Derber, C. 1982. *Professionals as Workers.* Boston: G.K. Hall.

Donegan, J. 1978. *Women and Men Midwives.* Westport, Conn: Greenview Press.

Donnison, J. 1977. *Midwives and Medical Men.* London: Heinemann.

Donnison, J. 1981. The Development of the Occupation of Midwife: A Comparative View. *Midwife is a Labour of Love* 38-53. Vancouver: Press Gang.

Eakins, P. 1986. *The American Way of Birth.* Philadelphia: Temple University Press.

Ehrenreich, B, and D English. 1973. *Witches, Midwives and Nurses.* New York: Feminist Press.

Field, M. 1980. The Health Care System and the Polity: A Contemporary American Dialectic. *Social Science and Medicine* 14A (5).

Flint, C. 1988. On the Brink: Midwifery in Britain. In S Kitzinger ed. *The Midwife Challenge,* 22-41. London: Pandora.

Freidson, E. 1970. *The Profession of Medicine: A Study in the Sociology of Applied Knowledge.* New York: Harper and Row.

Freddi, G, and J Bjoerkman eds. 1989. *Controlling Medical Professionals.* London: Newbury.

Hafferty, F. 1988. Theories at the Crossroads: A Discussion of Evolving Views on Medicine as a Profession. *The Milbank Quarterly* 66(2): 202–225.

Halpern, S. 1992. Dynamics of Professional Control: Internal Coalitions and Crossprofessional Boundaries. *American Journal of Sociology* 97(4): 994–1021.

Haug, M. 1973. Deprofessionalization: An Alternative Hypothesis for the Future. *Sociological Review Monograph* 20: 195–211.

Houd, S. 1988. Midwives in Denmark. In S Kitzinger ed. *The Midwife Challenge,* 176-196. London: Pandora.

Hughes, E. 1958. *Men and Their Work.* New York: Free Press.

Jordan, B. 1983. *Birth in Four Cultures.* London: Eden Press.

King's Printer 1971. Ordinances of the Province of Quebec 1763–91. Ottawa.

Kobrin, F. 1966. The American Midwife Controversy: A Crisis of Professionalization. *Bulletin of the History of Medicine* 40: 350–363.

Krause, E. 1988. Doctors, Partitocrazia, and the Italian State. *The Milbank Quarterly* 66(2): 148–166.

Laforce, H. 1990. The Different Stages of the Elimination of the Midwife in Quebec. In K Arnup et al. eds. *Delivering Motherhood,* 36-50. New York: Routledge.

Larkin, G. 1983. *Occupational Monopoly and Modern Medicine.* London: Tavistock.

Larson, M. 1977. *The Rise of Professionalism.* Berkeley: University of California Press.

Leavitt, J. 1986. *Brought to Bed: Childbearing in America 1750 to 1950.* New York: Oxford University Press.

Lefkowitz, M and M Fant. 1988. *Women's Life in Greece and Rome.* London: Duckworth.

Light, D. 1986. Corporate Medicine for Profit. *Scientific American* 255(6): 38–45.

Light, D, and S Levine. 1988. The Changing Character of the Medical Profession: A Theoretical Overview. *The Milbank Quarterly* 66(2): 10–32.

Litoff, J. 1978. *American Midwives.* Westport, Conn: Greenview Press.

Litoff, J. 1986. *The American Midwife Debate.* New York: Greenwood Press.

Lorber, J. 1984. *Women Physicians: Careers, Status, and Power.* London: Tavistock.

McKinlay, J, and J Arches. 1985. Towards the Proletarianization of Physicians. *International Journal of Health Services* 15: 161–195.

McKinlay, J, and J Stoeckle. 1988. Corporatization and the Social Transformation of Doctoring. *International Journal of Health Services* 18: 191–205.

Naylor, D. 1992. *Canadian Health Care and the State.* Montreal and Kingston: McGill-Queen's University Press.

Oakley, A. 1976. Wisewoman and Medicine Man: Changes in the Management of Childbirth. In J Mitchell and A Oakley eds. *The Rights and Wrongs of Women,* 17-58. Harmondsworth: Penguin.

Oakley, A and S Houd. 1986. Alternative Perinatal Services: Report on a Pilot Survey. In JML Phaff ed. *Perinatal Health Services in Europe: Searching for Better Childbirth,* 17-47. London: Croom Helm.

Oakley, A and S Houd. 1990. *Helpers in Childbirth: Midwifery Today.* New York: Hemisphere Publishing.

Okely, J. 1975. Gypsy Women: Models of Conflict. In S Ardner ed. *Perceiving Women.* New York: John Wiley and Sons.

Oppenheimer, J. 1983. Childbirth in Ontario: The Transition from Home to Hospital in the Early Twentieth Century. *Ontario History* 65(1): 36–60.

Park, K. 1992. Medicine and Society in Medieval Europe, 500–1500. In A Wear ed. *Medicine in Society: Historical Essays,* 59-90. Cambridge, England: Cambridge University Press.

Phaff, JML ed. 1986. *Perinatal Health Services in Europe: Searching for Better Childbirth.* London: Croom Helm.

Pizurki, H, A Mejia, I Butter, and L Ewart. 1987. *Women as Providers of Health Care.* Geneva: World Health Organization.

Reid, M. 1989. Sisterhood and Professionalization: A Case Study of the American Lay Midwife. In C Shepherd McClain ed. *Women Healers: Cross-Cultural Perspectives,* 219-238. Rutgers: The State University.

Relman, AS. 1980. The New Medical-Industrial Complex. *New England Journal of Medicine* 303: 963–970.

Riska, E. 1988. The Professional Status of Physicians in the Nordic Countries. *The Milbank Quarterly* 66(2): 133–147.

Riska, E, and K Wegar eds. 1993. *Gender, Work and Medicine: Women and the Medical Division of Labour.* London: Sage.

Roemer, M. 1991. *National Health Care Systems of the World. Vol 1.* New York: Oxford University Press.

Ruggie, M. 1992. The Paradox of Liberal Intervention: Health Policy and the American Welfare State. *American Journal of Sociology* 97(4): 919–944.

Ruzek, S. 1986. Feminist Visions of Health: An International Perspective. In A Oakley and J Mitchell eds. *What is Feminism?,* 184-207. New York: Pantheon Books.

Seward, R, J Seward, and V Natoli. 1984. Different Approaches to Childbirth and Their Consequences in Italy, Sweden and the United States. *International Journal of the Family* 14: 1–16.

Shorter, E. 1982. *A History of Women's Bodies.* New York: Basic Books.

Simmel, G. 1908. *On Individual and Social Forms.* D Levine ed. 1971. Chicago: The University of Chicago Press.

Stacey, M. 1988. *The Sociology of Health and Healing.* London: Unwin Hyman.

Starr, P. 1982. *The Social Transformation of American Medicine.* New York: Basic Books.

Stone, L. 1977. *The Family, Sex and Marriage in England 1500-1800.* New York: Harper and Row Publishers.

Strauss, A. 1978. *Negotiations.* San Francisco: Jossey-Bass.

Sullivan, D, and R Weitz. 1988. *Labor Pains: Modern Midwives and Home Birth.* New Haven: Yale University Press.

Sutherland, R, and J Fulton. 1988. *Health Care in Canada.* Ottawa: The Health Group.

Swartz, D. 1987. The Politics of Reform: Conflict and Accommodation in Canadian Health Policy. In D Coburn et al. eds. *Health and Canadian Society* 2nd ed, 568-589. . Toronto: Fitzhenry and Whiteside.

Torrance, G. 1987. Hospitals as Health Factories. In D. Coburn et al. eds. *Health and Canadian Society* 2nd ed, 479-500. . Toronto: Fitzhenry and Whiteside.

Van Teijlingen, E. 1992. Midwifery in the Netherlands: More than a Semi-Profession? Paper presented at the International Sociological Association Conference. Leicester, England. April 1992.

Valvanne, L. 1988. The Finnish Midwife and Her Renewed Challenges. In S Kitzinger ed. *The Midwife Challenge,* 214-234. London: Pandora.

Weller, GR. 1977. From 'Pressure Group Politics' to 'Medical-Industrial Complex': The Development of Approaches to the Politics of Health. *Journal of Health Politics, Policy and Law* 1(4): 444–470.

Weller, GR, and P Manga. 1983. The Push for Reprivatization of Health Care Services in Canada, Britain and the United States. *Journal of Health Politics, Policy and Law* 8(3).

Wertz, RW, and DC Wertz. 1977. *Lying-In: A History of Childbirth in America.* New York: Schocken Books.

Wertz, RW, and DC Wertz. 1990. Notes on the Decline of Midwives and the Rise of Medical Obstetricians. In P Conrad and R Kern eds. *The Sociology of Health and Illness: Critical Perspectives* 3rd ed., 148-160. New York: St. Martin's Press.

Wilsford, D. 1991. *Doctors and the State.* Durham: Duke University Press.

Witz, A. 1990. Patriarchy and Professions: The Gendered Politics of Occupational Closure. *Sociology* 24(1): 675–690.

Wolinsky, F. 1988. The Professional Dominance Perspective, Revisited. *The Milbank Quarterly* 66(2): 33–47.

21

Professional Ideology in Canadian Pharmacy[*]

Linda J. Muzzin, Gregory P. Brown, and Roy W. Hornosty

Ideology in an Interactionist Context

Although there are numerous and conflicting definitions of the term "ideology," Fine and Sandstrom (1993) have recently argued that the usefulness of this theoretical construct could be revived if it were built into a symbolic interactionist perspective. Specifically, they argue that the content and enactment of ideological beliefs could be explored empirically if this term were broadened to include "any linked set of beliefs about the social or political order ... connected to and produced within a wide variety of social institutions" (1993: 23). They point out that the concept of "doing ideology" fits naturally into a pragmatic, interactionist perspective, in capturing one of the central assumptions of this approach, that people profess and enact sets of ideas or symbolic representations in order to realize their interests and purposes in everyday situations. This flips the traditional usage of the term from one in which sets of ideas emerge as rationalizations for the status quo (e.g., Marx and Engels 1846; Bendix 1956) to one which emphasizes the activities of small groups in creating, developing and maintaining the philosophies that guide (as well as justify) their everyday activities. This reversal of emphasis opens the concept to be "grounded" through the study of how groups use their ideologies to recruit members, influence outsiders, promote group solidarity and mobilize resources.

The term "professional ideology" has already been used in this way by a few researchers who investigate how professional groups demarcate their areas of monopoly and attempt to garner resources for it. Gieryn (1983), for example, illustrates how spokespersons for science emphasized different, and sometimes contradictory, characteristics of science when they were demarcating its boundary with competing areas of non-science and defending its autonomy from the state. Freidson describes the concept of disease and its extensions as part of an ideology used by medical spokespersons to justify the expansion of medical authority into boundary areas to medicine, such as "mental disease" (1970: 5-8). Becker and Carper term the explanations used by engineers to define themselves and their

[*] Reprinted from *Health and Canadian Society*, Vol. 1, No. 2, Linda J. Muzzin, Gregory P. Brown, and Roy W. Hornosty, 'Professional Ideology in Canadian Pharmacy,' pp. 319-45, 1993, with permission of the publisher.

work an "ideology" (1970c: 180). Larson (1977) describes the defining of new markets by professions in terms of developing professional ideology. Others do not use the words "professional ideology" consistently, but clearly deal with the same set of phenomena in discussing the claims made and strategies pursued by members of professions that compete for jurisdiction over areas of expertise (e.g., Abbott 1988: 121; Birenbaum 1990).

An outline of the application of the concept of ideology in understanding the process, or natural history, of the health professions, can be found in Bucher's posthumously published article, in which she identifies strategies pursued by members of emerging or transforming occupations (1988). These include "discovering colleagueship" through identification with a new professional ideology, securing an institutional niche within which it can be practised, putting out the "call" for a new formal organization, developing leaders, tactics for recruiting, a "slogan" to attain legitimacy, building up consensus, and negotiating relationships for members within organizations. Key among these strategies for the professionalizing occupations has been "gaining space within the curriculum of the university or hospital system" (1988: 139). According to Bucher, leaders of professionalizing occupations express a great deal of concern that there is a "fit" between the curriculum and the proclaimed new ideology of the group. It is also essential that the group can place students within institutional niches where they may become what she terms "showcases" for the emerging or transformed occupation. Eventually, she argues, "everyday work ... leads to changes in the work itself and in its associated ideology" (1988: 141), which signals the development of specialties.

Becker's term, "situational adjustment," refers to the differing enactment of ideologies by work setting (1970b). Becker suggested that, while this concept needs more analytic elaboration, we could get a sense of the phenomenon by examining the so-called "cultures" or "subcultures" of particular groups and how they change over time. Examples that he used were those of prisoners who adapted to "prison culture" while incarcerated, and students who adapted to "student culture" while in medical school. These groups were found to orient towards new reference groups when they got out of prison and medical school, respectively. Kronus (1976) has used the idea of "situational adjustment" to explain how pharmacists choose their reference groups. Based on a study of 53 pharmacists, she argued that hospital pharmacists were physician-oriented, community pharmacists were colleague-oriented, and chain pharmacists were client-oriented, with each group focused towards what she called the "power structure of the work setting." It is important to emphasize here the point of Fine and Sandstrom that each small group does not create its own ideology, but only enacts it differently (1993: 33). Battles over these alternative interpretations of new ideology often occur within socializing institutions, which can become, in Bucher's terms, "bloody ideological battlegrounds" (1988: 142).

This paper examines these social processes for pharmacists, whose continuously challenged position in the medical hierarchy makes them theoretically interesting. First, the history of their development of professional ideologies, mainly within their socializing institutions, is analyzed, using the theoretical framework suggested by Fine and Sandstrom (1993) and by Bucher (1988). The emphasis of the first part of the paper is on the construction of curricula by pharmacy educators and their success and difficulties in finding "showcases" for these ideologies. In the second part of the paper, we use Becker's concept of "situational development" to explain divergent enactments of these ideologies by pharmacists. In the past three years we have conducted three studies of Ontario pharmacists that show evidence of ideological situational adjustment. Data showing divergence among pharmacists on the importance of patient counselling are presented here and we speculate briefly about the consequences of this fragmentation. The emphasis is on "doing ideology" and the perspective of pharmacists, rather than the views of other stakeholders or the larger environment within which the ideology unfolds. Since half of all practicing pharmacists in Ontario are now women, we examined the possibility that gender as well as situational adjustment affected the interpretation of the ideologies.[1] The fact that women have disproportionately chosen to practice hospital rather than community pharmacy suggested the hypothesis that gender, rather than work setting, influenced ideological interpretation in pharmacy. Thus we explored the effects of both gender and work setting on ideological interpretation.

The "Professionally-Challenged" Position of Pharmacy

It has been speculated that, before the turn of the century, "... druggists [in North America] were closer to the public ear than the doctor and were increasingly sought for advice in therapeutic matters" (Haller 1981: 268). This was particularly true for the poor and in areas without doctors (Coburn et al. 1983). When the medical profession tried to win regulatory control over Canadian pharmacists in the post-Confederation period, pharmacists had enough support that they not only resisted this medical takeover, but went on to achieve self-regulation in Ontario and Quebec via legislation in the 1870s (Canadian Pharmaceutical Association 1971). Since that time, however, they have faced progressive encroachment from other groups.

This process of "losing ground" has been characterized in sociological writings as a failure to attain or maintain status as a profession. As Becker points out, Flexner (1915) decided that pharmacy was not a profession because it "had no primary responsibility but only carried out the physician's orders" (1970a: 88). This was later echoed by Denzin and Mettlin (1968) who dismissed it as a profession because, as they put it, "pharmacy has not developed an ideology to limit the manner in which its members will view the drug" (1968: 376). That is, it has no control over its "social object," drugs, which are chosen for patients by physicians. Ackers and Quinney (1968) identified another problem: in a comparative analysis of five U.S. health professions, they found that, although pharmacy had a long history compared to other professions (with the exception of medicine), it was the most fragmented internally, with a separation and competition between commercial and professional elements. McCormack (1956) had also termed Canadian pharmacy a "marginal" profession because of its emphasis on commercialism. Somewhat later, Robbins (1979) described pharmacy as a "profession in search of a role," referring to the progressive loss of its jurisdiction over the production and packaging of drugs, which is now largely done by the pharmaceutical industry. In summary, pharmacy has been analyzed by sociologists as an occupation with a number of problems of jurisdiction and internal organization; these observations, however, have not yet been built into any theory of professions or organizations.

One might start by asking how a profession with so many problems has been able to survive for over a century in Canada. In answering this question, it is useful to examine the struggle of North American pharmacists to construct professional ideologies to counter the challenges that they faced. These ideologies are easy to locate, because they are disseminated *via* formal published curricula and professional journals and associations, and are publicly available. As Bucher (1988) and Gieryn (1983: 781) point out, the enactment of professional ideologies is routinely accomplished when new courses or new curricula are established. That is, the establishment of new curricula can be taken as attempts to enact a new ideology to define group membership, change the image of a group, and mobilize resources for the use of the group. Examination of pharmacy curricula and professional journals and newsletters reveals that there have been three different such ideologies in North America over the past 60 years, with the third largely a reformulation of the second. The first, emphasizing the scientific underpinning of the profession, clearly failed as a bid to improve the fortunes of pharmacy. The second, called "clinical pharmacy," which emphasizes the technical expertise that the pharmacist could offer physicians in the hospital setting, was not successful in community pharmacy, but survives in the hospital environment. The third, emphasizing the profession's commitment to "pharmaceutical care" for the patient, is a contemporary reformulation of the "clinical pharmacy" ideology which hinges on the ability of the pharmacist to counsel patients directly on their medications.

Transforming the Profession: The Fate of the Three Ideologies

The earliest of the attempts to halt the downward slide of pharmacy can be found in the hiring of science faculty in pharmacy schools and the establishment of a science-oriented curriculum, which included a proliferation of chemistry courses. This was achieved with the lengthening of formal university training to four years in the U.S. in 1932, and in Canada at the University of Toronto, in 1952 (Hepler 1987; Stieb 1983). Other schools soon followed suit. However, this early strategy backfired in that, as Hepler puts it, "society did not seem to need a scientist on every streetcorner" (1987: 3). The emphasis on acquiring highly scientific/technical knowledge (which was not directly related to practice), rather than buttressing the profession, actually led to the popular conception of the pharmacist as a "highly educated pill counter." The lowest point was reached in the early 1960s when academic leaders in the U.S. criticized the wall between professional practice and science-oriented education.

In Canada, numerous commissions and inquiries pointed to the gap between the pharmacist's scientific training and preoccupation with retail matters (e.g., Hall Commission 1964). The number of pharmacies steadily decreased and it was difficult to attract students into the discipline. As the dean of pharmacy in Toronto, F.N. Hughes, pointed out in a paper subtitled "The Eleventh Hour" (1967), pharmacy was, at that time, excluded from a $500 million fund that had been established for upgrading educational facilities. Although the Faculty had recommended to the Hall Commission the establishment of a second faculty of pharmacy in Ontario, where the largest number of pharmacists in Canada practised, this was not felt to be necessary. Indeed, Hughes cited other reports suggesting that pharmacy should be reduced to a three-year programme or even that a university-level education was not necessary for all pharmacists. With the failure of this ideological foray, pharmacy appeared to have actually lost ground. In Bucher's terms, the ideology had transformed the curriculum but pharmacy leaders failed to attain a niche in which it could be practised. There was no "showcase" to illustrate its legitimacy.

"Clinical" pharmacy, as it was called, was the second professional ideology that was used in the late 1960s[2] as the answer to the failure to establish an image of the "pharmacist as scientist." In this new vision, the pharmacist became a therapeutic advisor. The construction of this new version of the pharmacist was made possible by a number of developments. First, patient drug "profiles" began to be routinely collected by pharmacists in hospitals and in business, which made it possible for them to engage in what they call "drug monitoring" (Hepler 1987: 4). The proliferation of large hospitals in

Canada and the establishment of pharmacists in those settings were fortuitous developments that provided an institutional niche for the enactment of this ideology.[3] In university curricula, the scientific discipline of pharmacology, traditionally part of the pharmacy curriculum, was applied in the new area of pharmacy therapeutics. The most important new course that was introduced in pharmacy at this time was "pharmacokinetics," or the study of drug dosage – absorption, distribution, metabolism and elimination of drugs from the body. In Toronto, the coverage of this subject in the medical curriculum is not as comprehensive as in the pharmacy curriculum, where it constitutes a 52-hour course in the senior year. This subject has thus become an important point of demarcation between pharmacy and medicine.

The dream of North American pharmacy educators who supported the clinical pharmacy movement was that hospital pharmacists could advise doctors in this highly technical area, and thus stake a secure jurisdictional claim. In 1960 in Ontario, hospital pharmacy residency programmes were established in order to prepare pharmacists for their new role. These programmes, consisting of a series of rotations through various hospital departments, are similar to medical internships. They have produced 500 graduates who have become leaders within the profession in Canada in terms of the research they have published, their contributions to hospital inservice and university education (for physicians, nurses and others), and their restructuring of pharmacy work in hospitals (Muzzin et al. unpublished). In the U.S., at the University of California, a six-year programme leading to a Pharm.D., or doctor of pharmacy degree, was established to produce these highly-trained specialists. In that country, a heated and continuous debate rages about copying the successful California curriculum, in various forms, as an entry level programme in their 73 pharmacy schools.

At the same time that pharmacokinetics and therapeutics became one of the cornerstones of the North American pharmacy curriculum, there was growing recognition of the high rate of medication errors in hospitals and advocacy for a pharmacist-watchdog (Broadhead and Facchinetti 1985). Although the expansion of hospital pharmacy had already occurred, the mysterious deaths of infants with high levels of digoxin at the Hospital for Sick Children in Toronto in 1981 brought the dangerous situation of a lack of hospital medication monitoring home to the general public in Canada and helped to maintain an institutional niche for the pharmacist in large teaching hospitals. HSC itself received a million dollars to implement the "unit dose" system of prepackaging medications for patients as a safeguard (HSC Annual Report 1982). This safeguard has been strongly advocated and partly-enacted by hospital pharmacists in Toronto teaching hospitals over the past decade. Students in Toronto now rotate though placements in these "showcase" institutions. This linking of the new "clinical" role of the pharmacist in hospitals to a timely social issue was highly successful until the recent economic downturn in Canada, in that hospitals were the largest growing employment sector for pharmacists, now employing more than 25 percent of the 18,000 pharmacists in this country (Conklin 1991).

Nevertheless, this second professional ideology enjoyed limited success in the more populous community pharmacy arm of the profession in North America. Numerous studies in the 1960s and 1970s showed that community pharmacists in the U.S. had neither the time nor the inclination for counselling of patients or their physicians on their medications (e.g., Knapp et al. 1969; Wertheimer et al. 1974; Rowles et al. 1974; Nelson et al. 1976). For some time in the U.S., laws, in fact, restricted such activities by pharmacists. Further, spending time with patients is commercially inefficient when systems of reimbursement are tied to sale of a product. Thus the clinical pharmacy ideology went nowhere in this setting for two decades. Perhaps reflecting the irrelevance of the clinical pharmacy ideology for commercial practice, Toronto pharmacy graduates of the 1960s and 1970s have rated much of their undergraduate preparation for practice poorly as compared to graduates who both preceded and succeeded them (Muzzin and Hornosty 1993; Cockerill and Williams 1990). Similar evidence for the failure of the clinical pharmacy ideology was reported in studies of American pharmacy students during the late 1960s and 1970s (Manasse et al. 1975; Kirk 1976; Schwirian and Facchinetti 1975). This phenomenon was also observed among Israeli pharmacy students who encountered a curriculum which was a confusing mix of science and clinical courses, with only a small exposure to business (Shuval and Adler 1977).

Within the past five years, the professional ideology called "pharmaceutical care," has emerged. This term is buried in a 1987 article by Hepler that describes the new ideology as the "third wave in pharmacy education," but has since become the official designation of the new movement. Pharmaceutical care is defined by Hepler, in an appendix to a recent text as, "the responsible provision of drug therapy for the purpose of achieving definite outcomes that improve a patient's quality of life" (Smith and Knapp 1992: 282). Setting aside what this is taken to mean by practitioners (since this is still being hotly debated), some of the initial evidence of its success can be noted. In the cited text, students are urged not to wait for their pharmacy organizations to adopt the ideology before implementing it themselves as practitioners. The umbrella organization for colleges of pharmacy in the U.S., the American Association of Colleges of Pharmacy, has produced a series of papers proposing adoption of the pharmaceutical care model as the organizing principle of the curriculum in schools of pharmacy. The official journal of the A.A.C.P., the *American Journal of Pharmaceutical Education,* routinely publishes articles on applications and successes of this new role for the pharmacist as do other pharmacy journals. The studies show how pharmacist intervention improves physician prescribing, rationalizes treatment in nursing homes, and supplements medical and nursing care in the community (e.g., Soumerai and Avorn 1987; Ranelli 1991).

In the past two years, of the nine schools of pharmacy in Canada, the Universities of British Columbia and Toronto have established post-baccalaureate Pharm.D. programmes organized around this new professional ideology (as the pharmacy equivalents of MD programmes). At the same time, baccalaureate pharmacy curricula across Canada have been upgraded from four to five years post high school. In Toronto, Pharmacy has finally been successful in wrestling resources from the University to implement "the third wave." Its five year undergraduate programme, beginning in 1994, is composed of "professional practice" courses at each level around the theme of pharmaceutical care. In current texts, students are introduced to the profession of pharmacy by emphasizing the new role of pharmacy, professional ethics and self-regulation, patient care-seeking and the future of the profession (e.g., Wertheimer and Smith 1989).

How successful will this ideology be? Within the university itself, two studies of American pharmacy students show that they are still disillusioned, although the studies may have been conducted too soon for the new movement to have "caught on" (MacKeigan and McGhan 1988; Smith et al. 1991). In Canada, 1980s graduates give higher ratings to their pharmacy education than do any previous graduates back to the 1930s (Muzzin and Hornosty 1993) and one class that has been studied intensively remains positively-oriented to their new clinical role several years after graduation (Hornosty et al. 1992).

It is too soon to determine the success of this new wave of ideology beyond the walls of the university, but pharmaceutical care appears to have a better chance of wide-spread adoption than the original clinical pharmacy ideology. In the first place, the role of the pharmacist "as therapeutic advisor" is stated in general enough terms that it can be applied to both hospital and commercial settings. It may leave a door open for com-munity pharmacy to participate this time around by becoming a therapeutic advisor to the patient. Second, rather than opposing the movement, commercial pharmacy organi-zations are promoting it, or at least, its "patient counselling" component. The best indi-cation that the clinical pharmacy/pharmaceutical care ideology has been successful in representations to the outside world are pilot experiments in Washington State, Florida and California, which now allow pharmacists to "prescribe" from a restricted formu-lary (Selya 1988). Similarly, in Canada, since 1978, Quebec pharmacists have been able to claim financial compensation when they counsel patients without selling drugs. The important point about this development in Quebec is that it represents the first structural change allowing commercial pharmacy to move in the direction of clinical pharmacy/pharmaceutical care.[4] Professional associations and advertising by the phar-maceutical industry alike now encourage the practice of getting patients to "ask your pharmacist" across North America. This professional slogan appears on posters in pharmacies everywhere.[5] In Ontario, the most recent government inquiry into the phar-macy profession, the Lowy Commission (1990), strongly advocated pharmacist coun-selling of patients. In this report, pharmacists were urged to build counselling rooms in their pharmacies. More recently, the Ontario government's Drug Programs Reform Secretariat has endorsed the "pharmaceutical care" model (Ontario MOH 1993). There are thus numerous indications in Canada that this new reformulation of the role of the pharmacist may hold the much sought after key to refurbishing the pharmacist's image, and establishing a more secure professional jurisdiction, where previous attempts have failed.

Variations in the Enactment of a Professional Ideology

Thus far it has been argued that renewed curricula, official documents, and changes in public, institutional and clinical policies are attempts to enact new professional ideolo-gies in this troubled profession. In addition, a measure of their success can be surmised by changes or lack of change in laws regulating the jurisdiction of pharmacists. Fine and Sandstrom (1993), however, challenge us to document in much more detail how ideologies are adopted, maintained and used to capture resources and legitimacy. In the second part of this paper, we move in this direction by exploring how pharmacists with different educational and professional histories, working in different settings, react to statements about patient counselling, a key activity in their new professional ideology.

A reading of the pharmacy literature shows that there is little recognition that profes-sional ideologies such as "clinical pharmacy" and "pharmaceutical care" might be received and enacted differently by practitioners in different settings. The ideologies are typically presented as if they were unidimensional, or at least, as if they constituted an internally consistent framework for practice that could be transmitted unproblemati-cally to future practitioners. Pharmacy educators have expressed frustration in curricu-lum committees that community pharmacy lags behind in adoption of new professional ideologies without working out exactly how the practitioner is to enact the philosophy. As suggested by our analysis of the fate of the "clinical pharmacy" ideology, however, an assumption of internal consistency in practice is not warranted. We suggested that clinical pharmacy probably failed as a unifying ideology precisely because practitioners in the community setting could not see how they could become the advisor to the physician – with whom they seldom interacted except occasionally over the telephone. Further, their commercial organizations failed to see the relevance of this vision and failed to support it.

One problematic component of the North American clinical pharmacy/pharmaceutical care philosophy that is present in some, but not other, key documents is the concept of "patient-centred practice." The original vision of clinical pharmacy was somewhat paternalistic, placing the pharmacist as the technical advisor to the doctor, with the patient nowhere in sight. A few pharmacy educators feel that, despite lip service to patient-centredness, the pharmaceutical care ideology shows the same paternalism (e.g., Buerki and Vottero 1991) – that, in terms of our discussion, it is still "stuck" in the hospital setting. An examination of key documents describing pharmaceutical care shows that they gloss over what the exact relationship between the pharmacist and "patient" (not "client") is supposed to be in the new approach (e.g., Hepler and Strand 1989; Poston 1992). This fuzziness might actually serve to broaden the ideology so that it can be applied beyond the hospital setting. The problem is that studies of what community pharmacists are doing in practice, do *not* gloss the point. They look directly at whether the community pharmacist is counselling the patient (e.g., Carroll and Gagnon 1983; and Kirking 1984, in the U.S., and Laurier et al. 1989; Canadian Pharmaceutical Association 1990; and Willison and Muzzin 1992, in Canada).

The self-proclaimed aim of studies of pharmacist counselling has been to isolate particular situational variables and pharmacist characteristics that predict the extent of counselling, such as gender, prescription volume and size of pharmacy. In the process, they have turned up another problem – they have demonstrated that "counselling" can be enacted differently, ranging from putting a warning label on a drug vial to several minutes of history-taking and patient instruction. They have inadvertently provided evidence for the "situational adjustment" characteristic of professional life, by displaying the disparity in orientations towards this key component of the pharmacist's role. It is this situational adjustment that we wish to pursue in this part of the paper.

Natural History of Our Research on Professional Orientation

Our work on this topic grew out of a project undertaken by one of the authors (RWH) in the early 1980s. In the tradition of interactionist socialization studies of the professions, one class of 120 pharmacy students was followed in the last three years of their university programme; they were surveyed, interviewed, and studied via participant observation (Hornosty 1989). The major finding was that they graduated with what Hornosty called a "visionary, utopian ideology," prepared to transform the profession they were entering. When they were surveyed again seven years later they had maintained and even strengthened this ideological commitment despite the disappointments they faced in attempting to realize their new role in everyday practice (Hornosty et al. 1992). The intensity of their commitment was evidenced in 40 follow-up interviews conducted with members of the class (by LJM). At the same time, the interviews revealed a difference between how those employed in hospital pharmacy interpreted their professional ideology as compared to their colleagues in commercial pharmacy. As confirmed by analysis of responses by 93 graduates to survey questions about various aspects of their professional role, those in hospital pharmacy downplayed the importance of direct patient counselling, emphasized the importance of technical competence and expressed their preference for being a therapeutic advisor to the doctor rather than a counsellor of patients. This stance is reminiscent of the original clinical pharmacy ideology described above. On the other hand, those employed in commercial pharmacy felt that counselling and communication were more important than technical skills, and expressed their preference for patient counselling as compared to advising physicians (Muzzin et al. 1993).

The fact that possessing one orientation or the other is related only to the current position of the pharmacist was discovered the hard way, when the quantitatively oriented member of our team (GPB) spent several weeks trying to relate some composite of the sequence of career positions held by members of the class to each orientation (e.g., hospital position upon graduation but a switch to commercial pharmacy vs. commercial pharmacy then hospital pharmacy exposure vs. consistency of work setting over the seven years). A strong relationship between the cluster of attitudes and preferences and work setting emerged only when current work setting, i.e., the work setting the pharmacist was in *at the time of filling out the questionnaire*, was taken as the independent variable. This suggests "situational adjustment" in the extreme, and predicts that these pharmacists will "change their minds" about the importance of patient counselling if they move to a different setting!

These unexpected results also raise a number of questions. The first that might be asked is, what remains of one's original professional socialization after numerous "situational adjustments?" For example, graduates prior to the clinical pharmacy movement, in the 1930s, '40s, and even '50s, were often instructed *not* to talk to the patient. How do such graduates manage to reconcile the conflict between prior socialization and current professional ideology? Further, how do they "enact" a professional ideology which they have not been trained to perform? Finally, much has been written about the possible influence of the social origins of health professionals on the performance of their duties, including communication with patients. In pharmacy, little is known about the relationship between social class and role performance. However, it is known that women report more patient counselling (Laurier et al. 1989; Willison and Muzzin 1992). Do women have different orientations than men across all settings, or does "situational adjustment" wipe this out as well?

We embarked on two larger projects from 1990 to 1992 which will allow us to begin to answer these questions about situational adjustment, at least with respect to orientations towards patient counselling. The first of these studies aimed to explore the relationship between pharmacy education and practice during distinct periods of pharmacy education in Ontario: pre-1929, 1929-1954, and each of four decades post-1952, when a four-year programme was instituted. The details of the survey design and methodology have been reported elsewhere (Muzzin and Hornosty 1993). In open-ended follow-up interviews, conducted with 144 of the 302 respondents, participants were further questioned about their attitudes towards counselling. These interviews provided insights and hypotheses about how professional ideologies were acquired and reinforced in these groups. The second large study that we undertook focused on the hospital residency graduates referred to in the preceding discussion about the initiation of the clinical pharmacy ideology in Canada.[6] The main purpose of the study was to compare contributions to the profession made by residency graduates and non-graduates as well as to compare the professional orientations, contributions and career advancement for the two groups.

In all three of our studies, the same 42 attitudinal questions, derived from the original research done by Hornosty, have been used. Respondents were asked to indicate, on a five-point Likert scale, the extent to which they agreed or disagreed with each of a series of statements concerning their professional orientation. Correlation coefficients among the items were low, discouraging the construction of scales, and encouraging exploration of the determinants of differential responding. For purposes of this paper, only the seven questions specifically focusing on counselling were analyzed. (The other 35 questions related to gender issues, business orientation, perceptions of the image of the pharmacist and the relevance of pharmaceutical education.) Two of the questions probed the extent of pharmacists' acceptance of the patient counselling role:

(1)   The single most important function of the pharmacist is to counsel patients regarding prescription-related matters and OTCs (over-the-counter medication).

(2)   Drug counselling is really not feasible as a general practice in most community pharmacies.

Another two asked them to evaluate the competence and performance of pharmacists in the patient counselling role:

(3)   The average pharmacist in practice today is more competent to counsel patients regarding prescription medications and OTCs than the doctor.

(4)   The average pharmacist in practice today does a good job counselling patients regarding prescription medications and OTCs.

Two questions pitted the technical competence and physician consulting role which was part of the clinical pharmacy ideology against the patient counselling role:

(5)   To be a good pharmacist it is more important to be able to communicate effectively with patients than to possess extensive knowledge about the latest developments in the pharmaceutical sciences.

(6)   I think that I would rather counsel patients than be a drug consultant to the doctor.

Finally, one probed perception of the success of the clinical pharmacy role:

(7)   More and more doctors are becoming aware that the pharmacist is a highly qualified expert in the field of drug therapy and are more and more willing to consult them for advice.

The design of the historical study lent itself to analysis of the relationship between period of schooling and attitudes towards patient counselling. The hospital pharmacy study lent itself to finer analysis of the relationship between attitudes towards counselling, gender and the main independent variable of interest, current position.

Acceptance of Patient Counselling and Period of Socialization

Pre-1929

The oldest pharmacists in Ontario emphasized that formal pharmacy education of their time was narrowly focused on compounding, which was the major responsibility within the jurisdiction of pharmacists when they began practising. These 1920s graduates claimed not to have knowledge of current teaching in pharmacy school or whether pharmacists did a good job counselling. However, most had high praise for the young pharmacists in their community, whose behaviour, they felt, reflected an appropriate emphasis on communication with the patient. A few recalled that they indeed served as the "poor man's doctor" during the early part of the century. The pharmacist in the corner drugstore might do everything from diagnosis and preparation of medicine to psychological counselling and socializing with clients. This is probably why the largest single category of spontaneous comments about pharmacists whom they considered to be highly professional referred to dealing with or caring for people. They described the good pharmacist as treating people with respect, being sensitive, compassionate, a good communicator or personable and amiable. (See Muzzin and Hornosty 1994, for more details.)

Post-1929

Figure 1 summarizes the mean scores of male and female Ontario pharmacists representing the decades post-1929 on the two questions regarding acceptance of the patient counselling role. These means are close to neutral for the graduates of the two-year programme (1929-1954). Examination of average ratings across the 60-year period suggested that there were no differences among the responses of the men and women, and that they could be pooled across genders.[7] T-tests comparing each group's mean response with the next decade's graduates showed only one significant difference over the 50-year time period: between the 1930s/1940s graduates and 1950s graduates on two of the seven questions: the one regarding counselling as the most important function of the pharmacist (t=2.23, p=.03), which is illustrated in Figure 1; and the question regarding the importance of communication vs. technical knowledge (t=2.60, p=.01). There were no other differences among graduation groups on any of the other questions, i.e., in the other 26 comparisons made, suggesting a consensus across all but the 1930s and 1940s groups about the importance and feasibility of patient counselling, and its success as a component of the role of the pharmacist.

It is unlikely that the significant differences between 1930s and 1940s graduates and 1950s graduates occurred by chance, as analysis of our interviews with these pharmacists show. Graduates made it clear why they felt that patient counselling was less important than technical skill as compared to their colleagues: they pointed out repeatedly that they were not competent to counsel patients in the way that young graduates have been trained to do. A significant minority expressed mixed feelings about counselling patients at all, since their apprenticeship had taught them not to speak with the patient about the prescription – and that it was the legal responsibility of the *physician* to advise patients. They were conscious of the possibility of losing the physician's business if they encroached on her/his territory. Consistent with their training, they informed us that the major responsibility of the pharmacist is to check the prescription and make sure that it is accurate.

The enthusiasm of the 1950s graduates for the patient counselling role was also evident in interviews, and it was as strong as that expressed by more recent graduates. Although these graduates were socialized to a "scientific pharmacy" ideology, it may be that the failure of their scientific ideology in practice left them ready to embrace the clinical ideology that followed. Despite their enthusiasm, most graduates of this decade also admitted that they do not have the same skills as young graduates. They received no training in drug side effects, nor in how to communicate them, and they assess continuing education as inadequate to address this shortcoming in their education. It was not surprising to find that more recent graduates were accepting of the patient counselling role, and that, in interviews, they questioned the "commitment" of their seniors to clinical ideals and to the idea of patient counselling. It was somewhat surprising, however, to find out that these graduates were only as enthusiastic about the concept as their colleagues who had graduated in the 1950s and 1960s, as shown in Figure 1.[8]

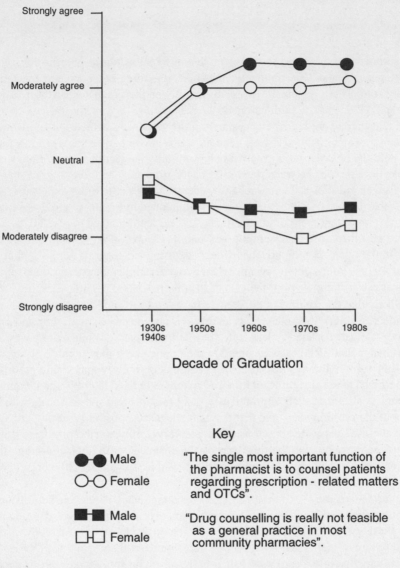

Decade of Graduation

Key

●—● Male
○—○ Female

"The single most important function of
the pharmacist is to counsel patients
regarding prescription - related matters
and OTCs".

■—■ Male
□—□ Female

"Drug counselling is really not feasible
as a general practice in most
community pharmacies".

Figure 1
Acceptance of patient counselling

What significance do these observations have? First, they suggest at least some survival of the old technical professional ideology that preceded the scientific era, which
specifically conflicts with the ideology currently in vogue on the point of patient counselling. The finding that those taught not to talk to the patient about prescriptions are
coolest about patient counselling now, illustrates this point. However, where there is no
ideological contest, as with training in scientific pharmacy without formal teaching of
counselling (as in the 1950s to 1970s), attitudes towards counselling are positive. Fur-

ther, the proportion of young graduates in practice has been growing, which means that commitment to patient counselling has also been growing over time.[9] However, it is difficult to explain the less than 100 percent acceptance of patient counselling that is evident in Figure 1. What is going on?

"Situational Adjustment" and Orientation Towards Counselling

Two possible explanations for the pattern of responding in Figure 1 that we explored were (1) that social background, specifically gender, influences orientation towards counselling; and (2) that particular work settings, or both, are important. The historical sample was too small to investigate the effects of both of these variables, since so many respondents were retired, but their significance could be examined when the responses to the seven questions for both the historical and hospital studies were pooled. Of 738 respondents in the two studies who were surveyed (a few were in both studies), 266 were eliminated because they were retired, held a position outside pharmacy, or were employed in a pharmacy setting other than hospital or community practice, thus yielding 472 cases for analysis.

Two-way analysis of variance (Table 1) showed that work setting was the most important independent variable in orientation towards counselling, as compared to gender. (Gender appears to be important only when respondents are evaluating their competence to counsel and their effect on physicians, with women more optimistic in their evaluations than men.) The main trend was for more community pharmacists than hospital pharmacists to agree with the statements regarding the paramount importance of patient counselling and the importance of effective communication as compared to technical knowledge. Conversely, more hospital pharmacists would rather be drug consultants to the doctor than counsellors of patients. They are more convinced, particularly the women among them, than their community colleagues that physicians respect them enough to consult them. This is a replication of our findings with the Class of 1983, as well as an extension of the work of Kronus (1976). The division of opinion on patient counselling that is evident in these findings is not difficult to understand in view of the virtual exclusion of the community pharmacist from face-to-face contact with the physician, while the hospital pharmacist must negotiate with physicians daily, often face-to-face (see Mesler 1989).

What is the significance of this divergence of enactment of pharmacy's new professional ideology? One might speculate that the tendency of hospital pharmacists to downplay the importance of counselling vis-á-vis other activities, technical, administrative and inter-professional, counters the educational ideology now in place in the formal education system as well as in community practice. For the future, it can be predicted that these ideological contradictions will continue in Canadian pharmacy. If the differences do not provoke "bloody battles," we think that there will at least be "bruising" between the subcultures of pharmacy. In the long run, the outcome of this ideological "adjustment" in the profession will be critical in determining the extent to which pharmacy can protect and enhance its professional jurisdiction.

TABLE 1
Effect of work setting and gender on orientation towards patient counselling (2-way ANOVA showing mean squares and p-values)[*]

	Work Setting	Gender	WS X G	
Question (see text)				
(1) Most Important Function	47.873 (.000)	0.508 (.533)	0.029 (.881)	1.302
(2) Counselling Not Feasible	0.350 (.632)	0.054 (.850)	1.076 (.401)	1.524
(3) Competence to Counsel	0.838 (.338)	7.799 (.004)	1.523 (.197)	0.913
(4) Good Job Counselling	25.375 (.000)	0.076 (.796)	1.382 (.271)	1.140
(5) Communication More Impt.	15.122 (.000)	0.104 (.760)	0.088 (.779)	1.112
(6) Prefer Counselling	111.384 (.000)	.292 (.054)	0.191 (.683)	1.145
(7) Doctors are Aware	14.976 (.000)	4.145 (.045)	0.541 (.467)	1.023

*   Tests for interaction effects were nonsignificant for all items
    Numbers beside items refer to designation of question in the text

Summary and Conclusions

In this article, pharmacists have been described as members of a profession with a beleaguered jurisdiction, that has been trying to transform itself over the past 60 years in North America. These attempts have involved developing a series of "professional ideologies" in the sense that this term was used by the interactionist Bucher (1988). She described how a professional ideology could be used to unify a profession, legitimize its new role and negotiate resources.

There have been three major curriculum revisions in pharmacy education in the past few decades in Canada, the U.S., and other jurisdictions. Since curricula in these jurisdictions still reflect, to some extent, these different ideologies, it is not surprising that some research has turned up descriptions of pharmacy education as "ambiguous," "disillusioning," and "vague" with respect to the future role of the pharmacist. However, it is argued here that in Canada the major problem is not that students are confused about their new role at the time that they graduate. Instead, the problem is that practising as they do in two distinct settings in hospitals and community pharmacies across the country, graduates try to adapt the ideologies to their respective settings and, in the process, derive somewhat conflicting perspectives. Ultimately, this may compromise their efforts to mobilize resources for their cause because they do not present a united front to those with whom they negotiate for resources.

The dynamics of this fragmentation were evident when we examined one specific aspect of their new clinical role, patient counselling. We found moderately positive acceptance of the idea, suggesting that, whether or not pharmacists actually engage in counselling, and how, this idea has acceptance in this part of North America. The question of how this came to be is of interest because counselling has only recently been taught as part of the formal curriculum. Our analyses show that the community work setting has been most influential in the acceptance of the idea of patient counselling by pharmacists. The diffusion of this idea, not only through the curriculum, but through the media and professional organizations, is pervasive. However, there is evidence that enthusiasm for this activity is blunted somewhat by lack of training for how to counsel (and what to counsel about) among some older pharmacists and preferential emphasis on other tasks, such as physician consulting, among hospital pharmacists. Most important, this analysis of orientations towards this one aspect of the philosophy of pharmaceutical care/clinical pharmacy suggests that, while pharmacists may be in favour of the new role of the pharmacist in principle, they differ on how it is to be realized. In the long run, this may undermine their cause.

More research is needed to clarify how beliefs about practice evolve, and how they are played out. In the case of pharmacy in Ontario, it appears that new graduates and business interests have combined to champion the pharmacist as patient counsellor. However, the preference of hospital pharmacists for being a team player with the physician is an alternative role for the pharmacist. How these different orientations, reflecting "situational adjustments" to developing professional ideologies, can be accommodated, remains to be seen.

Notes

1 For the reader interested in the backdrop against which the developments in this paper occur, there is virtually no Canadian literature that deals in a comprehensive way with the history of pharmacy. Stieb's account of pharmacy education (1983) and Hornosty and Coulas' (1988) analysis of feminization of Canadian pharmacy provide introductions to these two subjects. There are also brief historical accounts scattered in publications by licensing boards, the Canadian Pharmaceutical Journal and the Canadian Pharmaceutical Association (e.g., 1971). For a more complete account of broad trends within the profession, we are thus forced to rely on the American pharmaceutical and sociological literature, at least for the moment. The best American sources are Kremers and Urdang's History of Pharmacy (Sonnedecker 1976) and, more recently, sociological analyses by Phipps in the book edited by Reskin and Roos (1990). They document the steady account of growth of chain pharmacies in North America and the rapid feminization of the profession since 1970. The reactions of other health professionals (particularly physicians and administrators) and government are mentioned very briefly here, since the emphasis in the paper is on how pharmacists themselves have interpreted and enacted the ideologies. Very little research has been published on pharmacist-physician relationships and government-pharmacist relationships even in the U.S., although Mesler (1989, 1991) has made a beginning by documenting how hospital pharmacists negotiate jurisdictional turf with physicians in everyday practice in two American hospitals. Birenbaum (1990) also discusses these trends.

2 The idea of clinical pharmacy can be found much earlier in pharmaceutical publications, but the implementation of the ideology in the Canadian curriculum did not occur until this time (Norman Hughes, personal communication 1993).

3 The Statistics Canada List of Canadian Hospitals and Special Care Facilities shows that, while the number of small to mid-sized hospitals remained constant from 1965 to 1980, the number of hospitals with 200+ beds increased from 150 to 203 during this period. This was reflected in an increase in the total number of beds from 101,775 in 1965 to 125,592 in 1980 (while the number of hospitals was 852 in 1965 and 862 in 1980). In Toronto, an agreement between the large teaching hospitals and the University resulted in a radical expansion of pharmacy departments beginning in the late 1960s (N. Hughes, personal communication 1993). The history of Canadian hospital pharmacy has yet to be written.

4 Pharmacists had been slow to use this opportunity in Quebec until very recently, when the requirement that they "justify" such claims was dropped in an agreement between the government and pharmacy associations. The number of claims has now started to climb (C. Laurier, Pharmacy, University of Montreal, personal communication 1993).

5 One strong source of influence on the attitudes of pharmacists towards counselling in Ontario that was raised spontaneously in our interviews with pharmacists is the extensive advertising coverage of the new role of the pharmacist. On television and radio, pharmacists are portrayed as being approachable to patients, pleasant to deal with, professional, person-oriented and competent. In fact, it appears that the business community has discovered the benefits of selling the image of the pharmacist as a patient counsellor. Practising pharmacists in this province are now also exposed to a daily stream of commentary on patient counselling and the new role of the pharmacist through publications of their local, federal and international professional associations, the Faculty of Pharmacy, distributors and industry. The coverage of "pharmacist as counsellor" is so pervasive here that it would be remarkable indeed if a pharmacist were able to hold onto a negative orientation towards this particular activity. It would take a lifetime of commitment to another orientation, as well as isolation from professional and business influences.

6 The study was a follow-up of all graduates of hospital residency post-graduate programmes in Ontario. Their names were collected from participating hospitals since the inception of the programmes in 1960. The 500 individuals were paired with yoked controls who were of the same gender and year of graduation, had pursued hospital pharmacy, but had not done a residency. Of 901 individuals who could be located, 465 responded, of which 175 were pairs. Fifty were interviewed.

7 This was confirmed by performing regression analyses for each question, looking for a gender effect across graduation periods. For example, a model including gender of graduate, period of graduation, and their interactions (i.e. a full model) for the question regarding counselling as the single most important function of the pharmacist did not differ significantly from a model including only main effects (F=0.59, d.f.=4,237). Further, a model including only period of graduation did not differ significantly from one including gender and period of graduation (F=0.36, d.f.=1,238).

8 These results differ somewhat from those reported by R. Cockerill and P. Williams in a study that they conducted for the Lowy enquiry (1990, vol. 2 Appendices). In their study, 622 of 688, or 95 percent of Ontario Pharmacists surveyed reported that they "approved" of "new or greater responsibilities for counselling patients." This included over 90 percent of those graduating before 1970 (Table C4.4). The more positive orientation of pharmacists towards counselling reported in that study is probably due to the collapsing of the Likert scale into three categories, instead of the calculation of means, as we did in Figure 1. The question posed by Cockerill and Williams is also different from those posed in our studies. (Cockerill and Williams also reported that 61.5 percent of their sample approved of greater responsibilities "counselling prescribers" – 44 percent graduating before 1970 and 78 percent after 1980; they did not link approval of these statements with setting of practice.)

9 Data compiled at the Ontario College of Pharmacists in the mid-1980s showed that about a third of those practising were under 33, that is, had graduated in the mid-1970s or later (Des-Roches 1984). The 30 percent of practising pharmacists who were between 44 and 65 at that time, and the 10 percent over 65, are now nearing retirement, if they are not already retired. In this study, they are represented by graduates of the 1940s and 1950s, who saw the coming changes in pharmacy education and practice during their lifetimes, but who were not fully prepared for them. As they are succeeded by the next generation, most provide their enthusiastic support for the new ideology. The slightly older group, who are not as enthusiastic, probably retained their focus on technical expertise because many, including most of the women, retired before the advent of the emphasis on patient counselling.

Acknowledgements

We would like to acknowledge funding to support this research from the Social Sciences and Humanities Research Council of Canada, Grants #410-90-1221 and #484-90-0023. An earlier version of the first part of this paper was presented at the annual meetings of the Canadian Sociology and Anthropology Association, University of Victoria, Victoria, B.C., May 27 - 30, 1990.

References

Abbott, A. 1988. *The System of Professions: An Essay on the Division of Expert Labour.* Chicago: University of Chicago Press.

Akers, RL, and R Quinney. 1968. Differential Organization of Health Professions: A Comparative Analysis. *American Sociological Review* 33(1): 104–121.

American Association of Colleges of Pharmacy. 1991. *Commission to Implement Change in Pharmacy Education.* Background paper II. Washington D.C.

Becker, HS. 1970a. The Nature of a Profession. In HS Becker. *Sociological Work; Method and Substance.* Chicago: Aldine.

Becker, HS. 1970b. Personal Change in Adult Life. In HS Becker. *Sociological Work; Method and Substance.* Chicago: Aldine.

Becker, HS, and J Carper. 1970c. The Elements of Identification With an Occupation. In HS Becker. *Sociological Work; Method and Substance.* Chicago: Aldine.

Bendix, R. 1956. *Work and Authority in Industry; Ideologies of Management in the Course of Industrialization.* New York: Wiley.

Birenbaum, A. 1990. *In the Shadow of Medicine: Remaking the Division of Labour in Health Care.* New York: General Hall.

Broadhead, RS, and NJ Facchinetti. 1985. Drug Iatrogenesis and Clinical Pharmacy: The Mutual Fate of a Social Problem and a Professional Movement. *Social Problems* 32(5): 425–436.

Bucher, R. 1988. On the Natural History of Health Care Occupations. *Work and Occupations* 15(2): 131–147.

Buerki, RA, and LD Vottero. 1991. The Changing Face of Pharmaceutical Education: Ethics and Professional Prerogatives. *American Journal of Pharmaceutical Education* 55: 71–74.

Canadian Pharmaceutical Association. 1971. *Pharmacy in a New Age: Report of the Commission on Pharmaceutical Services.* Toronto: Canadian Pharmaceutical Association.

Canadian Pharmaceutical Association. 1990. *Patient Counselling, a Survey Among Community Pharmacists.* Upjohn Company of Canada. Ottawa.

Carroll, NV, and JP Gagnon. 1983. The Relationship Between Patient Variables and Frequency of Patient Counselling. *Drug Intelligence and Clinical Pharmacy* 17: 648–652.

Coburn, D, GM Torrance, and JM Kaufert. 1983. Medical Dominance in Canada in Historical Perspective: The Rise and Fall of Medicine? *International Journal of Health Services* 13(3): 407–432.

Cockerill, R, and P Williams. 1990. *1989 Survey of Pharmacists.* Pharmaceutical Inquiry of Ontario, Appendices Volume 2.

Conklin, DW. 1991. *Human Resources and Hospital Pharmacy.* The Canadian Society of Hospital Pharmacists, Ontario Branch.

Denzin, N, and CJ Mettlin. 1968. Incomplete Professionalization: The Case of Pharmacy. *Social Forces* 46: 375–381.

DesRoches, B. 1984. *Women in Pharmacy.* Unpublished manuscript, Ontario College of Pharmacists.

Fine, GA, and K Sandstrom. 1993. Ideology in Action: A Pragmatic Approach to a Contested Concept. *Sociological Theory* 11: 21–38.

Flexner, A. 1915. *Is Social Work a Profession?* Proceedings of the National Conference of Charities and Correction. Chicago: Hindmann Printing.

Freidson, E. 1970. *Professional Dominance: The Social Structure of Medical Care.* Chicago: Aldine.

Gieryn, TF. 1983. Boundary-Work and the Demarcation of Science from Non-Science: Strains and Interests in Professional Ideologies of Scientists. *American Sociological Review* 48: 781–795.

Hall Commission Report. 1964. *Royal Commission on Health Services.* Ottawa: Queen's Printer.

Haller, JS. 1981. *American Medicine in Transition 1840-1910.* Urbana, Ill.: University of Illinois Press.

Hepler, CD. 1987. The Third Wave in Pharmaceutical Education: The Clinical Movement. *American Journal of Pharmaceutical Education* 51: 1–17.

Hepler, CD, and LM Strand. 1989. Opportunities and Responsibilities in Pharmaceutical Care. *American Journal of Pharmaceutical Education* 53: 8S–15S.

Hornosty, RW. 1989. The Development of Idealism in Pharmacy School. *Symbolic Interaction* 12: 121–137.

Hornosty, RW, and G Coulas. 1988. The Feminization of Pharmacy: Is the Analysis Right? *Canadian Pharmaceutical Journal* Feb.: 93–98.

Hornosty, RW, LJ Muzzin, and GP Brown. 1992. Faith in the Ideal of Clinical Pharmacy Among Practising Pharmacists Seven Years After Graduation from Pharmacy School. *Journal of Social and Administrative Pharmacy* 9: 87–96.

Hospital for Sick Children. 1982. *Annual Report.*

Hughes, FN. 1967. The Practice of Pharmacy: The Eleventh Hour? *Bulletin of the Ontario College of Pharmacy* XVI: 65–72.

Kirk, KW. 1976. Pharmacy Students Revisited as Pharmacists. *American Journal of Pharmaceutical Education* 40: 125–128.

Kirking, DM. 1984. Evaluation of an Explanatory Model of Pharmacists' Patient Counselling Activities. *Journal of Social and Administrative Pharmacy* 2: 50–56.

Knapp, DA, HH Wolf, DE Knapp, and TA Rudy. 1969. The Pharmacist as Drug Advisor. *Journal of the American Pharmaceutical Association* NS9(10): 502–505.

Kronus, CL. 1976. Occupational Versus Organizational Influences on Reference Group Identification. The Case of Pharmacy. *Sociology of Work and Occupations* 3(3): 303–330.

Larson, MS. 1977. *The Rise of Professionalism.* Berkeley: University of California Press.

Laurier, C, A Archambault, and A Contrandriopoulos. 1989. Communication of Verbal Information by Community Pharmacists. *Drug Intelligence and Clinical Pharmacy* 23: 862–867.

Lowy Commission. 1990. Pharmaceutical Inquiry of Ontario: Role of the Pharmacist. *Pharmaceutical Inquiry of Ontario.* Fourth interim report, Jan. 25.

MacKeigan, LD, and WF McGhan. 1988. Person-Role Conflicts in Pharmacists: Its Relationship to Job Scope, Need for Achievement and Propensity to Leave an Organization. *Journal of Pharmaceutical Marketing and Management* 2: 3–22.

Manasse Jr., HR, JE Stewart, and RH Hall. 1975. Inconsistent Socialization in Pharmacy – a Pattern in Need of Change. *Journal of the American Pharmaceutical Association* NS15: 616–622.

Marx, K, and F Engels. 1846. *The German Ideology.* New York: International Publishers (1970).

McCormack, T. 1956. The Druggists' Dilemma: Problems of a Marginal Occupation. *American Journal of Sociology* 61: 308–315.

Mesler, MA. 1989. Negotiated Order for the Clinical Pharmacist: Ongoing Process of Structure. *Symbolic Interaction* 12(1): 139–157.

Mesler, MA. 1991. Boundary Encroachment and task Delegation: Clinical Pharmacists on the Medical Team. *Sociology of Health and Illness* 13(3): 310–331.

Muzzin, LJ, and RW Hornosty. 1993. Assessments of the Value of 80 Years of Formal and Practical Pharmacy Education in Ontario, Canada. *American Journal of Pharmaceutical Education* 57(4): 319–324.

Muzzin, LJ, and RW Hornosty. 1994. Formal and Informal Training in Pharmacy, Ontario, Canada, 1917-1927. *Pharmacy in History* 36(2): in press.

Muzzin, LJ, GP Brown, and RW Hornosty. 1993. The Effect of Hospital and Community Work Settings on Attitudes Towards Clinical Pharmacy. *Canadian Journal of Hospital Pharmacy* 46(6): 243–248.

Muzzin, LJ, RW Hornosty, and GP Brown. 1993. Gender, Educational Credentials, Contributions and Career Advancement in Hospital Pharmacy. Unpublished paper.

Nelson Jr. AA, RA Hutchinson, D Mahoney, and J Ringstrom. 1976. Evaluation of the Utilization of Medical Profiles. *Drug Intelligence and Clinical Pharmacy* 10: 274–281.

Ontario Ministry of Health. 1993. *Drug Programs Framework for Reform.* Consultation paper, 36 pages.

Phipps, PA. 1990. Industrial and Occupational Change in Pharmacy: Prescription for Feminization. In BF Reskin and PA Roos eds. *Job Queues, Gender Queues, Explaining Women's Inroads into Male Occupations.* Philadelphia: Temple University Press.

Poston, JW. 1992. Mission Statement for Pharmacy. *Canadian Pharmaceutical Journal* 125: 219–220.

Ranelli, P. 1991. Exploratory Study of Caregivers' Need for and Perceptions of Pharmaceutical Care for Elder Care-Recipients. *Journal of Geriatric Drug Therapy* 6(1): 75–84.

Robbins, J. 1979. *Pharmacy: A Profession in Search of a Role.* Stamford, Conn: Navillus.

Rowles, B, SM Keller, and PW Gavin. 1974. The Pharmacist as Compounder and Consultant. *Drug Intelligence and Clinical Pharmacy* 8(May): 242–244.

Schwirian, PM, and NJ Fachinetti. 1975. Professional Socialization and Disillusionment: The Case of Pharmacy. *American Journal of Pharmaceutical Education* 39: 18–23.

Selya, RM. 1988. Pharmacies as Alternative Sources of Health Care: The Case of Cincinnati. *Social Science and Medicine* 26(4): 409–416.

Shuval, JT, and I Adler. 1977. Health Occupations in Israel: Comparative Patterns of Change During Socialization. *The Journal of Health and Social Behaviour* 20: 77–89.

Smith, MC, S Messer, and JE Fincham. 1991. A Longitudinal Study of Attitude Change in Pharmacy Students During School and Post Graduation. *American Journal of Pharmaceutical Education* 55: 30–35.

Smith, MC, and DA Knapp. 1992. *Pharmacy, Drugs and Medical Care,* 5th ed. Baltimore: Williams and Wilkins.

Sonnedecker, G. 1976. *Kremers and Urdang's History of Pharmacy,* 4th ed. Philadelphia: Lippincott.

Soumerai, SB, and J Avorn. 1987. Predictors of Physician Prescribing Change in an Educational Experiment to Improve Medication Use. *Medical Care* 25(3): 210–221.

Stieb, EW. 1983. A Century of Formal Pharmaceutical Education in Ontario: Part one. *Canadian Pharmaceutical Journal* 116: 104–107.

Wertheimer, AI, E Shefter, and RM Cooper. 1974. More on the Pharmacist as Drug Consultant: Three Case Studies. *Drug Intelligence and Clinical Pharmacy* 7(Feb): 58–65.

Wertheimer, AI, and MC Smith. 1989. *Pharmacy Practice; Social and Behavioural Aspects,* 3rd ed. Baltimore: Williams and Wilkins.

Willison, DJ, and LJ Muzzin. 1992. *The Clinical Problem Solving Skills of Community Pharmacists Using Trained Observers Visiting Community Pharmacies.* Submitted to the Canadian Foundation for Pharmacy, 36 pages.

22

Women's Perspectives on Informal Care of the Elderly: Public Ideology and Personal Experience of Giving and Receiving Care*

Jane Aronson

Introduction

As in other industrialised countries with comparable social welfare systems, Canada has evolved a pattern of response to the needs of old people that relies heavily on the domestic sphere. As people age and, in various forms and degrees, confront health problems and practical problems in their everyday lives, family members typically step in to support them. It is estimated that this world of 'informal care' of the elderly constitutes 90% of the total care provided in society, the remaining 10% being supplied by the formal health and social services (Abrams 1985; Walker 1981a). The majority of both the elderly receiving informal support and of family members providing it are women. Accounting for this are, on the one hand, older women's greater life expectancy and tendency to marry men older than themselves and, on the other, women's association with the domestic sphere and with caring and responsiveness to others.

This paper examines women's experiences in this context, aiming to understand how their realities fit into the social and cultural processes that have produced and sustain this broad pattern of response to the needs of old people. To explore this link, I shall draw on conceptual perspectives that offer ways of understanding how people's conduct is shaped by prevailing ideological forces and on empirical material from a qualitative study of women giving and receiving care (Aronson 1988).

Informal Care of the Elderly: The Present Context

Studies of 'social support' and 'informal networks' over the past 10 or 15 years have focussed on the way needs are met and support is given outside the publicly funded or 'formal' health and social services. Contrary to conservative rhetoric about irresponsible families, studies reveal consistently that families feel an obligation towards and assume responsibility for the care of older relatives (Brody 1974; Marshall et al. 1987; Shanas 1979; Storm et al. 1985). They also suggest that, even in situations of what Lewis and Meredith describe as 'semi-care,' (Lewis and Meredith 1988) providing care

* Reprinted from *Ageing and Society*, Vol. 10, Jane Aronson, 'Women's Perspectives on Informal Care of the Elderly: Public Ideology and Personal Experience of Giving and Receiving Care', pp. 61-84, 1990, with the permission of Cambridge University Press.

can be a stressful experience. The focus of much of this literature on caregiver stress has tended to feed policy assumptions and preoccupations which aim to shore up informal care and facilitate the adjustment and coping of caregivers. The basic pattern and division of care between public and private spheres has gone largely unexamined.

There is some research that has made its assumptions clearer and looked more openly at the experiences and welfare of caregivers in their own terms – that is, as individuals rather than as essential labour in the care of others. The processes by which female kin – usually daughters, daughters-in-law and wives – assume responsibility for the care of elderly relatives have been identified in a very preliminary way. Research has also begun to clarify the social pressures that associate women with caring and make their apparently 'natural' designation to these roles difficult to resist (Evers 1985; Finch and Groves 1983; Hooyman and Ryan 1987; Qureshi and Walker forthcoming; Ungerson 1987). Qualitative studies are revealing the complexity of caregivers' experiences which may simultaneously include strongly held wishes to support a relative, stress, and resentment. Two recent studies of caregivers portray them as 'profoundly ambivalent' (Lewis and Meredith 1988) and 'often in self-contradiction and hence full of tension' (Ungerson 1987).

There has been relatively little systematic enquiry into elderly women receiving care. Women confront old age with considerable economic disadvantage (Dulude 1981; Neysmith 1984) and are relegated to a marginal social status that they experience as precarious and vulnerable (Cohen 1984; Ford and Sinclair 1987; Matthews 1979). That most research on informal care has focussed on caregivers has tended, implicitly, to objectify the elderly recipients of their care. Evers' important examination of elderly women's experiences of receiving care – both formal and informal – suggests the complexity of desired and tolerable levels of independence and dependence (Evers 1981; 1984; 1985). In her study of mothers receiving the care of daughters, she found simultaneous experiences of warmth, satisfaction, conflict and ambivalence (Evers 1985).

There is little opportunity for women receiving or giving care to translate such ambivalence into action by making other choices about securing needed support. The overall patterning of care arrangement in which they find themselves is characterised by an absence of alternatives. Formal services are very much in the background and, with cuts in government spending on health and social services, becoming more so (Patterson 1987).

Personal Experience in Social Context: Conceptual Issues

To recognise the broad patterning of the world of informal care in this way is an abstract exercise unless the recognition can be translated into the real terms of women's experiences in giving and receiving care. If we can make this translation and become more attuned to the entanglement of individuals' realities and wide social processes, we will have a more informed and complete basis for working towards social policies and practices that benefit and enhance women over the life course. The challenge – conceptualising the interrelationship of social structure and individual experience – is one that lies at the core of theorising in the social sciences.

Mills articulated the task of the 'sociological imagination' as understanding the intersection of biography and history in a particular society (Mills 1959). This intersection of forces has been expressed in terms of bridging differently nuanced polarities – micro and macro, self and social structure, individual and culture, personality and ideology. Each of these dimensions conceptualises how structural forces frame individual lives and how people are, at once, subject to social forces and the subjects of their own social worlds. Consideration of the development of this thinking in the fields of social welfare and social gerontology is important here as these fields bear most directly on analysis of the social status of old people and societal arrangements for meeting their needs.

Both fields have been characterised by a dominant focus on individual rather than structural forces. Countering the largely individual or 'micro' focus of much practice and education in the health and social services have been analyses of social problems and social welfare that stress the force of economic and social structures, including the welfare state, in shaping people's lives (Leonard 1984). The two perspectives, often expressed in simplified and oppositional terms as 'policy' and 'practice,' have tended to be separate spheres of study and intervention. A similar picture of theoretical development can be identified in social gerontology. The emergence of a 'political economy' of ageing over the last ten years (Estes et al. 1982; Guillemard 1983; Walker 1981b) has gone some way to offset the markedly social psychological orientation of the field.

The schism between these orientations to thinking about ageing and social policy continues to be striking; each selects different foci of study and posits different origins of the problems encountered by old people and, hence, different solutions for them. For example, writing from a social psychological standpoint, Hagestad describes the impact of population ageing on intergenerational relations and suggests that, with newly emerging family structures, people have considerable leeway 'minimal cultural guidance' (Hagestad 1981) – in creating and negotiating the nature of their ties and their conduct. She calls for increased focus at the level of interaction, suggesting that '... we are seeing socialisation not primarily as the transmission of expectations, but the creation of them' (Hagestad 1981). In outlining a political economy of ageing, Estes and associates call for a focus on the '... effects of social history, the world economy, capitalism and social class on the ageing process and the aged and the policies designed for them' (Estes et al. 1982). They would suggest, in contrast to Hagestad, that the ageing process is shaped by maximal 'cultural guidance' in the form of surrounding structural forces.

By juxtaposing these two theoretical emphases, I do not mean to create artificial oppositions or to repeat critiques of the limitations of interpretive and structural perspectives. Rather, I want to highlight the need for joining them into an approach that permits us to understand more completely the realities of people's lives. Increasingly, scholars are calling for such bridges between perspectives. Ryff, for example, cautions against confining theoretical and empirical development to the social psychological realm:

The key challenge ... becomes that of finding the balance, of putting together the inner experiences and intentional activities of the individual with the options and limits of the surrounding world. It is a task of joining the inside realm with the outside realm (Ryff 1986).

It is to this task that this paper is addressed: joining the personal experiences of women as both givers and receivers of care with the constraints of the social context to which they find themselves subject.

Offering some guidance for pursuing this task, analyses of gender relations have crossed the conventional disciplinary boundaries of the social sciences that have obscured our view of the forces in which everyday life is anchored (Finch 1987; Graham 1983; Westcott 1979). They have made revealing connections between individuals' psychological structuring, individuals' experiences of socialisation, analyses of the separate worlds of families and the public sphere, the relationship of paid and unpaid work, the economic and political order and the activities of the state. Dorothy Smith's work points to the fallacy of thinking that these various levels of analysis are separable (Smith 1987). Bridging the symbolic-interactionist conception of the dynamic relation of the individual to the social structure and Marxist analyses of power relations, Smith suggests the error of thinking of a person or single situation as merely an isolated or local phenomenon, arguing that:

Indeed, it is not a 'case,' for it presents itself to us rather as a point of entry, the locus of an experiencing subject or subjects, into a larger social and economic process. The problematic of the everyday world arises precisely at the juncture of particular experience with generalising and abstracted forms of social relations organising a division of labour in society at large (Smith 1986).

For women, the particular incongruities experienced at this 'juncture' derive from living in a social world in which they have been precluded from contributing to prevailing definitions of reality (Beeson 1975; Gilligan 1982; Smith 1987; Westkott 1979). Women generally experience their realities as awkward and incongruous, requiring contortion or suppression if they are to fit into the prescribed forms of available cultural meanings and symbols. Westkott captures the complexity of the strain produced by this split between personal experience and dominant cultural meanings, noting that it generates an internal process of self-criticism and 'estrangement' (Westkott 1979). The meaning given to this subjectively experienced estrangement and stress does not originate in a vacuum but, rather, is filtered through prevailing cultural forms and images (Cloward and Piven 1979). This paper examines this filtering process for women giving and receiving care, exploring how they incorporate prevailing ideological notions about need, care, family life and old age and attribute meaning and form to their experiences.

The Study

The empirical material in which this exploration of women's experiences of giving and receiving care is based is drawn from a qualitative study carried out in Toronto in 1987 and 1988. To locate women of various ages engaged in care relationships, I approached two Ontario women teachers' associations – one with a membership of currently working teachers, the other of retired teachers. Women responded to letters distributed by their association and to a newsletter announcement concerning the research. These initial respondents then introduced me, in a snowball fashion, to interested colleagues or acquaintances. They were invited to participate if they saw themselves as ageing mothers of adult daughters or adult daughters of such women.

Through this process, I located thirty-two women aged between 35 and 85. Of the women who identified themselves as ageing mothers, most were widows and lived alone, while younger respondents were more varied in terms of civil status and living arrangements. About half the subjects felt themselves or their mothers to be quite needy, experiencing health problems and difficulty in accomplishing everyday tasks. The others were conscious of their own or their mothers' ageing and developing needs and found themselves concerned in anticipation of the future.

The decision to include only professional subjects in the study was grounded in the expectation that women accustomed to some degree of economic independence and self-direction would, relative to less privileged women, have more developed expectations about their autonomy in middle and later life and be more likely to articulate strain or tension (Freeman 1973; Pinard 1967). While maximising the opportunity to explore this aspect of women's experience, this approach to sampling produced – predictably – a fairly homogeneous group of women. Almost all were white and none reported serious economic hardship. The members of the sample who were in the paid labour force at the time of the interviews received current Ontario teachers' salaries, and they and their older counterparts enjoyed occupational pension plans and other benefits.

In unstructured interviews lasting between 1 and 3 hours with the thirty-two women participating in the study, I explored: how their own or their mothers' needs for support emerged or were anticipated; their thoughts and feelings about themselves; the degree to which others – either friends, family or formal service providers – were involved in their situations; their general ideas about family ties and the place of public or formal service provision for the elderly; and key aspects of their biographies, work lives and family histories.

With respondents' consent, interviews were taped and transcribed so that the richness and detail of their accounts was preserved. Building on the conceptual perspectives outlined above, I regarded their accounts as both individual instances or 'cases' of caregiving and receiving and 'points of entry' into social processes far beyond subjects' realities (Smith 1986). Gathering and analysing data were simultaneous processes (Lofland and Lofland 1984) as themes in early interviews permitted an ongoing process of refocussing and reconceptualisation (Bulmer 1979). From this review of the transcripts I identified themes and patterns, refining them to develop an overarching conceptual picture of subjects' experiences. In presenting key aspects of this picture below, I have included extracts from interviews so that the analysis can be judged against the data from which it emerged, and because subjects' experiences can best be described in their own words.

Shared Assumptions About Giving and Receiving Care: The Ideological Context

Previous survey-style research on attitudes to family ties suggests that people subscribe to the general belief that family members have obligations and commitments to each other (Marshall et al. 1984; West 1984). The perceptions of the women who participated in the research reflected this broad attitudinal picture. Respondents who were confronting or anticipating their mothers' needs for support expressed a sense of responsibility toward them that was based variously in affection, reciprocity and duty. Older respondents dealing with their own emerging needs for assistance also referred to these general assumptions about families and many recalled having the same sense of obligation toward their own mothers in the past. Respondents of all ages recognised that female kin were the supporters of choice; younger respondents tended to see themselves rather than their brothers as the 'obvious' people to assist their mothers and older women spoke of 'taking comfort' from knowing they had daughters. These shared assumptions about families, obligation and gender can be understood as the key ingredients in the ideological context in which women find themselves; they constitute a commonly held understanding of what exists, what seems 'natural' and what is considered possible (Therborn 1980).

Alongside these general assumptions and values concerning obligations, a striking commonality in subjects' experiences was their efforts to set limits on the degree or manner in which they actually enacted them in giving or receiving help. Their limit-setting was concerned with establishing some control over their circumstances and it took such forms as: insistence on not sharing households with mothers or daughters; maintaining clear financial boundaries; limiting the amount of time devoted to assisting older mothers; and refusing to accept or ask for help from daughters under certain conditions. Women's efforts at determining their own situations, often expressed with difficulty, suggested resistance to forces perceived to be jeopardising or intrusive in some way. The underlying resistance and conflict for younger women resided in a sense that they should be doing more for their mothers, being more attentive and living up to an ideal of responsiveness and dutifulness, along with all the other activities in their lives. For older women – that is, for those in a position to be receiving assistance, tension derived from the strongly felt imperative that they did not want to burden their daughters, that they should 'let them live their own lives.' It was incumbent on them, therefore, to be self-reliant and undemanding – at a time when they were experiencing or anticipating need for support.

These tensions in respondents' lives were exacerbated by the realisation that they lacked alternatives for resolving them. For example, a 45-year-old daughter reflected sadly on her mother's deteriorating health and observed: "There's just me. Which is something else. There's no-one else for her to depend on." Another respondent, aged 79, spoke at length and adamantly of not going to live with daughter then added:

I almost made my daughter promise. I said, 'Please don't put me in a home.' I'm in that position where I just worry about the end of life. Who is going to ... ? If one's health fails ...

Comments like these represent the manifestations in individuals' lives of the broad patterning of care in society.

Respondents' descriptions of the degree to which others in their social contexts shared the responsibility for the care they gave or received suggested various degrees of isolation. Some sharing of responsibility with siblings was reported, generally with sisters. Less was expected of brothers – a situation that most respondents accepted unquestioningly. As a predictable corollary to this, two respondents expressed guilt and discomfort when this pattern was reversed – their brothers lived closer than they did to their mothers and did as much or more for them.

Sharing of responsibility with the formally provided health and social services was mainly with respect to medical services, for which the informal sphere cannot substitute, and, in a few instances, in regard to home care services. Women's reports of encounters with service providers varied, but were often uneasy and problematic. On the one hand, younger respondents asserted their entitlement to what they often felt to be grudgingly provided public help that could relieve them of excessive responsibility. On the other, they also felt the need to be watchful of the mothers' paths through the formal service system, concerned to protect them and advocate for their best interests. Based on their own experiences and those of other old people known to them, older respondents voiced apprehension about receiving formal care. Anxieties about poor care and, more fundamentally, about suffering the diminishment that comes with loss of control of basic life circumstances were expressed. Reporting encounters with service providers, many were acutely attuned to their devalued social status as old women.

The final element in respondents social contexts that could have been a potential avenue for supporting their care relationships was the workplace – schools for most of the study subjects. However, all saw work demands as inevitably conflicting with their supportive roles with mothers. A few noted, with appreciation, that school principals would bend or 'abuse' rules so that they could use a day of sick leave to take their mothers to an important appointment or to respond in an emergency.

In summary, the absence of alternatives for older women to secure support underscored the mother-daughter relationship as the key locus of care. While recognising and upholding the shared assumptions and cultural expectations underlying this pattern, respondents experienced awkwardness in translating them into the realities of their own lives. This awkwardness and tension was articulated in their efforts to set limits on their care giving and receiving – limits that were, essentially, in the service of protecting their own senses of integrity.

Reconciling Personal Realities and Ideology: Justifications and Accounts

Recognising that women's personal realities often did not fit easily into patterned assumptions about families, responsibility, need and old age, we turn to examining how women made sense of these discrepancies in giving and receiving care. Conceptual analyses of the processes by which people accomplish such cognitive order address the use of verbal statements of motives and accounts to explain conduct (Mills 1940; Scott and Lyman 1968). Explanations are informed by knowledge of cultural forms and prescriptions, which can be put to use to justify behaviour in terms acceptable to relevant audiences. Smith captures more graphically this image of working to fit together everyday experience and wider social processes, noting:

... how ideas and social forms of consciousness may originate outside experience coming from an external source and becoming a forced set of categories into which we must stuff the awkward and resistant actualities of our worlds (Smith 1979).

As the women studied described the limits they set on providing care, they engaged in this process by providing accompanying rationales for their behaviour or thinking. For example, after describing her mother's recent stroke, one respondent stressed:

It is really hectic. I've got twins of three and a daughter of five, so it's very hectic. So I really can't be involved in too much of it because I just don't have a lot of time ... Like, I could say that I'd do their groceries every week, but I couldn't say I'd be there to help them out.

The competing demands of husbands or children for time and energy were raised by many subjects, with an assumption clearly communicated that their claims took priority over their mothers. A single respondent expressed the reverse of this apparently obvious process:

From my point of view – I have no reason not to look after my mother. Like, I have no responsibilities – there's just me and my job.

Others were quite conscious of these processes of self-presentation and self-justification; a 47-year-old woman with adult children observed:

Work is also a release. I would imagine the woman who's not working and is at home and doesn't have the outlet and the other demands would find it sometimes even more overpowering. Like, I have lots of excuses and justifications for why I can't do more and don't do more so ... and I'm well aware of that.

Striking in respondents' approaches to aligning their conduct with prevailing norms was their difficulty or reluctance to raise their own wishes or aspirations as justifications for limiting their engagement with their mothers. In contrast, commitments to children, husbands and work were used, sometimes knowingly, to legitimate their limits or aspirations. One retired respondent raised her lack of time as a reason for not visiting her mother more, then reflected tentatively that it was an excuse; it was really her choice not to go more.

Older respondents' talk of aligning and reconciling their thoughts and behaviour with normative expectations was of a very different order. Unlike younger women, who were concerned with balancing and limiting the demands on their attention and time, they were concerned with setting limits on the claims and demands they made for assistance. In the interests of preserving their senses of worth and integrity, they sought to conform to the cultural injunction, noted above, that they do not impose burdens on their children. To make sense of their situations, they were, thus, balancing a wish for support and security with a wish to behave in accordance with norms of self-reliance and individualism. A common way of accounting for the limits they set on asking for daughters' help was to couch them in their daughters' interests, rather than their own, for example:

They would have me every weekend if I'd go ... but I think it's just too much burden on her. After all, she is carrying a full academic course and with a five-year-old, you know how much energy you have to have ... I feel that it's very wrong to, uh, impose myself on them because I feel they don't get too much time to be together – he's very busy and she's very busy.

This 78-year-old respondent mirrored younger women's acknowledgement of the primacy of the nuclear family. Some others recognised the marginality of their status across two generations – now, in their own old age and a generation before when they had been in a supportive position with their mothers:

As my son said to me at one point: 'Mum, I'll come and help you as much as I can, but my first obligation's to my own family – you know, to my wife and children.' And I thought that was kind of callous ... and then I thought afterwards: 'I did the same thing, you know, with my mother.'

These women's assumptions about families accord very closely with those of the caregivers in Ungerson's recent study (Ungerson 1987). She noted the discrepancy between, on the one hand, subjects' recognition of the relatively low priority of older women in their extended families and, on the other, the assumptions underlying government policies that invoke the extended family as the most suitable and available source of support.

The shared assumptions about older women's relatively low priority in their families were paralleled in older respondents' low expectations of society's response to them. Many identified the growing number of old people and government financial problems, taking on the negative portrayals of the elderly as an expensive burden to society – portrayals which have been criticised for their victim-blaming and destructive imagery (Minkler 1983). These appraisals of the 'facts' of their situations were, however, presented as if in the natural order of things. Limiting the demands they would make on others thus fitted with this general sense of marginality and low expectation.

The importance to older women of sustaining this alignment with cultural assumptions about self-sufficiency and independence was further revealed in the way they compared themselves with other people – real or abstract. They drew comparisons that were favourable to themselves, thus both bolstering their own self-esteem (Singer 1981) and revealing the importance of adhering to cultural prescriptions for older mothers:

I don't want to be one of those possessive mothers that just ... will act the martyr or ... play dependent, you know, at all. I like to be able to live my own life and see them in a nice social way.

I don't feel that I should impose myself on them. Now, his mother is just the opposite ... She's the kind, she's very fearful, afraid to stay alone, fearful of this and fearful of that.

These patterns of social comparisons among older subjects and the tendency to set their daughters' interests ahead of their own can be seen to signal a deprived social status. Hochschild notes how the identification of the powerless with the powerful (blacks with whites, old with young, women with men, poor with rich) supports the *status quo* and the existing maldistribution of resources and rewards (Hochschild 1973). Her research and these subjects' experiences suggest the considerable weight of ideological support that sustains this process. For the older women in this study, these ideological forces can be seen to stifle their pursuit of security and needed interdependence and to militate against a positive identification with other old women.

In summary, it is evident that women's efforts to align their personal realities with prevailing ideologies are qualitatively different for older and younger women. For women in potentially supportive positions, the tension that they strive to balance is between responsiveness to competing others and responsiveness to themselves – between self-enhancement and self-denial. For women in the position of needing care, the basic tension lies between their wish for security and confidence that their needs will be met and their wish to conform to the cultural imperative to be self reliant, undemanding and self-possessed. This section has explored the processes by which women try to make sense of these dilemmas; the next addresses the feeling dimensions of these cognitive processes.

The Feeling Side of Ideology: Shame and Guilt

Contributors to the emerging sociology of feeling move consideration of the fit between culture and individual experience to the realm of emotions (Hochschild 1975; Hochschild 1979; Shott 1979). Their work calls attention to the normative underpinning of the nature and expression of feelings, which Hochschild suggests are 'the bottom side of ideology' (Hochschild 1979). Articulating how this takes place in the inner world, Shott identifies a range of 'reflexive role-taking emotions' – e.g., guilt, shame, pride – which arise when an individual considers how his or her self appears to specific or abstract others (Shott 1979). The process of self-judgement and resulting motivation to repair a negative self-conception constitute a powerful form of internalised social control. Effectively, individuals' ideas and behaviour are shaped by the incorporation of prevailing views and assumptions to produce a self-regulating kind of self-criticism.

Women speaking of being, now or in the past, in potentially supportive positions in relation to their mothers often expressed guilty feelings – an emotion well-recognised in the literature on parent care (Brody 1985). Their guilt was heightened when they experienced most strongly the conflict discussed above, between making self-directed choices and being responsive to others' needs. Guilt can be understood as the incorporation of prevailing moral codes, in this instance the shared assumptions about obligation and caregiving. It signals their internalisation in such an effective way that they are levelled against the self, producing a kind of estranged self-criticism.

The experiences of Ms P S, a 53-year-old unmarried respondent, illustrate this complex and painful process. For many years, she had felt concerned about her mother's welfare, especially since she lived overseas, in Holland, from where Ms P S had emigrated after leaving school. At one time, at the urging of her brother and an uncle, Ms P S had contemplated bringing her mother to live with her in Canada, but had finally decided against it, feeling it would constrain her career and life unbearably. Ms P S described this process as a painful struggle, especially since she also held a very idealised view of family life and of what family members owed each other, and was saddened that her own family did not live up to this image. The limits she imposed on her engagement with her mother were, thus, accomplished with extreme guilt. She described this conflict, in all its complexity, when she compared herself with a woman friend who also had an elderly mother:

And Alice will say to me: 'Well, I can't play tennis, you know how it is: mother "expects".' And here I am saying to myself. 'Well, I'm really surprised at your coldness, you know, you really ought to be more dutiful, you should understand your mother more.' This is going through my head. Yeh, I'm surprised when other people are tougher than I am and don't give way to the 'shoulds' so fast. I mean, I always did. I was very weak. I could be easily manipulated ... She is so strong, she is so able to say: 'I do this much and no more. I have my own life to live and I have my duty to myself too.'

This internal dialogue captures acutely the divided sense of self and internalised self-criticism articulated by Westkott 1979 and Shott 1979. It reflects a contradiction that has already been described in the developing literature on women's psychology (Baker-Miller 1976) and women's moral development:

... while society may affirm publicly the woman's right to choose for herself, the exercise of such choice brings her privately into conflict with conventions of femininity, particularly the moral equation of goodness with self-sacrifice. Although independent assertion in judgement and action is considered to be the hallmark of adulthood, it is rather in their care and concern for others that women have both judged themselves and been judged (Gilligan 1982).

These judgements of self and others and their effects not only on behaviour, but also in the realm of feelings and inner experiences, are indicative of the profound embedding of ideology and cultural forces in individual realities and interpersonal relations – of the entanglement of public and private worlds.

For younger women, some conceptual form has already been given to this entanglement. Older women's experiences, however, have received less attention. As we have seen, permeating the accounts of older women was a cultural injunction to be independent, self-reliant and undemanding, while, in reality, they were confronting or anticipating a time of diminished physical ability, material resources and social ties. Despite being a relatively privileged group of older women, this contradiction was compounded by their accurate perception of their precarious social situations – a marginal social status in the contexts of both their families and the wider world. To reconcile these normative pressures with their own realities, we have seen that they employed various strategies: limiting their demands on others, bolstering their self-esteem by looking after their daughters' interests, and by identifying negatively with old women who were failing to live up to norms of individualism and independence that they adhered to themselves. Using the notion of reflexive role taking emotions, we can pose questions about the feelings associated with these processes – about how these older women feel about themselves when they take on these culturally induced self-appraisals.

The experiences of a 74-year-old woman with serious chronic health problems sheds light on these questions. Mrs E S worried about her ability to continue living alone and regretted that her daughter, her only child, lived at some distance and had little spare time:

Once in a while, I get kind of depressed, low-spirited, and I miss them, not seeing them. I think: 'Oh, grow up, will you, you know, they can't be running over here at night to see me or after their work'... but I feel that they're doing all they can do.

I asked Mrs E S if she ever shared this low-spirited mood with her daughter. She replied with a nervous laugh: 'I wouldn't dare show it to her. I'd be ashamed, kind of ashamed.' Shott describes shame, like guilt, as a reflexive role-taking emotion that is '... provoked by the realisation that others [or the generalised other] consider one's self deficient' (Shott 1979). Thus, to preserve a socially acceptable sense of self and protect herself from shame, Mrs E S contains her low spirits, masks her anxieties and bolsters her self-esteem by distancing herself from women who do not live up to this standard of behaviour. Remembering Westkott's and Gilligan's formulations of estrangement and the divided self (Gilligan 1982; Westkott 1979), Mrs E S can be seen as a harsh critic of her own experience, her incorporated beliefs permitting no compassion for her own difficulties.

The antithesis of feeling shame or fending off shame was preserving pride. Mrs A C remembered her own, now dead, mother's inability to speak to her of her needs and worries as she aged – an inability that irritated Mrs A C considerably. Now a widow and in poor health herself, she reflected how her mothers reserve had come to make sense to her. She understood that her mother was 'protecting her pride' and finds herself doing the same thing, setting limits on how much she reveals of her anxieties or asks of her daughters. Shott notes that pride derives from knowing one has behaved in accordance with normative expectations (Shott 1979). For older women, satisfaction at knowing this comes at the cost of self-denial and stifling needs for security. On the other hand, exposing insecurity comes at the cost of losing face by violating cultural expectations associated with being an older woman. A 59-year-old respondent, in poor health, seemed to have the detachment to articulate this dilemma. She made the socially appropriate assertions about not wanting to burden her daughter, but then reflected:

I don't want to be any sort of burden to her, in any way. That includes an emotional drain on her time, as well as the physical. Now, am I just saying that – just paying lip service to it? This is what I know I should say and I should feel. Do I really feel that way? I don't know. Perhaps ... when the time comes, I'll be a real clinging vine. You know, it appalls me – the thought – but, however, maybe I would be ... I'd certainly try not to be.

These painful contradictions in women's feelings of shame and pride can be seen to represent the manifestations in individuals' lives of ideological forces concerned with dependence and individualism that have their roots in wider economic and social structures.

In summary, the feelings – guilt and shame – associated with women's concerns at not living up to socially approved ideas about giving and receiving care reflect their profound internalisation of cultural prescriptions. Their incorporation and the resulting self-criticism and self-control represent highly effective – and invisible – forms of social control. Motivated to reduce feelings of guilt and shame, women implicitly suppress assertion of their own needs, so that the broad pattern of care of old people goes unchallenged – rather, it is sustained and reproduced.

Conclusion

The exploratory nature of the research reported in this paper and the complexity of some of the issues raised cannot generate firm conclusions. The study does, however, illuminate the contradictory character of giving and receiving care for women and draws attention to the underlying entanglement of personal meaning and prevailing ideology. Reflections and questions that the study raises about social change processes and social policies are discussed in this concluding section.

As noted earlier, the analysis developed here requires expansion through comparative study of other groups (e.g., poor women, women of different racial backgrounds, women without children, women who never married). Greater attention could also be usefully directed to exploring individual variations in women's management of the contradictions they experience in needing or providing care. The growing literature on women and ageing and women's caring over the life cycle provides grounding and direction for ongoing research on some of these themes.[1]

The Entanglement of Personal Experience and Public Ideology

To return to the questions posed at the beginning of the paper, the picture emerging from this study suggests that, rather than having 'minimal cultural guidance' (Hagestad 1981) about giving and receiving care between generations, women's experiences are firmly patterned by social forces that are constantly enacted in their lives. These forces are deeply embedded in their realities, shaping inner experiences of selfhood and feeling. This picture accords with conceptual frameworks that point to the unity of personal experience and wide social and ideological forces: people do not make their way idiosyncratically through uncharted social experiences any more than social structures exist as rarified abstractions far outside their social worlds. Structural forces are constantly enacted and reproduced in everyday life and, depending upon their particular biographies and resources, individuals may actively organise their social worlds.

The accounts of the women described in this paper are, therefore, understandable not simply as individual adaptive styles but as the complex products of personal experiences and wider contextual forces. If the broad social context were one that valued old people, communicated entitlement to needed supports and provided for individual and collective sharing of their provision, Mrs E S's low spirits and sense of jeopardy might have been much less. If straightforward statements of need were easily speakable, she would not have had to fend off shame, and Mrs A C and her mother would not have had to preserve pride at the cost of denying their real needs. Ms P S would have struggled less if prevailing ideologies made possible a wider sharing of responsibility for the care of others, instead of singling her out as an unmarried daughter and pressing her into a caregiving position.

With this appreciation of the interplay of social and ideological forces with individual biographies, the origins of some respondents' accounts of difficulties in their relationships with their mothers become clearer. Some women spoke of their resentment of their mothers' needs and felt unfairly manipulated and controlled by them. However, having noted, above, how older women struggle between needing security and the imperative to appear strong and undemanding, it is, perhaps, to be expected that – like all subordinate groups – they might resort to indirect means to get their needs met (Baker-Miller 1976). Similarly, in a pattern of care in which female kin are generally made responsible for solutions to older women's needs, it should not be surprising to find that younger women resent the absence of choice and target their resentment at its immediate or apparent cause – their mothers. Thus, while such interpersonal tension certainly has its individual character, it can also be understood as a socially structured patterning of relationship.

Within the structured constraints that shaped their lives, women were, of course, not simply passive actors. Rather, their efforts to set limits on giving and receiving care can be seen as active attempts to establish some control of their situations and make manageable the patterned tensions they experienced. These efforts were local responses to conflicts which, as we have seen, derived from structural processes. Confined to their immediately experienced worlds, they could have no impact on the broader social forces in which they originated. The possibility that these private difficulties might become expressed tension and, in the future, disturb the status quo is considered in the next section.

Reflections on Social Change

The accounts of the women who participated in the research were characterised, to varying degrees, by the experience of estrangement and inner contradiction. As we have seen, this sense of inner division generated a kind of internalised social control and privately borne tension. Theoretically, it is suggested that while the experience of such tension can be alienating and stifling – as evidenced here – it also holds the potential for social change (Leonard 1984; Margolis 1985). In Margolis' terms, the key transition in the emergence of this potential is accomplished when individuals move from sensing a privately experienced contradiction to expressing a publicly voiced challenge of a taken-for-granted meaning or assumption.

Analyses of the early stages of social movements and early expressions of social strain point to the associated processes by which stressful circumstances come to be seen as injustices to be protested rather than misfortunes to be endured (Turner 1969) and as social problems rather than personal problems (Freeman 1975; Margolis 1985; Spector and Kitsusc 1977). For this process to occur, articulated unease and a collective identification with others who share the discontent are necessary conditions. The women who took part in this study showed only limited signs of either condition. Their often strained experiences were filtered through an ideological frame that cast them as individual failings, occasioning feelings of guilt and shame and rendering them difficult to speak about. Further, there was no evidence of identification with others in the same position. In fact, many older respondents were at pains to distance themselves from other old women.

Looking ahead, it is sometimes speculated that as future cohorts of women grow old, they will bring the experiences of more independent work lives and more resources to old age, becoming a significant political force (Cohen 1984; Peace 1986). Thus, social change is envisioned as an emerging process, unfolding with the passage of time. As a cross-sectional picture of women's experiences, this research clearly cannot deal systematically with such future speculation, but it does offer an interesting retrospective view of older subjects' lives.

The older women in this study were, relative to other women of their generation, a privileged group who had worked outside the home and had a clear occupational identity. In fact, their life experiences correspond to those of the coming cohorts of women thought to herald a different old age for women (Cohen 1984; Peace 1986). However, looking at them over their lifetimes, there was no evidence to suggest empowerment and a disposition to collectivity in later life. Despite their relative material and social advantages, they were experiencing their later years as precarious and marginal. Two respondents who had been teachers all their working lives and, by virtue of early widowhood and divorce, were accustomed to being independent, illustrate this pattern. Both recalled their mothers, whom they had cared for in various ways as they aged, and reflected that: 'I thought it would be different for me.' That is, from the viewpoint of their middle years, they did not expect to experience the vulnerability and diminishment of their mothers – they thought they would have more control over their circumstances.

The experiences of these women do not, therefore, lend support to the notion that change and improvement in women's experiences of old age will simply come about in a progressive way as successive cohorts of women enter later life. Rather, the marginal social and economic status associated with being female and being old, the negative construction of need and frailty, and low levels of societal support appeared to be highly determining of the realities of later life. For them, these forces outweighed individual experiences at earlier stages of the life course and individual efforts in old age to achieve security and a positive social identity. These observations suggest that future public policy intervention, recognising the combined effects of age and gender, will be crucial if there is to be change and improvement in women's situations.

Implications for Social Policy

The accounts of the women studied revealed the deep embedding in their experiences of the image of families and, specifically, women as the key locus of care and of the notion of old women's individual responsibility and marginal status. The strongly individualistic cast of these internalised ideologies was reinforced by subjects' perceptions of the scarcity of alternatives in the form of public services and programmes for older people. These cultural assumptions and material realities work to sustain the existing pattern of care, keeping the major portion of responsibility outside the public realm and outside the concerns of men. However, as we have seen, sustaining this pattern comes at a high cost to women; it introduces contradictions and strains into their lives that stifle and suppress their pursuit of need-meeting behaviour and opportunities for self-enhancement. This suppression is testament to the power of the ideologies and assumptions that frame the existing pattern of care. That they are seen by women in their everyday lives as 'natural' or inevitable phenomena means that countenancing other possibilities seems implausible or unthinkable. Recognising the ways in which the existing pattern of care constrains women and works to their detriment over the life course, the challenge for the future is to render thinkable other societal responses to old people's needs that do not operate at the expense of women.

The central objective of such alternative responses will be to give women a solid and assured grasp on security, self-determination and independence at all ages. Continued emphasis on policies and programmes that shore up the existing division of responsibility between formal and informal care will not achieve these ends. Even if this pattern of service provision were more adequately funded, it would still rest on the assumptions internalised by this study's subjects: that families, especially female kin, are the proper context of care and that individualistic notions of self-sufficiency must be upheld. Reluctance to claim entitlement to public services or to acknowledge need and inability to 'cope' is a logical corollary to the espousal of these values. For women to identify their needs and wishes and translate them into action, not only would they require an array of available supportive services, but also a breaking down of these ideological barriers to using them.

In thinking of alternative types of supportive provisions, it must be remembered that security does not derive only from the presence of one-to-one care relationships. Needs for support may be met by adaptations to housing and environments, rehabilitation services, flexible community supports, provision of adequate income and so on; they do not necessarily translate into individualised caregiving responses and dependencies (Croft 1986; Finch 1984). That said, it is important that they are designed and introduced in ways that recognise the particular character of individuals' biographies and social ties. While care relationships were not, as such, the focus of this study, the complexity of the nature and capacity of ties between respondents and their mothers and daughters was evident and, from caregivers' perspectives, has received attention in recent research (Lewis and Meredith 1988).

In conclusion, this paper has focused consideration of the current pattern of care of the elderly on the experiences of those most affected by it – on women as both givers and receivers of care in the informal sphere. Appreciation of the deeply embedded linkages between their experiences and contemporary ideologies clarifies a two-fold task for the future. It will be important to challenge prevailing cultural assumptions about care, responsibility, old age and gender that effectively disadvantage women, stifling and individualising their experiences. Reduction of these ideological constraints must be accompanied by the development of alternative public responses to women's concerns that enhance their independence and security over the life course. Working towards such changes in the conceputalisation of social policies and practices can contribute to freeing women to express their needs and pursue solutions to them without the spectre of guilt and shame to which they are presently subject.

Note

1   For example: concerning research on variability in care relationships see Lewis and Meredith 1988, Quereshi and Walker (forthcoming), Ungerson 1987, Wenger 1984. For studies of older women located outside prevailing conceptions of families see Kehoe 1989, Simon 1987. Studies of the meanings and security derived from friendships in later life are dealt with in Jerrome 1981. On the significance of friendship for women in later life, see Jerrome 1981 and Matthews 1986. Reconceptualisations of patterns of care and assistance especially as they affect women are discussed in Allan 1988, Croft 1986, and Dalley 1988.

Acknowledgements

The work reported in this article was supported in part by the National Health Research and Development Programme of Health and Welfare Canada through a National Health Fellowship to the author, and also by the Programme in Gerontology at the University of Toronto through a seed money grant. For their advice and comments at different stages of the project, I would like to thank: Victor Marshall, Sheila Neysmith, David Locker, Carolyn Rosenthal, Judith Globerman and Janet Finch.

References

Abrams, P. 1985. Edited by M Bulmer. Policies to Promote Information Care: Some Reflections on Voluntary Action, Neighbourhood Involvement and Family Care. *Ageing and Society* 5: 1–18.

Allan, G. 1988. Kinship, Responsibility and Care for Elderly People. *Ageing and Society* 8: 249–268.

Aronson, J. 1988. *Women's Experiences of Giving and Receiving Care: Pathways to Social Change*. Ph.D. dissertation, University of Toronto.

Baker-Miller, J. 1976. *Toward a New Psychology of Women*. Boston: Beacon Press.

Beeson, D. 1975. Women in Studies of Aging: A Critique and Suggestion. *Social Problems* 23.

Brody, EM. 1985. Parent Care as a Normative Family Stress. *The Gerontologist* 25.

Brody, EM. 1974. Aged Parents and Aging Children. In P Ragan ed. *Aging Parents*. Berkley: University of Southern California Press.

Bulmer, M. 1979. Concepts in the Analysis of Qualitative Data. *Sociological Review* 27.

Cloward, RA, and FF Piven. 1979. Hidden Protest: The Channeling of Female Innovation and Resistance. *Signs* 4.

Cohen, L. 1984. *Small Expectations: Society's Betrayal of Older Women*. Toronto: McLelland and Stewart.

Croft, S. 1986. Women, Caring and the Recasting of Need: A Feminist Reappraisal. *Critical Social Policy* 6.

Dalley, G. 1988. *Ideologies of Caring*. London: MacMillan.

Dulude, L. 1981. *Pension Reform with Women in Mind*. Ottawa: Canadian Advisory Council on the Status of Women.

Estes, CL, JH Swan, and LE Gerard. 1982. Dominant and Competing Paradigms in Gerontology: Towards a Political Economy of Ageing. *Ageing and Society* 2.

Evers, H. 1985. The Frail Elderly Woman: Emergent Questions in Aging and Woman's Health. In E Lewin and V Oleson eds. *Women, Health and Illness*. New York: Tavistock.

Evers, H. 1984. Old Women's Self Perceptions of Dependency and Some Important Implications for Service Provision. *Journal of Epidemiology and Community Health* 38.

Evers, H. 1981. Care or Custody? The Experiences of Women Patients in Long-Stay Geriatric Wards. In B Hutter and G Williams eds. *Controlling Women: The Normal and the Deviant*. London: Croom Helm.

Finch, J. 1987. Family Obligations and the Life Course. In A Bryman et al. eds. *Rethinking the Life Cycle*. London: Macmillan.

Finch, J, and D Groves. 1983. *A Labour of Love: Women, Work and Caring*. London: Routledge and Kegan Paul.

Ford, J, and R Sinclair. 1987. *Sixty Years on: Women Talk About Old Age*. London: Women's Press.

Freeman, J. 1975. *The Politics of Women's Liberation*. New York: Longman.

Freeman, J. 1973. The Origins of the Women's Liberation Movement. *American Journal of Sociology* 78.

Gilligan, C. 1982. *In A Different Voice: Psychological Theory and Women's Development.* Cambridge, Mass: Harvard University Press.

Graham, H. 1983. Caring, a Labour of Love. In J Finch and D Groves eds. *A Labour of Love: Women, Work and Caring.* London: Routledge and Kegan Paul.

Guillemard, AM. 1983. The Making of Old Age Policy in France: Points of Debate, Issues at Stake, Underlying Social Relations. In AM Guillemard ed. *Old Age and the Welfare State.* London: Sage.

Hagestad, GO. 1981. Problems and Promises in the Social Psychology of Intergenerational Relations. In RW Fogel, E Hatfield, SB Kiesler, and E Shanas eds. *Ageing: Stability and Change in the Family.* New York: Academic Press.

Hochschild, AR. 1979. Emotion Work, Feeling Rules and Social Structure. *American Journal of Sociology* 85.

Hochschild, AR. 1975. The Sociology of Feeling and Emotion: Selected Possibilities. In M Millman and RM Kanter eds. *Another Voice: Feminist Perspectives on Social Life and Social Science.* New York: Anchor.

Hochschild, AR. 1973. *The Unexpected Community: Portrait of an Old Age Subculture.* Berkeley: University of Southern California Press.

Hooyman, NR, and R Ryan. 1987. Women as Caregivers of the Elderly: Catch 22 Dilemmas. In J Figueira-McDonough and R Sarri eds. *The Trapped Woman: Catch 22 in Deviance and Social Control.* Newburn Park: Sage.

Kehoe, M. 1989. *Lesbians Over Sixty Speak for Themselves.* New York: Harrington Park Press.

Jerrome, D. 1981. The Significance of Friendship for Women in Later Life. *Ageing and Society* 1: 175–198.

Leonard, P. 1984. *Personality and Ideology: Towards a Materialist Understanding of the Individual.* London: MacMillan.

Lewis, J, and B Meredith. 1988. *Daughters Who Care: Daughters Caring for Mothers at Home.* London: Routledge.

Lofland, J, and LH Lofland. 1984. *Analyzing Social Settings: A Guide to Qualitative Observation and Analysis,* 2nd ed. Belmont: Wadsworth Publishing.

Margolis, DR. 1985. Redefining the Situation: Negotiations on the Meaning of 'Women'. *Social Problems* 32.

Marshall, VM, CJ Rosenthal, and J Daciuk. 1987. Older Parents' Expectations for Filial Support. *Social Justice Research* 4.

Matthews, SH. 1979. *The Social World of Old Women: Management of Self-Identity.* Beverly Hills: Sage.

Matthews, SH. 1986. *Friendships Through the Life Course: Oral Biographies in Old Age.* London: Sage.

Mills, CW. 1959. *The Sociological Imagination.* Oxford: Oxford University Press.

Mills, CW. 1940. Situated Actions and Vocabularies of Motive. *American Sociological Review* 5.

Minkler, M. 1983. Blaming the Aged Victim: The Politics of Scape-Goating in Times of Fiscal Conservatism. *International Journal of Health Services* 13.

Neysmith, SM. 1984. Poverty in Old Age: Can Pension Reform the Needs of Women? *Canadian Women Studies* 5.

Patterson, J. 1987. Winding Down Social Spending: Social Spending Restraint in Ontario in the 1970s. In A Moscovitch and J Albert eds. *The 'Benevolent' State: The Growth of Welfare in Canada.* Toronto: Garmond Press.

Peace, S. 1986. The fForgotten Female: Social Policy and Older Women. In C Phillipson and A Walker eds. *Ageing and Social Policy: A Critical Assessment.* Aldershot: Gower.

Pinard, M. 1967. Poverty and Political Movements. *Social Problems.*

Pinch, J. 1984. Community Care, Developing Non-Sexist Alternatives. *Critical Social Policy* 9.

Qureshi, H, and A Walker. Forthcoming. *The Caring Relationship.* London: MacMillan.

Ryff, CD. 1986. The Subjective Construction of Self and Society: An Agenda for Life Span Research. In VW Marshall ed. *Later Life: The Social Psychology of Aging.* Beverly Hills: Sage.

Scott, MB, and SM Lyman. 1968. Accounts. *American Sociological Review* 33.

Shanas, E. 1979. The Family as a Social Support System in Old Age. *The Gerontologist* 17.

Shott, S. 1979. Emotion and Social Life: A Symbolic Interaction Analysis. *American Journal of Sociology* 84.

Simon, BL. 1987. *Never Married Women.* Philadelphia: Temple Unviersity Press.

Singer, E. 1981. Reference Groups and Social Evaluations. In M Rosenberg and RH Turner eds. *Social Psychology: Sociological Perspectives.* New York: Basic Books.

Smith, DE. 1987. *The Everyday World as Problematic: A Feminist Sociology.* Toronto: University of Toronto Press.

Smith, DE. 1986. Institutional Ethnography: A Feminist Method. *Resources for Feminist Research* 25.

Smith, DE. 1979. A Sociology for Women. In JA Sherman and E Torton Beck eds. *The Prism of Sex: Essays in the Sociology of Knowledge.* Madison: University of Wisconsin Press.

Spector, M, and J Kitsusc. 1977. *Constructing Social Problems.* Menlo Park: Cummings.

Storm, C, T Storm, and J Strike-Schurman. 1985. Obligations for Care: Beliefs in a Small Canadian Town. *Canadian Journal on Aging* 4.

Therborn, G. 1980. *The Ideology of Power and the Power of Ideology.* London: Verso.

Turner, RH. 1969. The Theme of Contemporary Social Movements. *British Journal of Sociology* 20.

Ungerson, C. 1987. *Policy is Personal: Sex, Gender and Informal Care.* London: Tavistock.

Walker, A. 1981a. Community Care and the Elderly in Great Britain: Theory and Practice. *International Journal of Health Services* II.

Walker, A. 1981b. Toward a Political Economy of Old Age. *Ageing and Society* I.

Wenger, GC. 1984. *The Supportive Network: Coping with Old Age.* London: George Allen and Unwin.

West, P. 1984. The Family, the Welfare State and Community Care: Political Rhetoric and Public Attitudes. *Journal of Social Policy* 13.

Westkott, M. 1979. Feminist Criticism of the Social Sciences. *Harvard Educational Review* 49.

Part V
Hospitals

The readings in this part of the book deal with one of the major health organizations, the hospital. Hospitals are one of the most interesting and currently volatile parts of the health care system. After a long period of uninterrupted growth, they have begun to undergo drastic change. Despite cutbacks however, they still employ the largest group of people working in health care.

The first reading in this section by David Gagan, a historian, discusses the rise of the modern hospital in Ontario from 1880 to 1950. The article touches on a number of themes that have contemporary relevance. One is the role of community, ethnic and professional pride in the founding of the institutions. Another is how innovations in medical and organizational technology changed the functions of the hospital, attracting new clienteles, creating and changing occupations, and, ultimately, raising the cost of care beyond the point where the local community could pay for it. A third theme is the tension between provincial governments and local authorities over funding and control of the hospitals.

With data from all general hospitals in the province as a backdrop, Gagan presents a portrait in depth of one community hospital, the Owen Sound General and Marine Hospital. Gagan shows that until the end of the nineteenth century hospitals mainly cared for the indigent, with middle-class patients finding care at home to be "infinitely preferable" to care in the hospital. Then, in a relatively short period up to the end of the First World War in 1918, hospitals underwent a radical transformation. Both in their treatment methods and in their "hotel" services, they became acceptable to middle-class patients, particularly women. Doctors were won over to use hospitals, rather than their own offices, as the site of many work activities.

But seeds of trouble were sewn at the same time, however. The new technology of laboratories, X-ray machines, antiseptic surgery, and hospital childbirth was expensive. The provincial government insisted that hospitals continue to care for indigent patients, but the allowance they paid for these patients was insufficient to meet the real costs. Middle-class patients who paid for their own care were charged more and more to cover the cost of subsidizing care for the poor. The increased charges strained the patients' capacity to pay.

Gagan shows how the hospitals' fiscal problems shaped the development of government health insurance. Provincial subsidies remained insufficient and pressure for relief of the hard-pressed middle-class persisted. This eventually led to hospital-sponsored voluntary prepaid health insurance schemes, then later to universal government-sponsored health insurance. Gagan states: "It is sometimes argued that government-administered health insurance in Canada arose out of political necessity, after 1945, to provide a 'social wage' for working class Canadians. Much of the evidence associated with the social history of hospitals in Ontario suggests that the debate also focused significantly on the threatened medical impoverishment of the middle class after 1930." Gagan's article should be seen in relation to those by Donald Swartz and the sociohistorical introduction to this volume.

The second chapter, by George Torrance, describes ways in which the industrial analogy ("health factories") applies to modern Canadian hospitals as workplaces. Updating his article from the first two editions, Torrance notes that drastic changes have taken place since the earlier versions. He documents the steady historical change in hospitals up till the late 1980s in size, structure, and technology, as well as the effects of these changes on the organization and content of hospital work. Then, using two case studies, he gives special attention to the large category of hospital workers outside direct patient-care settings, that is, the lower and middle-level people who make up the majority of hospital workers. Torrance concludes that in the non-clinical areas at least, hospital work and other kinds of work are now much more similar than they used to be. And, because there is little difference now between hospitals and other organizations of similar size and complexity, hospitals face similar problems: "... alienation among lower-level and semi-professional employees, an instrumental orientation to work, and industrial conflict between management and labour."

In the earlier versions of his article, Torrance predicted that, despite efforts to cut costs, hospitals would retain their centrality in the health care system. This now appears less certain as cost cutbacks penetrate deeper. Hospitals and beds have been closed, services have been converted to an out-patient basis, housekeeping functions have been contracted out, and treatment staff have been reduced. Lower-level hospital workers continue to bear the brunt of change, but nurses, therapists, technologists and even physicians and administrators have also felt its impact.

Sociological research on Canadian hospitals and related institutions has remained scarce since the last edition of this book. One exception is the work by Pat and Hugh Armstrong (1996) which critiques the "wasting away" of Canadian health care resulting from the cutbacks. These authors see downsizing as a response to the fiscal crisis of the state and to an international corporate agenda to reduce social benefits, roll back gains made by mainly female workers in the public sector, and increase the scope for private sector products like drugs and medical supplies.

It is the supportive, caring aspects of hospital work rather than "high-tech" interventions that are under heaviest attack as campaigns to cut costs are pushed forward. Women workers in middle-and lower-level hospital occupations were major beneficiaries of the modernization of hospitals over the last fifty years. Through participation in unions, they achieved considerable success in improving control over work, fringe benefits and wages. This operated to the advantage of patients as well as the workers since a well-trained, secure work force with adequate time and back-up provides superior care. However, recognition of the value of the work is still limited, leaving it vulnerable to campaigns to subdivide and delegate tasks to less-trained workers or to export them outside the hospital to unpaid household workers.

Undoubtedly, some work practices in hospitals were antiquated and ripe for change. Hospitals have always been recognized by sociologists as peculiar institutions, with a veneer of technological and organizational sophistication overlaid on an old organizational model. Earlier studies puzzled at the "two lines of authority" and the combination of bureaucratic and professional features. Later theorists saw hospitals' complex organizational structures as a rational adaptation to the differing states of treatment technology in different fields. However, the myth that medical care and hospital organization are scientific, rational and functionally optimal has been punctured by studies consistently revealing how much variation there is among physicians in rates of hospitalization and in treatment patterns for the same condition (see Roos 1992, among others). Many traditional hospital practices such as the emphasis on bed rest rather than active rehabilitation, regimentation of patients (and staff), and excessively long stays have been revealed as unnecessary or even harmful to recovery. While occupational restrictions on who can do what within the hospital have positive features, many are excessive, serving more to protect jobs and professional interests than to benefit patients.

The causes of hospital decline must be sought both in external factors like the actions of states and corporate elites, and in internal factors like the dynamics of changing disease distributions, diffusion of new technologies, and organizational and occupational obsolescence. That the changes are not just due to Canadian conditions is suggested by the changes also taking place in American hospitals over the same period. As Robinson (1994), Ginzburg (1995) and Stoeckle (1995) note, new technology enabling more to be done outside of hospital walls, plus pressures for cost containment from third-party payers, has reduced admissions, occupancy rates, beds and hospitals in the United States. Stoeckle in particular has argued that much of the decline can be attributed to the replacement of outmoded practices.

These developments underscore the need for more Canadian research on hospitals at several levels of analysis: as actors (or pawns) within a community, provincial, national and international political economy; as arenas for occupational development and conflict; as places of patient care; and as work settings. The range of patient care and work settings that emerged prior to the changes of recent years has scarcely begun to be described and analyzed. We still lack analyses of many types of nursing and allied health profession settings within acute-care hospitals. Moreover, studies of related institutions like rehabilitation centres, modern mental hospitals, nursing homes, and various kinds of residential care facilities and clinics remain rare.

As the preceding makes clear, the recent changes also raise a host of questions. How did an institution which seemed so powerful and central to modern health care change so suddenly? How did communities which used to take fierce pride in their hospitals, as places to receive care, to employ sons and daughters, to provide facilities for talented professionals, come to tolerate closures and downsizing? How have staff cutbacks affected everyday work and the balance of power among occupations? What is the social topography of work in the expanding settings like out-patient clinics and day surgery, or for new categories of workers like the patient care aides? Studies using a variety of methodologies, from qualitative ethnographies to cross-national comparative studies, are needed to shed light on these issues.

REFERENCES

Armstrong, P and H Armstrong. 1996. *Wasting Away: The Undermining of Canadian Health Care*. Toronto: Oxford University Press

Ginzberg E. 1995. Hospitals: From Center to Periphery. *Inquiry* 32: 11-13

Robinson, JC. 1994. The Changing Boundaries of the American Hospital. *The Milbank Quarterly* 72: 259-275

Roos, NP. 1992. Hospitalization Style of Physicians in Manitoba: The Disturbing Lack of Logic in Medical Practice. *Health Service Research* 27: 361-384

Stoeckle, JD. 1995. The Citadel Cannot Hold: Technologies Go Outside the Hospital: Patients and Doctors Too. *The Milbank Quarterly* 73: 3-17

23

For 'Patients of Moderate Means': The Transformation of Ontario's Public General Hospitals, 1880-1950*

David Gagan

The social history of medicine seeks to understand society's historical response to disease, especially in relation to the interaction between those in need of health care and those who provided it, as a microcosm, perhaps even a paradigm, of modern society. As one historian of medicine has explained, 'all those factors that have made the modern world modern – increases in scale, the domination of professional elites, the bureaucratization of human relationships, the tendency toward technological approaches to social problems ... [and] the legitimation of social roles and policies in terms of that technology' are to be found in the social history of medicine (Rosenberg 1981; cf Rosen 1967). Within this context, the history of the development of the modern hospital has attracted particular attention, because it was in the increasingly 'atomistic' (Rosenberg 1981) world of the evolving primary health-care centre that the dialogue between scientific medicine and social medicine, between social need and social policy, largely took place.

The history of the emergence of the modern system of hospital care in Britain and the United States is now fairly well understood, at least in broad outline, as the result of recent research. Well into the late Victorian era, before the advent of Listerism, professional standards of nursing care, or modern diagnostic and surgical techniques, hospitals were places more to be dreaded than valued or trusted. Essentially custodial facilities maintained as secular charities by wealthy patrons who in turn determined who should be admitted for care, hospitals were instruments for the social control of the working and destitute urban poor, better equipped to promulgate Victorian social virtues than to treat sickness in the urban-industrial societies that gave birth to them (Abel-Smith 1964; Vogel 1980; Rosenberg 1977). The better classes neither sought nor required treatment in these institutions, admission to which carried the stigma of poverty and dependency without the promise of medical improvement. The middle-class home with its clean environment, domestic servants, familial care, and attending private physician at hand was an infinitely preferable milieu for the convalescent.

* This chapter is excerpted from a longer article originally published in *The Canadian Historical Review*, Vol. LXX, No. 2, David Gagan, "Patients of Moderate Means": The Transformation of Ontario's Public General Hospital, 1880–1950, pp. 151–79, 1989. It is reprinted by permission of the University of Toronto Press Incorporated.

Around the end of the nineteenth century, however, the image of the hospital began to undergo a radical transformation. Antiseptic and aseptic procedures, the profession-alization of nursing and, more importantly, of hospital administration wrought by Flo-rence Nightingale and her disciples after 1870, the advent of new diagnostic technology (for example, the X-ray machine), improved surgical techniques, and the clustering in one place of a steadily widening range of medical expertise all contributed to the growing perception among both physicians and their private patients that the hos-pital, not the home, was the preferred place for the treatment of acute sickness (Starr 1982). This transformation was essentially complete by the end of the First World War, and was symbolized by the growing preponderance in hospitals of private rooms and semi-private wards. The differentiated and more costly care they represented signified the middle class's discovery of hospitals as no longer charitable institutions, but rather as the unequivocally necessary 'embodiments of modern medical science,' (Vogel 1980) and, consequently, the middle class's willingness and ability to pay the full costs of medical treatment. It was in this way that a market economy for health care was cre-ated where none had existed before (Starr 1977). It was an economy, however, which soon threatened not only to reduce medical care to a series of commercial transactions, but also to discriminate, on the basis of ability to pay, among the potential beneficiaries of its increasingly costly productivity; hence, the prolonged modern debate among medical scientists, practitioners, hospital administrators, boards of trustees, patients, and governments over the purpose, funding and control of, and access to hospital facil-ities.

The debate has produced different conclusions in different constituencies. In Can-ada, provincially administered universal hospital insurance schemes jointly funded by the federal government were first implemented in 1958. This followed a decade of intermittent federal-provincial negotiations in response to a health-care crisis which had been identified and studied intensively in the aftermath of the Great Depression and which subsequently became the focus of the federal Liberal government's plan for postwar social reconstruction (see Taylor 1978).

In the province of Ontario, at least, universal hospitalization insurance and the health-care system it was intended to sustain displaced in 1959 an earlier system that was a classic example of the transformation of the hospital from a Victorian secular charity for the indigent and working poor into a 'workplace for the production of health' (Starr 1982) for all members of the community. Most importantly, that earlier transformation had involved a redefinition of the relationship of the middle class to the voluntary public general hospital. Once merely patrons of the sick poor, providing material and moral support for the Victorian hospital, the middle class by the 1920s had become essential, as consumers of hospital care, to the new economics of medical progress. In this new situation, the costs of providing modern care to all sectors of the population had to be unevenly distributed between those who could afford to pay for hospital care and those who could not. The willingness of the middle class to bear this burden was the product not only of their recent perception of the inestimable promise of modern medical science, but also of the tangible evidence, in the form of preferen-tial accommodation and care at affordable rates, that they could avoid the Victorian stigma of poverty and dependence associated with the public wards and their non-pay-ing clientele.

Even as this transformation was taking place, however, its promises threatened increasingly to slip from the grasp of the middle class. The community general hospi-tal, statutorily bound as it was to treat, in return for public support, every citizen seeking medical care, could not divest itself of its historical identity as a charitable enterprise. At the same time, government social policies continued from the 1870s until the 1950s to define the hospitalization of indigents as a community responsibility primarily dependent on the deployment of hospital resources for medical philanthropy well below the rapidly escalating costs of providing 'scientific' medical care to all patients, and sharply differentiated care to some. As those costs mounted, public hospitals, unable to recover their fees for maintaining indigent patients, responded by repetitively increasing the tariff for paying patients. By the onset of the Depression, Ontario's hospitals claimed that they could no longer deliver efficient, social-structurally, differentiated care to the 'great middle class of self-respecting people' at prices they could afford (see Ontario Royal Commission on Public Welfare 1930) and as these preferred clients increasingly resisted hospitalization on those terms, the hospitals and their middle-class supporters became increasingly voluble proponents of any scheme that would preserve the benefits of modern hospital care for 'patients of moderate means.' It is sometimes argued that government-administered health insurance in Canada arose out of the political necessity, after 1945, to provide a 'social wage' for working-class Canadians (Coburn et al. 1983). Much of the evidence associated with the social history of hospitals in Ontario suggests that the debate also focused significantly on the threatened medical impoverishment of the middle class after 1930.

The timing of this transformation of the hospital from a one-class custodial-care facility into the temple of scientific medicine and the source of medical well-being for all social classes is a matter for debate. Among other factors, cultural biases and local circumstances, as much as sweeping scientific or technological change, dictated the pace of modernization. For example, judging by the preference among women for home births, the maternity ward was not a popular alternative before the end of the Second World War. It was not until the end of the Great Depression that even half the babies born in Ontario represented hospital births (Strong-Boag 1988). But some general developments had begun to make an impact on Ontario's emerging system of public general hospitals even before the end of the nineteenth century. For example, as early as 1885 the inspector of prisons and charities noted that 'there are now available in this country ladies of ability and experience, who have been systematically trained in nursing and the domestic management of hospitals' and who were more capable hospital administrators than either physicians or politicians (Ontario Legislative Assembly 1885). The inspectorate worried that nurses were receiving an excessively technical education which risked 'training out the woman and the nurse, and leaving behind a mischievous woman doctor' (Ontario Legislative Assembly 1890) but for all that, the professional hospital administrator, in the person of the lady superintendent, and the professional graduate nurse, some of them already highly specialized, were fixtures in the Ontario hospital system by 1890, promoting an administrative and patient management revolution essential to the emergence of the modern hospital. Similarly, well before the end of the nineteenth century, the inspectorate noted that at least some new hospitals were being erected according to the "modern and scientific principle of hospital construction," which included eliminating overcrowding by restricting public wards to a maximum of six patients, incorporating toilet and bathing facilities into the ward, and, in particular, providing a limited number of single private rooms for paying patients (Ontario Legislative Assembly 1896).

Safer hospitals offering professional care in an atmosphere of comfort and privacy while the patient convalesced were not in themselves a powerful inducement to the potential middle-class paying patron. Combined with the promise of the latest advances in scientific medical intervention, however, the social attributes of the modern hospital offered an increasingly attractive alternative to home care to the private patients of physicians who saw in this developing concentration of scientific expertise, medical skill, material resources, and efficient management a fitting focus for their own emerging professionalism.[1] Thus, as early as 1881, private physicians in Toronto began clamouring for the right to treat their private paying patients in the province's largest hospital, the Toronto General, with its newly organized medical departments staffed by consultants from the university's medical faculty and its recently inaugurated School of Nursing. The Hamilton Civic Hospital underwent a similar transition fifteen years later, when private physicians succeeded in overcoming the outright hostility of the hospital's appointed medical attendants to any intervention in their exclusive control of medical treatment in the institution (Crosbie 1975).[2]

The size and sophistication of these metropolitan institutions probably made them exceptional and, therefore, inaccurate gauges of the timing of this transformation of hospital care as it was experienced by the majority of the province's population. If we look for supporting evidence of the advent of the modern hospital in a smaller regional town, the timing of the transition, albeit delayed, seems nevertheless to fall well within the first two decades of this century. For example, the Owen Sound (population 10,000) General and Marine Hospital was established in 1893 as a charity for the sailors, travellers, teamsters, and westward-bound emigrants whose presence made the town one of the busiest ports on the Great Lakes between 1885 and 1912. By affording the community an opportunity to exercise its Christian obligations to the homeless sick, the hospital, according to its founders, was an instrument of collective happiness through the promulgation of good works (*Owen Sound Times* 1893). The rules governing the admission of patients and their behaviour while residents of the hospital (including the requirement that ambulatory patients would serve as the hospital's domestic servants) had more to do, however, with anticipating the threat of institutional social disorder posed by Owen Sound's 'great floating population' of homeless persons than with promoting an environment conducive to their effective treatment and convalescence (Owen Sound General and Marine Hospital 1891).[3]

This definition of 'The G&M' as fundamentally a charity for the custodial care of the sick poor, managed by a voluntary board of lay trustees, largely dependent on public goodwill for the success of the hospital's mission persisted at least until the eve of the First World War. But by 1914 the nature of the enterprise no longer conformed in fact to the rhetoric of selflessness the board of trustees routinely employed to convince citizens and their political leaders that the institution required and deserved ever larger public and private subventions to carry on its work. By 1905 the fees of paying private patients already had become the hospital's single most important source of income, contributing more to defraying the hospital's annual operating costs than the total income generated from municipal and provincial grants and private subscriptions (see Figure 1). The hospital's growing access to and dependence on income from patients' fees appears to reflect, in turn, three related developments: the rapid increase after 1900 of surgical and obstetric cases which became the hospital's *raison d'tre* by 1914; improvements in patient management which reduced the length of hospital stays by nearly 40 per cent between 1893 and 1908 and allowed the hospital to treat many more patients without increasing its actual capacity; and the developing perception, on the part of the town's physicians, that the Hospital was the preferred location for the treatment of their acutely ill private patients.

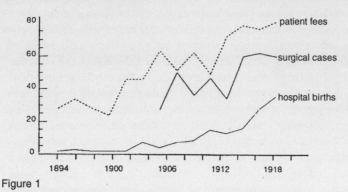

Figure 1
Income and admissions, Owen Sound General and Marine Hospital, 1894-1920

As early as 1904, Owen Sound's medical men had begun to lobby for the redefinition and restructuring of the hospital as a modern 'centre for the treatment of disease' with vastly improved operating facilities (*Owen Sound Times* 16 December 1904). Five years of inaction finally led them to vent their frustration not on the board of trustees, but on the lady superintendent (who was forced to resign) and her nursing students who stood accused of being both ignorant of, and incapable of implementing, the standards of antisepsis essential for 'scientific surgical techniques' (Owen Sound General and Marine Hospital, 4 May 1909). The doctors' newly articulated scientific imperative was a reflection of their developing professionalism which included, among other factors, the idea of the hospital rather than the physician's surgery or the patient's home as the most appropriate medical workshop. In Owen Sound, beginning about 1901 after the local surgeon returned from a sabbatical in Europe where he had studied the latest developments in modern surgery, the number of operations performed in the hospital each year began to increase dramatically. By 1908, more than half of the adult patients admitted to the G&M annually were surgical cases representing the recent (since 1890) advances made possible by an aseptic, or at least antiseptic, environment. Appendectomies, herniotomies, ovariotomies, mastectomies, and thyroidectomies became increasingly common procedures for the hospital's lone resident surgeon, a clear indication that even community hospitals staffed largely by general practitioners were now identified with up-to-date surgical intervention in cases of acute illness (Meade 1968).[4] Among the G&M's attending physicians, it became a matter of professional principle, after 1904, that scientific surgery was the business of the hospital.

At about the same time (1904), the women of Owen Sound, through a recently organized Ladies' Hospital Auxiliary, began to lobby as well for the inclusion of an obstetrics ward in the hospital, arguing that the G&M's medical ward, which lacked private accommodations and a separate nursery, was an unacceptable environment for maternity cases (Owen Sound General and Marine Hospital, 10 February 1904). Although nearly a quarter of a century would pass before even half of the births occurring in Owen Sound were hospital births, hospital maternity care, especially in difficult cases, was already an important option for those middle-class women who were active in hospital matters in the early part of the century. The extent of their commitment was reflected in the major addition to the G&M which was completed in 1911 and which contained private and semi-private accommodations for maternity patients offered at double the weekly rate for public-ward patients. In fact, the most conspicuous attributes of the newly refurbished hospital, which was heralded as the best 'evidence of progress' in one of Ontario's most progressive towns (*Owen Sound Times*, 6 July 1911) were its preponderance of private and semi-private rooms, its state-of-the-art surgical flat, its obstetrics ward, and its new schedule of differential fees emphasizing the preferential care available to paying patients in its private wards. This included special food from the hospital's new diet kitchen and greater individual attention from the G&M's staff of student nurses. The School of Nursing had been founded in 1901 to provide the hospital with a perpetual supply of inexpensive labour. During a decade of service earning much-needed extra income for the hospital as private-duty nurses in patients' homes, the students had helped to establish the advantages of professional over domestic nursing care in spite of the limitations of their own training.

By 1914, in short, the Owen Sound General and Marine Hospital had become an essentially 'modern' hospital in the sense that its transition from a socially useful to a medically indispensible institution was virtually complete.

By 1914, the G&M was advertising itself as 'the Best Hotel in the County,' an institution patronized by "the best citizens in every community," a hospital where those accustomed to private domestic care could receive 'All the Care a Home Can Provide, Without the Errors of Love' (Owen Sound General and Marine Hospital, 1920). It was also an institution which collected, after 1911, a week's fees in advance from all paying patients and retained a professional bill collection agency to recover the debts of any paying patient who continued to believe that the hospital was still a charitable enterprise (Owen Sound General and Marine Hospital, 21 December 1910 and 9 September 1914). Its board of trustees continued to insist, of course, that the G&M was still a medical charity. The fact that the well-to-do patient and the middle-class 'patient of moderate means' now patronised the hospital simply meant that the G&M was no longer a one-class institution; but the hospital's obligation to treat the poor remained, as did the community's responsibility to insure that the hospital continued to be accessible to the poor by providing the levels of support required to meet the full cost of their care and treatment (*Owen Sound Sun,* 2 April 1918).

In sum, the available evidence seems to suggest that the transformation of hospitals in Ontario, even those in rural areas, from refuges for the sick poor into citadels of scientific medicine took place over the course of no more than thirty years and was substantially complete by 1920, if not sooner. One might even choose the appearance in 1912 of the *Hospital World*, the first Canadian journal for hospital superintendents and lay trustees, as the symbolic demarcation of the modern from the historical era of hospital service. Its editor introduced the first issue with a random catalogue of questions which 'hospital workers the world over' needed to resolve. Who should pay for hospitals? Where, ideally, should hospitals be located? What was the preferable internal management structure for hospitals and their medical services? Should rich and poor patients be treated under the same roof? What was the most appropriate flooring for hospitals? Did physicians, graduate nurses, or laymen make the best superintendents? What was the optimum size for an operating room? Was the patient a 'person' or a 'case'; and what was the effect of 'institutionalism' on the patient's 'real self?' (*Hospital World,* January 1912). The journal, in short, was a public forum for the concerns of hospital professionals charged with managing a health-care revolution.

At the heart of that revolution was the developing social, economic and cultural interdependence of hospitals and their new paying middle-class patrons. Just how important this clientele had become to Ontario's 101 public general hospitals by 1920 may be inferred from the available provincial data on hospital finances and hospital usage (see Table 1). In 1880, total general hospital income in Ontario was just over $120,000, of which patient fees accounted for less than 10 per cent. By 1900, total income was approaching $600,000, of which patient fees contributed about one-third. By 1915, income had leaped to nearly $2.5 million, more than half of it representing the fees of pay patients. This exponential increase in total income obviously reflects the rapid diffusion of public general hospitals throughout Ontario after 1900 in response to public demand. But the growing proportion of that income attributable to patient fees, and the steadily declining annual number of provincially subsidized indigent patient-stay days suggest a hospital system undergoing a significant change of clientele as well as demand – a system, in fact, dependent for its survival on an imbalance of paying patients. (Interestingly, the steadily downward trend in average patient stays, undoubtedly the result of more efficient patient management, may also reflect the shorter stays of a predominantly paying, as opposed to a predominantly dependent, clientele.) Demand, including the demand for a higher quality of hospital service, engendered higher operating costs. Alternatively, the need to attract paying patients, in order to finance 'modernization,' involved expensive upgrading. In either case, push or pull, the result was the same. Average operating costs per patient day began to escalate dramatically around 1900 and continued to do so until the early 1920s. The growth in patient fees as a proportion of both total income and total contributions to annual operating costs reflects the hospitals' success in generating the revenue necessary to sustain this process of modernization. It seems reasonable to conclude that in the course of just two decades the dependence of the sick poor on the benevolence of the hospital's charity had been superceded by a much more symbiotically dependent relationship between the hospital as provider, and the middle-class patient as consumer, of the new medicine.

By the end of the First World War, Ontario's public hospitals had come to regard the widening gap between the rate of increase of their annual expenditures for maintenance and the much slower growth of public funding for the care of the indigent and working poor as a serious liability resulting from an anachronistic interpretation of their role in society. To make matters worse, in the mid-1920s the proportion of patient days attributable to patients subsidized at the statutory rate, after declining from 90 per cent to less than 45 per cent between 1890 and 1920, underwent a significant reversal. Widely regarded as a period of general prosperity, the 1920s, judged by the reversal of the trend in free admissions to Ontario's hospitals, must have exacerbated the structures of inequality in provincial society. Whatever the reason, although hospitals experienced a major increase in the number of admissions per 1000 of population between 1925 and 1930 (see Figure 2), the increase represented larger numbers of patients to be maintained at or below cost rather than at the hospitals' preferred rates based on the costs of maintaining full-pay patients. After several years of modest annual operating surpluses across the system, the hospitals in the early 1920s began to incur deficits. At the same time, municipal contributions, as a proportion of total hospital income, declined nearly 15 per cent. Private subscriptions and donations followed a parallel course (see Figure 3). Neither event was offset by a modest increase in provincial funding after 1925. Hospital administrators and trustees swiftly concluded that the process of fiscal and medical modernization that they had set in motion thirty years earlier was in jeopardy (*Canadian Hospital* 1927).

TABLE 1
Admissions, patient stays, income and expenditures
Ontario public general hospitals, 1880-1950

	1880*	1890	1900	1910	1920	1930	1941	1946
Number of patients admitted	5,302	9,094	29,572	52,321	130,459	215,623	254,598	408,551
Admissions per thousand pop'n	2.8	4.3	13.6	20.9	45.1	63.8	60.4	75.1
Average stay (days)	35	30	24	20	15	14	14	12
Avg. cost per patient day ($)	0.57	0.71	0.76	1.30	2.84	3.65	3.47	5.03
Avg. income per patient day ($)	0.66	0.82	0.81	1.25	2.82	3.97	3.84	5.58
Sources of annual income (%)								
municipalities	25.5	25.4	16.2	20.1	17.6	14.9	16.3	10.5
province	18.3	10.6	6.3	10.6	6.0	8.2	6.3	4.7
subscriptions/gifts	15.8	16.5	26.4	13.4	9.5	6.7	4.9	5.1
investments/interest	10.4	8.6	3.6	4.2	2.1	2.2	2.9	2.2
patients' fees	9.0	18.1	35.3	51.7	64.8	68.0	69.6	77.5
Proportion of patient days subsidized by province (%)	84.8	90.7	79.3	63.5	44.7	51.7	37.2	10.5
Patients fees as % of maintenance costs	10.4	20.8	37.7	49.6	64.2	74.0	77.1	86.0

*Data for years up to 1939 are for twelve months preceeding 30 Sept. of year noted.
Source: Province of Ontario, Legislative Assembly, *Sessional Papers*, Annual Reports of Returns to Inspector of Prisons and Charities and Department of Health, 1880-1946

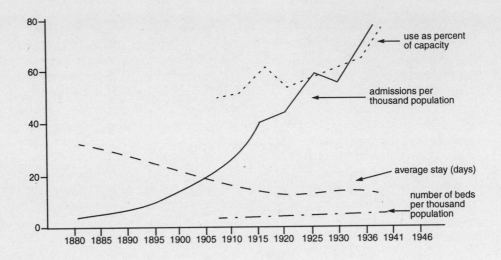

Figure 2
Admissions and utilization, Ontario public general hospitals, 1880-1946

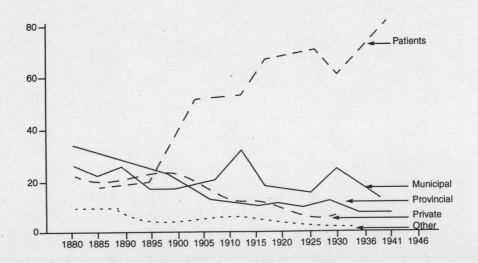

Figure 3
Contributions (%) to total annual income by source, Ontario public general hospitals, 1880-1946

Not only were the fees charged to paying patients subsidizing the maintenance of free patients, but total income from all sources was only adequate to fund an essentially static, not an improving, enterprise in an era of medical progress. Further improvement demanded either higher user fees or higher levels of municipal and provincial government subsidization of the costs of maintaining indigent patients.

It is especially important to recognize that these developments took place well before the Great Depression of the 1930s, because it is too often assumed that the Depression itself was responsible for both the crisis in hospital financing and the ensuing debates over social and economic responsibility for health care in general, and for the care of charity patients in particular (Taylor 1978; Taylor 1957). In fact, on the eve of the First World War it was already recognized, among hospital administrators and their boards of trustees, at the very least, that the revolution in hospital usage and hospital-based medical services demanded a parallel revolution in hospital funding. Speaking to his colleagues in 1912, the president of the Canadian Hospital Association (founded in 1906) accurately anticipated the modern health-care crisis and understood both its source and its long-range solution. 'Step by step patients have been gaining confidence in hospitals,' he noted, and 'the end is not yet [in sight]. The closing years of this century ... will be marked by an enormous increase in the number of institutions for the care of the sick ... In order to maintain this ever increasing number of institutions, larger and still larger sums of money will be needed. This will necessitate the educating of the people ... into more liberal support of hospitals ... If hospitals are to advance and keep up their present standard of efficiency there must be more money forthcoming.' (*Hospital World* 1912b) The rest of the speech repeated what had already become a familiar theme in the discourse of American hospital administrators: if hospitals became models of institutional economy and efficiency as well as purveyors of the most advanced medical treatment available, they could not fail in their humanitarian, scientific, or financial objectives. What is of particular significance, however, is that it was still possible, in 1912, for the speaker to assume that a combination of fiscal responsibility and social utility – the hallmarks of the Victorian charitable hospital – would continue to prove attractive to both government and private philanthropists as the historical and future sources of the hospitals' economic security (*Hospital World* 1912b; Rosenberg 1981).

Fifteen years later, all of the available evidence seemed to suggest to the president of the Ontario Hospital Association that it was neither realistic nor useful to continue to perceive hospital economics in this traditional context. The idea of the hospital as an object and dispenser of charity was as obsolete, he contended, as the government department (Prisons and Charities) to which it reported. The purpose of the modern hospital, he insisted, was to provide the best diagnostic and therapeutic facilities available at cost to those patients who paid the full cost of their care. Medical philanthropy was no longer the only, nor even the most significant aspect of a hospital's mandate, he argued; but it decidedly had become the principal hindrance to the achievement of the hospital's legitimate goals. Government's refusal to subsidize the full cost of treating the indigent forced hospitals to overcharge paying patients and to divert the additional income to the support of charity cases. The result, higher costs for the hospitals' largest group of clients, 'people of moderate means,' threatened to make health care inaccessible to them and, consequently, to deprive hospitals of their preferred patients and their most important source of income (*Canadian Hospital* 1927a).

Clearly, in the intervening fifteen years between these two commentaries, the middle classes' demand for, or susceptibility to the promise of, preferential care based on the ability to pay had become, in the minds of hospital professionals at least, not only a critical factor in hospital economics but a powerful new engine of medical progress. To unleash its potential, however, hospitals first had to rid themselves of the financial burden imposed by their historical social obligation to those unable to pay for medical care at any price, and for whose care municipal and provincial governments provided inadequate compensation. The Ontario Hospital Association estimated in 1926 that the cost to its member hospitals of subsidizing the care of non-pay patients was $1.3 million (*Canadian Hospital* 1928). The objective was not to deny them access to hospitals. Instead, the hospitals set out to appeal to middle-class self-interest in order to bring about statutory changes in government social policy, changes that would explicitly acknowledge that hospitals were no longer charitable enterprises. Rather, they were centres for the scientific treatment of disease among all classes of the population at a fair price in relation to the value of their product and the ability of the consumer to pay the full cost of non-profit treatment. As one hospital administrator put it, 'legitimate business principles should ... be applied to our hospitals ... The hospital has [a] very necessary service to render ... and the recipient must pay.' If this seemed out of character with the ideal of hospital service, he suggested, then it was time that hospitals clearly distinguished between the idealism reflected in the hospitals' commitment to scientific professionalism and the realities of hospital economics. In practical terms, this meant that the full cost of caring for those who could not pay was the community's, not the hospital's nor the paying patient's, responsibility (*Canadian Hospital* 1926).

Coincidentally, the Canadian Medical Association took up the same line of argument on behalf of the hospitals. 'I am convinced that we have gone about far enough in the direction of free treatment,' its president announced in 1927. Drawing a distinction between the 'provident' and the 'non-provident' sick, he argued that the 'Robin Hood' principal of 'supertaxing' the paying middle-class patient to support the sick poor was 'inadequate for the distribution of scientific medical care' in the twentieth century, and was specifically responsible for hospitals that were 'half filled with people who cannot, or will not, or do not pay.' The effect was to distract the hospital, once 'the dispenser of charity to the few,' from 'becoming a dispenser of medical science to all' through the transference of sickness from the home to the 'specially-equipped centre,' just as the industrial revolution had transferred the workshop to the factory, and compulsory education had displaced learning from the home to the public school. The 'team-work of the well-equipped hospital' and the 'efficiency of specialism' were valueless while hospitals remained refuges 'for the poor and the rich, but impossible for all between.' Consequently, the most difficult problem of modern social administration, he contended, was ensuring that 'more hospitals became real community health centres' for the 'ordinary sick citizen' (*Canadian Medical Association Journal* 1927).

Physicians' concerns about these matters arose from somewhat different, albeit related, sources from those of hospital administrators. The medical profession now accepted that hospitals were 'the agents through which the latest achievements of science are made available in the treatment of the sick by the profession' and that doctors denied access to the 'group practice' made possible by up-to-date hospitals laboured under a severe professional handicap (McKenty 1927). Hospitals rendered inaccessible to the private physician's paying patients as the result of either a shortage of beds or inflated charges attributable to the hospitals' charitable obligations were equally inaccessible to the physician himself except as a dispenser of charity. There were no easy answers, and the CMA had even supported the idea of state medicine in the past; but in the mid-1920s private enterprise was in the ascendant among doctors who found themselves in agreement with the solution put forward by hospital administrators (Naylor 1986). Government should entirely subsidize basic hospitalization and medical care for the deserving poor so that what 'the middle-class people are looking for' – a hospital 'where medical skill would be adequate, the accommodation comfortable and the patients would not be haunted with the spectre of 'the cost''' – would serve the self-interest of the doctor, the paying patient and the hospital alike (*Canadian Hospital* 1927b). As Charles Rosenberg has amply demonstrated, questioning the moral basis of medical charity on the grounds that its recipients were improvident and, therefore, 'undeserving malingerers' who distracted the hospital from its appointment with destiny, was the last stage in the transformation of the American hospital from a social to a medical institution (Rosenberg 1981).

With the Depression in full sway, municipal responsibility for a guaranteed minimum standard of health care for every citizen was scarcely a proposal whose time had arrived. Between 1928 and 1929 alone, the number of indigents seeking free medical care in general hospitals had increased 10 per cent (*Canadian Hospital* 1931a). Then, in 1931, the provincial government repealed the Hospital and Charitable Institutions Act and replaced it with the Public Hospitals Act. Essentially, the new act repeated most of the provisions of its predecessor; but in fourteen detailed and lengthy clauses it spelled out a far more rigorous set of municipal obligations for the maintenance in hospital of sick municipal indicants and their dependents, clearly compounding the already crushing burden of depression-induced municipal relief. By 1936, the proportion of patient days for which hospitals claimed municipal subsidies had risen to 63 per cent. Municipal statutory payments to general hospitals doubled. Ironically, in spite of the fact that total hospital revenues declined marginally between 1930 and 1936, a higher proportion of subsidized patient days together with depression-induced institutional economies produced the kind of year-end balance sheets that administrators and trustees preferred, and to some extent demonstrated the validity of the hospitals' arguments regarding government funding. Nevertheless, the hospitals had surrendered, even if only temporarily, their much-publicized image as scientific, not social, institutions and they became even more insistent on additional public funding to subsidize the full cost of maintaining indigent patients in order to provide more economical care for, and to retain the patronage of, the paying 'patient of average means' (see *Canadian Hospital*, 1931b; 1936). By 1936, according to hospital professionals, this person, unable and unwilling to subsidize indigents by paying higher fees and unwilling to accept charity as a public-ward patient, appeared to be avoiding hospitals at any possible cost.

Again, the experience of the Owen Sound General and Marine Hospital during the Depression illustrates many of the problems encountered by both hospitals and their patients. At the height of the Depression, in 1933, more than 2000 men, women, and children – 17 per cent of the city's population – were on relief (*Owen Sound Daily Sun-Times* 7 January 1933). From the earliest days of the Depression the city's costs of medical relief had frequently run to 50 per cent of monthly expenditures on welfare and, by 1933, annual municipal payments to the G&M for the care of indigents were 66 per cent higher than they had been in the years immediately preceding the Depression (*Owen Sound Daily Sun-Times* 15 November and 12 December 1930; Ontario Inspector of Hospitals 1929-35). One result was that the hospital's total annual income in 1933 was virtually the same as its income in 1929, in spite of a 12 per cent decrease in annual admissions and, much more importantly, in spite of a 21 per cent reduction in annual income from fees attributable to paying patients (Ontario Sound General and Marine Hopsital 1919-33). Patterns of hospital morbidity during the Depression offer similar evidence of a departure from the patterns of hospitalization established before 1929 and the G&M's reversion to the role of custodian of the sick poor. As Table 2 illustrates, the proportion of patients admitted annually to the hospital during the Depression with unspecified or undetermined illnesses was significantly higher than normal, and a very limited range of acute illnesses accounted for a much higher proportion of total admissions in 1931 and 1936 than in 1941. These observations suggest a hospital increasingly used by physicians as a convenient refuge for patients seeking medical charity, and by paying patients only in cases of urgent medical necessity. When admissions patterns and income began to return to normal in 1936-7, the G&M's legacy from the Depression was an accumulated deficit of about $16,000, most of it ($12,900) representing, not the price of treating indigents below cost, but the uncollectible accounts of 'paying' patients (Owen Sound Daily Sun-Times 24 October 1956).

A formal study undertaken by the Ontario Department of Health in 1936 and concluded in 1940 indicates that the experience of the G&M had been shared by Ontario's public hospitals generally. Among a province-wide sample of more than 50,000 patients discharged from general hospitals in 1938, self-pay patients comprised only 56 per cent.

TABLE 2
Patterns of hospital morbidity (%) selected diseases, G&M Hospital, 1930-40

	1930-1	1935-6	1941
Nervous/sensory system	5	3	6
Respiratory disease	17	19	17
Digestive system	12	11	13
Genito-urinary	5	7	8
Pregnancy/puerperium	15	15	24
Accidental injury	8	2	10
Not stated	30	37	4
Total	92	94	82

Source: General and Marine Hospital, Admissions Registers, 1930, 1935, 1941

'The financial control applied voluntarily or involuntarily to themselves by paying patients ... is undoubtedly important in keeping hospitalization among them to the present level,' the analyst reported, noting that the average length of hospital stay among paying patients had also declined significantly, while the same statistic for indigent patients had increased markedly during the 'recession.' (Ontario Survey of General Hospitals 1940) He conceded that demographic factors such as population ageing, medical considerations including physical debilitation, and even social variables such as a 'weak psychological stimulus for recovery' were all responsible for the increase in the duration of hospital stays among the poor, which was the source of the hospitals' reversion to the role of custodial care facilities and of municipal governments' mounting expenditures on medical relief (Ontario Survey of General Hospitals 1940). This phenomenon was to be interpreted, however, primarily as a consequence of temporary economic conditions which would shortly be alleviated. What was needed in the interim, the study concluded, was, first, the imposition of longer waiting periods for eligibility and shorter periods of support for patients seeking medical philanthropy, and, second, municipal regulation and policing of the hospitals themselves to eliminate waste, inefficiency, and the 'long-stay' indigent (Ontario Survey of General Hospitals 1940). These conclusions confirmed the hospitals' worst fears. In general, hospitals were accused by patients of being too business-like, even heartless and mercenary; by the government, of being wasteful and inefficient; by the poor, of being institutions for the rich; and by the middle class, of being designed only for the poor or the wealthy. In this situation, mere public relations, a new aspect of hospital work in the 1930s, was no longer an adequate response (Canadian Hospital 1937).

All of these factors promoted a growing interest among various constituencies in national, provincial, or private health-insurance schemes. Each of these solutions was widely canvassed during the Depression.   The federal government, the Ontario Hospital Association, and the Canadian Medical Association's Committee on Economics, among others, investigated the merits of health insurance, and generally supported the idea (Naylor 1986; *Canadian Hospital* 1932; 1939). Indeed, as early as 1932 a spokesman for the Ontario Department of Health anticipated an imminent 'workable scheme of national health insurance' as 'the next, and let us hope final, stage of [the hospitals'] transition' (*Ontario Health* 1934). But another decade passed before Prime Minister WLM King created an Advisory Committee on Health Insurance to consult widely on the matter. The Heagerty Committee's Report included a draft health insurance bill which provided, among its other benefits, for a full range of hospital services (Canada Advisory Committee on Health Insurance 1943). The proposal was welcomed, at least in principle, by the Canadian Hospital Council, whose objective was to preserve the autonomy and advance the mission of Canada's non-profit, voluntary, and 'democratic' public hospitals. Their trustees, the council's spokesman contended, had become 'discouraged' by the controversy over who should pay for indigent patients, and their 'patients of moderate means' had become handicapped, in the face of the escalating costs of hospital care, by their inability to budget for unanticipated sickness (Canada Special Committee on Social Security 1943). In an interesting refinement of these arguments, the expert adviser to the House of Common's Special Committee on Social Security, Leonard Marsh, subsequently concluded that while the improvement in national efficiency that would result from better health care for low-income Canadians represented the 'general case' for a national scheme of health insurance, the well-documented inability of the average wage-earner ... to provide adequate medical care for ... his family' constituted the 'special case' for a program of national health insurance (Canada Special Committee on Social Security 1943).

The Heagerty Committee's report did not bear fruit until 1955, when a federal-provincial conference finally promoted political agreement on a national hospital insurance scheme. In the meantime, private carriers such as Associated Medical Services (whose program was launched during the Depression) and non-profit insurance schemes such as Blue Cross (organized by the Canadian Hospital Association) had begun to provide voluntary group hospitalization insurance coverage through employers. By 1948 one in every five patients – one in every four paying patients – admitted to a public general hospital in Ontario carried some form of hospitalization insurance (Ontario, Ministry of Health 1950: Table A7, 23). One apparent effect can be seen in the proportion of private and semi-private ward patients – 50 per cent – admitted to public general hospitals in 1948. Their average per diem room charges, in a typical Toronto hospital for example, were subject to average surcharges of 44 per cent for extra services (Ontario, Ministry of Health 1950 Table A4, 21). In Owen Sound, where contributory group hospital insurance was identified as the cause of 'an appalling short-age' of hospital beds by 1950 (*Owen Sound Daily Sun-Times* 10 April 1950; Owen Sound General and Marine Hospital, 1949), surcharges for pharmaceuticals, laboratory services, and medical/surgical sundries added 35 per cent to the accounts of paying patients who might pay an additional surcharge of 21 per cent for delivery or operating room services. Together with the hospital's basic maintenance charges, these fees comprised 96 per cent of the G&M's annual revenues by 1955. (Calculated from data reported in *Owen Sound Daily Sun-Times* 6 April 1956) The newly insured patient of average means and his insurer continued to subsidize, to an even greater extent than before, the cost of conducting the hospital's business and, for 10 per cent of its patients, its philanthropic obligations as a still charitable enterprise.

The Ontario Health Survey Committee appointed to investigate 'the state of hospital business in Ontario' reported in 1950 that a critical shortage of acute-care beds had developed because the mechanisms for financing the work of the province's general hospitals had failed to keep pace with the public's perception of the social and medical utility of hospitals 'in recent years.' 'Both patients and physicians have come to depend increasingly upon hospital service... Doctors prefer working in hospitals because they provide a wider range of modern laboratory techniques and procedures than was previously available, and in hospitals they have the benefit of consultation with specialists. Patients are more inclined to seek hospitalization today because overcrowding and other circumstances in many homes combine with a shortage of suitably-trained help to make home nursing care impracticable' (Health Survey Committee 1950). The major problem confronting Ontario's public general hospitals in the face of this new demand for their services, the committee concluded, was the unfair system of provincial and municipal grants which forced hospitals to overcharge paying patients in order to subsidize the costs of maintaining public ward patients (Health Survey Committee 1950: 32).

It seems remarkable that these themes should have been rehearsed in 1950, as new phenomena, to explain a problem that had been a subject of open and often vigorous debate between the province's general hospitals, the public, and their elected representatives at least since the mid-1920s. The transformation of Ontario's public general hospitals – from one-class custodial-care facilities promoting a form of social control in response to the conditions of a rapidly urbanizing and industrializing population, to centres of scientific medicine for the treatment of acute disease, at a price, among all classes of the population – was virtually complete on the eve of the First World War. At the outset of that transitional process, hospital administrators and trustees had deliberately courted the paying middle-class patient as the source of hospital modernization with the promise of efficient, efficacious, social-structurally differentiated health care based on the ability to pay. By the 1920s, however, maintaining accessibility, in terms of the cost of differential care, for the paying middle-class patient had become a difficult proposition in the face of mounting operating losses driven by the growing demand for hospital care, by the price of medical innovation, and above all by the failure of governments to accept full responsibility for the hospitalization of the sick poor. Both the morality and the practical economics of taxing their principal benefactors in order to perpetuate the hospitals' charitable obligations rather than to provide more 'efficient' hospital service seemed, to hospital professionals and lay trustees at least, entirely inconsistent with their aspirations to maintain the hospital as an appropriate institutional embodiment of the progress of scientific medicine in modern society. Consequently, long before the Great Depression brought the question into bold relief as a matter of national social policy, hospitals and their paying patients had begun to ask, as a matter of self-interest, whether those consumers who could not pay for good health would become charges against the public purse or remain dependent on the hospital's fast-fading identity as a once charitable institution whose paying 'patients of moderate means' would bear the costs of perpetuating this anachronism. Those costs might include soaring hospital maintenance charges for differential care, less progressive treatment, and the stigma, ultimately, of undifferentiated, subsidized public-bed care.

. The social circumstances created by the Depression exacerbated the question of the hospital's responsibility for medical philanthropy, just as improved social and economic conditions during and after the Second World War, and the resultant demand for affordable hospital care, reopened the debate over the relative claims of the poor, the rich, and those in between on a system straining to accommodate all. As the foregoing analysis suggests, whatever else it did, the advent of national health insurance in the 1950s preserved the self-respect of the middling classes. They had invented the Victorian hospital, supported its mission through their voluntary subscriptions and managerial participation, supervised its transformation into a modern community health-care centre, and nurtured its aspirations to become the principal source for all classes of the population, not least of all themselves, of the humanitarian benefits of scientific medicine. By 1930, their 'moderate means' had ceased to guarantee them access, on social, cultural, and economic terms acceptable to them, to the first-class health care that the transformation of the public general hospital between 1890 and 1920 had promised.

Notes

1 Historians disagree on the sequence of events. Vogel argues that the middle class discovered the hospital in advance of any medical necessity to resort to hospital care. David Rosner in 'Business at the Bedside: Health Care in Brooklyn, 1890-1915,' *Health Care in America: Essays in Social History*, ed. Susan Reverby and David Rosner (Philadelphia 1979), argues that hospital facilities attracted physicians who in turn referred their patients in exchange for hospital privileges.

2 The Toronto General and Hamilton Civic hospitals make an interesting contrast in the history of the development of large inner-city hospitals in the period. For the Hamilton Civic see, in addition to the annual reports of the inspector of hospitals, the *Hamilton Spectator*, 1890-1900, and the Minutes of the Hamilton City Council, 1885-1900.

3 I am grateful to the board of trustees of the Grey and Bruce Regional Health Centre for giving me access to the historical records of the now defunct Owen Sound General and Marine Hospital (OSGMH).

4 By 1915 the hospital had begun to list in its annual reports the surgical procedures carried out each year.

Acknowledgements

I wish to acknowledge the generosity of the Canadian Studies in Wales Group who provided me with a happy milieu in which to explore the social history of medicine in the fall term of 1986. My colleagues, Dean Peter George and Dr. Rosemary Gagan, commented on the original draft of this paper but cannot be held responsible for its continuing shortcomings. The essay first appeared as an informal working paper of McMaster University's Research Consortium for Quantitative Studies in Economics and Population.

References

Abel-Smith, B. 1964. *The Hospitals, 1800-1948: A Study in Social Administration in England and Wales.* Cambridge: Harvard University Press.

Canada Advisory Committee on Health Insurance. 1943. Ottawa: Canada House of Commons, Special Committee on Social Security, Health Insurance: Report of the Advisory Committee on Health Insurance.

Canada Special Committee on Social Security. 1943. Minutes of Proceedings and Evidence, No 6, 9 April, 174–175.

Canadian Hospital. 1926. A Hospital Problem. Survey 3 (February):12.

Canadian Hospital. 1927a. Hospitals Handicapped by Meagre Grants. 4: 11–12.

Canadian Hospital. 1927b. Paying the Hospital Bill. 4 (November) 9.

Canadian Hospital. 1928. Representative Deputation Presses Claims at Parliament Buildings. 5 (February): 14.

Canadian Hospital. 1931a. Rates and Index Numbers of Hospital Charges Throughout Canada. 8 (May): 10.

Canadian Hospital. 1931b. Hospital Service to the Patient of Average Means. 8 (August): 12–18.

Canadian Hospital. 1932. Health Insurance Survey Completed by McGill Expert. 9 (June):11.

Canadian Hospital. 1936. Hospital Current Revenues. 13 (May): 11–13.

Canadian Hospital. 1937. Public Relations. 14 (October): 64.

Canadian Hospital. 1939. The Proposed Hospital Care Plan for Ontario. 16 (June): 28.

Canadian Medical Association Journal. 1927. The Care of the Sick. 17 (January): 94–97.

Coburn, D, G Torrance, and J Kaufert. 1983. Medical Dominance in Canada in Historical Perspective: The Rise and Fall of Medicine. *International Journal of Health Services* 13: 407–432.

Crosbie, WG. 1975. *The Toronto General Hospital, 1819-1865: A Chronicle.* Toronto, 68-113.

Health Survey Committee. 1950a. Report of the Ontario Health Survey Committee. 1950: 57.

Health Survey Committee. 1950b. Report of the Ontario Health Survey Committee. 1950: 32.

Hospital Care in Canada. 1960. Recent Trends and Developments, Health Care Series Memorandum No 12, Ottawa.

Hospital World. 1912a. Salutatory. 1 (January): 1–5.

Hospital World. 1912b. President's Address. 1 (May): 307, 311.

McKenty, J. 1927. The Relations of the Medical Profession to Hospitals. *Canadian Medical Association Journal* 17: 151–152.

Meade, RH. 1968. *An Introduction to the History of General Surgery.* Philadelphia: Saunders.

Naylor, CD. 1986. *Private Practice. Public Payment. Canadian Medicine and the Politics of Health Insurance, 1911 -1966.* Kingston, Ont: McGill-Queen's University Press.

Ontario, Department of Health, Division of Medical Statistics. 1940a. *A Survey of General Hospitals.* Toronto.

Ontario Department of Health. 1934. *The Hospitals of Ontario: A Short History.* Toronto, 19–20.

Ontario Inspector of Hospitals. *Annual reports, 1929–35.*

Ontario Legislative Assembly. 1880. *Sessional Papers. Annual Reports of the Provincial Inspector of Hospitals and Charities, 1880–90.*

Ontario Legislative Assembly. 1885. *Sessional Papers.* 39, OSP.

Ontario Legislative Assembly. 1890. *Sessional Papers.* 14: 52.

Ontario Legislative Assembly. 1896. *Sessional Papers.* 36: np.

Ontario Ministry of Health. 1950. *Report of the Ontario Health Survey Committee.* Vol. 1, Toronto.

Ontario Royal Commission on Public Welfare. 1930. *Report.* Toronto, 15.

Owen Sound Daily Sun-Times. 1930. 15 November; 12 December.

Owen Sound Daily Sun-Times. 1933. 7 January.

Owen Sound Daily Sun-Times. 1936. 24 October.

Owen Sound Daily Sun-Times. 1950. April.

Owen Sound Daily Sun-Times. 1956. Calculated from revenue breakdowns reported in auditors report to annual meeting, 6 April.

Owen Sound General and Marine Hospital. 1891. *Bylaws and Regulations,* 11 April.

Owen Sound General and Marine Hospital. 1904. *Minutes,* 10 February.

Owen Sound General and Marine Hospital. 1909. *Board of Trustees, Minutes.* 4 May.

Owen Sound General and Marine Hospital. 1910-27. *Annual Reports, 1910–27.*

Owen Sound General and Marine Hospital. 1910b. *Board of Trustees, Minutes.* 21 December.

Owen Sound General and Marine Hospital. 1914. *Board of Trustees, Minutes.* 9 September.

Owen Sound General and Marine Hospital. 1920. *Annual Reports.*

Owen Sound General and Marine Hospital. 1949. *Annual reports 1919–33,* as reported in Daily Sun-Times and OSGMH, Board of Trustees, Minutes.

Owen Sound Times. 1893. 22 June.

Owen Sound Times. 1904. 16 December.

Owen Sound Times. 1911. 6 July.

Owen Sound Sun. 1918. 2 April.

Report of Medical Staff. 1949. *Owen Sound General and Marine Hospital Miscellaneous Reports,* for 1949 (undated 1950).

Rosen, G. 1967. People, Disease and Emotion: Some Newer Problems for Research in Medical History. *Bulletin of the History of Medicine* 41: 8–9.

Rosenberg, CE. 1977. "And Heal the Sick": The Hospital and the Patient in 19th Century America. *Journal of Social History* 10 (June).

Rosenberg, CE. 1981. Inward Vision and Outward Glance: The Shaping of the American Hospital, 1880-1914. In DJ Rothman and S Wheeler eds. *Social History and Social Policy.* New York.

Starr, P. 1982. *The Social Transformation of American Medicine.* New York: Basic Books.

Starr, P. 1977. Medicine, Economy and Society in Nineteenth-Century America. In P Branca ed. *The Medicine Show.* New York: Science History Publications/U.S.A.

Strong-Boag, V. 1988. *The New Day Recalled: The Lives of Girls and Women in English Canada, 1919-1939.* Toronto, 155–161.

Taylor, MG. 1978. *Health Insurance and Canadian Public Policy: The Seven Decisions that Created the Canadian Health Insurance System.* Montreal: Queen's University Press.

Taylor, MG. 1957. The Hospital Challenge For the Future. *Canadian Hospital* 54 (January): 33.

Vogel, MJ. 1980. *The Invention of the Modern Hospital: Boston, 1870-1930.* Chicago: University of Chicago Press.

24

Hospitals As Health Factories[*]

G. Torrance

Introduction

The previous version of this paper predicted that "... hospitals will continue to hold their own, as centres not only of highly specialized inpatient treatment but also as locations for significant amounts of outpatient care." This prediction has been challenged by subsequent developments. A dramatic change is taking place, appearing to slow or even reverse 100 years of growth in size, technology and budgets. As Ginzberg notes there is a perception that "... the hospital sector is about to undergo a catastrophic change, one that will dislodge the acute care hospital from the centre of the health care delivery system to the periphery" (Ginsberg 1995: 11).

Nevertheless, hospitals still remain the largest component of the Canadian health-care system. They employ two-thirds of all the workers in the health industry and account for a high proportion of total expenditures on health. They are a big industry in the Canadian economy. In over 1,200 separate "plants" scattered across the country, hospitals employ approximately 468,000 full- and part-time workers. This represents a bigger part of the labour force than that employed in many primary and secondary industries – for instance, more than are employed in auto manufacturing, iron and steel mills, and pulp and paper mills combined. If institutions closely related to hospitals, such as nursing homes, homes for the aged, and homes for special care are added the total is even more impressive.

In 1967, Freidson applied the term "health factories" to large hospitals and referred to studies of their operations as "the new industrial sociology." In using the industrial analogy, Freidson (1967) was particularly concerned with what the rationalization of services did to patients who became objects of depersonalized care. Our concern in this chapter is to explore in a simpler sense how the industrial analogy applies to modern general hospitals. The emphasis is on their changing character as workplaces, rather than as people-processing institutions, and we focus particularly on the large category of hospital workers outside patient-care settings.

The purpose of this chapter is to provide a brief overview of some rarely discussed aspects of the hospital work world. Two theoretical themes underlie the analysis. One is the transformation of hospitals in size, technology, and structure – factors affecting the intrinsic aspects of work – from small, simple organizations to large, bureaucratized, technologically complex industries. The second theme involves the staffing system, the social mechanisms used to recruit, retain, and

[*] Revised from the second edition for this volume.

obtain compliance from their workers, and the hospitals' transition in this sense from what Etzioni (1961) calls "normative organizations" to "utilitarian organizations." This directs attention to the extrinsic as well as the intrinsic aspects of hospital work.

The chapter is composed of two main parts. The first part, reviewing some historical background on hospitals as workplaces in Canada and providing a brief description of the structure of the contemporary hospital industry, is based on existing secondary sources.[1] The second part consists of two case studies of how the industrial analogy applies to hospital workers in two areas: the service departments where the "non-professionals" are employed, and the hospital laboratories. These accounts are based respectively on the author's PhD and MA dissertations (Torrance 1978; 1970).

Historical Background

Canadian general hospitals were usually founded by religious orders, groups of prominent citizens (non-profit lay corporations), or by municipalities, while mental hospitals were established by provincial authorities. However, the state of the medical art before the turn of the century was such that, in Canada as elsewhere (see Rosen 1963), even the general hospitals were often merely places of shelter for the chronically ill poor, while the rich and the middle classes received care at home or at the doctor's office. The big teaching hospitals attached to medical schools might exhibit some complexity in functions and structure, but the smaller community hospitals were likely to consist of little more than several beds in a large house donated by the town's rich family and staffed by a few nurses.

Not much is written on the process by which new technology was incorporated in the general hospitals or on how doctors and patients came to use it more. It is clear, however, that by the 1920s hospitals were the locales for medical and surgical procedures that were either new or had been previously performed mainly in doctors' offices or patients' homes. Middle-class and upper-class patients were being admitted to the private and semi-private rooms that were being added to the old public wards. A perusal of hospital journals indicates that new technological equipment was being acquired. By the 1920s X-ray machines were found in all large and most medium-sized hospitals in Canada. In the 1920s and 1930s hospital laboratories spread from the large teaching hospitals to the smaller institutions.

Despite the expansion of technology and functions, hospitals of the 1920s were still relatively primitive. This was particularly true of their staffing mechanisms. They continued to rely heavily on various forms of voluntary or unpaid labour to meet their growing needs. Nuns in religious institutions and unpaid student nurses did most of the work required to make an increasingly complex institution run. In the nursing area, the pattern was for a small permanent staff of graduate nurses to supervise the work of a large rotating cadre of student nurses who not only provided most of the bedside care, but also did many of the domestic chores as well (Coburn 1974). Domestic staffs were small and undifferentiated, often consisting of a few cooks, kitchen helpers, cleaning women and janitors, many of whom "lived in" at the hospital residence. By today's standards, Canadian hospitals of the era were thinly staffed and had extremely low labour costs.

The residential system was a remarkable feature of the hospital work world. Nursing matrons and instructors, students, and some domestic workers tended to live together in the hospital residence. (All of the permanent nursing staff were required to remain single and to live in.) The conjuncture of work and residence gave hospitals the character of total institutions for their staff (Goffman 1961). To a large extent, life was regulated off the job as well as on. Long hours, night work, and split shifts demanded a devotion or subservience to the institution that is hard to imagine today. A sacrificial ethic prevailed – an ideology of service and obedience - that reflected the religious, military, and Nightingale influences of the hospitals' origins.

Hospital wages and payrolls were very low. Since most of the permanent staff and students were provided with "full maintenance" – free meals and rooms – cash wages could be kept to a minimum. As late as 1942, the cash salaries of general-duty nurses and maids in larger hospitals across Canada averaged only about $60 and $26 a month respectively, while student nurses were given an allowance of about $7 a month (Canadian Hospital Journal Oct-Nov 1942: 44–50; 34–40). While the free room and board had considerable value, the cash wages were far below rates for equivalent work outside.

Despite the Depression, Canadian hospitals exhibited a fair amount of growth and differentiation during the 1930s. Although the hospitals pleaded financial crises, money was found for some things, if not for staff. Although nursing schools in smaller hospitals began to decline in the 1920s and the Weir Report of 1932 advocated the employment of graduate nurses, the old system showed a remarkable persistence. The hospitals' response to the Depression was not to lay off staff, but to lower wages and continue the residential system. For their part, many of the hospitals' permanent employees preferred low wages in a sheltered job to the uncertainties of life outside. It was claimed that hospitals were charitable organizations fundamentally different from other employers: that they provided "more than just jobs" for their workers (Burling et al. 1956: 160).

The Second World War marks a transition point in the hospitals' evolution from relatively simple, quasi-charitable organizations to large modern industries. The mobilization of nurses and the availability of war work for other employees disrupted the traditional staffing system whereby hospitals had been guaranteed a stable, compliant work force (see Canadian Medical Procurement and Assignment Board, 1945, for examples). Although hospitals opposed their employees' inclusion in unemployment insurance and in legislation encouraging collective bargaining passed during the war, they were not exempted, and the special status of hospitals outside the mainstream of modern industry was eroded. Hospital employees joined unions, gained shorter hours, made new wage demands, and showed a degree of mobility that was unprecedented in the security-conscious Depression years.

After the war the Canadian hospital industry was transformed. The pent-up demand for new facilities and technology exploded. Doctors and patients began to use hospitals as never before. In the eight years following the war, total hospital expenditures in Ontario grew by 250 per cent, wages and salaries by 300 per cent (Taylor 1978: 111). The federal hospital construction grants of 1948 helped to fuel the wave of hospital capital expansion, while programs of government hospital insurance – Saskatchewan's in 1947, followed by several other provinces and by a national program in 1957 – financed hospital operating costs and especially wages and salaries. The transformation of the industry is starkly reflected in the increase of total hospital operating costs in Ontario from $130 million in 1948 to $4.8 billion by 1973, an increase of 37 times over 25 years; wages and salaries accounted for less than 50 per cent of this total at the start of the period, but more than 70 per cent by the end of it.

Two massive changes took place in hospital staffing patterns. The first was an increase in the intensity of staffing. In 1934, the total number of staff in Canadian public general hospitals, including student nurses, was only about 34,000, a ratio of 67 staff per 100 hospital beds. By 1991-92, the number of full-time staff was over 299,000, a ratio of 185 employees per 100 beds. Thus the number of full-time staff in Canadian hospitals had not only increased almost nine-fold over forty years, but the numbers needed to staff the same 100 beds had almost tripled. And these statistics underestimate the real change since the use of part-time staff had also grown steadily.

The second change was a great increase in occupational differentiation and specialization. In the nursing ranks, graduate nurses replaced student nurses. From small beginnings during the war, a new assistant category, that of Registered Nursing Assistants, grew rapidly in the 1950s and 1960s (Russell 1970: 142). New auxiliaries, like ward clerks, rose to take on tasks delegated by nursing, joining the traditional non-professional nursing workers such as nurse's aides and orderlies.

The most dramatic change, however, was in the ranks of allied professional and technical workers who chiefly work outside the traditional nursing settings. Although some pharmacists, physiotherapists, social workers, and technicians were found in prewar hospitals, their numbers proliferated in the 1950s and 1960s. The speed of growth can be illustrated by the example of X-ray and laboratory technicians in Ontario public general hospitals. In 1948, the Ontario Health Survey reported only 480 lab technicians and 456 X-ray technicians. By 1982, the number of lab technicians had risen to over 4,000 and X-ray technicians to over 1,800. Although reliable prewar figures are not available, it appears that the broad category of "Special Services," which encompasses these allied professional and technical workers and their auxiliaries, rose from less than 5 per cent of the hospital labour force to over 21 per cent at the present time.

Although change among the domestic workers was less dramatic, there was still some differentiation. Separate departments of dietetics, housekeeping, laundry, linen service, and engineering and maintenance emerged along with full-time administrators and supervisors. To administer an increasingly complex institution and deal with the paper work generated by it, the number of clerical and administrative employees rose substantially. The growth of university programs of hospital administration and the need for specialists in such areas as finance, personnel, and public relations gave an increasingly professionalised cast to the administrative ranks.

Growing size and the infusion of new technology were two factors behind the postwar changes in staffing. Bigger hospitals were being built, and into them were pouring the flood of innovations which have made modern hospitals the centre of high-technology medicine. New diagnostic tests and equipment, new monitoring machinery for critically ill patients, new therapies and surgical techniques were introduced at an unprecedented rate. These not only required more staff, but a more highly trained and specialized staff. The new technologists staffed units such as emergency services, intensive care, diagnostic laboratories, and rehabilitation medicine which were arising both within and outside the traditional four-service structure of medicine, surgery, obstetrics, and pediatrics.

A precondition for these changes, however, was change on the part of the community and community elites about the resources to be devoted to hospitals. In this sphere of the political economy of hospitals, a drastic change had taken place. Partly through piecemeal decisions at the level of individual hospitals, partly through provincial and national decisions like government hospital insurance, Canadian society had opted for a large-scale collective investment in hospitals rather than leaving them to be run on a quasi-charity basis. As in the prewar years, however, resources devoted to training and paying staff lagged behind investments in physical plant and new technology. Hospitals continued to retain the system of operating their own training schools and making use of the work of unpaid trainees in nursing and technical fields. As late as 1961, the Royal Commission on Health Services (1964: 227) found that, in hospitals with nursing schools, student nurses were still providing almost a third of the bedside care. But this system was to prove increasingly incapable of keeping up with change. As in other areas of the economy, Canadian hospitals had to rely heavily on skilled immigrants from Europe, and later from Third World countries, to fill the demand for nursing and technical personnel. Continuing low wages deterred greater numbers of Canadians from entering the training programs and taking these technical positions. It was only by the mid-1970s, when most hospital-based training programs had been disbanded and replaced by community college programs and wages had been substantially increased, that the transition to a modern staffing system was relatively complete.

The extent to which the hospital industry caught up to other industries in wages and salaries is a matter of doubt (see Evans 1975; and Swartz 1977). The huge increases in hospital labour costs since the war reflect such things as the phasing out of the residential-training system and the changing composition of staff as well as wage gains by individual hospital occupations. However, a comparison between hospital wages and the average industrial wage from 1942 to the present time indicates that substantial improvements indeed occurred. Even allowing a fairly generous allowance for room and board, nurses' salaries and those for the unskilled categories of hospital maids were well below the average industrial wage in 1942. They had gained little relative to it by 1962, reflecting the rapid rise in all labour incomes over this period. Between 1962 and 1977, however, nurses had surpassed the average industrial wage and maids had moved up from less than 50 per cent to about 75 per cent of the industrial composite. This rise coincides with the era of government hospital insurance and the growth and militancy of hospital unions. Despite continuing disparities within the hospital wage structure – as, for instance, between doctors or administrators and other workers and as between men and women doing similar work – Canadian hospitals moved from a decidedly low-wage industry to a middle-rank position among other industries.

In both their internal structure and technology, then, and in the social mechanisms used to recruit, train, and motivate staff, Canadian hospitals had undergone drastic transformations from the prewar years to the mid 1980s. However, the stage was set for a reaction. Hospitals had become very costly, and although still popular with the public, were obvious targets for the neoliberal wave of cost-cutting. Before looking at reasons for the change, let us turn to examine briefly some aspects of the contemporary structure of the hospital industry.

Aspects of the Current Structure of Canadian Hospitals

Even excluding nursing and other homes, the contemporary hospital industry is heterogeneous, being composed of a variety of types and sizes of institutions. In Canadian hospital statistics, three main ownership groups are distinguished, public, proprietary, and federal, with the vast majority being public hospitals. Within this group, hospitals are further classified as being general, specialty (including pediatric and short-term psychiatric), rehabilitation, extended care, and long-term psychiatric. Table 1 shows the distribution of hospitals and beds among these types of institutions in 1991-92. Public hospitals account for 96 per cent of hospital bed capacity, and within that general hospitals account for almost three-quarters.

TABLE 1

Distribution of operating hospitals and beds by type of hospital, Canada 1991-92

	Hospitals		Hospital Beds	
	Number	Percent	Number	Percent
Public				
General	832	68.8	127,974	74.4
Specialty	36	3.0	5,448	3.2
Rehabilitation	20	1.7	2,657	1.5
Extended Care	88	7.3	17,632	10.3
Psychiatric Long-Term	21	1.7	11,828	6.9
Other	64	5.3	208	0.1
Sub-Total, Public	1,061	87.7	165,747	96.4
Proprietary	57	4.7	3,590	2.1
Federal	92	7.6	2,567	1.5
Total - All Hospitals	1,210	100.0	171,904	100.0

Source: Statistics Canada, *Hospital Annual Statistics* 1991-92, Catalogue no. 83-242

The mix of types of hospitals has changed over time. In 1953, tuberculosis (TB) hospitals represented 10 per cent of all hospital bed capacity but these have now vanished altogether as a separate entity. Mental hospitals in 1953 accounted for a third of all Canadian hospital beds; they have now shrunk to a fraction of that. These institutions declined in the sixties, partly because of new drugs which encouraged treatment outside, partly because of the deinstitutionalization movement, but also because of the trend to incorporate psychiatric units in general hospitals. Their decline affects the nature of hospital employment because they tended to be large custodial institutions – in effect "warehouses" rather than "health factories" – with a distinctive sociological character as workplaces documented in many studies (see, for instance, Belknap 1956; Roth 1963).

Another source of heterogeneity lies in the ownership and control of hospitals. The major bodies owning and operating hospitals in Canada in order of importance include: non-profit lay corporations, religious organizations, provincial governments, municipalities, the federal government, and proprietorial interests. Although the direct source of ownership is probably of declining significance to what hospitals actually do, a few points should be noted. One is the small role of profit-making proprietorial hospitals on the Canadian scene as compared to the United States. A second is the comparatively large, but currently declining, role of religious institutions, in part a reflection of Canada's large Catholic population and the role of religious orders serving this population. Historically, if not at the present time, religious affiliation definitely appears to have affected the work environment.

A more important variable currently affecting hospitals as workplaces is that of size. Here we restrict our description to public general hospitals, the real object of our investigation as the centre of technological change. Again we note considerable diversity in the structure of the contemporary industry. What initially strikes the eye is the prevalence of small hospitals: almost six out of ten public general hospitals in Canada in 1991-92 were small institutions of fewer than 100 beds, hardly large bureaucratic organizations. Another 14 per cent are in the range from 100 to 199 beds, again not giant bureaucracies. But when we look at the proportion of beds and number of employees each size group contains (Table 2), a different picture emerges. The larger institutions, the teaching hospitals and those with over 200 beds, although making up only 25 per cent of all public general hospitals, have about 73 per cent of the total bed capacity and 80 per cent of the full-time staff.

Table 2 also shows the number of full-time equivalent (FTE) employees per 100 beds for each size group of hospital. This gives an indication of the increase in the intensity of staffing as hospitals grow larger. The small hospitals under 100 beds have 181 FTE employees per 100 beds; the ratio increases to 209 among those from 100 to 200 beds. Hospitals with more than 300 beds have 225 FTE employees per 100 beds. Clearly, staff size does not merely reflect bed size; it also indicates the increased technological complexity and the concurrent need for integration that accompanies it. This becomes more apparent in what follows.

The largest hospitals are behemoths which overstride the hospital world. Most of the really big general hospitals in Canada are teaching hospitals affiliated with university medical schools. These include such institutions as the Vancouver General in British Columbia, and Health Science Centre in Manitoba, the Toronto Hospital in Ontario, and the Montreal General or Hospital Notre-Dame in Quebec. Some have over 1,000 beds, sprawl over several city blocks, and employ over 3,000 workers. Whereas the largest public general hospitals have 225 FTE employees per 100 beds, the full- and partial-teaching hospitals among them have 336. This reflects the extra personnel required by the teaching, research, and more specialized services concentrated in these elite hospitals.

The size distribution of hospitals varies by province, regions within a province, and community size. Not surprisingly, for instance, heavily urbanized provinces like Ontario and Quebec alone have 91 of the 139 largest public general and teaching hospitals, while the Atlantic provinces together have only 11. The combination of community characteristics and hospital size provides a variety of distinctive work and social milieux for hospital workers.

The degree of occupational differentiation, as suggested earlier, is one of the most striking current characteristics of public general hospitals. Table 3 shows the distribution of hospital workers among the four main services identified by Statistics Canada. The nursing units account for 37 per cent of all full-time employees. Diagnostic and Therapeutic Services (formerly "Special Services") is the category including most of the allied health professionals and technical workers and their auxiliaries whose entry in force to the hospital has added to organizational complexity since the 1930s. This group now accounts for 25 per cent of full-time personnel. Educational services, those involved with nursing and technical training programs, were once much larger but now account for five per cent. Administrative and Supportive Services, which includes administrative, clerical, trades, and service workers, has the remaining 33 per cent of full-time employees. What is striking about this table as a whole is that three out of five of the hospital labour force works outside the nursing service, the main production line of the health factory.

Wow!! why is nursing so underrepresented

TABLE 2

Distribution of reporting hospitals, beds and employees by hospital type and bed-size, Canada 1991-92

Size Group	Hospitals		Beds		Full-time Employees		Part-time Employees		Full-time equivalent		FTE Employees / Hospital	FTE Employees / 100 Beds
	No.	%	No.	%	No.	%	No.	%	No.	%		
1-99	501	46.7	18,564	11.1	23,076	7.6	21,173	12.9	33,662	8.7	67.2	181.3
100-199	111	10.3	15,496	9.3	24,620	8.1	15,514	9.5	32,377	8.4	291.7	208.9
200-299	58	5.4	14,121	8.5	25,402	8.4	15,124	9.2	32,964	8.5	568.3	233.4
300 +	88	8.2	39,657	23.8	69,112	22.7	40,330	24.6	89,277	23.1	1014.5	225.1
Teaching	58	5.4	38,861	23.3	107,619	35.4	46,116	28.1	130,677	33.9	2253.1	336.3
Specialty	32	3.0	5,355	3.2	17,822	5.9	6,246	3.8	20,945	5.4	654.5	391.1
Rehabilitation	19	1.8	2,539	1.5	3,823	1.3	1,931	1.2	4,788	1.2	252.0	188.6
Extended Care	87	8.1	17,395	10.4	16,967	5.6	11,050	6.7	22,492	5.8	258.5	129.3
Psychiatric (LT)	17	1.6	10,121	6.1	11,389	3.7	3,949	2.4	13,363	3.5	786.1	132.0
Other	8	0.7	35	0.0	97	0.0	49	0.0	121	0.0	15.1	345.7
Proprietary	51	4.8	3,355	2.0	2,460	0.8	2,540	1.5	3,730	1.0	73.1	111.2
Federal	43	4.0	995	0.6	1,444	0.5	142	0.1	1,515	0.4	35.2	152.3
Total	1,073	100.0	166,494	100.0	303,831	100.0	164,164	100.0	385,913	100.0	359.7	231.8

Source: Statistics Canada, Hospital Annual Statistics 1991-92, Catalogue no. 83-242

The classification by service in Table 3 does not do justice to the proliferation of occupational specialties. The largest single occupational group is, of course, registered nurses, who make up over one-quarter of the total full-time workers. The three other largest groups within the nursing area are qualified nursing assistants (RNAs, LPNs) who account for just under 10 per cent, the miscellaneous ward aides and unlicensed assistants, and the male orderlies. Diagnostic and Therapeutic Services includes a host of specialties – laboratory and radiology scientists, technologists and technicians, physiotherapists and occupational therapists, pharmacists, social workers, psychologists, audiologists, speech therapists, and many other specialties. The largest component is laboratory technologists, followed by radiology technologists and physiotherapists. Within the Administrative and Supportive category are the management specialists, clerks, typists, etc.; the dieticians and food service supervisors; the medical records librarians and technicians; the tradesmen such as plumbers, electricians and stationary engineers; and the service workers in the dietary, housekeeping, laundry and linen service departments. Since many of the major occupations are further divided both hierarchically and by sub-specialties, even this listing is far from complete.

TABLE 3

Personnel employed by service, reporting public general hospitals, Canada, 1991-92

Service	Full-Time		Part-Time	
	Number	Percent	Number	Percent
Nursing	92,422	37.0	72,574	52.5
Diagnostic & Therapeutic	61,928	24.8	28,791	20.8
Educational Programs	12,777	5.1	681	0.5
Administrative & Support	82,702	33.1	36,211	26.2
Total	249,829	100.0 (64.4)	138,257	100.0

Source: Statistics Canada, Hospital Annual Statistics 1991-92, Catalogue no. 83-242

The larger the hospital, the more specialized personnel it has. In particular, the full-teaching hospitals have a diversified staff. Nursing accounts for only 36 per cent of the full-time staff in these hospitals, less than are in administrative and supportive services, with proportionately more as well in the special services and in education. These hospitals employ the majority of all scientists, researchers and department heads with postgraduate degrees working in hospitals.

Size and complexity implies a large administrative cadre to ensure coordination of activities. One indication of this from the nursing area is that one in five of the graduate nurses employed full time are in some sort of administrative role as directors, supervisors, head nurses, or assistant heads. Looking at other areas, including the medical, it is of interest to cite the specific example of one hospital, the Health Science Centre in Winnipeg which in 1985 had four member hospitals with approximately 1,100 beds, a budget of over $147 million, almost 4,000 staff, and 579 students. It had a corporate form of organization which, according to the Canadian Hospital Directory listing (1985), included a president, three senior vice-presidents, two other vice-presidents, an assistant to the president, four administrators and 39 departmental or service directors.

Large teaching hospitals, as typified by the Health Science Centre, clearly carry the industrial analogy to its fullest extent in their advanced bureaucratic and technological base. Although they are extreme cases, they illustrate the distance the hospital industry has travelled towards becoming a modern, rationalized, technologically complex one. Nor is this invalidated by the apparent diversity revealed above in hospital size or in ownership and control, since it masks the extent to which hospitals are knit into systems (Hall 1970: 5). This is manifest at the level of planning, in formal and informal referral systems, and especially at the level of industrial relations and collective bargaining. Since government hospital insurance brought provincial authorities into the hospital industry in the 1960s, central or regional coordination and control of hospitals has become more formalized. Smaller hospitals can thus realistically be viewed as satellites of the larger system. In industrial relations, the trend towards regional and provincial collective bargaining has brought similar wage levels, fringe benefits, and conditions of work to workers in large and small, rural and urban hospitals. In effect the employer is a very large organization controlling many separate plants; hospital workers are essentially quasi-government employees.

This was the scene up to the mid-eighties. Although hospital rationalization and cost-cutting had been talked about since the late 1960's, the speed of change when it came in the late 1980's and especially the 1990's was startling. The most dramatic manifestation is the closure of hospitals and beds in virtually all provinces. Since the last revision of this paper in 1987, the following events have occurred.

- B.C. became the first province to successfully close an acute care hospital (the Shaughnessy Hospital) in a major city.
- Saskatchewan closed 52 small rural hospitals.
- In Alberta, between March 1993 and 1995, the Klein cutbacks meant a loss of 2,200 acute care beds. Three major city hospitals were to be closed (Holy Cross and Grace in Calgary and Camsell in Edmonton.) There were plans to convert seven acute care hospitals to long-term care and 10 to community health centres providing family health services, emergency care and maternity services. Some 204 hospital boards were to be reduced to 17 regional boards.
- In Ontario, 20% of beds have been cut since 1986 – Metro Toronto has seen 30% closed or transformed. Between 1989 and 1994, Ontario closed 8,631 beds. On top of this, a report in the fall of 1995 recommended the closure of a dozen hospitals in Metro Toronto, reducing beds by 13 per cent. The number of emergency rooms would be reduced from 21 to 14, the number of operating rooms from 184 to 154. Similar reductions were posited for other Ontario cities including Ottawa.
- New Brunswick wiped out 51 separate hospital boards and created eight regional boards.
- Quebec is closing seven hospitals in Montreal, nine across the province. It has concluded there are 4,000 too many acute care beds. Ten thousand people attended a rally to save a Quebec City Hospital and there was a candlelight vigil for the Queen Elizabeth Hospital in Montreal.
- Nova Scotia announced plans in November 1995 to buy out 2,000 health care workers over three years to meet the target of reducing health care expenses by 12 per cent over five years.

Hospital unions also suffered. From a prewar situation in which unions were virtually unknown and hospital strikes unthinkable, the industry moved to comparatively heavy unionization and frequent strikes by the late 1970's. Soderstrom (1978: 84) estimates that in 1978, 43 per cent of hospital employees were unionized as compared to

32 per cent of the total non-agricultural labour force. By 1978, the large majority of Canadian hospitals had one or more unions representing their employees. The service workers are the most heavily unionized but nurses and technical personnel also flocked to unions.

Hospital strikes also became commonplace. The number of strikes increased steadily until by the seventies they were averaging about six a year. Although some provinces imposed restrictive legislation, hospital workers, like industrial workers elsewhere, adopted the strike as the normal means of expressing their demands.

Since the 1990's, the hospital unions have been on the defensive. Wage freezes, staff cutbacks, contracting out and contract-breaking have become common, with resistance seemingly futile. The result has been depleted staffing patterns, increased work stress, burnout, and a growth in work situations that threaten patient safety. Only recently, with the successful resistance in November 1995 of some Alberta hospital workers to the loss of their jobs, have some signs of the unions' old power begun to reappear.

At the macro level, the various indices we have examined show some of the ways the industrial analogy applies to Canadian hospitals. We now turn to the micro level to examine through two case studies other resemblances between hospitals and factories. How has the growth in size, bureaucratization, and technology affected the experience of work in hospitals? Have similar problems of fragmentation, alienation, and an instrumental orientation to work observed in traditional industries (Blauner 1964) developed in the hospital? In seeking answers, it is particularly pertinent to concentrate on large hospitals and to focus on such groups as the lower-level hospital workers who resemble the blue-collar workers in other industries and on the growing category of laboratory technicians, who represent the new wave of middle-level non-clinical personnel. Keep in mind that these vignettes represent the situation prior to the recent changes.

Two Case Studies of Work in the Hospital

Lower-Level Hospital Workers[2]

Sociologically, there are three main "castes" of hospital workers with virtually impenetrable status and mobility barriers between them. The top caste is composed of the doctors who are "in but not of" the hospital and a few high-ranking administrators; the second caste includes semi-professionals and technicians such as nurses, dieticians, physiotherapists, and lab personnel; and the third is formed of non-professional service workers who constitute the invisible underside of the industry. Although this last group make up one-third to one-half of the hospital labour force, little is known about them. It is to them that the industrial analogy most strongly applies.

A case study of these workers in two large metropolitan hospitals in Ontario revealed that they were recruited heavily from recent immigrants to Canada. Many had little knowledge of languages other than their native Portuguese, Italian, Spanish, Yugoslav, or Greek although others, from the West Indies or Asia, had more education and a greater fluency in English. After very limited orientations, they were placed in service jobs in the dietary, laundry, or housekeeping departments or were appointed as nursing auxiliaries, these last being drawn chiefly from those with experience or fluency in English. From then on, the workers had little chance for further mobility. The departmental organization was highly segmented. To a large extent, the different departments constituted separate worlds where the workers remained as long as they stayed with the hospital.

In the two Toronto hospitals included in this case study (Torrance 1978), the dietary departments were the largest department outside nursing employing non-professionals. Situated in both cases in the hospital basements, they physically resembled the largest and best-equipped of institutional kitchens, occupying suites of rooms filled with modern machinery. The organization of these departments was complex, involving two main divisions, a production division and a therapeutic one. Like the hospital as a whole, there tended to be dual lines of authority, one involving the professional dieticians, engaged in producing special diets, and in research and teaching; the other involving production managers and those having responsibility for the preparation of most of the meals. The main work of the departments revolved around the preparation of upwards of 5,000 staff and patient meals a day. To accomplish this, a coordinated routine had been worked out. This involved breaking tasks down into their smallest components, rotating workers among these repetitive jobs, and relying on close supervision to ensure that the final product was of uniform quality.

Although there were a fair number of skilled jobs in the kitchens (cooks, bakers, butchers, etc.), most of the jobs were semi-skilled and unskilled and were delegated to female dietary aides and male cleaners, porters, and dishwashers. The food service aides rotated among ingredient-preparation jobs and took part in the regular operation of a conveyor belt on which were assembled the meals for the patients on the floors. These jobs were physically and mentally demanding – the women were on their feet all day and close concentration was required to make sure no mistakes were made.

In their reactions to the work, the dietary workers resembled those of assembly-line workers in industry. Complaints about bad working conditions, a hectic pace, and unnecessary and harassing supervision were common. Terms like "animals," "machines," "slaves," and "robots" were used to describe their situation.

Except for those who delivered meals to the wards and who worked on special therapeutic diets, the sense of participation in the role of healing the sick was minimal. Some of the kitchen workers were almost completely oblivious to the fact they were working in a hospital – it could have been an institutional kitchen anywhere. One long-term veteran claimed that he had never been upstairs to the patient-care settings in all the years he had worked in the hospital. Doctors and senior administrators might be served in the cafeteria, but they were conceived as a remote and aloof group who had nothing to do with the kitchen workers' activities.

Structurally, the workers in the housekeeping departments have a much closer contact with the patient-care settings because most of them actually work in and around patients. In these two hospitals, the housekeeping departments were the second largest non-clinical unit employing non-professional workers. They had their own executive heads, assistant heads, and supervisors in charge of the housekeeping workers in various parts of the hospital. The janitors and female aides had two sources of supervision: their supervisors and the head nurses on the units where they were stationed.

The work of the housekeepers had not been as rationalized as that of the kitchen workers. It used the traditional technology of vacuum cleaners, dusters, and elbow grease. The tasks had to be fitted around the ward routines and the patients' situation. As a result there was less direction and more flexibility. Additionally, there was a fair bit of spectator interest in observing life on the wards.

The housekeepers were less prone to alienation than the kitchen workers. While the work was experienced as physically tough, there was little of the sense of depersonalization that existed in the kitchens. There was more of a sense of involvement in the task of patient care – even if mainly as a spectator. However, too active an interest was discouraged. The housekeepers were expected to know their place and keep it.

The nature and organization of work for the non-professionals in nursing is as varied as the settings in which they work. Some of them found the work challenging and involving; others found it routine, repetitive, and alienating. In one of the hospitals studied, unlicensed nursing auxiliaries still played a big part in patient care. In the other, they were a small and declining group with all the patient-care functions being restricted to registered assistants and graduate nurses.

An example of the extension of rationalization to the nursing area is the central supply rooms and the central dispatch system, which has been implemented in one of the hospitals. The former's function was to prepare trays of sterilized instruments, which were used in the operating rooms, nursing units and clinics. Aside from the sterilization of instruments, the preparation of trays involved bench work in a self-contained, enclosed room. The nursing auxiliaries worked here sitting on stools and standing up, assembling the trays. Since each tray must contain exactly the right instruments, the workers operated under the close supervision of graduate nurses. A high degree of concentration was required. The work was generally regarded as less interesting than that in the nursing units. Here, too, despite the nursing backgrounds of the staff, it was easy to lose sight of the wider mission of the hospital and to develop a sense of isolation and alientation.

The central dispatch system in operation at one of the hospitals was highly regarded as the latest model of efficiency. It used male dispatchers and porters. Carts were assembled for replacing the stocks of equipment used on the wards, and the porters changed these carts regularly during the day. They were also on call to deliver emergency orders to the wards. Close supervision ensured that they did not spend too much time on calls. By centralizing the porter service in this way, the hospital had clearly separated the tasks done by the porters and orderlies and confined the former to a small and simplified job. Their old role as participants on the wards was diminished, and this tended to heighten alienation.

The reactions of the nursing nonprofessionals to their work was mixed. Some were deeply involved and highly satisfied there was nothing they would rather be doing. Others, especially those whose work was subdivided, routine and tightly supervised, approximated the kitchen workers in their alienation. This feeling was exacerbated because they tended to be more highly educated and more ambitious than the other service workers. A strong complaint of many who had previous experience was that their skills and potential contribution were underutilized.

Given the restricted tasks, the routine work, the isolation of their units from the mainstream of the hospital and their recruitment base, it is not surprising that most of the non-professional workers expressed a strictly instrumental attitude toward their jobs. For most it was "just a job," distinguished only on the positive side by the lighter, steadier work it offered over the available alternatives and on the negative side by the shift and weekend work entailed by the hospital's operation. Only a small minority had been able to salvage some intrinsic meaning from their work.

The hospitals had made very limited initiatives to involve this group of workers. Although some administrators had good intentions, they simply did not have the resources to do much. Instead, they largely used the cheapest way of organizing the work, the line of least resistance, which relied on unskilled workers, job simplification and close supervision in short a classic bureaucratic-rational mode of administration.

Given the reliance today on utilitarian incentives to maintain compliance among these workers, a final point of interest is to inquire how well these incentives actually functioned. The workers had benefited from a large wage increase won after a threatened strike by the Canadian Union of Public Employees in Ontario hospitals. They now earn well above the minimum wage. In general, they expressed moderate satisfaction with their current pay in relation to the "sweat" involved in the work and to their education and skills. One strong reason why most were able to get by was that there was more than one money earner in the family. Those who were sole earners supporting dependents – a minority in the sample – had a harder time.

Even for the better off, the pattern of two earners working long hours for modest pay was regarded as a hard life. However, a series of questions designed to tap their sense of relative deprivation compared to the incomes of higher-status groups within the hospital and to outside workers revealed little envy or sense of injustice. They simply did not compare incomes. Their concern, above all, was to stay abreast of inflation. Through hard, unstinting work and doing without amenities that most Canadians took for granted, they had attained a measure of security and now struggled to hold on to it.

Economic considerations were important to these workers and affected their reactions to their jobs. The more satisfied they were with the pay, the more likely they were to express satisfaction with their jobs. Whatever intrinsic satisfaction they were able to gain from the work was secondary; for the majority utilitarian considerations took first place. Despite the supposed large relative wage gains by hospital workers over the previous decades, these workers still saw themselves as living on the financial margin.

The Hospital Laboratories[3]

Laboratory personnel now account for about 40 percent of the Diagnostic and Therapeutic Services category of hospital workers. Hospital laboratories have evolved greatly since prewar days when a typical lab might involve a few assistants helping the pathologist with such tests as were then available. The development of new technology in the field of diagnostic testing has been rapid. Its diffusion to the routine laboratories and increasing use by hospital physicians have caused the rapid rise of the laboratories with specialized staffs in various fields. Aside from histology and cytology – the traditional core areas of the pathologist's expertise – separate units have split off in clinical biochemistry, haematology, microbiology and blood banking. Larger hospitals may have further laboratories for specialties like electron microscopy, nuclear medicine and ultrasound scanning. All these laboratories may have separate heads, although in smaller hospitals the pathologist may assume responsibility for the full range. Organizational complexity is added by the range of qualifications found among laboratory personnel. At the upper end are found MDs with specialist qualifications in the specific field and post graduate scientists. A middle level, itself consisting of several tiers, is formed by the technologists and technicians. Finally come the unlicensed assistants and cleaners.

The actual technology and organization of work is highly varied according to field. The clinical chemistry laboratories are the largest in terms of volume of work processed and the number of staff employed. The second largest are usually microbiology labs, followed by haematology, blood banking and cytology and histology. Because of the large volumes and nature of the work, work in clinical biochemistry is the most rationalized and routine. It is now highly automated. Work in other fields is less routine and varies from the craft technology emphasizing delicate manual skills as required in cytology and histology to the machine-tending skill required in haematology.

There are, however, some common elements across the laboratories. The first is that they work mainly with disembodied specimens, things rather than people, and have very little contact with patients. The departments are physically and socially isolated from the patient-care settings, and there is little chance to develop a personal involvement with particular patients and their illnesses. A second common element is the extreme care necessary to avoid mistakes. A high degree of concentration is required, and there is close supervision by the charge technicians.

To illustrate the nature of work in hospital labs, we use the example of clinical chemistry, the largest and most rationalized field. At the time of the study, clinical chemistry was partly but not completely automated. Routine assays had been almost completely automated using big multichannel autoanalysers; special assays, however, still had to be done on a custom, one-at-a-time basis. The labs were divided into a series of benches around which the technicians rotated in a regular cycle. The routine technicians had become mainly machine tenders, checking to see that the autoanalysers were functioning properly, and transcribing the results. The special chemistry tests were handled by the more highly qualified personnel. These involved a lot of sequential laboratory procedures done manually and provided more opportunities to utilize skills and knowledge.

For the routine technicians, if not for the others, then, work was repetitive and subdivided with little challenge once the basic routines had been learned. Even the introduction of automated equipment posed few challenges in terms of learning how to maintain complex equipment. This function had devolved to special electronics technicians employed by the manufacturers. The closely supervised work thus offered little opportunity for autonomy or creativity.

The administrative career ladder provided the only opportunity to move up. But the rungs on the supervisory ladder and the salary differentials were very truncated. Moreover, the top jobs were monopolized either by university-trained chemists or by charge technicians with years of experience. For the women and immigrants who predominated in routine technicians' jobs, there were definite barriers to mounting the administrative career ladder.

Given the lack of challenge in their work and the absence of mobility opportunities into supervisory and administrative roles, it is no surprise that many of the routine technicians had developed an instrumental orientation to work. Interest in taking technical courses was low. Turnover rates were high as technicians moved to other hospitals or dropped out of the occupation. The instrumental orientation was also reflected in their attitudes toward their professional association, the Canadian Society of Laboratory Technologists (CSLT).

Like many of the paramedical associations, the CSLT at the time was a fairly weak vehicle, not exercising any real control over entry or training in the occupation and little able to influence technicians' conditions of work or salaries within the hospital. The technicians appeared to be indifferent to its educational role and wanted it to become more of a bargaining agency. A limited subgroup of mainly male technicians, however, saw it as a means for individual upward mobility. Holders of advanced CSLT credentials were disproportionately active in association affairs.

Future technological developments seem to favour more and more automation in the laboratories. Undoubtedly, the volume of laboratory work will increase as new tests are continually developed and diffused. The future of the technicians remains in doubt *hospitals are very industrial.*

however. Continued automation would seem to imply increased simplification of their skills. At the same time, new technologies introduce new equipment outside the routine areas and create opportunities for new specialties. The laboratories, therefore, exhibit dual trends: on the one hand, they are at the cutting edge where new technologies are introduced into routine use in patient care; on the other, the rationalization of work moves in the opposite direction.

While factory conditions of work and reactions to it might be predictable among lower-level service workers in the hospital, they are less expected among a semiprofessional occupation that shares some of the glamour of medical science and research. This is not surprising, however, when we recognize that the professionalization of technicians was largely "professionalization from above" (Goldner and Ritte 1967), fostered by the employers and the senior professionals to ensure a supply of competent auxiliaries who would remain satisfied with their place. With little real control over their work, the technologists have been subject to the processes of proletarianization encountered by many professionals or semiprofessionals who work in large industrial organizations.

Conclusion

This chapter has attempted to show some of the ways the industrial analogy applies to modern hospitals as workplaces and to chart out the change this represents from the hospital's historical origins. We have focussed primarily on the large hidden categories of hospital workers who are outside the most visible areas of nursing and medical care. We looked both at the content and organization of work – the intrinsic aspects – and at some of the extrinsic aspects as well – wages, mobility opportunities and their meaning. In brief, the conclusion is that, in nonclinical areas, the difference that may once have existed between hospital work and other kinds of work has now diminished. The larger hospitals in particular are rationalized modern bureaucracies with little to distinguish them from others of similar size and complexity. As such, they face – or engender – the same problems other industries are subject to: alienation among both lower-level and semi-professional employees, an instrumental orientation to work and industrial conflict between management and labour.

Several qualifications should be added to this conclusion. Despite convergence on many traits, hospitals are still varied in size, technological complexity, degree of bureaucratization and community setting. Conditions in the small and medium-sized hospitals in smaller communities are likely to differ from those in the large metropolitan hospitals from which our examples are taken. They draw on different recruitment pools for their workers, and their more human scale may make a sense of participation and identification with the central purposes of the institution easier. A second qualification is that, even within the large hospitals, the work settings are highly diverse. In selecting material for these case studies, we have admittedly chosen rather extreme cases. Hospital work groups in most settings – nursing and non-nursing – are relatively small, seldom exceeding ten to fifteen people, so the extremes of mass production and impersonality are not found here. If they are to be conceived as factories, general hospitals are best visualized as a series of small, specialized workshops all housed within the same organization rather than as a single production line. Trends in the nursing area reinforce the diversification: increasingly, specialization and design changes have broken down nursing units into smaller enclaves from the large, open wards that once prevailed.

Discussion of nursing settings raises the issue that Freidson (1967) was chiefly concerned with when he applied the term "health factories" to large hospitals: the consequences of rationalization of services for patient care. Our limited focus on nonclinical settings does not allow any generalization to this area. Since most of the service and laboratory workers we examined had little contact with patients, only gross incidents such as severe understaffing or strikes could have a direct impact on patient care. It is the nursing settings one would have to examine to look for the more subtle ways in which cutbacks and rationalization of work might affect the quality of care.

Several sociological studies provide indications that the situation in these settings bears some resemblance to the nonclinical areas. There is considerable variation in worker involvement and alienation among different units – between active treatment and chronic wards, between medical and surgical services.

Canadian studies of hospitals as workplaces and as patient-care settings remain rare. Given its importance, it is to be hoped that the hospital industry will attract more attention from sociologists. Such contributions may be particularly appropriate when the role of the hospitals in our health system is being increasingly questioned under the stimulus of mounting health costs.

Notes

1   Statistical references in the text are based mainly on Statistics Canada *Hospital Statistics* for the appropriate years. Where Ontario statistics are cited, they are from the annual reports of the Ontario Hospital Services Commission or the Hospital Statistics of the Ontario Ministry of Health.
2   Based on a random sample of 118 lower-level hospital workers in two Toronto hospitals (Torrance 1978).
3   The study of hospital laboratory technicians on which the author's M.A. dissertation (Torrance 1970) was based was part of a larger study of hospital-based paramedical personnel in five Ontario hospitals directed by Oswald Hall. For additional information on this study, see Hall (1970).

References

Belknap, I. 1956. *Human Problems of a State Mental Hospital.* New York: McGraw Hill.

Blauner, R. 1964. *Alienation and Freedom.* Chicago: University of Chicago Press.

Burling, T, EM Lenz, and RN Wilson. 1956. *The Give and Take in Hospitals.* New York: Putnams.

Canada. 1964. *Report of the Royal Commission on Health Services.* Ottawa: Queen's Printer.

Canadian Hospital Association. 1985. *Canadian Hospital Directory.* Ottawa: Canadian Hospital Association.

Canadian Medical Procurement and Assignment Board. 1940. *Report of the National Health Survey.* Ottawa: King's Printer.

Coburn, J. 1974. I See and Am Silent: A Short History of Nursing in Ontario. In J Acton, P Goldsmith and B Shepard eds. *Women at Work, Ontario 1850-1930.* Toronto: Canadian Women's Educational Press.

Etzioni, A. 1961. *A Comparative Analysis of Complex Organizations.* New York: Free Press.

Evans, RG. 1975. Beyond the Medical Marketplace. In S Andreopoulos ed. *National Health Insurance: Can We Learn From Canada?* New York: Wiley.

Freidson, E. 1967. Health Factories: The New Industrial Sociology. *Social Problems* 14: 493–500.

Ginzberg, E. 1995. Hospitals: From Center to Periphery. *Inquiry* 32: 11–13.

Goffman, E. 1961. *Asylums*. Chicago: Aldine.

Goldner, FH, and R Ritti. 1967. Professionalization as Career Immobility. *American Journal of Sociology* 73: 86–94.

Hall, O. 1970. *The Paramedical Occupations in Ontario*. A Study for the Committee on the Healing Arts. Toronto: Queen's Printer.

Ontario Ministry of Labour. 1974. *The Report of the Hospital Inquiry Commission.* Toronto.

Rosen, G. 1963. The Hospital: Historical Sociology of a Community Institution. In E Freidson, ed.. *The Hospital in Modern Society*. New York: Free Press.

Roth, JA. 1963. *Timetables*. New York: Bobbs-Merrill.

Royal Commission on Health Services. 1964. *Report.* Volume II. Ottawa: Queen's Printer.

Russell, MG. 1970. The Emergence of the Nursing Assistant. In MQ Innis ed. *Nursing Education in a Changing Society*. Toronto: University of Toronto Press.

Soderstrom, L. 1978. *The Canadian Health System*. London: Croom Helm.

Swartz, D. 1977. The Politics of Reform: Conflict and Accommodation in Canadian Health Policy. In L Panich ed. *The Canadian State: Political Economy and Political Power*. Toronto: University of Toronto Press.

Taylor, MG. 1978. *Health Insurance and Canadian Public Policy*. Montreal: McGill-Queen's University Press.

Torrance, GM. 1970. *Hospital Laboratory Technicians: Specialization and Career Patterns in a New Occupation*. Unpublished M.A. dissertation, University of Toronto.

Torrance, GM. 1978. *The Underside of the Hospital: Recruitment and the Meaning of Work Among Non-Professional Hospital Workers*. Unpublished Ph.D. dissertation, University of Toronto.

Weir, GM. 1932. *Survey of Nursing Education in Canada.* Toronto: University of Toronto Press.

Part VI
The Health Care System

In common-sense terms health care systems are readily envisioned as composed of hospitals, health care professions, paramedicals, public-health units, and other organizations and occupations with a formal public mandate for healing. Sociologically, however, viewed as encompassing those actions taken relative to health, the system would look much bigger, more complex, and with fuzzier boundaries. The latter would include, for example, those individuals, organizations, and actions relating to non-prescription and well as to prescription drugs, possibly to sports and other "health-enhancing" activities, as well as to care given within the domestic sphere. It might also include health care businesses, the hospital supply industry, and Ministries of Health. It is difficult to draw the borders between health matters, well-being, or notions of "the good society" generally. Most often, the former, more restrictive definition has been used, with a rather stultifying effect both on our conceptions of what actually produces health and on our views of the structure of health care systems, nationally and internationally. For example, if there are varying boundaries between formal health care and domestic health care, difficulties arise in international comparisons of the amount of time and resources different countries are actually devoting to health care.

Still, it is easier, and more immediately comprehensible to see health care as meaning hospitals, doctors, and nurses, other "paramedical" occupations, and even drug companies. We have already noted these components of health care. Of greater political and practical importance is the social arrangements of these components, that is, their interrelationships and the way the system is organized relative to those it is supposed to serve. Such matters as whether the system is organized as a health service under state auspices or as a health insurance system under state or private insurers have obvious implications for access to health care and for national levels of health status. Indeed, much that has been written about health care systems is about equality or equity in access to services. The health care system may be viewed either "from below," by patients, or "from above" by, for example, the state.

Much of the relationship between health care and politics in the twentieth century has revolved about public access to health care. This care was viewed both as needed and as not being adequately provided through private health care. Major political struggles led to state involvement in health care, this state involvement varying in nature and extent amongst different countries. Canada likes to place itself somewhere between the United States, with a mostly market dominated system, and the United Kingdom with a mostly state-run system. As Naylor (1986) has noted, Canada has public payment but private practice, with the latter now under pressure to become more "public," while the former is being pushed to become more private.

The components of the system and their interaction with patients and with the state are shaped by their placement in social formations with different economic, political, and social structures. Although some have viewed governments as introducing various public health measures in the face of opposition by a laissez-faire oriented medical profession, the introduction of health insurance needs to be placed within broader class

[Handwritten note at top of page:]
what is the health care system
 - it is definitely > hospitals / physicians.
 - it is addressing social determinants of health
   i.e. poverty, education

struggles and welfare state developments. Medicine itself, once all-powerful, is now facing challenges on many fronts, primarily from payers.

Certainly systems with one or a few payers have different dynamics than those with many payers. And, if the state is involved as paymaster, the trends are a movement from simply paying the bills to managing the system.

At the same time as the system was becoming increasingly rationalized, doubts arose as to the efficacy of health care systems. Did formal health care actually improve national levels of health status? The conclusion now is that there are many social determinants of health, with health care systems simply one of these, and, perhaps not even the most important. Thus, new policies or orientations to health emerged, not only from the "health promotion" movement, and, more recently, from those espousing "population health," but also from provincial and federal Ministries intent on cutting expenditures.

In the meantime all of the interrelationships within the system were being shaken by the introduction of a mass market in health care, that is, universal or almost universal access to care by Canadians. These interrelationships were also dramatically influenced by Ministry of Health cost-cutting, and by demands from various quarters for more effective or humane care. Old alliances, between the medical profession and state/bureaucratic elites, and between the profession and business elites, were undermined. The actions of those pushing for evermore expenditures in a provider- and drug-driven system were called into question. Public involvement in health care organizations or decisions was viewed by some as not only more democratic, but also as helping to balance state, professional, or health care organization interests.

In Canada, since the introduction of insurance for physician services in the early 1970s, state involvement in health care has increased step by step, as has state resistance to the apparently open-ended increases in the costs of care. In the early years of medicare there were dozens of provincial and federal committees and commissions on the financing of care and on the reorganization of services in a system now with public financing. Most recently have come federal and provincial concerns with costs, with management of the system, and with efficacy. The general trends in public policies have been to fund only those forms of care which were of demonstrated efficacy. The use of health care systems, and particularly the most expensive component of that system, hospitals, was viewed as an action of last resort. Nearly every province closed hospital beds, or closed hospitals. The watchwords have been "Do more with less." The squeezing of health care brought debates about whether this simply dumped care back into the lap of women in the home, or actually was a good way of bringing health care back to the community in a more patient-oriented sense. And, the increasing intensification of work in health care adversely effected lower status health care workers.

In This Part

Mhatre and Deber examine issues emerging from the "relative success" of the Canadian health care system. The new challenges include issues of access to high technology care and the fact that health care does not necessarily mean improved health. There are, in addition, issues emanating from such matters as economic trends and an aging population. Mhatre and Deber note the contents of provincial reports on health policy in this changing environment. Most of the reports have common elements, particularly regarding an increasing emphasis on health promotion or prevention, attempts to downsize the hospital sector in favour of community based care, regionalization, and increased public participation in decision-making. But these policies are emerging at a time of social and economic uncertainty. Even given a real desire to move to prevention and community based care, the authors note the uncertainty of implementation.

Joel Lexchin has spent many years studying the drug industry. Not only is the drug industry one of the major shapers of health care but drug costs have been the costs escalating most rapidly. Although the Health Protection Branch of the federal government is supposed to regulate the drug industry "in the public interest," Lexchin notes what many other observers have also reported – that the relationship between the drug industry and its government regulators is far from being at arm's length. In fact, most analysts, like Lexchin, see a powerful industry influencing or controlling a relatively weak government department. Who is regulating whom?

Boudreau and O'Neill both tackle emerging governance strategies in health care. On the one hand Boudreau analyzes the notion of "partnership" in the Quebec mental health system while on the other, O'Neill examines community participation. Boudreau shows how the term "partnership" became a new mantra within the Quebec mental health system. The term arose as a response to loss of faith in government and in professional knowledge and to the complexity of demands on the state. Partnership promised to alleviate some of the abuses of the past, such as the overbearing power of providers, by instituting a new regional planning system involving consumers, community groups, and government alongside professionals and public sector unions. Boudreau indicates a certain skepticism about the eventual outcome, given the highly unequal balance of power between the putative partners. O'Neill similarly indicates how community participation is co-opted or subverted in actual practice in the Quebec case. The rhetoric of participation was actually used by Quebec state technocrats in order to gain control in health care. In fact, given the current power structure in health care and differences in expertise between the public and providers, can community participation actually be realized in practice? While there are exciting developments in community participation and community empowerment, O'Neill argues that only by rethinking these terms within the context of social theory can we understand their possibilities and their limits.

Reference

Naylor, CD. 1986. *Private Practice, Public Payment: Canadian Medicine and the Politics of Health Insurance, 1911-1966.* Kingston and Montreal: McGill-Queen's University Press.

25

From Equal Access to Health Care to Equitable Access to Health: A Review of Canadian Provincial Health Commissions and Reports[*]

Sharmila L. Mhatre and Raisa B. Deber

Canada's system of universal medical and hospital insurance, now known generically as Medicare, is considered to be one of the best in the world. It has achieved high levels of health status with minimal restrictions on patients or providers, and enjoys wide public support. Like many other health care systems, however, it faces increased challenges from changes in the social, political, and economic environment.

As Aaron Wildavsky has pointed out, the solution of one set of problems leads to the creation of new dilemmas; the challenge for policymakers is to select which set of problems they prefer (Wildavsky 1989). The original objective of Canada's health care system was equality of access to medical care. This objective has largely been achieved. However, class disparities in health status remain, although these have been substantially reduced from the pre-Medicare period. This policy success has forced Canadian policymakers to recognize the limits of medical care in achieving health. Consequently, a 'new' policy goal has been proposed – achieving equity of access to health.

Equality and equity, although sometimes used interchangeably, are not equivalent. Political scientists such as Stone (Stone 1988) define an *equal* distribution as one involving *identical* or similar treatment of two or more entities, and an *equitable* distribution as conferring a *fair* treatment, which may require unequal treatment to respond to unequal needs. The language of equality, however, is often used to address the concept of equity. The Panel on Health Goals for Ontario, for example, wrote that equity in health "implies that members of all population groups have equal opportunities to achieve and maintain health" (Ontario Ministry of Health 1987: 45).

[*] Reprinted and revised from *International Journal of Health Services*, Vol. 22, No. 4, Sharmila L. Mhatre and Raisa B. Deber, 'From equal access to health care to equitable access to health: A review of Canadian provincial health commission and reports', pp. 645–68, 1992, with permission from Baywood Publishing Company, Incorporated, Amityville, New York.

What are the policy options being proposed in order to achieve access to health? A series of extensive reviews have been conducted by provincial royal commissions since 1987 on the future of their respective health care systems. This article will briefly review the Canadian health care system, highlight its qualified success, note current concerns, categorize the policy options advocated by the commissions, and analyze the recommended policies.

A Brief History of the Canadian Health Care System

The saga of the establishment of Canadian Medicare has been recorded elsewhere (see for example Deber and Vayda 1985; Taylor 1987). As defined by the Constitution Act of 1867, health care is constitutionally a provincial responsibility. Thus, Medicare developed incrementally from two voluntary cost-shared programmes – the Hospital Insurance and Diagnostic Services (HIDS) Act (1957) and the Medical Care Act (1966-67) – wherein the federal (national) government provided funds to provincial plans as long as those plans complied with specified terms and conditions. These terms entrenched access to health care as a 'merit good' which should be, by right, available to all. To qualify for federal funds all provincial insurance plans had to comply with five principles. They had to be *universal*, *comprehensive* (covering all "medically necessary procedures"), and *accessible* (including a requirement that "reasonable access" not be impeded or precluded, "either directly or indirectly, whether by charges or otherwise." In 1984, this was clarified in the Canada Health Act as prohibiting any direct charges or deductibles for insured services; see Heiber and Deber 1987). To enable Canadians to be covered anywhere in Canada, the plans were required to be *portable*. Finally, the role of private insurers was limited by a requirement that the insurance plans be *publicly administered*, since the private alternative was seen as more expensive and less effective. Accordingly, each Canadian province has a single payer for insured health services (i.e., the government-run insurance plan). In most provinces, the provincial plans have been financed through general revenues, although premiums or designated payroll taxes may also be used by some to cover a proportion of the costs. Federal support for provincially run social welfare programmes, many of them health related, was consolidated in another shared-cost programme, the *Canada Assistance Plan* (CAP) of 1966. Unlike Medicare, CAP was means-tested. CAP can be used by the provinces to subsidize a range of health related services and benefits, e.g., homemaker services, casework, counselling, and services for the disabled (Manga and Angus 1989).

Federal ability to influence health care thus rested primarily on administrative arrangements under the funding mechanisms. It was further weakened by the post-1977 change in funding arrangements (the Federal-Provincial Fiscal Arrangements and Established Programs Financing Act (EPF), since renamed the Federal-Provincial Fiscal Arrangements and Federal Post-Secondary Education and Health Contributions Act 1977), which replaced the old cost-sharing formulae with a combination of tax points transfers plus block grants, indexed to growth in population and gross national product (GNP). This new financing arrangement gave the provinces greater flexibility over spending, and gave them full fiscal responsibility for all above-inflation increases in health spending (Hastings 1986; Vayda and Deber 1984). Subsequent revisions to the EPF formula have further decreased the growth in federal transfers, shrunk the proportion of those transfers paid in cash (rather than tax transfers), and placed even greater responsibility for spending and its control on the provinces (Barker 1988; Manga and Angus 1989).

A momentary effort to strengthen federal control came in April 1984, when the HIDS Act and the Medical Care Act were replaced by the Canada Health Act. The Canada Health Act was a reaction to fears that Medicare was being "eroded" (Health and Welfare Canada 1983). It reaffirmed the five principles of Medicare and established financial penalties for provinces allowing direct charges to patients for insured services (e.g., extra-billing and hospital user fees). Parliament, however, did not choose to take the opportunity to reform the future system or address key questions regarding the delivery of health services (Heiber and Deber 1987).

Having one insurer per province, rather than the multiple health plans found in the United States, has had several salutary effects: administrative costs are far lower, there is little incentive to shift costs to other insurers, and the costs are shared across the economy rather than loaded onto the manufacturing sector (United States General Accounting Office 1991; Woolhandler and Himmelstein 1991). The historical evolution of the system, however, has also left Medicare with two major problems.

First, although the federal government has taken responsibility for partial funding of the system and for setting national standards, constitutional responsibility for health continues to rest with provincial governments. Health policy accordingly often becomes entangled with federal-provincial relations. As will be noted below, decreasing financial contributions produces a lowered capacity to enforce national objectives, and Medicare may thus fall victim to policy forces outside of the health sphere.

Second, the fact that the cost-shared programmes from which the current system has arisen had restricted their coverage to those medically necessary services provided in hospitals (HIDS) or by physicians (Medical Care Act) has skewed subsequent patterns of service delivery. Although these restrictions were formally removed in 1977 when the funding formula shifted from cost-sharing to block funding (Van Loon 1978), the inertia of the existing resource infrastructure continued to exert an influence. Canada's system is far more physician and hospital intensive than planners would consider optimal.

Canada's Qualified Success Story

The Canadian health care system can be considered a qualified success. It is able to provide universal and comprehensive coverage. With the exception of the United States, health expenditures are roughly comparable with those of other advanced industrial nations, while health status measures (e.g., life expectancy and infant mortality) are quite favourable. Canadians also indicate a high rate of satisfaction and pride in their system.

Although Canada's health expenditures are markedly lower than those of the United States, which does not have a universal plan (Evans et al. 1989), they are relatively high in international terms. In 1991 Canada had the second highest health expenditures relative to gross domestic product and the second highest per capita health expenditures (measured in U.S. dollars using gross domestic product purchasing power parities) (Organisation for Economic Co-operation and Development 1993; Schieber et al. 1992). Both these rates are greater than the Organisation for Economic Cooperation and Development (OECD) mean (Table 1). The glass may be interpreted as being half empty or as half full. Evans has suggested that the main reason for cost escalation is poor economic growth (i.e., the denominator) rather than exploding costs (Evans 1993).

TABLE 1

Total health expenditures as a percentage of gross domestic product, selected OECD countries - 1970-1991

	1970	1975	1980	1985	1987	1989	1991
United Kingdom	4.5	5.5	5.8	6.0	6.1	6.1	6.6
Japan	4.4	5.5	6.4	6.6	6.8	6.7	6.6
Italy	4.8	5.8	6.8	6.7	6.9	8.3	8.3
Germany	5.5	7.8	7.9	8.2	8.2	8.3	8.5
Sweden	7.2	8.0	9.5	9.4	9.0	8.6	8.6
France	5.8	6.8	7.6	8.6	8.6	8.7	8.9
Canada	7.2	7.3	7.4	8.4	8.6	9.0	10.0
United States	7.4	8.4	9.2	10.9	11.2	11.6	13.4
Mean[a]	5.3	6.5	7.0	7.4	7.3	7.5	7.9

Source: Schieber and Poullier 1989; Schieber et al. 1992; OECD 1993

[a]   Mean of all 24 OECD countries

Optimistically, Canada's rate of increase is relatively small as compared to the other major industrialized countries, and Culyer (1988) has demonstrated that Canada has a comparatively good record of cost control in the period since 1971, when Medicare was fully implemented. Pessimistically, one notes that although Canada's real expenditure growth from 1980 to 1990 was lower than the OECD mean, its rate of excess health care inflation was greater (Table 2; see also Coyte 1990). Schieber and Poullier (1989) suggest that the high excess inflation for both Canada and the United States reflects the fee-for-service reimbursement system prevalent in these two countries, resulting in looser controls on physician incomes. Not surprisingly, as noted below, physician reimbursement methods have accordingly been one major target of proposed reforms.

TABLE 2

Per capita health expenditures (1991), real growth, and excess inflation in seven major OECD countries - 1980-1990

	Per Capita Health Expenditure 1991, $[a]	Real Expenditure Per Capita Growth 1980-90, %[b]	Excess Health Care Inflation 1980-90, %[c]
United Kingdom	1,043	1.9	1.2
Japan	1,267	3.0	0.7
Italy	1,408	n/a	n/a
France	1,650	4.5	-1.1
Germany	1,659	1.1	0.4
Canada	1,915	2.3	1.9
United States	2,867	2.1	2.2
Mean	1,687	2.5	0.9

[a]   This is in Purchasing Power Parities (PPPs) in US dollars. PPPs are the rate of currency conversion which eliminate the differences in price levels between countries. Source: OECD 1993

[b]   This is adjusted for population growth and health care inflation, which then represents the growth in volume and intensity of services. Source: Schieber et al. 1992

[c]   Source: Schieber et al. 1992

TABLE 3
Life expectancy at birth (by sex) and infant mortality rates in the seven major OECD countries

| | Life Expectancy at Birth, 1991, Years | | Infant Mortality Rate per 1,000 Live Births |
	Female	Male	
Japan	82.1	76.1	4.6[a]
France	81.1	73.0	7.3
Canada	80.4[a]	73.8[a]	6.8[a]
Italy	80.0[b]	73.5[b]	8.3
Germany	79.0[b]	72.6[b]	7.1[a]
United Kingdom	78.8	73.2	7.4
United States	78.8[a]	72.0[a]	8.9
Mean	80.0	73.5	7.2

Source: OECD 1993
[a] 1990
[b] 1989

Table 3 demonstrates Canada's favourable health status among the seven major industrialized OECD countries. Canada has the second highest life expectancy rate at birth for males and has the second lowest infant mortality rate, next to Japan. It should be noted that these traditional health status indicators are based on the medical model, in which health is regarded narrowly as the absence of disease, and hence give only a partial picture of 'health.'

Income-related barriers to access have been largely eliminated. Studies from the 1971 to 1984 period reveal few differences in admission rates among income groups, and a reduction in the gap in life expectancy rates between the highest and lowest income groups (D'Arcy 1988; United States General Accounting Office 1991).

Canadians' level of satisfaction with the system has been documented by Blendon and Taylor (1989). Their data from surveys conducted in the fall of 1988 among adults in the United States, Canada, and Great Britain indicated that Canadians were the most satisfied with their national health insurance system (56 percent) whereas Americans were the least satisfied (10 percent). Over 90 percent of Canadians expressed a preference to remain with their current system rather than adopt a U.S. or U.K. system; in contrast, 61 percent of Americans surveyed indicated preference for adopting a Canadian type system and 29 percent a United Kingdom type system. In 1990, seven additional countries were surveyed – the Netherlands, Italy, West Germany, France, Sweden, Australia, and Japan (Blendon et al. 1990). Among the ten nations, Canadians were the most satisfied with their current health care system and Americans the least satisfied. Another study compared Canadian consumer satisfaction with six government services – fire protection, Medicare, garbage collection, police, education, and postal service. Eighty-nine percent believed they received good value from fire protection, and 87 percent believed they received good value from Medicare (Roth et al. 1990).

As in other health care systems, there are acknowledged inefficiencies in service delivery. For example, faulty population growth projections led to expansions in medical schools, and a resulting growth of physician supply which exceeds population growth (by 2.3 percent per year from 1961 to 1986) and has led to population-physician ratios richer than desired by many health planners (Barer et al. 1989). Guaranteed fund-

Examples of inefficiency + potential waste.

ing to hospitals reduced the pressure for innovations (e.g., day surgery, ambulatory treatment); consequently, length of stay and admission rates did not drop as quickly as they did in the post-DRG U.S. (Newhouse et al. 1988; Rachlis and Kushner 1989). Liability concerns and uncertainty-adverse practice patterns have led to similar (if less dramatic) possible overuse of radiographs, laboratory tests (Hazelton 1986) and surgical procedures (Anderson and Lomas 1989; Roos 1984; Vayda et al. 1984). Subsidized or free drugs for seniors have led to over-prescription of drugs for the elderly (Ontario Ministry of Health 1990). The lack of mechanisms to assess the effectiveness, efficacy, and cost-efficiency of new technologies and drugs have resulted in some unnecessary and inappropriate use, with potential hazards to patients (Deber et al. 1988; Linton 1990). Lastly, there is a comparative lack of mechanisms to assure quality of care among physicians in independent solo practice (Lomas 1990; Rachlis and Kushner 1989). These organizational and management problems are finally receiving the needed attention from providers and government to improve the efficiency of a basically healthy system.

The Qualified Success: Emerging Issues

Examination of current concerns reveals that Canada's health care system is a *qualified* success story. Can this success be maintained? Two strands of challenge within the health policy domain can be noted: that there is insufficient access to high technology care, and that access to health care itself is insufficient for health. In addition, four challenges have emerged from outside health policy: economic trends, demographic projections, federal-provincial disputes, and ideological beliefs.

Access to Technology

The issue of access to "state-of-the-art" technology in Canada has received considerable attention in recent years. The disaggregated management of the system makes comprehensive data on access to services difficult to obtain; arguments on this issue have used anecdotes and perceptions more than hard facts (Senate of Canada 1990). A report from the United States General Accounting Office discusses the limited access to diagnostic technologies such as magnetic resonance imaging and computed tomography (CT) scanners in Canada; however, the report indicates that patients with immediate or life-threatening needs rarely wait for services (United States General Accounting Office 1991). A widely cited study conducted by Rublee (1989) on the availability of six technologies in the United States, Canada, and Germany noted that the United States had nearly eight times more magnetic resonance imaging and radiation-therapy units per capita and over six times more lithotripsy centres per capita than did Canada (the study was conducted using Canadian data from 1988 and U.S. data from 1987). Two caveats, however, must be recognized before one can conclude that Canada is under serviced with technology. One, noted by Rublee, is that not all use is appropriate, and the U.S. figures may reflect some unnecessary diffusion. Less widely recognized is the difference between the number of units and the number of procedures; in contrast with the U.S., Canada has made deliberate efforts to regionalize high technology units, and ensure that each would have sufficient volume to ensure quality care. For example, Anderson et al. (1989) compared the number of procedures for cardiovascular disease in Canada with the rates in the United States, and concluded that with the exception of coronary bypass surgery, a procedure which is often deemed to be

EBP may help to ↑ efficiency of medicine

performed unnecessarily in the U.S. (Braunwald 1983; Winslow et al. 1988), elderly Canadians indeed had *higher* rates than did Americans for other complex but potentially beneficial procedures.

For the most part, allegations of waiting lists, once investigated, have usually proved to result either from organizational bottlenecks or from the rapid changes in practice patterns. The bottlenecks are a result of poor referral procedures which lead to a lack of knowledge of the available capacity coupled with waiting lists for particular providers. Subsequently, this is managed by the establishment of registries or hotlines. Providers and government have also been slow in reacting to changes in practice patterns such as the increased use of radiotherapy rather than surgery for certain cancers (see Naylor 1991). Such problems could well be considered growing pains as governments attempt to plan and manage a formerly disaggregated non-system. The extent of the waiting list problem is difficult to ascertain, but based on available evidence, to date it appears to have been greatly overstated by U.S. opponents of Canadian-style health care.

A second issue highlighted by technological advances is whether access to care should be governed by medical need or by ability to pay. The close proximity of the U.S. offers a simple alternative for sufficiently affluent Canadian patients dissatisfied with the position assigned to them in the queue. Canadian governments have taken the position that access should be governed by need, and that 'two tier' medicine is categorically unacceptable. To the extent that services must be offered to everyone or to no one, this view has tended to lead to everything eventually being available to everyone, and resulting cost pressure; in a universal system, the alternative would entail denying individuals the right to purchase services which might benefit them. In the long run, there is considerable concern that cost constraint measures, if these result in rationing, will lead to pressure to allow private insurance/private payment and hence undermine the universality of Medicare.

The Limits of Medical Care

Social determinants of health.

Health is not simply the absence of disease; increasingly, it is being defined as a "resource for everyday living" (World Health Organization 1984). Indeed, environmental awareness has resulted in linking the health of the individual to the health of the planet (Nelson 1989). As noted, this expansion of the definition of health has shifted the emphasis from equality of access to medical care to equity of access to health. Given that most policies have health implications, this broad definition presents the health care system with the challenge of determining and defining their boundaries in fulfilling this goal. Health is affected by poverty; does this mean that health policy should shift its attention from hospital and medical services to income distribution, housing, diet, education, environment, and employment? An example of taking such a broad definition can be seen in the *Health For All Ontario – Report of the Panel for Health Goals for Ontario* (Ontario Ministry of Health 1987). This report concludes that "society has a collective responsibility to ensure equity through its public policies and its allocation of resources" (p. 45), and draws from this a powerful agenda for action, stating that "government action is required to reduce the unacceptable risks to health which are experienced by many Ontarians." Among the programmes advocated are "affirmative action to enable the disadvantaged to reach their potential" (p. 48); "provision of affordable housing, rigorous enforcement of pollution controls, and ensuring of safe workplaces" (p. 49); elimination of all user fees and reduction of other barriers to access; and empowerment of local communities and transfer of decision making authority to the local level.

Conversely, if we choose to accept that inequalities in the quality of housing, diet, or education available are appropriate (i.e., that social justice requires provision of a 'minimal' standard, but allows 'Cadillacs and steaks' for the more affluent), how can the case for a universal one-tier medical care system be maintained once we recognize that medical care is less important to health than are these other factors? To date, these questions have only partially been dealt with by the advocates of equity of access to health.

Economic Trends

An additional complication results if one recognizes the link between social programmes and an economy healthy enough to generate the necessary economic surplus (Mustard 1990). A major challenge to Canadian health policy thus comes from Canadian economic trends, as well as their impact on federal-provincial transfer payments.

At the present time, Canada is facing relatively high unemployment and inflation rates, and is running large government deficits. In fact, Canada has the largest public debt, per capita, in the world (Editorial 1993). The OECD has warned that this large debt could slow the pace of Canada's economic recovery (Canadian Press 1993). In comparison to the G-7 OECD countries, Canada had the highest unemployment rate in 1993 (11.3%) next to Italy (11.5%) (Conference Board of Canada 1994; Nevison 1993). On an encouraging note, the Conference Board of Canada forecasts that the unemployment rate will decline to 10.7% in 1994. Furthermore, Canada is forecasted to have the strongest growth among the G-7 economies in 1994 (3%) (Nevison 1993).

Pressured by a less than healthy economy and a massive ($34.6 billion in 1991-92) (Canada Department of Finance 1993) federal deficit, Canada's federal government has adopted a policy goal of reducing its financial commitment to the provinces. This practise of reducing transfers to provinces by a greater proportion than other federal programme spending has been termed "off-loading." According to the C.D. Howe Institute, the federal government's off-loading practise has reduced health care transfers by $1.7 billion in the fiscal year 1991/92 (Boothe and Johnston 1993). Boothe and Johnston conclude that "the health care system has been targeted as one of the main areas to bear the burden of federal deficit reduction" (Boothe and Johnston 1993: 10).[1] The effects of the cut backs will be further compounded by the federal Government Expenditure Restraint Act which came into effect February 1, 1991. If unchanged, the resulting modifications of the spending formula were predicted to lead to the elimination of the cash portion of federal transfer payments under EPF within 15 years, and the consequent elimination of its financial levers to enforce national standards for Medicare (Bryce 1991). In partial response to the resulting uproar, the federal government introduced Bill C-20 which has been enacted as the Budget Implementation Act, 1991. This act has maintained the federal power to withhold federal cash transfers from the provinces in non-health areas if they violate the Canada Health Act.

This attempt by the federal government to reduce its financial commitment to Medicare comes at a time when the growth rate in utilization of medical services has exceeded the rate of growth in population, and the growth in costs has exceeded the growth in provincial revenues. Consequently, health care spending has been absorbing an increasing share of provincial budgets. For example, in the industrial heartland of Ontario, the cost of health care in the decade ending in 1988 rose by 63.4 percent while the provincial economy grew by 42.7 percent (Ontario Ministry of Health 1989). Economic forces have thus placed pressure on the provinces to find innovative approaches to meeting the health needs. Since cost-shifting is simpler than cost-containment, fears for the future of Medicare have revived (Rachlis 1991). In fact, Boothe and Johnston conclude that "as EPF transfers decline, greater decentralization of and disparity in health care is inevitable" (Boothe and Johnston 1993: 9).

Demographic Projections

The demographic shift to an older population and the shift from infectious diseases to chronic and degenerative diseases as the major medical problem of Canadians poses another challenge to the current delivery of health services (Jackson 1986). Canada currently has the youngest population among the seven OECD nations (Organisation for Economic Co-operation and Development 1993). Changes in medical patterns of practice, sparked by technological improvements, have resulted in an increased use of medical interventions among the elderly (Barer et al. 1987). Projections therefore suggest that unless changes are made in the way services are delivered and financed, the system will become unmanageable as the proportion of elderly in Canada increases to European levels.

Federal-Provincial Disputes

At the political level the relationship between the federal and provincial governments is strained as a result of the reduced financial commitment on part of the federal government and past discussions as to the future of the Canadian confederation, which to date are still unresolved. As noted, Canada's constitution clearly placed health care under provincial jurisdiction. During the constitutional discussions and subsequent political debates at the party levels, Medicare continues to be debated; the main issues being universality, and the role of the federal government.

Medicare is an extremely popular programme, to the extent that it has been mentioned as "a modern-day equivalent of the Transcontinental railway: a tie that binds from coast to coast" (Courchene 1991), and was cited by the Citizens' Forum on Canada's Future[2] as a key element of the Canadian identity (Minister of Supply and Services Canada 1991). Nonetheless, there are voices suggesting that the federal government should withdraw completely from the health field and transfer the additional revenue to the general funds of the provinces (The Group of 22 1991). Such suggestions have been welcomed by advocates of greater provincial power, particularly in Western Canada and Quebec, and attacked by the defenders of Medicare. Given the popularity of Medicare, advocates of federal withdrawal have carefully insisted that Medicare would not be endangered by the removal of national standards, since provinces would tamper with Medicare at their peril. Others are not reassured. Indeed, in 1991, a massive health action lobby, HEAL, was formed to defend national standards.[3]

Ideological Beliefs

Evans has referred to ideas that should be dead, but still walk around and do damage as "zombies" (Evans 1992). U.S.-influenced market concepts have suggested that 'free' services will inevitably be 'abused.' Accordingly, the debate over user fees has refused to die. Despite a consensus among Canadian health economists that patient-based direct charges are not a good way to control costs (Stoddart et al. 1993) and their elim-ination after the passage of the Canada Health Act with all party approval (Heiber and Deber 1987), the erosion of federal transfer payments and the resulting pressure on provincial budgets have reawakened provincial proposals to transfer costs out of pro-vincial budgets to reduce the need for tax increases. One form these pressures have taken is increased use of alternative revenue generation methods, e.g., charging annual premiums which cover only a small percentage of health costs, but which augment pro-vincial general revenues. Alberta and British Columbia currently charge such fees and Nova Scotia is considering them; Ontario has replaced its premiums with a payroll tax. Another form is more careful scrutiny of which health services will be defined as 'med-ically required' and hence insured under Medicare, and deinsurance of procedures deemed marginal (Alberta and Ontario have done this). The third form, explicitly penalized under the Canada Health Act, is the introduction of user charges for insured services; Quebec has nonetheless proposed such charges (e.g., $5 per 'unnecessary' emergency room visit) as part of its ongoing challenge to federal authority over areas they perceive to be constitutionally under provincial control. Also there are user fees for non-insured services, such as prescription drugs. If proposals for a vastly reduced federal role are adopted (The Group of 22 1991), it is likely that provinces will con-tinue such efforts to transfer costs, even though they may violate the Canada Health Act, with consequent erosion of Medicare.

Provincial Commissions: Policy Options for More Success

Given the changing environment, it is notable that seven of the ten Canadian provinces have recently conducted extensive reviews of their health systems. In this analysis, we consider these reports:

* British Columbia: *Closer to Home* (British Columbia Royal Commission on Health Care and Costs 1991);
* Alberta: *Rainbow Report: Our Vision For Health* (Alberta Premier's Commission on Future Health Care for Albertans 1989);
* Saskatchewan: *Future Directions For Health Care In Saskatchewan* (Saskatchewan Commission on Directions in Health Care 1990);
* Quebec: *Commission D'Enquête Sur Les Services De Santé Et Les Services Sociaux* (Quebec: Commission d'Enquête Sur Les Services de Santé et Les Ser-vices Sociaux 1987);
* New Brunswick: *Report of The Commission On Selected Health Care Programs* (New Brunswick Commission on Selected Health Care Programs 1989);
* Nova Scotia: *The Report of the Nova Scotia Royal Commission On Health Care: Toward a New Strategy* (Nova Scotia Royal Commission on Health Care 1989);
* Ontario Ministry of Health: *Toward A Shared Direction For Health In Ontario* [Evans Report] (Evans 1987), *Health For All Ontario: Report of the Panel On Health Goals For Ontario* [Spasoff Report] (Ontario Ministry of Health 1987), *Health Promotion Matters In Ontario* [Podborski Report] (Podborski 1987), and *Deciding The Future Of Our Health Care* (Ontario Ministry of Health 1989);
* Ontario Premier's Council on Health Strategy, which was established in response to the Evans, Spasoff, and Podborski reports: *A Vision Of Health: Health Goals for Ontario* (Premier's Council on Health Strategy 1989a), *From Vision To Action* (Pre-mier's Council on Health Strategy 1989b), *Nurturing Health* (Premier's Council on

Health Strategy 1991a), *Local Decision Making For Health and Social Services* (Premier's Council on Health Strategy 1991b), and *Achieving the Vision: Health Human Resources* (Premier's Council on Health Strategy 1991c).

In June 1991, Prince Edward Island released a non-comprehensive study focusing on hospitals in the community. This study has not been included in the subsequent discussion.

Health Policy Themes Mentioned in Provincial Reports

A review of the reports reveals several recurring themes (Table 4):

1. Broadening the definition of health with the collaboration of multiple sectors.
2. Shifting emphasis from curing illness to promoting health and preventing disease.
3. Switching focus to community based rather than institution based care.
4. Providing more opportunity for individuals to participate with service providers in making decisions on health choices and policies.
5. Devolution or decentralization of the provincial systems to some form of regional authorities.
6. Improved human resources planning, with particular emphasis on alternative methods for remuneration of physicians.
7. Enhanced efficiency in the management of services through the establishment of councils, co-ordinating bodies, and secretariats.
8. Increasing funds for health services research, especially in the areas of utilization, technology assessment, programme/system evaluation, and information systems.

TABLE 4
Health policy themes mentioned in provincial reports

Common Themes	BC	AB	SAS	ONT	QUE	NB	NS [a]
Broad definition of health		X	X	X	X	X	X
Intersectoral planning	X		X	X	X		X
Health promotion and disease prevention	X	X	X	X	X	X	X
Shift from institution to community	X	X	X	X	X	X	X
Increased participation	X	X	X	X	X	X	X
Regional authorities	X	X	X	X	X	X	X
Improved human resources planning	X	X	X	X	X	X	X
Alternative methods of physician renumeration		X	X	X	X	X	X
Premier's Council	X			X		X	X
Research	X	X	X	X	X	X	X

[a] Province abbreviations: BC = British Columbia; AB = Alberta; SAS = Saskatchewan; ONT = Ontario; QUE = Quebec; NB = New Brunswick; NS = Nova Scotia.

1. Broadening the Definition of Health

With the exception of the B.C. Commission,[4] all of the reviews accepted a broad definition of health, corresponding to the World Health Organization's definition of health as being a resource for everyday living, not just the absence of disease. In practice, this definition requires addressing issues other than medical care (e.g., education, housing, unemployment, food production, equity, social justice, and the environment) which play a major role in creating a healthy society. Policy initiatives which address these issues are termed 'healthy public policy,' and require the collaboration of multiple sectors. Healthy public policy advocates also stress the importance of public participation in policy formulation and implementation (Hancock 1985; Milio 1985; Pederson et al. 1988).

The healthy public policy approach occurs frequently in the provincial reviews. Quebec's recommendations would extend this concept into service delivery, for example it was proposed that the regional authorities be given power over both health and social services. Multisectoral initiatives in the other provinces concentrated on planning. Saskatchewan recommended an "Enriched Housing Committee" and a "Social Policy Secretariat" which would facilitate communication, co-ordination, and planning of common programmes and services; suggested representation would include the Departments of Health, Social Services, Education, Human Resources, Labour and Employment, Alcohol and Drug Abuse Foundation, Housing Corporation, and the Saskatchewan Family Foundation. Nova Scotia similarly recommended inter-sectoral co-ordination of such departments as Health, Community Services, Education, Environment, Housing, and Labour, under the aegis of a Cabinet Secretariat. British Columbia recommended that the "regional ministries" work with the Ministry of Housing and Social Services for better planning. The British Columbia Commission made a number of recommendations addressing issues such as poverty, employment, and the environment, and even went as far to recommend that all proposed provincial programmes or legislation be reviewed by the Ministry of Health to identify the possible health effect. Ontario set up a multisectorial Premier's Council on Health Strategy with representation from six government ministries, plus professional, labour, business, and community representatives.[5] Its Healthy Public Policy Subcommittee published a 1991 report, *Nurturing Health*, with the theme that access to medical care does not necessarily mean that there is equal access to health, and that "even more significant improvements in health can result from policy initiatives outside the arena of the health care system proper" (Premier's Council on Health Strategy 1991a: 2).

2. Promoting Health and Preventing Disease

The reports reflect a partial rejection of the medical model, and a wish for increased emphasis on health promotion and disease prevention. The Alberta Commission recommended reallocating a minimum of one percent of the health budget to health promotion and illness/injury prevention activities. Nova Scotia's Commission recommended the establishment of a Community Health Initiatives Fund in support of health promotion and illness prevention projects at the community level. Saskatchewan's Commission recommended that the total provincial health promotion fund should be determined on the basis of $10 per capita. (The other provinces emphasized the importance of health promotion, but did not make specific budget recommendations.) The shifting of emphasis to health promotion and disease prevention was one of the five health goals set by Ontario's Premier's Council on Health Strategy. British Columbia's Commission expressed a need to spend more money on the prevention of illness or injury and on protecting health, and made recommendations about illness and injury prevention initiatives (bicycle helmets and paths, alcohol limit, and truck braking systems), immunization, and sexually transmitted diseases. New Brunswick's Commission recommended that their provincial council on health review existing health promotion and education programmes and determine future needs.

3. Community Based Care

The reports all echoed a desire to shift emphasis from institution based to community based care. One of Saskatchewan's six proposed "directions for the future" is an emphasis on community and supportive living services. According to the report, this would involve the development of a comprehensive, co-ordinated, and integrated programme of community health by each of the division councils (regional authorities), and establishing user fees for home care services (e.g., home maintenance, meals on wheels, and personal emergency response systems). Acute care facilities would be reclassified to serve community needs and ensure the most appropriate services are available at various levels.

British Columbia, Ontario, and Nova Scotia identified the need to allocate resources to community based services. This was evident in British Columbia Commission's recommendations of decreasing beds and improving on care in the community. New Brunswick's Commission praised the Extra-Mural Hospital programme, established in New Brunswick in 1981 to provide hospital care in the home, as exemplifying the switch from institutional to community based care, and recommended its expansion.

4. Increased Participation

Involving individuals in the planning and management of the health system is one of the major principles advocated by all the reviews. The devolution of power through regional authorities is one of the major avenues recommended to translate the participation principle into practice. Other routes include ensuring the membership of community members on planning committees, and education of consumers on how to use the system more effectively.

Only Alberta's Commission suggested shifting fiscal caps from the province or community level to the individual; it recommended the introduction of a "smart card" which would allocate a fixed quota of health resources to each Albertan, and give the individual the responsibility for "disbursing, managing and monitoring the funds required for their health care needs" (Alberta Premier's Commission on Future Health Care for Albertans 1989: 35).

The Alberta Commission also recommended the introduction of legislation to enable Albertans to provide enduring power of attorney and advanced directives. Other provinces (e.g., Ontario) are also investigating these issues, but did not include them in their reports.

5. Regional Authorities

How can community based care, consumer participation, equity of services, and improved efficiency and effectiveness be achieved? All the provincial reports recommend the development of regional authorities. However, there is variation in how much power they believed should be devolved.

The reports differed in their recommendations for how the proposed regional authorities should be funded, membership and appointment of boards, range of services offered, and responsibilities of both the regional authority and provincial government. New Brunswick's formula of regional authority would consist of "Area Health Planning Councils" which would primarily function to co-ordinate and rationalize services in their respective areas and regularly report to the Premier's Council. The proposed regional authorities in British Columbia, Alberta, Saskatchewan, Quebec, and Nova Scotia would be globally funded, based on population. The British Columbia Commission recommended that the budget would take into account local service need and broad base health risk indicators and the process would involve consumers and providers. Quebec and Saskatchewan recommended that their regional authorities also be given limited power to raise funds through municipal levy; Saskatchewan limiting this to a maximum of five percent of the provincial allocation, and Quebec to financing deficits.

With the exception of British Columbia, the proposed regional authorities would all be governed by a board which British Columbia's Commission recommended, that the board would play an advisory role, and that its membership should be determined locally. The other provinces, with the exception of Nova Scotia all recommended that the board would be locally elected. Alberta proposed the mandatory inclusion of one youth representative on the board. Nova Scotia advocated an appointed board comprised of consumers and providers.

It should be noted that the British Columbia Commission's recommendation of decentralization is one more of the formation of "regional centres" whereby there is Ministry staff at the regions who are accountable to senior management in the Ministry of Health. The regional centres will be responsible for area-specific health services planning and resource allocation.

Alberta, Saskatchewan, Quebec, and Nova Scotia all proposed that their respective regional authorities provide an extensive range of health services including health promotion, primary and secondary acute care services, ambulance services, long term care, and community based care. Alberta explicitly stated that its regional authorities would not be responsible for social services; whereas Quebec's proposed regional bodies would be responsible for both health and social services and the British Columbia Commission recommended the creation of cross-ministerial regional teams (i.e. Housing and Social Services). Saskatchewan's version of regional authorities, called "health services division councils," would also be responsible for mental health. Nova Scotia's regional health authority, according to the Commission, would also be responsible for Pharmacare. In addition to actual delivery of services the regional authorities would be expected to be responsible for planning, administration, budget allocation, human resources planning, and in some cases evaluation. Quebec and Nova Scotia's models also gave considerable authority with respect to physician remuneration. Ontario to a certain extent had already decentralized planning with the gradual introduction of District Health Councils since 1973. These voluntary bodies, with consumer, provider, and local government representation, continue to serve as advisory bodies to the Ontario Ministry of Health, but have no budgetary authority.[6]

6. Human Resources Planning

All of the commissions recommended that planning for numbers, roles, distribution, and mix of health professionals must be improved. Suggestions were also made for the training of future health professionals which incorporates the future directions of the system. Ontario recommended the creation of a planning agency at the provincial level whereby the planning process would achieve consensus based on population health needs, include consumer participation, and be open to public scrutiny (Premier's Council on Health Strategy 1991c).

British Columbia, Saskatchewan, Ontario, Quebec, New Brunswick, and Nova Scotia all suggested the need to review the current fee-for-service remuneration method and introduce other methods such as capitation, salary, or a mixed reimbursement system. Nova Scotia's and British Columbia's Royal Commission recommended reducing undergraduate medical school enrollment. It should be noted that in June 1991, a report entitled, *Toward Integrated Medical Resource Policies For Canada,* was submitted to the Steering Committee of the Conference of Deputy Ministries of Health which focused on physician resource policy in Canada. A number of recommendations were made including reducing medical school enrollment to maintain current population:physician ratio and the replacement of fee-for-service as a payment mechanism for physicians where this method "aligns poorly with the nature or objective of the service being provided" (Barer and Stoddart 1991: 26).

One controversial recommendation made by the British Columbia Commission was its rejection of the policy – advocated by professional nursing – to make the baccalaureate the minimal entry level requirement for nursing. According to the Commission, this recommendation was based on the idea that the level of training should not exceed the skills necessary to perform the required tasks and there was concern of the increasing costs associated with the upgrading. *Want to maintain status quo. Does this relate to BC commission not looking ahead to a greater definition of health?*

7. Provincial Planning and Co-ordination

In order to define and achieve desired outcomes the commissions have emphasized efficient management through the establishment of provincial councils, regional authorities, and co-ordinating bodies. Alberta's Commission recommended the establishment of a Research and Technology Council and an "Advocate for a Healthy Alberta" to review the efficiency, effectiveness, and suitability of the health system. The Saskatchewan Commission recommended the reclassification and redefinition of the mandates of acute care facilities, and the establishment of approximately seventeen new committees, boards, and secretariats. In Ontario, a provincial council, chaired by the Premier has been established since 1987. A similar council has been recommended in British Columbia, New Brunswick and Nova Scotia. The Quebec Commission suggested a refocused central authority, creation of a Centre for Public Health, and a Council on Health and Welfare. The health council recommended by the British Columbia Commission made it very clear that the council should report to the Legislative Assembly, not the Ministry of Health. In order to improve on the organization and administration of the system the New Brunswick Commission recommended (in addition to a health council and an area planning council) improvements in the organization and operation of hospitals in: the division of labor, role of physicians in hospital management, and measures for controlling costs. Nova Scotia's Commission recommended a new planning dynamic which would be comprehensive, multisectoral, and have an ecological perspective. Specifically, it recommended merging of various current commissions into one department, and establishing a Health Policy and Management Research Centre. Both New Brunswick and Nova Scotia recommended the establishment of interprovincial co-ordination for tertiary care, health professionals, health services research, and medical technology assessment.

8. Research

Although the commissions implicitly, and in some cases explicitly, were oriented to 'healthy public policy' they also expressed concern about the efficiency and effectiveness of the current medical system. Alberta, Saskatchewan, Quebec, New Brunswick, and Quebec all recommended increasing funds for research on health care utilization, cost effectiveness and efficiency of delivery systems and medical practices, health services research, and technology assessment. Alberta proposed to do this by expanding the mandate of the Alberta Research Council; Saskatchewan recommended establishing a Health Analysis and Development Centre; New Brunswick recommended the expansion of the capacity of the Planning and Evaluation Division of the Department of the Health and Community Services and ensuring that a part of the health budget (1/4 of 1 percent) would be set aside for programmes or facilities to improve their effectiveness; and Nova Scotia proposed a standing committee of the Health Council to examine the acquisition and use of technology. The British Columbia Commission made numerous recommendations to improving data bases and make them more accessible in order to ensure that the services were meeting the needs of the people. In fact, one of its recommendations was to expand the mandate of the British Columbia Office of Health Technology Assessment to include quality assurance and utilization management activities and change its name to the British Columbia Office of Health Care Evaluation. In Ontario, the Health Care System Committee of the Premier's Council on Health Strategy recommended a doubling of provincial funding for such outcome oriented research, and the since disbanded Ontario Task Force On the Use and Provision of Medical Services, recommended the creation of a Technology Assessment Council and a guidelines committee to develop effective approaches to the provision of care and use of resources within the health care system.

9. Other Recommendations

An assortment of other recommendations are included in particular reports. For example, Alberta and Saskatchewan in their reports each suggested the establishment of an Ethics Centre. British Columbia, Saskatchewan, and Quebec were the only provinces to address the issue of the health of Canada's First Nations People (aboriginal people) in the major review of their health care system, although other provinces have prepared other specific reports addressing the issue of First Nations People's health.

Discussion of the Policy Options

The policy options of incorporating a broader definition of health, health promotion and disease prevention, community based care, consumer participation, and improved efficiency and effectiveness in the health care system are neither new nor original ideas. The qualified success of Medicare in largely solving access issues has given Canada the luxury of recognizing and acknowledging them, while the current political, social, and economic climate indicate that their time to come to fruition may finally have arrived.

Implications of a Broader Definition of Health

Canada may have largely solved one set of problems – ensuring equality of access to medical care. By recognizing the limits of medical care and broadening the definition of health, however, it has created another problem to solve – ensuring equity of access to health. This goal, however desirable, cannot be addressed by the health sector alone. As Evans and Stoddart state: "the WHO definition is difficult to use as the basis for health policy, because implicitly it includes all policy as health policy" (Evans and Stoddart 1990: 3). They conclude, however, that by only focusing on health care, rather than health, "we may find that we are as a society both poorer, and less healthy, than we could otherwise be" (Evans and Stoddart 1990: 58).

Examination of the provincial reports does reveal that the provinces do recognize that access to health cannot be accomplished by the health sector alone. However, their operational suggestions as to how other elements can be mobilized are, not surprisingly, tentative and incomplete. For example, although the environment clearly plays an important role in attaining access to health, only Alberta and Ontario explicitly identify the impact of the environment on health, and their recommendations are modest. Alberta has subsequently recommended developing an Alberta Code of Health and Environmental Ethics and encouraged research in environmental health and protection. Ontario's document *Nurturing Health* (1991a) addresses the issue of the necessity of a cleaner and safer environment in order to be healthy, but deals only with air pollution; water pollution, for example, is ignored, even though Ontario borders four of the five Great Lakes, which supply much of the province with drinking water. The Saskatchewan Commission recognizes the harmful effects of environmental pollutants on health, yet no recommendations were made to deal with this issue. The British Columbia Commission does discuss the environment in terms of the healthy communities movement. Its recommendations primarily deal with ensuring that health effects are considered in any environmental impact analysis and provision of safe drinking water.

Although the commissions do make some recommendations to translate this broad definition of health into practice, it could be argued that these still are not concrete enough. Ironically, the British Columbia Commission report explicitly stated that it did not use the broad definition of health, but had recommendations which better translated the broad definition of health than did the other commissions. For example, legislation of bicycle helmets, licensing standards for child care programmes, increasing level of welfare payments for families with children, and reducing violence in television programmes all speak to health in the broadest sense.

The broad definition of health also implies reallocation of resources, and potential cross country collaboration to deal with externalities and spillovers. Given the 'unhealthy' state of the Canadian economy, the growing fiscal burden on the provinces, and the political battle over federal-provincial responsibilities,[7] this will be a difficult task for the provinces to accomplish. In addition, current federal government determination to reduce transfer payments essentially eliminates a potential source of seed money for new initiatives.

Acceptance of the broad definition of health would require major policy changes. As Brown has noted, such policy "breakthroughs" become difficult as they are overshad-

owed by a need to deal with the maintenance and improvement ("rationalizing politics") of current policy initiatives. This "rationalizing" approach of current policies
(improving their efficiency, management, coherence, and co-ordination) "challenge,
constrain, and hold hostage visions of breakthroughs" (Brown 1983: 66). Sparked by
economic difficulties and constitutional uncertainties, Medicare itself is being challenged. For example, provinces seeking to shift costs are again speculating about user
fees, while the attack from the right (particularly powerful in the U.S. and in the U.K.)
has suggested that universal programmes, however desirable and popular, may no
longer be affordable in current tough economic times (Deber 1991). These ideas trade
on 'popular wisdom' which holds that 'free programmes,' by definition, will be
'abused,' and that the public sector is always less efficient than the private sector. As
Evans has noted, these ideas can be shown to be incorrect, but have proven remarkably
resilient (Evans 1992).

Paradoxically, broadening the definition of health can threaten the gains already
achieved. First, separating essential from marginal programmes may become more difficult. Second, as policy recommendations attempt to link health with such other areas
such as housing, for which there exists strong public support for an existing multi-
tiered system, health may become subjected to the same criteria. Healthy public policy
in effect requires that we rethink not only our health care system, but also society's values and priorities. The goal of access to health is thus likely to prove far more challenging than was access to medical care.

A New Organizational Structure: Regional Health Authorities?

The commissions all endorsed a shift in focus from doctors and hospitals to a community based, consumer participation model, involving the decentralization of planning
authority from the provincial to the regional level. This emphasis is not new; these concepts have long been advocated by Canadian health planners (e.g., see Health and Welfare Canada 1973; and Mustard 1974). What is new is that these recommendations
finally seem to have percolated into 'common knowledge' and are receiving more serious attention. Given that provincial governments, under the Constitution, retain ultimate accountability for health policy and expenditures, it is striking that the provincial
reports all recommended varying degrees of decentralization or even devolution (i.e.,
transfer of power) to regional health authorities. Both decentralization and devolution
involve some transfer of decision making from a larger unit to a smaller 'sub-unit'; in
devolved models, the province would also transfer some financial responsibility and
accountability.

It should be noted that an alternative approach for changing delivery models has
been reflected in experiments with managed care models based on voluntary enrollment of individuals within an organization. The organization in turn would receive cap-
itated funds, with which it would have to provide comprehensive care to its members.
Such managed care systems are not responsible for non-members outside their geographical catchment areas. Ontario has plans to test Comprehensive Health Organizations, Quebec has a system called Organisations de soins intégré de santé, and
Vancouver Vi-Care (Lamb et al. 1991). These models in theory can embody a broad
definition of health; their implementation requires devolution of management activities
to consumers and providers rather than to regional bodies. Although such models are
compatible with public competition approaches (Saltman and von Otter 1992), the ability of such models to co-exist with other regional planning structures is unclear. For

example, the Saskatchewan report called for regions with budgetary authority and made no reference to the Health Co-operative Models which have been in place in Saskatchewan since 1962, even though these organizations provide a similar set of services, and stress the principle of community based organization (rather than by region) and democratic control by their members.

Implementation of the recommendations is proceeding at various rates across the country. The government of Quebec, already the most regionalized province, has been most active. The 1989 report endorsed the Rochon Commission's recommendation of devolution by the formation of regional health and social services boards, but rejected its Commission's suggestion that the board be elected locally and given the ability to tax. Saskatchewan has also been very active in implementing regional authorities. The Health District Act, passed in May 1993, announced an elected and appointed board structure. The board would be responsible for allocating resources in its "health district" based on its assessment of health needs and ensure the delivery of core health services. The targeted date for district formation was August 1993. Region sizes vary between about 12,000 and 250,000 (in the major cities of Regina and Saskatoon). The reforms have been greeted with a combination of enthusiasm (because of the potential for enhancing community-based primary care) and public concern, particularly where hospitals would be closed down, resulting in loss of employment for a number of people.

New Brunswick in March 1992 legislated that 51 hospital boards and management committees in hospitals and health services centres were to be dissolved and replaced by eight new region boards. Members of the regions' boards would either be selected or appointed by the Minister of Health and the board itself. The boards' responsibilities would range from organizing, planning, and managing resources. The British Columbia Commission had also recommended a type of regional authority which they referred to as "regional centres." In the Fall of 1993, the provincial NDP government did introduce a similar concept, proposing 20 regional health boards. As of this writing, implementation has not yet taken place.

The government of Nova Scotia issued the report *Health Strategy for the Nineties: Managing Better Health* (Nova Scotia Department of Health 1990). Based on this report, Nova Scotia appears to be reluctant to cede the degree of authority recommended by its Commission. Rather than establishing regional health authorities, as recommended by the Commission, the government has decided to introduce Regional Health Agencies. These Agencies will serve as an advisory body to the Department of Health and will not have any fiscal authority. They appear to be similar to the District Health Councils in Ontario.

Ontario has not yet been as active in the development of regional authorities. In 1991 the Southwestern Ontario Comprehensive Health System Planning Commission put together a report (*Working Together to Achieve Better Health For All*) proposing a regional level of governance and funding (Southwestern Ontario Comprehensive Health System Planning Commission 1991). The focus in Ontario at the present seems more on rationalizing hospital services and improving efficiency of service delivery than on forming regional authorities, although experiments with regional budgets for targeted services (e.g., long term care) are being proposed and investigated.

The reports were hampered by a lack of clarity in defining the rationale for regional models. Generally, it was expected that regional authorities could serve multiple goals simultaneously – more responsive and democratic decision making, more equitable and appropriate services, and better cost control.

A review of experiences in other countries indicates that the multiple goals may not all be achievable. Although buffering plus global budgets may indeed be successful in achieving cost containment, the democratic gains may prove more elusive. Evaluation of the 1984 Norway reform – which decentralized primary health care services to the municipalities in an effort to achieve more equitable distribution of services and to enhance democracy by increasing local political control over the health services – concluded that these goals were not being achieved in practice. Elstad noted that inequities present between municipalities on such dimensions as staffing ratios and revenue levels were similar in 1983 (prior to the reform) and 1988 (after the reform). In addition, the reform's requirement of local participation merely replaced the old central hierarchies with "local hierarchies" dominated by professionals and bureaucrats (Elstad 1989). Similarly, preliminary results from a study underway in Quebec on the Healthy Cities Network reveals that the primary actors in the healthy cities projects are professionals rather than the local citizens (O'Neill 1991).

In contrast, democratic control and accountability is one of the major strengths of the Swedish system, in which elected local county councils are the primary agencies responsible for financing and managing health services; the weakness of the system lies in the lack of integration between primary care, hospital care, and social care. There also appears to be a strong emphasis on hospital care to the "neglect of primary and community health services" with limited choice for patients (Ham 1992: 136). Ham discusses the possibility of a "shift back from decentralization," primarily strengthening the policymaking role at the centre to enable it to monitor and review the performance of county councils (Ham 1992: 137).

The goal of better cost control theoretically does seem feasible. By capping the total funds available, the regional authority model does in theory have the potential to increase the effectiveness of resource allocation, including shifting funds from institutions to community based services and encouraging healthy public policy initiatives. On the other hand, regionalization may operate as a mechanism to allow higher levels of government to reduce health expenditures by shifting them (and the resulting struggles about resource allocation) elsewhere (Elstad 1989; Tsalikis 1989; Wildavsky 1989). As Evans has noted, health costs are also health incomes (1984); hence realizing the potential savings will require political battles with providers who may see lowered incomes as the consequence of lowered costs.

Can we expect that Canadian regional authorities, if implemented, will improve equity and increase consumer input? It seems unlikely. There also remains major issues of implementation.

Conclusions: Achieving Access to Health?

Having achieved its goal of providing access to health care for all Canadians, within its borders, can Canada take the next step and provide equitable access to health? Based on the provincial reviews, certainly current provincial health policy documents respond with a "yes;" they define health in the broadest context and emphasize community based care and consumer participation through a more devolved system. They also focus on improving the efficiency and effectiveness of the resources used by the medical system.

Policy, however, has become increasingly interdependent. Health policy issues can no longer be handled in isolation; they have moved outside the protected policy arena of the 'medical care system.' Canada's health goals must now operate in an environ-

Existing power structures õ in health care have deep cultural roots. How do we △ this?

Mhatre and Deber   479

ment of economic, political, and constitutional uncertainty. Policy prouncements are also not the same as the actual implementation of reform. At both the policy stages, but particularly at the stage of implementation the existing power structures of society, and of the health care system, are revealed.

Notes

1   EPF transfers, the largest single source of federal assistance to the provinces, had grown from $14.5 billion in 1984-85 to approximately $20 billion in 1990-91 (Canada Department of Finance 1991: 70). In 1990-91 total transfer payments (cash and tax) via EPF accounted for approximately 18.8 percent of federal programme spending. Although the original EPF formula had been scheduled to grow roughly in line with inflation and population growth, a series of unilateral federal modifications were announced. In 1986 the EPF formula was modified to limit the rate of growth of federal transfers to two percent less than the average nominal GNP growth in the preceding three years (Barker 1988). In 1989, this was further reduced to GNP less three percentage points. In February 1990, the per capita EPF transfers for 1990-91 and 1991-92 were frozen at the 1989-90 level (see Note 7). The 1991 federal budget extended the freeze on the per capita EPF entitlements and the 5 percent cap on the growth of the CAP payments to 1994-95 (Canada Department of Finance 1989, 1990, 1991; Health and Welfare Canada 1990). This freeze was reiterated in the 1993 federal budget (Canada Department of Finance 1993).

2   The Citizens' Forum on Canada's Future, chaired by Keith Spicer, was a forum established by the federal Progressive Conservative government on November 1, 1990 to go across the country and listen to what Canadians wanted and believed to be important to the future of their country. This dialogue involved forums across the country, a toll free telephone line, submission of briefs and letters, and participation in small informal discussion groups (Minister of Supply and Services 1991).

3   HEAL is a lobby of seven of Canada's largest health and consumer groups – the Canadian Hospital Association, Canadian Long Term Care Association, Canadian Medical Association, Canadian Nursing Association, Canadian Psychological Association, Canadian Public Health Association, and the Consumers Association of Canada. It was established in 1991 to develop and analyze options for a renewed health care system which will guarantee and protect the principles of Medicare.

4   The report states that it understands this broader definition of health, yet for the purpose of the report "[the Commission] have concentrated on the narrower fields set out in our terms of reference. [The Commission] believes that this focus is essential and that it has resulted in recommendations which are both pragmatic in nature and achievable in scope" (British Columbia Royal Commission on Health Care and Costs 1991: iv).

5   The Premier's Council's mandate is to examine policy options for the future direction of health and health care in Ontario; to establish priorities; and to build consensus for change in partnership with health care providers and community representatives. With the election of a New Democratic Party provincial government in 1990 the Council has been renamed to the Premier's Council on Health, Well Being, and Social Justice, and the membership altered to provide more "grass roots" membership. The impact of this restructing on its mandate is not yet clear. The reports from the old council, however, have been adopted.

6   Two possible governance models were proposed: a local government model and a special purpose body model. The local government model would involve a regional or upper tier of local government body to function as a committee of the municipal council. Members would be elected, thus ensuring accountability. This special purpose body model would build on the

expertise of such bodies as the District Health Councils; its members might be chosen through provincial appointment, direct election, or the combination of elected or appointed members.

7 The February 1990 federal budget also announced that the growth in Canada Assistance Plan (CAP) transfers to the three wealthiest provinces (Alberta, British Columbia, and Ontario) would be limited to 5% a year for the next two years. The Government of Canada's ability to make such unilateral changes to the shared-cost agreements with the provinces was upheld by the Supreme Court of Canada in August 1991 (British Columbia Reference 1991).

References

Alberta Premier's Commission on Future Health Care for Albertans. 1989. *The Rainbow Report: Our Vision for Health,* Vols. 1-3. Edmonton: Premier's Commission on Future Health Care for Albertans.

Anderson, GM, and J Lomas. 1989. Regionalization of Coronary Artery Bypass Surgery: Effects on Access. *Medical Care,* 27: 288–296.

Anderson, G, JP Newhouse, and LLJ Roos. 1989. Hospital Care for Elderly Patients With Diseases of the Circulatory System: A Comparison of Hospital Use in the United States and Canada. *New England Journal of Medicine* 321: 1443–1448.

Barer, ML, RG Evans, C Hertzman, and J Lomas. 1987. Aging and Health Care Utilization: New Evidence on Old Fallacies. *Social Science and Medicine* 24: 851–862.

Barer, ML, A Gafni, and J Lomas. 1989. Accommodating Rapid Growth in Physician Supply: Lessons From Israel, Warnings for Canada. *International Journal of Health Services* 19: 95–115.

Barer, ML, and GL Stoddart. 1991. Toward Integrated Medical Resource Policies for Canada. Vancouver: University of British Columbia Centre for Health Services and Policy Research.

Barker, P. 1988. The Development of the Major Shared-Cost Programs in Canada. In RD Oilling and MW Westmacott Eds. *Perspectives on Canadian Federalism,* 195–219. Toronto: Prentice Hall.

Blendon, RJ, R Leitman, I Morrison, and K Donelan. 1990. Satisfaction with Health Systems in Ten Nations. *Health Affairs* 9: 185–192.

Blendon, RJ, and H Taylor. 1989. Views on Health Care: Public Opinion in Three Nations. *Health Affairs* 8: 149–157.

Boothe, P, and B Johnston. 1993. *Stealing the Emperor's Clothes: Deficit Off-loading and National Standards in Health Care.* CD Howe Institute Commentary 41. Toronto: CD Howe Institute.

Braunwald, E. 1983. Effects of Coronary-Artery Bypass Grafting on Survival. *New England Journal of Medicine* 309: 1181–1184.

British Columbia Reference. 1991. re Constitutional Question Act (B.C.) *National Reporter* 127: 161–213.

British Columbia Royal Commission on Health Care and Costs. 1991. *Closer to Home: The Report of the British Columbia Royal Commission on Health Care and Costs,* Vols. 1 and 2. British Columbia: British Columbia Royal Commission on Health Care and Costs.

Brown, LD. 1983. *New Policies, New Politics: Government's Response to Government's Growth.* Washington: The Brookings Institution.

Bryce, GK. 1991. *Medicare on the ropes.* Cananadian Journal of Public Health 82: 75–76.

Canada Department of Finance. 1989. *The Budget.* Ottawa: Department of Finance.

Canada Department of Finance. 1990. *The Budget.* Ottawa: Department of Finance.

Canada Department of Finance. 1991. *The Budget.* Ottawa: Department of Finance.

Canada Department of Finance. 1993. *The Budget*. Ottawa: Department of Finance, February.

Canadian Press. 1993. OECD Warns of Debt Threat. *The Globe and Mail* 2 December.

Conference Board of Canada. 1994. *Key Economic Indicators*. Canadian Outlook, Winter.

Courchene, TJ. 1991. Compared With the U.S. Health System, Canada's Model Wins Handily. *The Globe and Mail* Toronto, 7 June (as cited by J Simpson).

Coyte, PC. 1990. Current trends in Canadian Health Care: Myths and Misconceptions in Health Economics. *Journal of Public Health Policy* 169–188.

Culyer, AJ. 1988. *Health Expenditures in Canada: Myth and Reality Past and Future*. Toronto: Canadian Tax Foundation.

D'Arcy, C. 1988. *Reducing Inequalities in Health*. Health Services and Promotion Branch Working Paper, 88–116. Ottawa: Health and Welfare Canada, 1988.

Deber, RB. 1991. Philosophical Underpinnings of Canada's Health Care System. *Canada-U.S. Outlook* 2: 20–45.

Deber, RB, GG Thompson, and P Leatt. 1988. Technology acquisition in Canada: Control in a Regulated Market. *International Journal of Technology Assessment in Health Care* 4: 185–206.

Deber, RB, and E Vayda. 1985. The Environment of Health Policy Implementation: The Ontario, Canada Example. In WW Holland, R Detels, and G Knox eds. *Oxford Textbook of Public Health Volume III: Investigative Methods in Public Health*, 441–461. Oxford: Oxford University Press.

Deber, RB, and E Vayda. 1990. *Summary of Models of Devolution in Ontario and Other Jurisdictions*. Unpublished Report. Department of Health Administration, University of Toronto, October.

Editorial. 1993. Hang Together or Hang Separately. *The Globe and Mail* 8 March, 1993.

Elstad, JI. 1989. Health Services and Decentralized Government: The Case of Primary Health Services in Norway. *International Journal of Health Services* 20: 545–559.

Evans, JR. 1987. *Toward a Shared Direction for Health in Ontario*. Report of the Ontario Health Review Panel. Toronto: Ontario Ministry of Health.

Evans, RG. 1992. U.S. Influences on Canada: Can We Prevent the Spread of Kuru? In RB Deber and GG Thompson eds. *Restructuring Canada's Health Services System: How Do We Get There From Here?* 143–148. Toronto: University of Toronto Press.

Evans, RG. 1993. Health Care Reform: "The Issue From Hell." *Policy Options* 14: 35–41.

Evans, RG, and GL Stoddart. 1990. *Producing Health, Consuming Health Care*. Centre for Health Economics and Policy Analysis Working Paper Series No. 90–6. Hamilton, McMaster University, May.

Evans, RG, J Lomas, ML Barer, RJ Labelle, C Fooks, GL Stoddart, GM Anderson, D Feeny, A Gafni, GW Torrance, and WG Tholl. 1989. Controlling Health Rxpenditure: The Canadian Reality. *New England Journal of Medicine* 320: 571–577.

Government du Québec. 1989. *Improving Health and Well-Being in Quebec*. Montreal: Ministère de la Santé et des Services Sociaux.

Gouvernement du Québec. 1990. *A Reform Centered on the Citizen*. Québec City: Ministère de la Santé et des Services Sociaux.

Ham, C. 1992. *Health Policy in Britain: The Politics and Organization of the National Health Service*, 3rd ed. Houndmills, Basingstoke: MacMillan.

Hancock, T. 1985. Beyond Health Care: From Public Health Policy to Healthy Public Policy. *Canadian Journal of Public Health* 76(Suppl): 9–11.

Hastings, JEF. 1986. Organized Ambulatory Care in Canada: Health Service Organizations and Community Health Centres. *Journal of Public Health Policy* 7: 239–247.

Hazelton, AE. 1986. Technology Assessment: How Effective is Medical Care? *Clinics in Geriatric Medicine* 2: 481–490.

Health and Welfare Canada. 1973. *The Community Health Centre in Canada.* Report of the Community Health Centre Project to the Health Ministers. Ottawa: Information Canada.

Health and Welfare Canada. 1983. *Preserving Universal Medicare: A Government of Canada Position Paper.* Ottawa: Minister of Supplies and Services Canada.

Health and Welfare Canada. 1990. *Canada Health Act Annual Report 1989-1990.* Ottawa: Health and Welfare Canada.

Heiber, S, and RB Deber. 1987. Banning Extra-Billing in Canada: Just What the Doctor Didn't Order. *Canadian Public Policy* 13: 62–74.

Jackson, RW. 1986. *Issues in Preventive Health Care.* Ottawa: Science Council of Canada (May).

Lamb, M., RB Deber, CD Naylor, and JEF Hastings. 1991. *Managed Care in Canada: The Toronto Hospital's Proposed Comprehensive Health Organization.* Ottawa: Canadian Hospital Association Press.

Linton, AL. 1990. The Canadian Health Care System - A Canadian Physician's Perspective. *New England Journal of Medicine* 322: 197–199.

Lomas, J. 1990. *Policy Commentary: Quality Assurance and Effectiveness in Health Care: An Overview.* Centre for Health Economics and Policy Analysis Working Paper Series 90–93. Hamilton: McMaster University.

Manga, P, and DE Angus. 1989. *Fiscal Federalism from the Perspective of Nova Scotia.* In The Report of The Nova Scotia Royal Commission on Health Care: Towards a New Strategy - Research Studies Vol. I. Halifax: The Nova Scotia Royal Commission on Health Care.

Milio, N. 1985. Healthy Nations: Creating a New Ecology of Public Policy for Health. *Canadian Journal of Public Health* 76(Suppl): 79–85.

Mills, A. 1993. *Decentralization and Accountability from an International Perspective: What are the Choices?* CHEPA's 6th Annual Health Policy Conference, Hamilton, Ontario, 21 May.

Minister of Supply and Services Canada. 1991. *Citizen's Forum on Canada's Future: Report to the People and Government of Canada.* Minister of Supply and Services Canada, June 27.

Mustard, JF. 1990. *Health and Prosperity.* Paper presented at the 3rd Annual Health Policy Conference, Niagara-On-The-Lake, Canada, May 25.

Mustard, JF. 1974. *Report of the Health Planning Task Force.* Toronto: Ministry of Health.

Naylor, CD. 1991. A Different View of Queues in Ontario. *Health Affairs* 10: 110–128.

Nelson, M. 1989. A Global Challenge: Health Promotion for People and the Planet. *Health Promotion* 28: 2–7.

Nevison, D. 1993. *World Economy Continues to Inch its Way Forward. World Outlook - Global Economic Trends and Prospects.* Ottawa: Conference Board of Canada, Autumn.

New Brunswick Commission on Selected Health Care Programs. 1989. *Report of the Commission on Selected Health Care Programs.* New Brunswick: Commission on Selected Health Care Programs.

Newhouse, JP, GM Anderson, and LLJ Roos. 1988. Hospital Spending in the United States and Canada: A Comparison. *Health Affairs* 7: 6–16.

Nova Scotia Department of Health. 1990. *Health Strategies for the Nineties: Managing Better Health.* Halifax: Nova Scotia Department of Health.

Nova Scotia Royal Commission on Health Care. 1989. *Report of the Nova Scotia Royal Commission on Health Care: Towards a New Strategy,* Vols. 1-3. Halifax: Nova Scotia Royal Commission on Health Care.

O'Neill, M. 1991. *Healthy Cities - Quebec Network.* Toronto: Presentation, University of Toronto, April 12.

Ontario Ministry of Health. 1987. *Health for All Ontario: Report of the Panel on Health Goals for Ontario.* Toronto: Panel of Health Goals for Ontario.

Ontario Ministry of Health. 1989. *Deciding The Future of Our Health Care.* Toronto: Ontario Ministry of Health, April.

Ontario Ministry of Health. 1990. *Pharmaceutical Inquiry of Ontario.* Toronto: Ontario Ministry of Health, July.

Organisation for Economic Co-operation and Development. 1993. *OECD in Figures: Statistics on the Member Countries.* Supplement to the OECD Observer No. 182. Paris: Organisation for Economic Co-operation and Development.

Pederson, AP, RK Edwards, M Kelner, VW Marshall, and KR Allison. 1988. *Coordinating Healthy Public Policy: An Analytic Literature Review And Bibliography.* Ottawa: Health and Welfare Canada, January.

Podborski, S. 1987. *Health Promotion Matters in Ontario. A Report of the Minister's Advisory Group on Health Promotion.* Toronto: Ministry of Health.

Premier's Council on Health Strategy. 1989a. *A Vision Of Health - Health Goals For Ontario.* Toronto: Government of Ontario, April 24.

Premier's Council on Health Strategy. 1989b. *From Vision to Action: Report of the Health Care System Committee.* Toronto: Government of Ontario.

Premier's Council on Health Strategy. 1991a. *Nurturing Health - A Framework on the Determinants of Health.* Toronto: Government of Ontario, March.

Premier's Council on Health Strategy. 1991b. *Local Decision Making For Health And Social Services.* Toronto: Government of Ontario, March.

Premier's Council on Health Strategy. 1991c. *Achieving the Vision: Health Human Resources.* Toronto: Government of Ontario.

Quebec: Commission d'Enquête Sur Les Services de Santé et Les Services Sociaux. 1987. *Quebec: Commission d'Enquête Sur Les Services de Santé et Les Services Sociaux (Summary).* Quebec.

Rachlis, M. 1991. *The Impact of the 1991 Federal Budget on Health Care, Public Health Programs and the Health Status of Ontario Citizens.* Paper prepared for the Toronto Board of Health, May 8.

Rachlis, M, and C Kushner. 1989. *Second Opinion: What's Wrong With Canada's Health Care System and How to Fix it.* Toronto: Collins.

Roos, NP. 1984. Hysterectomy: Variations in Rates Across Small Areas and Across Physicians Practices. *American Journal of Public Health* 74: 327–335.

Roth, VJ, L Bozinoff, and P MacIntosh. 1990. Public Opinion and the Measurement of Consumer Satisfaction with Government Services. *Canadian Public Administration* 33: 571–583.

Rublee, DA. 1989. Medical Technology in Canada, Germany, and the United States. *Health Affairs* 8: 178–181.

Saltman, RB, and C von Otter. 1992. *Planned Markets and Public Competition: Strategic Reform in Northern European Health Systems.* Philadelphia: Open University Press.

Saskatchewan Commission on Directions in Health Care. 1990. *Future Directions for Health Care in Saskatchewan.* Regina: Government of Saskatchewan, Commission (Chair, RG Murray).

Schieber, GJ, and J.P Poullier. 1989. International Health Care Expenditure Trends: 1987. *Health Affairs* 8: 169–177.

Schieber, GJ, J.P Poullier, and LM Greenwald. 1992. U.S. Health Expenditure Performance: An International Comparison and Update. *Health Care Financing Review* 13: 1–14.

Senate of Canada. 1990. *Accessibility to Hospital Services - Is There a Crisis.* Ottawa: Senate of Canada, Issue No. 23.

Southwestern Ontario Comprehensive Health System Planning Commission. 1991. *Working Together to Achieve Better Health For All.* Toronto: Ontario Ministry of Health.

Stoddart, GL, ML Barer, RG Evans, and V Bhatia. 1993. *Why Not User Charges? The Real Issues.* Toronto: The Premier's Council on Health, Well-Being and Social Justice, September.

Stone, DA. 1988. *Policy Paradox and Political Reason.* Glenview, Illinois: Harper Collins.

Taylor, MG. 1987. *Health Insurance and Canadian Public Policy: The Seven Decisions That Created the Canadian Health Insurance System and Their Outcomes.* Kingston: McGill-Queen's University Press.

The Group of 22. 1991. *Some Practical Suggestions for Canada - Report of The Group of 22.* Montreal: The Group of 22, June.

Tsalikis, G. 1989. The Political Economy of Decentralization of Health and Social Services in Canada. *International Journal of Health Services* 4: 293–309.

United States General Accounting Office. 1991. *Canadian Health Insurance: Lessons for the United States. Report to the Chairman, Committee on Government Operations.* House of Representatives, Washington, DC: GAO.

Van Loon, RJ. 1978. From Shared Cost to Block Funding and Beyond: The Politics of Health Insurance in Canada. *Journal of Health Politics, Policy and Law* 2: 454–478.

Vayda, E, JM Barnsley, WR Mindell, and B Cardillo. 1984. Five-year Study of Surgical Rates in Ontario's Counties. *Canadian Medical Association Journal* 131: 111–115.

Vayda, E, and RB Deber. 1984. The Canadian Health Care System: An Overview. *Social Science and Medicine* 18: 191–197.

Wildavsky, A. 1989. *Speaking Truth to Power: The Art and Craft of Policy Analysis.* New Brunswick, New Jersey: Transactions Publishers.

Winslow, CM et al. 1988. The Appropriateness of Performing Coronary Artery Bypass Surgery. *Journal of the American Medical Association* 260: 505–509.

Woolhandler, S, and DU Himmelstein. 1991. The Deteriorating Administrative Efficiency of the U.S. Health Care System. *New England Journal of Medicine* 324: 1253–1258.

World Health Organization. 1984. *Health Promotion: A Discussion Document on the Concept and Principles.* Copenhagen: WHO Regional Office for Europe.

26

Drug Makers and Drug Regulators: Too Close for Comfort. A Study of the Canadian Situation[*]

Joel Lexchin

Introduction

Canadian drug laws and regulations have had a steady evolution over the past 40 years. In 1951 specific regulations governing the sale and distribution of new drugs were promulgated, including requirements that a new drug submission must be filled prior to marketing the drug to support the safety of the drug. In 1963 companies were required to submit substantial evidence of effectiveness before they would be issued with a Notice of Compliance to sell their product. The 1970s saw the review of protocols for clinical trials in investigational drugs and the development of guidelines for New Drug Submissions (NDS). Within the past year (1989), the government has published a 10-volume report on nearly all aspects of Canada's Drug Safety, Quality and Efficacy Program.

The reason for the rules and regulations is to ensure that products reaching the Canadian market are safe and effective. No one would seriously argue that drugs should be proven to be 100% safe. No set of regulations could achieve that goal, because it is an impossibility; all drugs carry some risks. However, the kinds of regulations we have, and how stringently they are enforced, can determine how many of the hazards of a new drug we learn about before it appears on the drugstore shelves and also how quickly dangerous drugs can be removed from the market.

Canadian laws and regulations are some of the strictest in the world, but they still have major gaps that ultimately jeopardize the health of people taking medications. It is my view that these gaps are not just merely accidents or oversights, but that there is a systemic reason why they exist. In this paper I propose first to examine some of the most serious deficiencies and, where possible, show through concrete examples how these gaps either have directly or potentially endangered the health of Canadians. In the next section I will explore the underlying basis for these deficiencies and finally propose what I believe to be the only viable method for correcting them.

[*] Reprinted from *Social Science and Medicine*, Vol. 31, Joel Lexchin, 'Drug makers and drug regulators: too close for comfort. A study of the Canadian situation,' pp. 1257–63, 1990, with permission from Elsevier Science Ltd., Oxford, England.

Not Stringent Enough: Gaps in Canadian Drug Laws and Regulations

When Canada amended its Food and Drugs Act in 1963 in the wake of thalidomide, companies were required to demonstrate the effectiveness of new drugs before they could be licensed for sale. However, this requirement was not made retroactive for products already on the market. Some idea of the extent of the problem can be gleaned from an examination of the United States where the drug market closely resembles the Canadian one. In that country the Food and Drug Administration (FDA) struck special National Academy of Sciences and National Research Council (NAS/NRC) panels to review pre-1963 drugs. Out of 4000-odd products, 760 were categorized as 'ineffective' or 'ineffective as a fixed-ratio combination.' Approximately 600 were banned from the market and hundreds of others were approved but only with significant labeling changes (Silverman and Lee 1974).

As late as 1982 Canadian authorities suspected that about 450 products were either completely worthless or lacked meaningful medical benefits (Regush 1982a). One such drug is Albamycin T, known as Panalba in the United States. It is a combination of two antibiotics, tetracycline and novobiocin. Panalba was one of the more than 4000 drugs evaluated by the NAS/NRC panels. According to their report, combination products such as this "no longer belong in the therapeutic armamentarium" (Mintz 1969). About one in every five patients who receives the novobiocin component of Panalba would be expected to have an allergic or hypersensitivity type of reaction and a smaller proportion could experience temporary but very severe liver damage from exposure to the novobiocin component. On the question of whether drugs such as Panalba should be removed from the market, the head of the panel, Dr. Heinz F. Eichenwald of the University of Texas said: "There are few instances in medicine when so many experts have agreed unanimously and without reservation" (Mintz 1969). In the United States Panalba was taken off the shelves in 1970; in Canada in 1989 Albamycin T is still available.

Under Canadian law, companies are not obliged to inform the Health Protection Branch (HPB) of adverse reactions occurring with old (pre-1963) drugs, even if those reactions occur in Canada. One striking example of the danger of this loophole is the experience with clioquinol, marketed under the trade name Entero-Vioform by Ciba-Geigy since 1934 as a treatment for intestinal infections.

By the mid-1950s increasing numbers of people in Japan were becoming ill with a neurological disorder that produced degenerative and often irreversible changes leaving people paralyzed and blind. This new disease acquired the name sub-acute myelooptic neuropathy or SMON. Eventually an estimated 20,000 Japanese were afflicted (Hansson 1989). Despite mounting incontrovertable evidence that Entero-Vioform caused SMON, Ciba-Geigy denied the connection for years.

Both Norway and Sweden banned the drug by 1975. The Canadian reaction was to do essentially nothing and as a result Entero-Vioform remained available, on prescription, in Canada until 1985 when a campaign lead by the late Swedish neurologist Olle Hansson and the International Organization of Consumers Unions succeeded in forcing Ciba-Geigy to withdraw the drug from sale world wide. Why was the Canadian reaction so muted? One of Ciba's defences, once it had grudgingly admitted the connection between SMON and Entero-Vioform, was that SMON was a 'Japanese disease.' Careful documentation by Hansson shows that claim to have been untrue. While the majority of known cases occurred in Japan, Hansson gives details of people affected in Sweden, Switzerland and other countries.

Canadian officials seem to have completely accepted Ciba's claim. One senior HPB official was quoted as saying that Entero-Vioform and related drugs "really were not found to be causing any serious problems [in Canada]. This is what's so queer about it, it's all directly related to Japan" (Anonymous 1979). The basis behind that statement was apparently the fact that the HPB knew of only 10 minor and 2 serious reactions in Canada to Entero-Vioform. Were there more reactions? How many? How many were serious? The short answer is that we don't know. Entero-Vioform was marketed in Canada before 1963 and was therefore classed as an 'old drug' by the HPB.

Even with new (post-1963) drugs, companies do not have to report adverse reactions that occur outside of Canada or that are recorded with the parent company. The most recent widely-known example of non-reporting involved Oraflex (benoxaprofen) an anti-arthritic product from Eli Lilly. In 1980, this drug was marketed in Britain under the name of Opren. Shortly after the drug appeared on the shelves of British pharmacies, Lilly's British subsidiary informed British health officials of the first of eight deaths resulting from suspected adverse reactions to benoxaprofen. In February 1982, nine months after the first known British death, benoxaprofen was evaluated by the HPB as safe for use in Canada. In its submission, Lilly did not mention the eight deaths in Britain connected to benoxaprofen. Other omissions from Lilly's initial documentation included: suspected adverse drug reaction reports compiled by American doctors participating in Lilly sponsored tests with benoxaprofen; and the results of a Lilly sponsored study presented in Paris in June 1981 showing that dosages of benoxaprofen had to be modified for elderly patients.

Although Canadian officials approved the drug in February 1982, Lilly decided to delay the marketing until that September. Finally in early May Lilly informed the HPB about seven deaths in Britain, just prior to the appearance of an article in the British Medical Journal describing some deaths. At the same time Lilly gave the HPB a summary of data from the Paris symposium. The combination of the two pieces of information resulted in the HPB reversing its decision on the marketing of benoxaprofen in Canada. By the time the drug was finally removed from sale in Britain it was inconclusively linked to 61 deaths (Regush 1982b).

Canadian rules about trials of investigational drugs demonstrate major deficiencies. Once a firm gets approval to run clinical trials, there is no requirement for it to report the results to the HPB unless (a) a patient develops an unexpected adverse reaction to the drug or (b) the firm later files a NDS. If a firm does research on a drug, finds there is not sufficient reason to market it, and does not submit a NDS, HPB will rarely hear how the research turned out (Overstreet et al. 1989). The dangers of course are that there will be violations of the trial protocols. According to Dr. Ian Henderson, former director of the Bureau of Human Prescription Drugs at the HPB, "there are probably lots of protocol violations we know nothing about ... I don't place much faith in drug-company monitoring" (Hollobon and Lipovenko 1982a). Dr. Henderson recalled that when he was a clinical researcher, drug company monitors who came around to assess progress on a trial were mostly concerned with whether he was completing the forms properly.

When the results of drug trials are submitted to the HPB the facts in them are verified by re-examining the 'raw data' which must also be submitted. If there is doubt about the veracity of data an inspection of pharmaceutical premises can be carried out (Dr. Ian Henderson, personal communication). However, the HPB does not carry out detailed "for cause" audits similar to those done by the FDA. "For cause" audits are undertaken in a number of circumstances: if a routine data audit uncovers serious deficiencies; if the FDA receives a complaint about the clinician from the drug manufacturer; if a colleague or employee reports an investigator to the FDA; if the data in a study appear to be too 'clean'; if a clinician appears to have enrolled a larger number of subjects from his or her practice than seems realistically attainable; or if previous audits have uncovered problems with an investigator. These 'for cause' audits are conducted not only by a field investigator but also with a scientist from FDA headquarters. They go into greater depth and cover a larger number of individual case reports than do routine data audits and may involve a review of other studies which the clinical investigator has completed in the relatively recent past (Lisook 1982). Over the period June 1977 to April 1988 there were a total of 395 such audits completed. Forty-three (11%) led to the disqualification of the investigator, while in 19 others (5%) investigators agreed to some restriction in access to investigational drugs or in the conduct of studies (Shapiro and Charrow 1989). The magnitude of the problem in Canada is simply not known.

The results of routine data audits done by the FDA also point to another gap in Canadian regulations about clinical studies of investigational drugs. Out of 1955 audits from June 1977 to April 1988, 1002 (51%) showed problems with patient consent (Shapiro and Charrow 1989). In Canada, informed consent from patients is not required by law. It is almost always obtained, but because the HPB does not set any standards for consent, the degree to which patients are informed of the risks they face could vary widely. Approval of drug trials by ethics committees is also not required under Canadian law. Where ethics committees exist, and nearly all universities and hospitals have one, the committees set their own standards. Although the HPB asks for a certificate showing that a drug-trial protocol has been reviewed by an ethics committee, the document need not give details as to how the committee reached its decision. "I have suspected at times that it's rubber-stamping," said Dr. Henderson referring to some decisions of ethics committees (see Hollobon and Lipovenko 1982b). Asked about the lack of monitoring of drug trials, Dr. Thomas Clark, who administered the University of Toronto's ethics committee in the early 1980s, said: "You're putting your finger on a weakness in the system" (Hollobon and Lipovenko 1982a). The recent death of a patient involved in a clinical study of a new asthma medication reinforces these concerns about the ambiguities in the responsibilities of ethics committees in Canada. An investigation into the death was undertaken by a public affairs television show. On the show Dr. Gordon Johnson, the current head of the Bureau of Human Prescription Drugs in the HPB, stated that "they [drug trials] are constantly under the surveillance of the local ethics committee," while "the actual conduct of the trial is the responsibility of the sponsor." However, according to the head of the committee that approved the trial in question the committee does not do "as much [checking on compliance] as we would like because we don't have the resources." Finally, the opinion from a representative of the drug company sponsoring the trial was that "the actual responsibility for a given circumstance is going to depend on the specific case ... It could be any one of the parties concerned, it could be all the parties or it could be none of the parties."

When a manufacturer files a NDS with the HPB, one part of that document is the Official Drug Monograph which is basically a summary of the scientific information available on the product. This monograph is a key document in the provision of information to health professionals. It essentially forms the basis for the information that appears in the Compendium of Pharmaceuticals and Specialties (CPS), the most widely consulted source on therapeutic information in Canada (Hall and Parker 1976; Parker 1979). But the HPB undertakes no systematic monitoring to ensure that information in product monographs is current. Regulations under the Food and Drugs Act require manufacturers to annually furnish a notification confirming that all the information previously supplied by the manufacturer regarding a drug is correct. HPB narrowly interprets this regulation to require only information on whether the company is still marketing the product. HPB has not developed or implemented any mechanism to ensure that this regulation is adhered to and that current product information is provided to the HPB. Manufacturers do not, in fact, always advise the HPB even when a drug is withdrawn (Turriff et al. 1989).

One member of the Canadian Medical Association's subcommittee on drugs and pharmacotherapy suggested that "70% to 75% of Monographs published to date are now inaccurate, according to an informal university pharmacology study" (Berger and Johnson 1989). Some subcommittee members believe that inaccurate monographs are not only a poor source of information, they are potentially dangerous (Berger and Johnson 1989).

Two such instances involve the monographs for Slow K, a potassium replacement medication, and the heart drug digoxin. Slow K was introduced in Canada in 1970 and by 1983 was one of Ciba-Geigy's most successful products chalking up sales of almost $7 million annually (Supply and Services Canada 1985). Potassium replacements are actually seldom needed and if someone's potassium level drops too low the simplest and safest way of raising it is through dietary changes. When medication is required Slow K is not a good choice. Independent studies have shown that it can cause ulcerations in the stomach and intestines especially in elderly people.

The Medical Letter, a highly respected bulletin on drugs and therapeutics that accepts no advertising concluded that: "Slow-release potassium tablets such as Slow K ... are dangerous and should not be used. Supplementation of the regular diet with potassium-rich foods is the safest way to prevent hypokalemia [potassium deficiency] in patients taking diuretics." The Medical Letter went on to recommend potassium solutions rather than potassium pills if medication was required (see Anonymous 1978). The information about Slow K in the CPS doesn't say that potassium replacements are unusually necessary, nor is there any mention about dietary supplementation being the first choice if the potassium level is too low. The incidence of side effects such as stomach and intestinal ulceration from Slow K are compared with those caused by other types of potassium tablets not to those caused by the safer potassium solutions. The data in the CPS clearly contradict leading medical advice and give an erroneous impression about the usefulness and safety of Slow K.

The monograph on digoxin in the CPS does not recommend any alteration in dosage for the elderly despite the fact this drug is one of the most common causes of adverse drug reactions in this age group (Lexchin 1989).

Finally, the HPB does not have an adequate adverse drug reporting program. No systematic postmarketing surveillance is conducted; there is no encouragement for physicians or hospitals to submit adverse drug reaction reports; feedback to physicians who do report is virtually nonexistent; and what information that is collected cannot be analyzed and disseminated to health practitioners in a timely manner to educate them on hazardous drug products and hazardous use (Turriff et al. 1989).

PMAC and HPB: Clientele Pluralism

The HPB is not unaware of these deficiencies, indeed most of them are well described in the recently completed multivolume report on Canada's Drug Safety, Quality and

Efficacy Program. Officials in the HPB have, at times, sought to correct some of these problems. Over the years Dr. Henderson repeatedly requested money to conduct an evaluation of pre-1963 drugs, only to be turned down by the Treasury Board.

There are a variety of possible explanations for the deficiencies. One study written for the Federal Commission of Inquiry on the Pharmaceutical Industry identified major areas of bureaucratic inefficiency and poor organization in the HPB which precluded streamlining and updating Canada's drug laws and regulations (Goyer 1985).

I believe that the underlying factor is the collegial relationship between the Pharmaceutical Manufacturers Association of Canada (PMAC), the organization representing the major drug companies operating in the country, and the HPB. When HPB officials were being interviewed for a series of articles in a Montreal newspaper they repeatedly stated that they had opted for a co-operative and open door policy with Canadian drug company officials instead of a tough adversarial stance. They were proud of how friendly their relations were with representatives of Canadian drug subsidiaries of American companies (Regush 1982b). According to one HPB official, interviewed by political scientists Michael Atkinson and William Coleman of McMaster University, industry and government are on very good terms compared to most countries (Atkinson and Coleman 1989).

Before I continue, let me emphasize that by positing a close relationship between the pharmaceutical industry and the HPB I am not implying that there cannot be conflicts between the two. Indeed, PMAC has been strongly critical of the HPB for what it regards as the excessive delays in approving new drugs. I am also not suggesting any sort of conspiracy theory. What I will try to demonstrate is that the type of interaction between the PMAC and the HPB creates an atmosphere which allows major gaps in regulatory standards to come into existence and to be perpetuated.

Crossovers between government and industry are not unknown. In the mid-1960s, Dr. C.A. Morrell left his position as head of the Food and Drug Directorate (FDD), the predecessor to the HPB, for a spot on the board of directors of Ciba. Currently, the President of the Pharmaceutical Manufacturers Association of Canada is Judy Erola, who until 1984 was the Federal Minister of Consumer and Corporate Affairs. However, this interchange of individuals is not the major driving force behind the closeness of the two organizations. Moreover, crossovers of individuals are not always detrimental (Braithwaite 1984).

Government regulation of drug safety, quality and efficacy is almost solely the responsibility of the HPB. But, as Atkinson and Coleman (1989) point out, the state does not possess the wherewithal to undertake the elaborate clinical and pre-clinical trials required to meet the objective of providing safe and effective medications. Some authority must be relinquished to the drug manufacturers, especially with respect to information which forms the basis on which regulatory decisions are made. This is a situation which Atkinson and Coleman label as one where the state has a high degree of concentration of power in one agency (the HPB), but a low degree of autonomy. On the other hand, the association representing all of the multinational companies operating in Canada, the PMAC, is highly mobilized to assume a role in the making and implementing of drug policy through an elaborate committee structure, the ability to act on behalf of its members and the capacity to bind member firms to agreements. (There is an association of domestically owned generic pharmaceutical manufacturers, the Canadian Drug Manufacturers Association, but its members are responsible for less than 10% of drug sales in Canada.) The result is a method of interaction, a policy network, termed clientele pluralism. In clientele pluralism, the state relinquishes some of its authority to private-sector actors, who, in turn, pursue objectives with which officials are in broad agreement (Atkinson and Coleman 1989).

Not only does the state, in this case the HPB, turn over some of its authority, but the objectives that are being pursued are ones that are often jointly developed between PMAC and the HPB. In the classic pattern of clientele pluralism the regulations governing matters of drug safety, quality and efficacy are very general, leaving much open to negotiation and discussion. An official in the HPB described the situation in the following manner:

They [the regulations] are not that great now. There are about six or seven pages and that covers all there is in Canada about new drugs. In the usual way, following the old British tradition, we keep things very vague. For example, what is your regulation for testing the safety of a new drug? Well, what's asked for in our regulations is submission to us of details of the test carried out to establish safety. That's the extent of the regulation ... So we need to have and we do have a fair amount of guidelines explaining what we interpret that regulation to mean (Atkinson and Coleman 1985).

Officials from both groups meet on a regular basis about every 6 weeks in joint committees to work on regulatory changes and their accompanying guidelines. For example, at a meeting of the Bureau of Human Prescription Drugs/PMAC Medical R & D Section Liaison Committee in the fall of 1983, the need for guidelines on filing an Investigational New Drug (IND) submission was discussed, primarily at the PMAC's initiative (Goyer 1985). In addition, senior officials in the HPB, including the assistant deputy minister meet with the PMAC board of directors, elected from senior executives of 15 companies, at the PMAC's Annual and Semi-Annual meetings (Atkinson and Coleman 1989). At these events the HPB informs the industry of its plans for the following year. The informal nature of these discussions is highlighted by the lack of any minutes.

Another mechanism of communication between the two groups is via a formal 'information letter' in which the HPB publicly announces proposed changes to regulations and requests feedback from interested parties, including industry. The PMAC clearly prefers the informal meetings to information letters as can be illustrated by further consideration of the matter of the IND guidelines. The first draft document was, according to the PMAC, unexpectedly tabled at an October 23/84 Liaison Committee meeting for detailed discussion at the next Committee meeting scheduled for early January 1985. However, at a November meeting between HPB officials and the PMAC Board, the HPB announced that it was moving forward with the draft to the formal information letter stage without further preliminary informal discussion and input via the Liaison Committee. The PMAC was very upset by this move and strongly requested that the document be given thorough study and review via the informal Liaison Committee mechanism before regulatory change was initiated via the formal information letter procedure (Goyer 1985). This example, besides illustrating the importance of the PMAC/HPB meetings, also serves to underline my previous point that friction continues to occur between the two despite an overall close working relationship.

It may be necessary to work closely with the PMAC, but it is also not generally a difficult task. The HPB official interviewed by Atkinson and Coleman (1989) called it very easy to work with the PMAC because both groups talk the same language. Of course, both groups are using the same language because both groups have essentially the same composition – doctors, pharmacists and people with degrees in biological and medical sciences. Not only will they talk the same, but they will probably also share the same world view when it comes to the role of drugs in the health care system.

The informal relationship between the PMAC and the HPB extends even beyond liaison committees. For example, according to the Food and Drug Regulations, a manufacturer dissatisfied with an HPB decision about licensing a new drug could require the formation of a three-member new drug committee: one member selected by the manufacturer, one by the HPB and the third by the two previously selected members. The Minister of Health and Welfare, the ministry overseeing the HPB, may reconsider the decision on the findings and recommendations of the new drug committee. Yet very few manufacturers have used this procedure. Most companies will first discuss the matter with the senior officials in the HPB and reach a settlement. Although a dispute could be brought to court for a final decision, no multinational pharmaceutical company has used this approach in years (Mailhot 1986).

Industry officials also frequently approach the HPB in an informal manner to get advice about how best to conduct clinical research, problems they are encountering in running drug trials, or whether or not the evidence supports submitting an application to market a new drug for certain indications.

Two examples serve to show concretely how a clientele pluralist policy network operates in the field of drug policy. Since the Food and Drugs Act was promulgated in 1953, an inspection program has existed for all drug plants to ensure cleanliness and requirements such as dosage accuracy. Representatives of the PMAC worked with government in drawing up the standards for manufacturing and a number of PMAC member companies helped to train the inspectors who apply them (Pharmaceutical Manufacturers Association of Canada 1966). As a further refinement in regulating manufacturing practices a joint industry and government committee was struck which led to the development of Good Manufacturing Practices (GMPs) and these came into effect in 1981. The companies continue to be provided with a regular opportunity for input into refinements of GMP regulations in the form of an annual meeting between HPB officials and PMAC. Other interested parties such as workers in pharmaceutical plants and consumers are notably excluded from participation in such meetings. While there are a set of guidelines for inspectors to use to assess compliance with GMPs, they are published "by the authority of the Minister of National Health and Welfare" and carry no legal force. However, membership in PMAC is conditional upon acceptance of GMPs and so the association acts to enforce compliance with the guidelines. If companies break them they can be threatened with expulsion from the PMAC (Atkinson and Coleman 1985).

A second example of delegation of government authority to the industry is control of promotional practices. This area has had a long and contentious history, but also a long history of cooperation between government and industry. In the early 1960s, PMAC and the FDD jointly established definite requirements and standards for advertising material (Pharmaceutical Manufacturers Association of Canada 1966). In the mid-1970s, amid increasing controversy over industry marketing tactics, the PMAC was able to head off action by the HPB through the launching of the Pharmaceutical Advertising Advisory Board (PAAB). The PAAB has representatives from PMAC, advertisers' groups, medical and pharmacists' associations and the Consumers' Association of Canada (CAC). The HPB is represented in an exofficio, nonvoting capacity and acts as advisor and resource body to the board. The PAAB works by voluntary compliance, with no effective sanctions for companies that violate its rules. Its Code of Advertising Acceptance is so weak that advertising material that complies with it can still be deceptive (Lexchin 1987). Section 9 of the Food and Drugs Act prohibits the false advertising of drugs, so if the HPB wished to act in the matter of pharmaceutical promotion it has the legal authority, but instead it has delegated that responsibility.

One of the conditions for PMAC membership is acceptance of its Code of Marketing Practices which states that all PMAC members agree to abide by the PAAB's Code of Advertising Acceptance. Nonadherence to the PAAB's Code could lead to expulsion from the PMAC, so once again the association becomes a self-regulation agent (Atkinson and Coleman 1985). The threat of expulsion is not taken lightly. Membership in the association is extremely beneficial. Besides offering its members access to the HPB the PMAC also supplies member companies with valuable assistance and information which would often be prohibitively expensive, difficult to obtain, or otherwise unavailable (Pharmaceutical Manufacturers Association of Canada n.d.).

The joint state-industry development and implementation of GMPs appears to be relatively successful, as opposed to the control of promotional practices, but the issue here is not how well these examples of the operation of a clientele pluralist policy network are functioning. The issue is that in both cases the state and industry are co-responsible for the formulation of policy, and the state has largely ceded its responsibility for the implementation and enforcement of policy to the PMAC (Atkinson and Coleman 1989). As I showed earlier, this process of joint policy development has been institutionalized through the PMAC/HPB liaison committees. Despite the fact that the interests of consumers, workers and professionals are involved, the interests of business have assumed a privileged place in the definition and administration of policy (Atkinson and Coleman 1985).

Conclusion

Recently, the HPB has been given approval to increase its staffing levels, a much needed move in light of the increasing work requirements. This increase in resources should allow the HPB to perform its functions more rapidly and perhaps more efficiently, but if my thesis is right that it is a system of clientele pluralism which ultimately gives rise to the deficiencies in Canadian drug laws and regulations, then more resources are not the answer. Plugging the current gaps would obviously be a positive step, but inevitably the system will generate new problems.

This conclusion is reinforced by looking at the experience in other Western industrialized countries. For example, while the specific deficiencies in the Canadian laws and regulations are not present in the United States, the overall regulatory environment there is no stricter because other equally dangerous problems exist (Braithwaite 1984). I believe that this outcome is a reflection of the fact that Canada is not unique when it comes to the interactions between the industry and the regulatory authorities. There are strong similarities between the situation in the United Kingdom and the United States (Braithwaite 1984; Hughes and Brewin 1979) and Canada. The regulatory agencies in Australia and the U.K., like the HPB, have also turned over control of promotional practices to the pharmaceutical industry with predictable results (Harvey 1990; Herxheimer and Collier 1990). Because the underlying structural relationship between the pharmaceutical industry and the state is fundamentally the same in advanced capitalist countries, each country will have serious flaws in its regulatory system, although these flaws will not necessarily be the same from country to country.

I believe that basic changes are necessary in the way that pharmaceutical policy is formulated, implemented and enforced. However, restricting the interactions between

HPB officials and the drug companies is not a viable option. As long as the present arrangement is in place with privately owned companies being regulated by government, a situation that is likely to prevail for the foreseeable future, then it will be necessary for the two groups to have frequent and close contacts. The best hope we have for changing the ethos is by diluting the influence of the drug companies. Instead of just having regular informal meetings with PMAC there should be similar meetings with a wide range of interested parties ranging from the consumer groups, to women's health groups to professional associations. It might then be possible for these groups to influence the development of drug laws and regulations at their formative stage. This would have the effect of removing business from its privileged place in the definition and administration of policy. Currently, the first time these groups find out about policy changes, and the only stage at which they are able to intervene, is when the HPB makes a formal announcement in an information letter. However, by this time, as I have shown earlier, there have already been a long series of talks between the HPB and the PMAC. The PMAC's clear preference is to make itself felt at the informal negotiating period. While the PMAC has a legitimate claim, representing the companies who will be affected by any new rules, to want to be in on the ground floor of negotiations, people who will be consuming the products and professionals who will be prescribing and dispensing the products have an equally legitimate right to demand to be present from the beginning.

Similarly, a strong case can be made for opening up the drug approval process to involve groups outside of the HPB and the company wishing to market the drug. Information that is supplied by companies in favor of their application should be disclosed to the public so that people can judge for themselves the basis on which the HPB makes its decisions (McGarity and Shapiro 1980). Even more fundamentally, outside groups should be able to intervene in the approval process.

At this stage this hope for democratization of HPB decision making is just that, a hope. If it is realized there is still the long and arduous task of working out the details to make it functional. However, even convincing the government to explore this option poses major difficulties. In 1964, there existed a Consumer Advisory Committee formed from a representative sample of consumers. The mandate of the committee was to keep its members informed about HPB activities and to elicit their views on actual or proposed HPB initiatives. However, the committee was disbanded in 1968 for reasons which were never clearly stated. There is no indication that the government is willing to reconstitute any similar committee. The CAC, the largest and best organized of Canadian consumer groups, is not even on the list of those associations with whom the HPB meets regularly (Berger and Overstreet 1988).

Details of a drug evaluation carried out by the HPB are made available, when requested, to the submitting company but are not released to outside parties since they are viewed as trade secrets and therefore are exempted from the Federal Access to Information Law (Dr. Ian Henderson, personal communication). When the HPB was considering the approval of Depo-Provera, a controversial injectable hormonal contraceptive, there was a strong protest by women's groups across the country and a demand for public input into the decision. The only concession from the HPB was to appoint a panel to hold meetings in six cities to hear submissions about all methods of contraception. The hearings were not open to the public and presentations of briefs to the panel were by invitation only. Even a list of invited participants' names had scrawled across the top of it, "Do not release to the media or the public. The meeting is by invitation only" (Barnett 1986). HPB officials' defense was that people would not come forward if the meetings were public.

In January 1987, the government initiated the formation of a Working Group on Drug Submission Review with a mandate to review and recommend on Canada's regulatory process for drug submission review. The sole member not from government or industry, who was nominally the public representative, was from the Canadian Public Health Association. Finally, the only place that the 10-volume report on Canada's Drug Safety, Quality and Efficacy Program makes any mention about increasing public input to the system is when it records the results of the interview with the CAC (see Gerer and Overstreet 1988; Turriff, Berger and Overstreet 1989).

Unfortunately for the Canadian public, democratization in the field of drug policy seems a long way off.

References

Anonymous. 1978. Slow K Follow-Up. *Medical Letter* 20: 3031.

Anonymous. 1979. No Ban is Planned for Drug Blamed for Japanese Outbreak. *Globe and Mail*, 20 September, T2.

Atkinson, MM, and WD Coleman. 1985. Corporatism and Industrial Policy. In A Cawson ed. *Organized Interests and the State,* 41. London: Sage.

Atkinson, MM, and WD Coleman. 1989. *The State, Business and Industrial Change in Canada.* Toronto: University of Toronto Press.

Barnett, V. 1986. Drug Hearings Shouldn't be Held in Secret. *Calgary Herald,* 11 September, A8.

Berger, J, and V Johnson. 1989. *Information to Help Ensure Judicious Use. Technical Report No. 7.* Program Evaluation Study of the Drug Safety, Quality and Efficacy Program Health and Welfare Canada. Ottawa: Health and Welfare Canada.

Berger, J, and RE Overstreet. 1988. *Opinions of Stakeholder Associations. Technical Report No. 2.* Program Evaluation Study of the Drug Safety, Quality and Efficacy Program Health and Welfare Canada. Ottawa: Health and Welfare Canada.

Braithwaite, J. 1984. *Corporate Crime in the Pharmaceutical Industry.* London: Routledge & Kegan Paul.

Goyer, R. 1985. *Regulatory Aspects and Their Influence on Pharmaceutical Research and on the Introduction of Drugs in Canada. Background Study for the Commission of Inquiry on the Pharmaceutical Industry.* Ottawa: Supply and Services Canada.

Hall, KW, and WA Parker. 1976. Physician's View of the Pharmacist's Professional Role. *Canadian Pharmaceutical Journal* 109: 311–314.

Hansson, 0. 1989. *Inside Ciba - Geigy.* Paper read at International Organization of Consumers Unions, at Penang.

Harvey, K. 1990. Pharmaceutical Promotion. *Medical Journal of Australia* 152: 57–58.

Herxheimer, A, and J Collier. 1990. Promotion by the British pharmaceutical industry, 1983–88: A Critical Analysis of Self Regulation. *British Medical Journal* 300: 307–310.

Hollobon, J, and D Lipovenko. 1982a. Companies Gamble Money, but Public also has Stake. *Globe and Mail,* 20 October, 4.

Hollobon, J, and D Lipovenko. 1982b. No Protection for Human Guinea Pigs. *Globe and Mail,* 19 October, 1,2.

Hughes, R, and R Brewin. 1979. *The Tranquilizing of America. Pill Popping and the American Way of Life.* New York: HB Jovanovich.

Lexchin, J. 1987. Advertisement Scrutiny. *Lancet* 1: 1323–1324.

Lexchin, J. 1989. Prescribing to the Elderly: A Review of the English Language Canadian Literature. *Canadian Family Physician* 35: 1613–1617.

Lisook, AB. 1982. FDA Audit of Investigators and Sponsors. *Drug Information Journal* 16: 97–101.

Mailhot, R. 1986. The Canadian Drug Regulatory Process. *Journal of Clinical Pharmacology* 26: 232–239.

McGarity, T0, and SA Shapiro. 1980. The Trade Secret Status of Health and Safety Testing Information Reforming Agency Disclosure Policies. *Harvard Law Review* 93: 837–888.

Mintz, M. 1969. FDA and Panalba: A Conflict of Commercial, Therapeutic Goals? *Science* 165: 875–881.

Overstreet, RE, K Aitken, J Berger, et al. 1989. *Pre-Market Clearance of Drug Products. Technical Report No. 4.* Program Evaluation Study of the Drug Safety, Quality and Efficacy Program, Health and Welfare Canada. Ottawa: Health and Welfare Canada.

Parker, WA. 1979. The Compendium of Pharmaceuticals and Specialties as a Drug Information Resource for Treatment of Acute Drug Overdose. *Canadian Family Physician* 25: 211–215.

Pharmaceutical Manufacturers Association of Canada. 1966. *Submission to House of Commons Special Committee on Drug Costs and Prices.* Ottawa: PMAC.

Pharmaceutical Manufacturers Association of Canada. n.d. *Member Benefits and Services:* Ottawa: PMAC.

Regush, N. 1982a. Drug Dangers Elude our Safety Controls. *Montreal Gazette*, 23 October, A1, A4.

Regush, N. 1982b. How a Suspect Arthritis Drug Evaded Government Checks. *Montreal Gazette,* 23 October, A1, A6.

Shapiro, MF, and RP Charrow. 1989. The Role of Data Audits in Detecting Scientific Misconduct. Results of the FDA program. *Journal of American Medical Association* 261: 2505–2511.

Silverman, M, and PR Lee. 1974. *Pills, Profits, and Politics.* Berkeley, CA: University of California Press.

Supply and Services Canada. 1985. *Commission of Inquiry on the Pharmaceutical Industry.* Report. Ottawa.

Turriff, CL, J Berger, and RE Overstreet. 1989. *Program Roles and Responsibilities, Resources, Systems and Procedures. Technical Report No. 9.* Program Evaluation Study of the Drug Safety, Quality and Efficacy Program, Health and Welfare Canada. Ottawa: Health and Welfare Canada.

27

Partnership as a New Strategy in Mental Health Policy: The Case of Quebec*

Françoise Boudreau, Ph. D.

Introduction

Policymaking, very crudely defined, is largely a search for politically powerful words, words which in and of themselves stand as "self-evident truths" which electrify, convince, and serve well. It is a search for words which have the power to rescue in times of crisis, which can influence attitudes, change behavior and redirect action towards new goals, new ideals, and even towards the beginning of a new, "more progressive" era. As Václav Havel remarked, when awarded the Peace Prize of the German Booksellers Association on 15 October 1989, "We have always believed in the power of words to change history, and rightly so ... In the part of the world I inhabit, the word 'Solidarity' was capable of shaking an entire power block" (1990: 5). Yet, it always pays to be suspicious of words and to be wary of them, the president of Czechoslovakia continued. "The selfsame word can, at one moment, radiate great hopes, at another, it can emit lethal rays. The selfsame word can be true at one moment and false the next, at one moment illuminating, at another deceptive" (1990: 6).

New, politically powerful words which appear to make consensus and promise a solution to our current problems must be kept under careful and adequate observation. Our purpose here is to examine such a word, one which has permeated Canadian policymaking vocabulary and regularly finds its way on billboards, advertisement pamphlets, calls for contributions and public involvement of all kinds. The word is "Partnership" and its Quebec equivalent: *le Partenariat*.

A few examples will demonstrate the widespread popularity of this term in Canada. According to a 1989 poster put out by the Toronto Board of Education, parents are "Partners in Education;" the 1989 National Conference on the Role of Conservatory Music Training in Canada was entitled "Partners in Music;" the Canadian Physiotherapy Association called its 1990 National Physiotherapy week, "Your Partner in Action." On a recent publicity pamphlet, the Ministry of Energy, Mines, and Resources and its minister, Jake Epp, announced that CANMET (Centre canadien de la technologie des minéraux et de l'énergie) is a *partenaire* of the Quebec Mining Industry. The Seventh Annual Family Service Canada Conference held in

* Reprinted and revised, from *Journal of Health Politics, Policy and Law,* Vol. 16, No. 2, Françoise Boudreau, 'Partnership in a new strategy in mental health policy: The case of Quebec,' pp. 307–29, Summer 1991. Copyright Duke University Press, 1990. Reprinted with permission.

October 1989, in Moncton, New Brunswick, was entitled "In Partnership with Families." The results of a symposium, sponsored by the Canadian Real Estate Association and Canadian Mortgage and Housing Corporation and entitled *Housing the Homeless and Poor: New Partnerships among the Private, Public and Third Sectors*, have just been published in a book edited by George Fallis and Alex Murray (1990). Manitoba's Department of Health 1989 health promotion initiative was called "Partners for Health." In the early 1990's, outlining her vision of health care in the 1990's for *Hospital News* (Moralis 1990: 1), Ontario Health Minister Elinor Caplan declared, "What I foresee in the future is a better coordinated partnership" of health care professionals and consumers. At the Fifth International Conference on AIDS in Montreal, on June 2, 1989, Perrin Beatty, Minister of National Health and Welfare pledged the department's support of, and partnership with, community groups. For a final example, if we look at the priorities outlined in the Canadian Council on Social Development's newly released book, *Social Policies for the Nineties*, we will find that "Social organizations should develop new partnerships with labour, business and governments to solve specific problems, such as the growing number of poor mother-led families, or the demand for services for seniors" (Canadian Council on Social Development 1990: 2).

The notion of partnership has swept the imagination of Canada's image-makers and invaded our policy designers and politicians' conception of the desirable, the rational, and the marketable. This is particularly true in the field of mental health, which was, in fact, one of the first to initiate the trend and is now earnestly putting it into operation.

The word made its political debut in Canada in November 1985 at the Canadian Mental Health Association's national conference on mental health advocacy entitled "Empowerment through Partnership." While the concept of empowerment has shown itself to be too politically intimidating and remains a quasi exclusive, though influential, feature of grass-root and community support literature, the word *partnership* was destined for a much more glorious career. By 1987, the Harnois Report on Quebec's mental health services had integrated it into its title *Pour un Partenariat Élargi.*[1] A year later, Ontario's Graham Report (1988), *Building Community Support for People*, recommended that "Ontario's mental health system provides for a partnership between consumers, their families, service providers and government in the planning, development and delivery of services" (p. 6). That same year, a document published by Health and Welfare Canada, *Mental Health for Canadians: Striking a Balance,* informs us that "What we need is breadth of vision and a willingness to learn from one another in a spirit of partnership" (p. 10). On January 16, 1989, it had become the key concept and guiding principle of Quebec's official mental health policy. The same was true a few months later in Manitoba which issued its own mental health policy and called it, *"For a New Partnership."* And these, once again, are only a few examples.

What is the meaning of all this? Is it that our policymakers, in their avid search for paradigmatic consensus and for frictionless solutions, have seized on the notion of partnership because it annihilates, by definition, all adversaries, all contradictions? Is skepticism justified? Or is enthusiasm the more appropriate response? Before we subscribe entirely to the evident truth within this new concept, it is important that we reflect upon its full significance.

I have selected for my examination of partnership the case of Quebec, the province which has carried its faith in *partenariat* the farthest. I outline here how Quebec's recent mental health policy defines *partenariat* and point out the measures taken to operationalize it. I then identify the roots of this concept as used in the field of mental health and propose a number of reasons which may account for its sudden currency in mental health policy making in Quebec and in general.

Such an exploration will provide us with some unique insights into the meanings and implications of a concept which may very well dominate the political landscape of the new century.

Le Partenariat Élargi and Quebec's Mental Health Policy

My purpose here is not to summarize in detail the policy, with its identified priorities, objectives, and plans for action, but rather to concentrate on its notion of partnership and on the measures outlined to initiate it. The policy clearly maintained the Harnois Report's conception (1987: 5) of an "enlarged" or "extended" partnership between all actors involved as a "privileged method of action in mental health." The 1987 report and the 1989 policy which followed, both say that they are based on the recognition of the potential and on the concerted mobilization of "the person" in need, of his or her family, kin, friends, community, professional and nonprofessional parties, public resources and resources of the "natural milieu." Along with the Quebec Government, the Ministry of Health and Social services and other relevant ministries, such as justice and housing, these are the partners for whom the policy proposes (Quebec Government 1989: 26) "a recognition of respective potential, open lines of communication and the adoption of common objectives," always keeping "the person" at the center of preoccupations. This *partenariat*, says the policy in its introduction, "is not a regimented line of conduct, but rather an approach" (p. 27). It must characterize the mental health system's intervention, planning, organizational and managerial activities, at the local, regional and central levels.

The Local Level

By local level, the policy document refers to the mental health services provided within Quebec's health and social service institutions: local community service centers, hospitals, rehabilitation centers, long-term care centers and other protection centers (see diagram). At this level, says the policy document, the mental health service delivery system must focus primarily on the bio-psycho-social needs of "the person" through the obligatory preparation, in cooperation with all involved actors, of Individualized Service Plans for priority clients. The aim of these plans, the policy says, is to permit continuity and coordination of services provided for each client, within/between institutions and within the community. The Individualized Service Plans are also meant to permit a careful evaluation or monitoring of the individual services and their results for "the person." [2] The responsibility to initiate each plan must come from what the policy calls "the "principal resource" providing the services to "the person" and its coordination becomes the responsibility of a "pivotal person" chosen by all actors. It is important to note that the policy does not specify who this "principal resource" or this "pivotal person" are to be, nor their professional background. It could be any one of the partners involved as – to the great dissatisfaction of psychiatrists – leadership roles are not identified with professional status. The policy also delegates to the Regional Health and Social Services Boards (see diagram) the responsibility of financing local Groups for the Promotion and Defense of Consumer Rights from within their own regional budgets. Originally created in 1970 as Regional Advisory Councils[3] these boards' decision-making and executive responsibilities have been increasingly enhanced over the years and especially since 1991 as a result of what is known in Quebec as Bill 120. The Quebec mental health policy of 1989 was thus the first legislated step in a more global reform of the health and social service system carried out as "a Citizen Centered Reform" [4]; this reform is now being implemented.

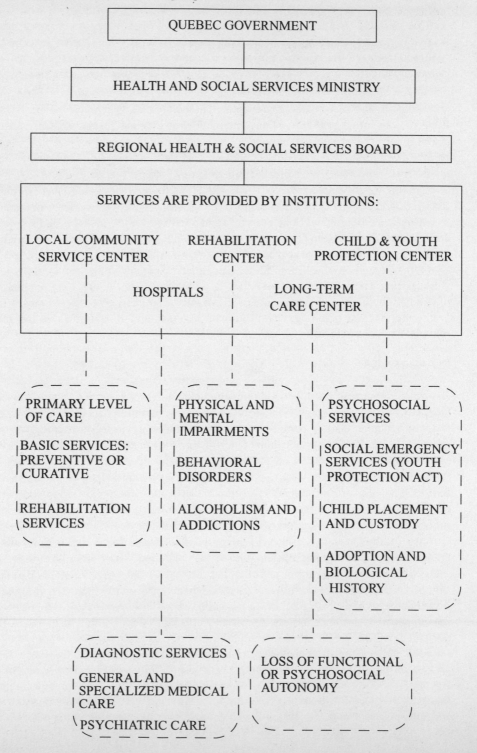

The Quebec mental health policy of 1989, also calls, at the local level, for the establishment of a companion service to assist "the person" in need; it also provides for the extension of the role of the public ombudsman to the settlement of cases of persons with mental problems. Committees of Beneficiaries, as key partners within institutions, are granted an annual budget equivalent to 0.1 percent of the institution's overall budget, i.e., not less than $20,000 and not more than $75,000.[5] Respite services are made available to families. Intent on finding solutions in the person's living environment, the policy recognized the key role played by community organizations carefully avoiding the term "alternative services," for how can alternatives be partners? Community organizations, in the language of the policy, are those directly offering diversified services to people in need and/or bringing together individuals who wish to find their own solutions in the form of support or self-help groups. Funds for such groups are to come from the region's budget package, to be made available for a three year period "in accordance with predetermined parameters" (p. 48). Psychiatric establishments are also required to develop, in collaboration with their regional partners in health, social, and other services, appropriate deinstitutionalization plans, due in April 1990, which would reallocate their resources on the outside in order to follow the persons returning to the community. A province-wide information campaign was launched to increase the community's awareness and its willingness to cooperate. A continuing education budget was established for staff and also for family and friends who are engaged in helping partnerships.

The Regional Level

It is in the context of system management at the regional level, says the policy document, that partnership is the most vital to mental health work. Here, partnership meant the decentralization of planning, budgeting and managing responsibilities of the Ministry of Health and Social Services. The policy delegated these responsibilities to the Regional Councils of the time, soon to become, in 1991, Regional Boards of Health and Social Services. Eighteen Regional Boards were thereby given the responsibility of regional subgovernments, with board members coming from a broad variety of partners in the system. Different regions having different strengths and different needs, the Ministry preferred, according to the policy documents, not to impose from the top down a uniform plan for action. Each region's first mandate was therefore the elaboration through "concertation" and "in a spirit of partnership," "harmony," and "equity," of a *Regional Service Organization Plan in mental health*, identifying the regional priorities, resources, needs and plans for the distribution of roles, mandates and responsibilities in mental health across the region. To help accomplish these tasks, each Regional Board had to appoint a *tripartite committee* of approximately twelve to eighteen members, depending on the region, composed of: 1) one-third representatives from the public network of   institutions offering mental health services (establishments, intermediate and half-way services ...); 2) one-third representatives from community resources active in mental health service delivery (such as alternative groups, self-help groups and organizations); and 3) one-third representatives from community resources at large which could have an influence on mental health promotion, on the prevention of illness, and on the social reintegration of patients (such as the police, families, union representatives, representatives from municipalities, from the school system, volunteer workers and ex-patients associations ...).[6]   Once approved by the ministry, if it conforms to seven given criteria,[7] the implementation and financial management of the plan becomes the regional council's complete responsibility. The tripartite committees will have fulfilled their mandate.[8]

The Central Level

This is the level of government, the Ministry of Health and Social Services and other relevant ministries (see diagram). At this level, the policy requires what it calls *un partenariat gouvernemental*.

While the Ministry of Health and Social Services remains the focal point, the goals of intersectoral cooperation, common objectives and compatible socioeconomic policies will be sought, says the policy document, through the creation of an intergovernmental committee with representatives from (1) the Ministry of Municipal Affairs and the Quebec Housing Corporation, (2) the Ministry of Education and the Ministry of Higher Education and Science, (3) the Ministry of Cultural Communities and Immigration, (4) the Ministry of Justice and Public Security, and (5) the Ministry of Labor and Revenue Security. The Ministry of Health and Social Services provides the leadership for this committee which will submit its recommendations directly to a permanent ministerial Committee of Cultural and Social Affairs.

The policy also contains provisions relative to research (15 percent of the Health Research Budget), training (of general practitioners in psychiatry), public information, promotion, evaluation of results (after five years of implementation) and so on – all to be carried out in this "spirit of partnership." Finally, to attach some dollar signs to its policy paper, the Province allocated an extra $32 million dollars to be spent during the next four years.[9] "The mental health policy," it is concluded, "must be seen as an opportunity for the Quebec government to provide concrete evidence of a genuine partnership and the possibilities offered by an intersectorial approach" (p. 55).

Partnership and the Social-Ecological Mindscape

A close examination of the mental health literature advocating partnership shows it to be, we believe, an offshoot of the community mental health movement of the 1960's and 1970's and of the disappointing outcome of the American community mental health centers. It is an attempt, inspired by the self-help, mutual-aid and citizen participation dialogues, to redefine the movement and to relocate it out of the mental health centers and into the neighborhoods and the natural living milieu of the person in need (Berger and Neuhaus 1977; Biegel 1979; Biegel and Naparstek 1979; 1982). A key reference point for projects both in United States and in Canada has also been the report of The President's Commission on Mental Health (1978) in the U.S. and its prescription:

Mental health services should be offered to individuals which would build first on their own assets and strengths, maintaining and cultivating their membership in social networks and natural communities in the least restrictive environment. This would mean developing methods which could identify and assess the functioning of an individual's natural support systems, and establishing, where appropriate, linkages between the natural support systems and the professional caregiving systems based on a respect for privacy and *on genuine cooperation and collaboration, not cooperation and control* ... Helping people where they are and assisting them to help themselves allows entry into the help giving and receiving systems without requiring that a person be labeled patient or deemed "sick" (Vol. 2, p. 154).

As Canadian psychologist Ben Gottlieb notes "the Presidential Commission's prescription for cooperation between professionals and lay helpers has been heeded by numerous health and welfare agencies in North America" (1983: 214). Many concrete experiences of such cooperation have been documented in the United States[10] and in Canada (Froland et al. 1981; Naparstek et al. 1982: 50; Gottlieb 1983). Whether under the label of "the Social Support model," the "Planned Support Network model," "the Social-ecological approach," "the Neighborhood Support Systems approach," "the Community Mental Health Empowerment model," or again, "the Community Network Support approach," the approach stresses the importance of placing "the person in need" at the center of concerns, of ending the imposed hegemony of professionals over the system and instead, of developing cooperative linkages between the professional and the natural helping networks (Naparstek and Biegel 1979). Such partnerships, according to advocates, must however be locality-based because their objectives are related to a specific neighborhood or subsection of a city. "A 'top-down' approach," they say, "proved unworkable because the government failed to provide mechanisms to devolve power to citizens at the neighborhood level" (Naparsteck et al. 1982: 85). It is within this particular mindscape that the Canadian Mental Health Association's 1985 call for *Empowerment through Partnership* acquires its full significance. Since the mid-eighties, the Canadian Mental Health Association (CMHA) with its provincial and municipal branches across Canada has greatly contributed to propagate this conceptual framework through a series of policy documents entitled "Framework for Support" (Church 1986), public messages on billboards and through its own local community empowerment programs.

It is within this social-ecological mindscape, that policy designers across Canada have discovered partnership. Now, they call it "the key to the future" in provincial mental health planning. In other words, they have elevated "partnership" from its basic roots in local neighborhood support ideology to "Partnership" as the conceptual basis for broader Province wide policy making. Quebec is right there, setting the pace, having made it an integral part of its mental health legislation and being involved already in implementation.

What is happening in Quebec is a true demonstration of the spirit of the times. Within the current economic and political landscape, partnership emerges as a promising solution to the multitude of crises, the remedy for government's most current strategic problems.

Partnership and the "Logic of the State"

While we cannot presume to get into the psyche of policy makers, we can recognize in the choice of the language of "Partnership" a certain logic of the State in response to key strategic problems: 1) the exhaustion of resources and allocation of losses; 2) the loss of faith in government and the consequent need to redefine the role of the State; 3) the loss of faith in professional knowledge and the increasingly forceful voice of alternative and "psychiatric survivor" groups; 4) the problem of overload in pluralist and competitive democracy and related to this, the ubiquitous search for consensus and frictionless solutions. Partnership, applied to state level policy making, borrows the language of neocorporatism. In their desperate search for a "third way" between competitive pluralism and monopolistic corporatism in mental health, policy cogitators and social engineers are being seduced by the potentials for salvation and rescue in neocorporatist ideas applied to the management of human services.

The Exhaustion of Resources

An economist told us, in 1980, that in the future, every economic gain for one interest group must mean fewer resources for another (Thurow 1980). Thurow was putting in very crude terms the acute problem of allocation of resources ... and what has become the allocation of losses. In this context, partnership is government's response to fiscal restraints.

For so long, resources for social expenditures had seemed limitless. When in the mid- and late-1970s the tide began to turn and governments found themselves in the midst of economic and political crises,. the resources they chose to allocate to social objectives were severely curtailed (Leseman 1988). Earlier objectives were qualified as unrealistic, beyond the ability of any democratic government to achieve at this time (Wildavsky 1979: 47). "Implementation of innovative programs in any area is difficult" (Marmor and Gill 1989: 463). In mental health, the lack of fit between objectives and resources was particularly poignant, as the fiscal logic behind the reform begun in the 1960s gained precedence over its therapeutic logic, creating what we know as the "deinstitutionalization crisis." To the rescue came models of intervention emphasizing self-help, mutual help and community support of the person in need in his or her own living milieu by his kin, friends and social network, *quasi* symbiotically. In Quebec, the "ecological model," as it was called, was so enticing that it rapidly made its way into government-published documents (Conseil des Affaires sociales et de la Famille 1984; Ministère des Affaires Sociales 1985) as the new conceptual framework for intervention in mental health: "Respect, dialogue and mutual help between Quebecers," the model said, "are not only the best safeguards of one's mental health but the essential tools to counter suffering, solitude, the aches and pains of living, and to help overcome the difficulties of life" (Ministère des Affaires Sociales 1985: 4). By a simple change of definition, resources which appeared insufficient had become potentially limitless. Though enticing, the model as such smacked of idealism and ran into severe criticisms (Boudreau 1987a; 1987b). A few years later, the model has now reappeared, revised, reformulated and with added requirements: state orchestrated cooperation between the informal and the formal networks along with a "spirit of partnership" at the local level between service givers and consumers, at the regional level with tripartite committees responsible for the elaboration of a regional service plan and at the Government level between relevant ministries.

What remains to be shown is whether such a spirit can be instilled "by decree" (Crozier 1979). There is cause for concern at all three levels, given the highly credible assumption which says that most people, most of the time, tend to act more or less as "rational egoists" (Axelrod 1981; 1984) working to maintain and improve their own individual or group situation.

The Loss of Faith in Government and Government's Need to Redefine and Restructure Itself

Not so long ago, says Richard F. Elmore, we believed in Government's ability to define problems, identify causes, design rational solutions and translate them into binding prescriptions (1983). We recognized central governments' right to use beneficent coercion to implement these prescriptions (Moynihan 1969; Crozier 1980). It was also believed, continues Elmore, that as long as a case could be made for intervention – by an appeal to data or political argument – government would provide the resources necessary to make intervention work. The story of social policy and of the technocratic efforts to construct rational systems of social intervention over the past 15 to 20 years, has proven these assumptions "wrong on all counts" (Elmore 1983: 213).

The Welfare State is in crisis not solely because of the tight money situation, but also because it has not been able to fulfill its promises when it had – or acted as though it had – the financial means to do so. Government's knowledge, judgement and ability to provide and to manage from the top has found itself seriously challenged by testimonies of thwarted expectations and serious rhetoric-performance gaps, uncontrolled spending and damaging unanticipated consequences, such as increases in the numbers of the homeless and the militant hostility shown by communities against integrated housing for the system's 'clients' or 'beneficiaries'. Testimonies also denounce the system's overwhelming bureaucracy, its "rigid organization, poor delivery of services, unsolved problems and neverending needs for expansion" (Oyen 1986: 6). In the United States and in Canadian provinces, the gigantic and costly bureaucracy responsible for managing the system found itself increasingly defined as the problem rather than the solution. Marmor and Gill speak of the disdain and suspicion of the American nation for its civil servants (1989: 463). As Paul R. Bélanger says of Quebec, "the prevailing image has shifted from that of a Welfare State to that of a highly bureaucratized system full of fatly paid civil servants who furthermore are indifferent to the people's problems" (1989: 107).[11] The Welfare State consensus, as it was called, has crumbled. "Something like a loss of innocence has occurred" says Elmore (1983: 229), a loss of innocence which indeed demands from government a redefinition of its role and responsibilities.

The knowledge, legitimacy, accountability and solvability problems facing governments are compounded by uncertainty about the future. In response to this loss of faith in Governments and to progressively forceful demands for a "minimum state" (Crozier 1979; Lemieux 1983), governments are increasingly opting to define themselves as "facilitators of local solutions" (Dahrendorf 1987), as partners in societal projects, rather that as providers and deciders. A Deputy-Minister in Quebec was recently reported as saying: "The time when the state acted and the community simply provided support is dead and gone; it is now time for the community to act while the state will provide the support" (Duplantie and Rodrigue 1989: 18).[12]

Governments, such as that of Quebec are, and will likely increasingly be opting for the more attractive option of writing legislation in general terms, of formulating global objectives, of organizing and mobilizing regional partners in representative tripartite committees and giving them the authority to "fill in the details and make whatever adjustments are necessary over time" (Chubb and Peterson 1989: 271). Decentralization with greater discretionary powers at the regional level in designing service organization plans, putting them into operation and managing the regional network of services, is thus becoming the ideal companion strategy for partnership.

Partnership coupled with decentralization is government's response to demands for "debureaucratization" of the system, for greater accountability of the administration (Aucoin and Bakvis 1988) and for involvement of regional and local people in the management of their own problems. The hopes are that partnership and decentralization together may lead government administration out of the present impasse while at the same time responding to regional diversity and providing more harmonious, responsive and equitable services.

From a more critical standpoint, however, some analysts of the situation (Maffesoli 1976,1982; Baudrillard 1982,1983; Renaud 1984) would likely suggest that this managerial philosophy may in fact serve to further consolidate government and technocratic dominance over an even more highly structured, programmed and accountable system where the stakeholders-made-partners are compelled to be involved, to cooperate and to play by rules they themselves, along with twelve to eighteen partners, are invited to establish.

Decentralization coupled with partnership is we believe, government's strategic response to chronic confrontations between all stakeholders over the allocation of roles and territory. A paradox in the Quebec experience is that while professional stakeholders resent and complain of excessive government involvement in their "affairs," they expect from government and the new policy, a clear-cut identification of their respective roles and territories. They want the Ministry to say, from the top and before everyone, who is to do what and when, and they are ready to fight with government at the provincial level if the assigned roles do not please them. In bowing out, the government postponed and transformed the fight into a regional issue where the actors, as members of regional tripartite committees, are more on their own, vulnerable to the demands of partnership and lacking the immediate and strong backing of their corporate bodies. All this is justified in the name of decentralization, regionalization and, of course, partnership. In specifically refusing to attach professional creed to the terms *"intervenants,"* "primary resource" and "pivotal person" in the management of the individualized service plans, the ministry has plainly notified all interested stakeholders that it was not about to take sides in local power struggles, either. Here again, this is left to the "spirit of partnership" of all the actors involved. Of course, in not taking sides, government has ignored the strongly voiced contention of psychiatrists that they are the only legitimate senior partners throughout the system. It has also left unaddressed the demands by the Quebec Association of Psychologists for a partnership that is "fully competitive with psychiatrists," that is, for a partnership where their services – as the other senior partners in the system – are equally covered by the universal health insurance plan. To a world which thinks in terms of senior and junior partners, government responded with a nonhierarchically specific definition of a partnership "between all involved actors" and repeatedly stressed that partnership is above all, a question of attitude.

The Loss of Faith in Professional Knowledge and the Increasingly Forceful Voice of Alternative and "Psychiatric Survivor" Groups

The "loss of innocence" (Elmore 1983) which ten years ago began to characterize attitudes towards the welfare state also modified attitudes towards professionals and professional knowledge. This is another reason for the strategic emphasis on "partnership." The "crisis of confidence in professional knowledge" (Schon 1983: 3) which hit the entire domain of social intervention has been particularly vigorous in the field of mental health.

Confronted by the glaring perversions of deinstitutionalization, and multiple demands for proof of effectiveness, claims of professional "skills" and scientific knowledge have fallen into disarray. They have been increasingly met with skepticism, cynicism and at times real hostility. Monopolies of knowledge and practice have been challenged and corporate interests denounced (Robitscher 1980; Breggin 1983; Burstow and Weitz 1988). Antipsychiatry groups have taken upon themselves to provide a representative voice and alternative mental health resources to "fellow survivors" of the system. They have done so with growing credibility and political clout insisting on their vital need for financial security and for an official recognition of their specificity and autonomy.

Blind faith in "superior knowledge" has given way to faith in "ordinary knowledge, skill and craft" as "ways of knowing that rely less on abstraction and precision than on close proximity to experience and simple rules of the thumb" (Lindbloom and Cohen 1979: 12–13). True solutions have increasingly been sought in the private and voluntary acts of individuals, in the lessons of experience, in the deprofessionalization of the field, the vulgarization of expertise. This new mindscape has also given rise to a call upon natural helpers (Elmore 1983) and, more particularly in Quebec, to this ecological model which calls upon each and every Québecer to contribute in his or her own milieu "human values such as ... what can I do for the welfare of ... my child, my parents ... my friends, my neighbors ... my fellow citizens" (MAS 1985: 3). The 1989 policy decision in favor of an "enlarged partnership" involving all actors may be understood as government's decision to promote a regionally designed and mutually agreed upon balance between ordinary and professional knowledge. It may also have provided policy designers with a convenient way out of taking a stance on the quality and effectiveness of these knowledges and on the conflicting claims of those who live by them. Hopefully the rules of the game for each region will be designed in such a way that the right kind of knowledge(s) will come into play at the right place and at the right time. To legislate partnership does not miraculously erase the inevitable tensions between the professional and the ordinary knowledge, between knowledge which claims it is "scientific and objective" and knowledge which is experiential, between knowledge which is impersonal and knowledge which is self-disclosing and which therefore may put its bearer in a position of discredit and vulnerability (Boudreau 1991).

One last point worth making on this issue is that while on the one hand refusing to endorse the medical model, Quebec policy makers have, on the other hand, neutralised the model's more vociferous opponents, the alternative groups. Mainly self-help and representative groups of ex-psychiatric patients who consider themselves survivors of the system, these were lumped by the policy into the global category of community groups, without recognition of their unique status. These groups of highly politicized survivors see their role in partnership, thus defined, as a form of co-opted integration into a system which, by their very existence, they reject. They are placed in the paradoxical situation of having to become "integrated alternatives," cooperating partners in a system which is responsible for the allocation of regional funds and thus for their livelihood and for the assignment of territorial responsibilities between service providers, including themselves.[13] An interesting question for our sociology students: would Durkheim, a century ago, have recognized in this "forced partnership" a pathological form of division of labour? Or would he have seen, in this attempt at partnership in the mental health field, early signs of the implementation of his personal vision of an ideal society, which pulled together in rule making and consensus oriented corporation-like associations, all mutually interdependent actors involved in the various spheres of labour? This was, in his mind, the only solution to a pathological division of labour and to the absence of "organic solidarity" in the highly differentiated and complex modern societies. Contemporary authors have called this the problem of overload in pluralist and competitive democracy.

The Problem of Overload in Pluralist and Competitive Democracy

The political attractiveness of the concept of partnership is also buttressed by what has been called, usually as part of neo-conservative discourse (Jalbert and Lepage 1986) the excessive vitality of democracy. "The demands on democratic government grow," they say, "while the capacity of democratic government stagnates" (Crozier et al. 1975: 9). From this standpoint, the resulting "crisis of democracy" or "crisis of governability" (Chubb & Peterson 1989) has arisen ineluctably from the inherent workings of the democratic process itself. In his broad-reaching book entitled *The Democratic Wish* (1990) James A. Morone specifically charges that recurring attempts to empower the people in America have paradoxically resulted in built-up bureaucracies and a less competent government which is more difficult for the people to control. "Democracy is killing democracy," says Sartori (1975). Here it is not the welfare state as above which is questioned but the decision-making and governing process in pluralist, democratic societies.

The difficulties are similar across democracies in Europe, Japan and North America: 1) the political systems are overloaded with participants and demands and they have increasing difficulty in mastering the very complexity which is the natural result of their economic growth and political development; and 2) the bureaucratic cohesiveness they have to sustain in order to maintain their capacity to decide and implement tends to foster irresponsibility and the breakdown of consensus, which increase in turn the difficulty of their task (Crozier et al. 1975: 12).

The resulting situation is one of "anomic democracy" say Crozier et al. (1975: 161), in which democratic politics becomes more an arena for the assertion of conflicts of interests than a process for the building of common purposes. Crozier's analogy to the "Babel tower" (Crozier 1979: 31) expresses very well the resulting confusion and disarray of a system where so many people and groups speak so many mutually incomprehensible languages each with such urgent tones.

In Quebec, the Rochon Report on Health and Social Services has painted a similarly disturbing picture of a "system taken hostage" (1988: 395), overcome by "ferocious competition" (1988: 419), "prisoner of the innumerable interest groups which crisscross it: groups of producers of services, institutions, pressure groups from the communities, unions etc." Here, they say, "the only law in operation is the law of the strongest," "conflict is omnipresent," "the democratic means of arbitration are no longer effective," "money goes to those who have more power," "there is no pursuit of a wider more fundamental common good" (1988: 407). The 1970 ruling which created professional corporations with reserved titles and areas of practice[14] has led, they say, to narrow and rigid corporatism, instead of the anticipated simplified relations among parties. It has prevented interdisciplinary cooperation and led to highly entrenched hierarchization of professions and a constraining judiciarization of work relations. Finally, the commission reports on the highly antagonistic legal entanglements between state administrators, professional corporations, and unions in the allocation of resources: "Everyone, or nearly, has the feeling of no longer being able to get any good work done" (1988: 415) – while people in distress are treated "like ping-pong balls" (1988: 419) at the mercy of territorial arguments. "Not only do we find a lot of confusion," says the Rochon Commission, "but also an expression of bad faith in the debates concerning everyone's particular mission. These debates cannot mask the ongoing maneuvers whereby every interest group attempts to broaden its own organizational empire"(1988: 419)[15].

This definition of the situation is not unique to the Rochon Commissioners: "Quebec society," says Paul R. Bélanger, "has lost its sense of collectivity; it has lost its whole-ness to self-centered individualistic autonomies" (1988: 109).[16] He could have added that Quebec is not unique in this situation.

Such a negative and telling diagnosis of the extra-parliamentary political process in action has called for a new method of orchestrating working relationships and of restructuring dialogues while compensating for the differentials among the parties involved. The policymakers' goal is ultimately to reach this much-wanting and -wanted, fair, and acceptable consensus on fundamental goals and procedures. This search for "consensus" or – as Québécois rational-technocratic rhetoric prudently calls it, "some form of consensus" – is understood to be, in Michel Crozier's words, "at the heart of democratic politics" (1975: 165). It is so, not just because general agreement makes life easier, and therefore is a "facilitating condition of democracy" (Sartori 1987: 90), not just because "where consensus exists, one of the most disagreeable and morally offensive features of human interaction – coercion – can be avoided" (Graham 1986: 108) but because "consensus equates with legitimation" (Pross 1986: 241). This is, indeed, a highly desired political good.

The solution proposed by Michel Crozier in a fascinating book entitled wisely *You Cannot Change Society by Decree* (1979) is to transform adversaries into partners, not by "destroying adversaries" but by facilitating experiences and offering occasions for cooperation, by organizing participation of citizens and stakeholders, involving actors in setting goals and in working towards mutual interests, developing new competences and ultimately "making a bet on human capacities" (1979: 272). This appears to be what the authors of the Quebec Mental Health Policy have elected to do in legislating the creation of regional tripartite committees pulling together the main stakeholders involved and giving them the responsibility of designing their own region's organiza-tional plan for mental health. If democracy is indeed self-destructing (Crozier et al. 1975), decentralized partnership, in the logic of the State, may be the way to save democracy by sharing responsibilities and reducing the political pressures on Govern-ment. As the last message of his book, *Corporatism and Welfare* (1982), Alan Cawson suggests that "in the final analysis, democracy means voluntary co-operation, in the sense of active rather than passive consent, in collective social arrangements. A demo-cratic struggle must be made up of an infinity of democratic acts, which means that democratic ends cannot be reached except by democratic means" (1982: 112). This is the role of the tripartite committees; they are temporary forums for carrying out the democratic process. This government delegated mission invokes John Dewey's compel-ling 1927 prescription: "The cure for the ailments of democracy is more democracy" – with caution highly recommended by Morone's conclusions in *The Democratic Wish* (1990: 322).

Partnership as Part of the Neo-Corporatist Mindscape

By bringing about some sort of cooperative regional sub-governments and by speaking of managing consensus as opposed to managing conflict, Quebec policy makers have attempted to create rules of the game which belong to what political theorists have called a "post-pluralist situation" (Pross 1986). By officially – though selectively – set-ting aside authoritarian modes of control of the mental health system, and taking on the role of active partner, by elevating the political status of non-professional community helping groups (Offe 1981), by adopting the language of tripartism and integrating three basic categories of interest groups as joint partners in the planning and coordination of the system, the Quebec Government followed and furthered its neo-corporatist tendencies (Panitch 1979; Archibald 1983, 1984).

Quebec is not alone in having taken this path. According to John H. Goldthorpe, Western societies over recent decades, especially those in which social-democratic parties[17] have played a dominant role in government, have rediscovered and renewed corporatist principles, which entail "a certain blurring of the line of division between the state and civil society" (1984: 324).

The ideal-typical definition of "neo-corporatism" has inspired many fascinating debates (Offe 1981; Lehmbruch and Schmitter 1982; Cawson 1986); so has the question of its applicability to social policy (Cawson 1982; Harrison 1984). We would like to suggest that the language of partnership, as adopted by a growing number of social policy makers, is translated from a neo-corporatist conception of economic management into the world of human service management. Instead of speaking of representatives from capital, labour and government at the negotiating table, the "partners" invited are representatives from the public service network and various levels of community groups, providers, and consumers.

As part of the tripartite committees, these partners, are given a say in the planning of their regional mental health service system. Yet, while they may have equal representation on the committee, a word of caution is necessary. In the same way power, as defined by Michel Crozier (1973), is not exclusively a question of relationships but also a question of strategies and process, partnership is not exclusively a matter of mapping out membership and creating relationships on a committee. Setting up temporary decision-making tripartite committees at the regional level with the mandate of creating a regional plan of services may not be sufficient for "true partnership" if especially powerful "partners" afterwards or at the local level still act the way they have always acted, that is, with mighty struggles against encroachment on territories, privileges, and prerogatives (Coburn et al. 1983). The structural constraints to a "true process of partnership" are many and resillient. They are imbedded in the restrictive Canadian health insurance plan which, by reimbursing only medical care, restricts access to alternatives and thus gives the medical profession a virtual monopoly in care, and guarantees its dominance over the entire mental health system; they are imbedded in restrictive collective conventions, which guarantee exclusivity of practice to various professional groups, wittingly or unwittingly setting limits and boundaries within which partnerships can be negotiated and enacted; they are inherent in the inequality of resources, of organizational ability and clout of the various partners, in the increasing tendency on the part of government to hire mainly part-time personnel in the health and social services, and in the network's difficulty in maintaining qualified personnel (Bélanger 1988a, 1988b; Bélanger and Lévesque 1990). Deeper structural changes than those introduced by Quebec's mental health policy are necessary if "true partnership" is to be a viable process. These changes are not impossible but will require a total reconsideration of the rules of the game which provide the context to partnership. Time will tell if the global reform of the health and social service system now being implemented in the Province of Quebec will provide this favorable context.

Partnership is a solution with many challenges. It is a solution which will require inspired nurturing, true commitment and the readiness to make sure that it is not just another politically appealing but empty and deceptive concept.

Conclusion

In answer to the often bemused questions of stakeholders affected by the new policy as to "where does this *partenariat* come from" I would like to suggest – in language perhaps as bemusing – that *partenariat* as defined and put into operation in Quebec's Mental Health Policy, is an improvisation with a strong neo-corporatist flavor which aims to be the middle point in a continuum. This continuum has at one end, "the open, competitive and fluid interplay of interests characteristic of pluralism" and at the other end, "the closed, monopolistic and relatively stable structure of interests best captured by the concept of corporatism" (Cawson 1986: 147). It is, I believe, an attempt to create at the regional managerial level, a "democratic" resolution to the highly objectionable and conflict-producing coexistence of "competitive corporatism for the powerful" – that is for the professional corporations and public sector unions – and "unbalanced pluralism for the weak," that is for community and alternative groups who demand a say in the system.

The language of partnership as a third way in the management of the Quebec Mental Health system presents itself as the language of fairness and equitability. The actual effectiveness of Partnership, however, rests on the firm belief that stakeholders will demonstrate, "their concrete willingness to stand on the proposition that the best hope for a stable and peaceful human existence is not envy, greed, competition, and inequality; but instead, cooperation, public spiritedness and the sentiment of equality" (Green 1985: 272).

In proposing that stakeholders become partners, the Quebec Mental Health Policy has accepted Crozier et al.'s (1975) bet in favor of human capabilities. It has not yet, however, sufficiently changed the rules of the game and the structural constraints that exist at all levels to put the odds on its side. Now is time to examine partnership in action. The next few years will require careful observation and will impose their own conclusions. Meanwhile, the term partnership regularly appears on policy documents of all sorts carrying hopes and expectations. For those who choose to put their trust in this language and its problem-solving abilities, it is my hope that they will do so with a reasonable understanding of the forces giving it life and propelling it towards political acceptance.

Notes

1   "For an Enlarged or a Broadened Partnership."
2   It is important to note here however that on March 3, 1993, the Rassemblement des Ressources Alternatives en Santé Mentale du Quebec, a committe which represents over 100 alternative groups and services in the Province, has voiced its official opposition to the Plans de Services Individualisés because, among other things, such plans meant that too much control will be exercised over the life and freedom of the person.
3   For an excellent discussion of the historical background of Quebec's experience with decentralization and regionalization, read Roger Gosselin's excellent article entitled: "Decentralization/Regionalization in Health Care: The Quebec Experience" (1984).
4   After many years of province wide consultation with stakeholders in the health and social services, the Province of Quebec introduced in 1991, with Bill 120, what it called "A Citizen Centred Reform" of its Health and Social Service System. Of direct relevance to us here, was, among other things, the transformation of the Regional Councils into actual Regional managerial Boards, called Régies Régionales in line with a policy of "true decentralisation to

the regions." The Boards' eight functions are 1) to plan, organise, implement and evaluate health and social services programs, 2) to formulate priorities in matters of health and welfare, 3) to allocate budgets, 4) to ensure economical and efficient management of human, material and financial resources, 5) to implement measures for the protection of public health and social protection of individuals, families and groups, 6) to establish and evaluate service organisation plans, 7) to ensure co-ordination of medical activities of physicians, institutions, community organisations and nursing homes, and 8) to ensure public participation and users' rights. Here again is emphasised the spirit of partnership and public involvement. This Bill is totally in line with the Mental Health Policy which preceded it (in 1987) as the first step in the global reform of Health and Social Services in the Province of Quebec.

5   In concrete terms, for instance, it means that an institution like Montreal's Louis Hippolyte Lafontaine Hospital will increase the budget of its patients' committee to $75,000 from about $40,000, 90% of which is now used for recreation.

6   The Regional Councils were to nominate the members of the tripartite committee from suggestions coming from these three sectors. The choice of the actual individuals was up to the Councils and, as we were told on many instances, of very judicious and strategic importance for the achievement of the desired consensus. Specific personality characteristics of the potential partners – such as the ability to make compromise – were looked for and, as we were told by several regional directors, often became the determining factors.

7   The criteria concern the plan's "conformity to the goals of the policy, and available budget; the reallocation of resources and identification of priority problems; the determination of responsibilities in the production and financing of services; the integration of deinstitutionalization plans for institutions; signed agreements concerning intraregional, interregional and intersectorial complementarity; and a schedule for implementation and subsequent evaluation of the plan." In fact, by 1993, all regional plans had been submitted but had not yet been accepted. This revealed itself to be a more difficult and lengthier process than anticipated.

8   A first evaluation of the performance of the tripartite committees, whose mandate was exclusively to prepare the regional plans, led the ministry to adopt the resolution that they be maintained as consulting committees to the General Director of each Regional Board on a long term basis.

9   At the time, the Province of Quebec had a $500 Million annual budget for Mental Health, and spent an annual $7.5 billion on health and social services.

10   In the United States, a large number of these initiatives were first sponsored by the National Institute of Mental Health, including Community Support Programs for chronic mental patients, Primary Health Care, Community Mental Health Centre linkage projects and the Most-In-Need Program for child mental health services (Naparstek et al. 1982: 50). Naparstek et al. also speak of the Baltimore, Maryland, and Milwaukee, Wisconsin tests of the Community Mental Health Empowerment model with all its imperfections – and all its promise (1982: 50).

11   Translated by the author of this chapter.

12   Translated by the author of this chapter.

13   For excellent discussions of this particular issue and of other aspects of Policy and Planning in the Quebec Mental Health System read White 1992 and White and Mercier 1991a and 1991b.

14   One of the recommendations of the December 1990 reform is to reevaluate, over the next two years, the professions' regulatory framework with a view to replacing exclusive fields of practice by exclusive acts or shared acts or reserved titles.

15   Quotations from the Rochon Report have all been translated by the author of this chapter.

16   Translated by the author of this chapter.

17 For an excellent analysis of the role of the Parti Québécois in favoring and furthering neo-corporatist ideas when in power, see Archibald 1983.

References

Archibald, C. 1983. *Un Québec Corporatiste?* Hull: Editions Asticou.

Archibald, C. 1984. Corporatist Tendencies in Quebec. In AG Gagnon ed. *Quebec: State and Society.* Toronto: Methuen.

Aucoin, P and H Bakvis. 1988. *The Centralization-Decentralization Conundrum: Organization and Management in the Canadian Government.* Halifax: The Institute for Research on Public Policy.

Axelrod, R. 1981. The Emergence of Cooperation Among Egoists. *American Political Science Review* 75(2): 306–318.

Axelrod, R. 1984. *The Evolution of Cooperation.* New York: Basic Books.

Barrel, Y. 1984. *La Société du Vide.* Paris: Seuil.

Baudrillard, J. 1982. *À l'Ombre des Majorités Silencieuses, la Fin du Social.* Paris: Denoel/Gonthier.

Baudrillard, J. 1983. *Les Stratégies Fatales.* Paris: Grasset.

Bélanger, J-P. 1990. Du Rapport Castonguay au Rapport Rochon; le développement du système de santé au Québec. *Revue Canadienne de Santé Mentale Communautaire* 9 (1): 143–155.

Bélanger, PR. 1988a. Les Nouveaux Mouvements Sociaux à l'Aube des Années 90. *Nouvelles Pratiques Sociales* 1(1): 101–115.

Bélanger, PR. 1988b. Santé et Services Sociaux au Québec; Un Système en Otage ou en Crise: De l'Analyse Stratégique aux Modes de Régulation. *Revue Internationale d'Action Communautaire* 20(60): 157–169.

Bélanger, PR and B Lévesque. 1990. Le Système de santé et de services sociaux au Québec: Crise des relations de travail et du mode de consommation. *Sociologie du Travail* 2 (90): 231–244.

Berger, P and R Neuhaus. 1977. *To Empower People: The Role of Mediating Institutions.* Washington, DC: American Enterprise Institute for Public Policy Research.

Biegel, D. 1979. *Neighborhood Support Systems: People Helping Themselves.* Keynote Address, Pittsburgh Conference on Neighborhood Support Systems, Pittsburgh.

Biegel, D and A Naparstek. 1979. Organizing for Mental Health: An Empowerment Model. *Journal of Alternative Human Services* 5(3): 8–14.

Biegel, D and A Naparstek. 1982. The Neighborhood and Family Services Projects: An Empowerment Moled Linking Clergy, Agency Professionals and Community Residents. In A Jeger and R Slotnic eds. *Community Mental Health and Behavioral-Ecology: A Handbook of Theory, Research and Practice.* New York: Blenmum Press.

Boudreau, F. 1984. *De l'Asile à la Santé Mentale, Les Soins Psychiatriques: Histoire et Institutions.* Montréal: Editions Saint-Martin.

Boudreau, F. 1987a. The Making of Mental Health Policy: The 1980's and the Challenge of Sanity in Québec and Ontario. *Canadian Journal of Community Mental Health* 6 (1): 27–47.

Boudreau, F. 1987b. The Vicissitudes of Psychiatric Intervention in Québec - From the Institutional to the Ecological Model, In EM Bennett ed. *Social Intervention, Theory and Practice.* Lewiston/Queenston: Edwin Mellin Press.

Boudreau, F. 1991. Stakeholders as Partners: The Challenges of Partnership in Québec Mental Health Policy. *Canadian Journal of Community Mental Health* 10(1): 7-28.

Breggin, PR. 1985. *Psychiatric Drugs: Hazards to the Brain.* New York: Springer.

Burstow, B and D Weitz. 1988. *Shrink Resistant, The Struggle Against Psychiatry in Canada.* Vancouver: New Star Books.

Canadian Council on Social Development. 1990. Social Policies for the Nineties. *Social Development Overview* 7(3): 2–3.

Cawson, A. 1982. *Corporatism and Welfare, Social Policy and State Intervention in Britain.* London: Heinemann Educational Books.

Cawson, A. 1986. *Corporatism and Political Theory.* New York: Basil Blackwell Inc.

Chamard, C. 1989. Le Nouveau Défi du Partenariat en Santé Mentale. *Artère,* (Association des Hôpitaux du Québec) 7(2): 2

Chubb, JE and PE Peterson. 1989. *Can the Government Govern?* Washington, DC: Brookings Institution.

Church, K. 1986. *Building a Framework for Support.* Toronto: Canadian Mental Health Association.

Coburn, D, GM Torrance, and J Kaufert. 1983. Medical Dominance in Canada in Historical Perspective: The Rise and Fall of Medicine? *International Journal of Health Services* 13(3): 407–432.

Conseil des Affaires Sociales et de la Famille. 1984. *Objectif: Santé, Rapport du Comité d' Etudes sur la Promotion de la Santé Québec.* Direction Générale des Publications Gouvernementales.

Crozier, B. 1979. *The Minimum State - Beyond Party Politics.* London: Hamish Hamilton.

Crozier, B. 1973. The Problem of Power. *Social Research* 40: 219.

Crozier, M, S Huntington, and J Watanuki. 1975. *The Crisis of Democracy Report on the Governability of Democracies to the Trilateral Commission.* New York: New York University Press.

Crozier, M. 1979. *On ne Change Pas la Société par Décret.* Paris:Bernard Grasset.

Crozier, M. 1980. *Le Mal Américain.* Paris: Fayard.

Crozier, M. 1987. *Etât Modeste, Etât Moderne.* Paris: Fayard.

Dahrendorf, R. 1987. *The Changing Role of Government. Interdependence and Cooperation in Tomorrow's World.* Paris: Organization for Economic Cooperation and Development.

Doughton, MJ. 1976. *People Power.* Bethlehem, Pa: Media America.

Duplantie, JP, and N Rodrigue. 1988. L' Entrevue: Les Lendemains du Rapport Rochon. *Nouvelles Pratiques Sociales* 1(1): 15–33.

Durkheim, E. 1960. *De la division du travail social.* Paris: Presses Universitaires de France.

Elmore, RF. 1983. Social Policymaking as Strategic Intervention. In E Seidman ed. *Handbook of Social Intervention.* Beverly Hills: Sage.

Fallis, G, and A Murray. 1990. *Housing the Homeless and Poor, New Partnerships among the Private, Public and Third Sectors.* Toronto: University of Toronto Press.

Froland,C, G Brodsky, M Olson, and L Stewart. 1979. Social Support and Social Adjustment: Implications for Mental Health Professionals. *Community Mental Health Journal* 15: 82–93.

Froland, C, D Pancoast, N Chapmen, and P Kimboko. 1981. *Helping Networks and Human Services.* Beverly Hills: Sage.

Goldthorpe, JH. 1984. The End of Convergence: Corporatist and Dualist Tendencies in Modern Western Societies. In JH Goldthorpe ed. *Order and Conflict in Contemporary Capitalism.* Oxford: Clarendon Press.

Gosselin, R. 1984. Decentralization/Regionalization in Health Care: The Québec Experience. *Health Care Management Review* (Winter): 7–23.

Gottlieb, BH. 1982. Mutual-Help Groups: Members' Views of their Benefits and of Roles for Professionals. *Prevention in Human Services* 1: 55–67.

Gottlieb, BH. 1983. *Social Support Strategies, Guidelines for Mental Health Practice.* Beverly Hills: Sage.

Graham, K. 1986. *The Battle of Democracy: Conflict, Consensus, and the Individual.* Totowa, NJ: Barnes & Noble

Graham Report. 1988. *Building Community Support for People: A Plan for Mental Health in Ontario.* The Provincial Community Mental Health Committee.

Green, P. 1985. *Retrieving Democracy, In Search of Civic Equality.* Totowa, NJ: Rowman & Allanheld.

Harnois Report. 1987. *Pour un Partenariat Élargi - Projet de Politique de Santé Mentale pour le Québec, Rapport du Comité de la Politique de la Santé Mentale.* Québec: Gouvernement du Québec, Ministère de la Santé et des Services Sociaux.

Harrison, ML. 1984. *Corporatism and the Welfare State.* Hampshire Gull, England: Gower.

Havel, V. 1990. Words on Words. *New York Review of Books,* January 18: 5–8.

Health and Welfare Canada. 1988. *Mental Health for Canadians: Striking a Balance.* Ottawa: Ministry of Supply and Services.

Huizinga, J. 1970. *Homo Ludens.* London: Paladin.

Jalbert, L, and L Lepage. 1986. *Néo-conservatisme et Restructuration de L'État.* Québec: Presses de l'Université du Québec.

Keohane, RO. 1984. *After Hegemony, Cooperation and Discord in the World Political Economy.* Princeton, NJ: Princeton University Press.

Lehmbruch, G, and PC Schmitter. 1982. *Patterns of Corporatist Policy-Making.* Beverly Hills: Sage.

Lemieux, P. 1983. *Du Libéralisme à l'Anarcho-capitalisme.* Paris: Presses Universitaires de France.

Leseman, F. 1988. *La Politique Sociale Américaine.* Montréal: Ed. Saint-Martin.

Lindbloom, C, and D Cohen. 1979. *Usable Knowledge: Social Science and Social Problem Solving.* New Haven: Yale University Press.

Maffesoli, M. 1976. *Logique de la Domination.* Paris: PUF.

Maffesoli, M. 1982. *L'Ombre de Dionysos, Contribution à une Sociologie de l'Orgie.* Paris: Méridiens/Anthropos.

Marmor, TR, and KC Gill. 1989. The Political and Economic Context of Mental Health Care in the United States. *Journal of Health Politics, Policy and Law* 14(3): 459–475.

Ministère des Affaires Sociales (MAS), Direction Générale de la Santé. 1985. *L'intervention En Santé Mentale: Du Modèle Institutionnel vers le modèle Ecologique,* Document de Consultation sur les Éléments d'une politique de Santé Mentale. Québec: Gouvernement du Québec.

Moralis, M. 1990. Key to Future is Co-operation, Consumer Empowerment. *Hospital News* 3(7): A1 and A7.

Morone, J. 1990. *The Democratic Wish, Popular Participation and the Limits of American Government.* New York: Basic Books.

Moynihan, PD. 1969. *Maximum Feasible Misunderstanding.* New York: Free Press.

Naparstek, AJ, and D Biegel. 1979. *Partnership Building in Mental Health and Human Services: A Community Support Systems Approach.* In *Community Support for Mental Patients.* Washington, DC: Subcommittee on Health and the Environment, Committee on Interstate and Foreign Commerce.

Naparstek, AJ, and D Biegel. 1982. A Policy Framework for Community Support Systems. In D Biegel and A Naparstek eds. *Community Support Systems and Mental Health: Research, Practice and Policy.* New York: Springer.

Naparstek, AJ, DE Biegel, and HR Spiro, with J Coffey and J Andreozzi. 1982. *Neighborhood Networks for Humane Mental Health Care.* New York: Plenum Press.

Offe, C. 1981. The Attribution of Public Status to Interest Groups: Observations on the West German Case. In S Berger ed. *Organizing Interests in Western Europe: Pluralism, Corporatism and the Transformation of Politics.* Cambridge: Cambridge University Press.

Oyen, E. 1986. *Comparing Welfare States and Their Futures, Studies in Social Policy and Welfare.* Aldershot, England: Gower Publishing Company Ltd.

Panitch, L. 1979. *Corporatism in Canada?* In R Schultz, OM Kruhlak and JC Terry eds. *The Canadian Political Process.* Toronto: Holt, Rinehart and Winston.

President's Commission on Mental Health. 1978. *Task Panel Reports* Vols 2-4 Washington, DC: Government Printing Office.

Pross, AP. 1986. *Group Politics and Public Policy.* Toronto: Oxford University Press.

Québec Government. 1989. *Mental Health Policy* - English translation. Québec: Gouvernement du Québec, Ministère de la Santé et des Services Sociaux.

Renaud, G. 1984. *A l'ombre du rationalisme, La Société Québécoise, de sa Dépendance à sa Quotidienneté.* Montréal: Ed. Saint-Martin.

Robitscher, J. 1980. *The Powers of Psychiatry.* Boston: Houghton Mifflin Company.

Rochon, J et al. 1988. *Rapport de la Commission D'Enquête sur les Services de Santé et les Services Sociaux.* Québec: Les Publications du Québec.

Sartori, G. 1987. *The Theory of Democracy Revisited.* Chatham, NJ: Chatham House.

Schon, DA. 1983. *The Reflective Practitioner, How Professionals Think in Action.* New York: Basic Books.

Seidman, H, and R Gilmour. 1986. *Politics, Position and Power, From the Positive to the Regulatory State.* Oxford: Oxford University Press.

Spiegel, D. 1982. Self-help and Mutual Support Groups: A Synthesis of the Recent Literature. In D Biegel and A Naparstek eds. *Community Support Systems and Mental Health: Practice, Policy and Research.* New York: Springer.

Thurow, LC. 1980. *The Zero-Sum Society: Distribution and the Possibilities for Economic Change.* New York: Basic Books.

Trainor, J, and K Church. 1989. *User Involvement in Mental Health Planning.* A Discussion Paper of the Alliance Development Committee prepared by the Working Party on Consumer and Family Involvement. Toronto.

White, D. 1992. (De)-Constructing Continjuity of Care: The Deinstitutionalization of Support Services for the People with Mental Health Problems. *Canadian Journal of Community Mental Health,* 2(1): 85-99.

White, D, and C Mercier. 1991a. Reorienting Mental Health Systems: The Dynamics of Policy and Planning. *International Journal of Mental Health,* 19(4): 3-24.

White, D, and C Mercier. 1991b. Coordinating Community and Public-Institutional Mental Health Services: Some Unintended Consequences. *Social Science and Medicine,* 33(6): 729-739.

Wildavsky, A. 1979. *Speaking Truth to Power: The Art and Craft of Policy Analysis.* Toronto: Little, Brown.

Wilensky, HL. 1976. *The New Corporatism, Centralization and the Welfare State.* Beverly Hills: Sage.

Wilensky, HL. 1981. Democratic Corporatism, Consensus and Social Policy. In HL Wilensky ed. *The Welfare State in Crisis.* Paris: Organisation for Economic Co-operation and Development.

Williamson, P. 1985. *Varieties of Corporatism: Theory and Practice.* Cambridge: Cambridge University Press.

28

Community Participation In Quebec's Health System: A Strategy To Curtail Community Empowerment?*

Michel O'Neill

Introduction

Since the middle of the 1980s, there has been a revival of interest in approaches oriented toward structural sociopolitical changes to improve the health of populations. This interest has mainly been rekindled by the World Health Organization's vision of health promotion, developed in its European Office based in Copenhagen (World Health Organization 1984; Kickbusch 1986; World Health Organization 1986; Kickbusch 1988). Concepts such as "community participation," "community empowerment," "healthy public policy," or "new public health," to name but a few, are now part of the discourse of public health professionals, policy-makers, and politicians, whereas similar concepts were popular in North America during the 1960s and 1970s (O'Neill 1986) but were downplayed when Reagan came into power in the early 1980s.

Quebec chose almost 20 years ago to institutionalize community participation in a health and welfare system that was then thoroughly reformed and came under the direct control of the provincial government. In this article I will first review whether or not this institutionalization has really led to community empowerment in Quebec, then describe the significant revisions of the health system that are currently proposed in this province and describe how the issue of community participation is dealt with in these proposals. Finally, I will discuss a few central issues raised by what has happened in Quebec over the past 20 years. Promoting "community participation" has proven to be a means by which, without empowering the community in general, the technocrats and professionals of Quebec's new francophone middle class, in the health and welfare sector as in the rest of society, were able to develop and maintain their own power base at the expense of anglophone or traditional francophone elites. People currently willing to develop community participation as a means to foster community empowerment, in the wake of the "new public health movement" encouraged by WHO's approach to health promotion, are

* Reprinted from *International Journal of Health Services*, Vol. 18, No. 2, Michel O'Neill, 'Community participation in Quebec's health care system: A strategy to curtail community empowerment?,' pp. 237–54, 1992, with permission from Baywood Publishing Company, Incorporated, Amityville, New York.

thus likely to be interested by the lessons learned in this province after two decades of formal experimentation.

A Brief Overview of Quebec's Health System

General Context

Quebec is the second most populated province of Canada, after Ontario. It is especially characterized by its French-speaking population: about 80 percent of its 6.5 million people have French as their first language. The francophone population of Canada constitutes roughly 20 percent of a total of about 25 million people; 80 percent of French-speaking Canadians are concentrated in the province of Quebec, the rest being scattered elsewhere in this enormous country, especially in the maritime provinces (notably New Brunswick and Nova Scotia) and in Northern Ontario. The linguistic characteristic, and all the related elements pertaining to values, way of life, access to economic and political power, etc., may seem a strange way to introduce a place. In the case of Canada, however, it has surely been a central, if not the major, determinant of the country's past.

The recent history of Quebec, since the election of a liberal provincial government that launched in 1960 the modernization period called the "revolution tranquille" (the "quiet revolution"), is thus mainly the history of the emancipation of its French majority, using the provincial state as a key tool to develop its society. The fast expansion of the provincial governmental bureaucracies after 1960 enabled francophones to gain access to jobs and power that were not available to them in the anglo-dominated Quebec economy in which, after World War II, U.S. capital progressively replaced British capital to exploit the vast natural resources of the province (especially wood and mining products, most notably iron). This utilization of the state apparatus as a key tool for the economic and social development of its French majority is probably the major feature of Quebec's recent evolution, as many analysts have shown (Renaud 1978; Simard 1979).

The Recent Evolution of Quebec Health and Welfare Services

In Quebec, the delivery of health care and social work services was radically transformed during the early 1970s (Lesemann 1981; Renaud 1977; Renaud 1984), in line with the significant reforms prompted by the provincial state in the spirit of the "revolution tranquille." The conclusions of a sociologist who has devoted much time to scrutinizing this reform are worth quoting at length (Renaud 1977: 138–139; the author's free translation):

When they got access to political power, Castonguay and his team – using the ambitious, coercive and authoritarian style which was characteristic of all the reforms of the Quebec government since 1960 – passed, in less than four years, laws that reformed the professions and the delivery of health services as well as their management on a scale which was unparalleled in North America. Agencies were abolished (Unites sanitaires). Others were created: Local Community Service Centers (CLSC), Community Health Departments (DSC), Regional Councils of Health and Social Services (CRSSS), Quebec's Board of Professions (OPQ), Quebec Health Insurance Board (RAMQ). Others saw their roles and functions redefined: the Ministry of Social Affairs

(MAS) and the professional corporations. Finally, the general structure of the system was clarified, on paper at least. In brief, a major reorganization took place.

This reform, which has been heralded by many as the one of the fastest and most comprehensive undertaken in Western capitalist countries, has created a centralized state-controlled health and welfare system, funded almost 100 percent by the provincial government, which is in turn refunded in part by the federal government. The federal contribution was about 50 percent when the reforms were implemented but dwindled to about 39.7 percent in 1987-88 (Government of Quebec 1988: 390), the rest of the money coming from various taxation schemes of the provincial government.

But for a few private nursing homes, the health and welfare facilities are owned and operated by public corporations, which are legally independent from the ministry of health and social services (MSSS; Ministere de la sante et des services sociaux). How-ever, these bodies are entirely funded by the Quebec government and are bound by very strict legal and administrative regulations, especially because the collective contracts regulating the working conditions of these bodies' employees (whose salaries account for over 80 percent of the agencies' expenditures) are negotiated and signed centrally between unions and the government. The reform of the early 1970s has consolidated into five types of agencies and facilities the thousands that existed before 1970. These types are: (a) several categories of hospitals; (b) social work agencies; (c) rehabilitation centers; (d) nursing homes of various kinds; (e) local community service centers (CLSC; Centre local de services communautaires). The CLSCs, described in more detail below, have often been seen as the most original part of the whole reform. Also, as a result of this reform, 32 hospitals were given, by the government, a very peculiar mandate: to create a Community Health Department (DSC; Departement de sante communautaire). This other series of community health agencies, in addition to the CLSC network, is thus composed of 32 hospital departments. It covers the whole prov-ince for the planning of public health interventions and the monitoring of the popula-tion's health status, both at the subregional level. The reform finally integrated geographically, over ten regions, all the health and social work facilities under a central planning agency, the CRSSS (Conseil regional de la sante et des services sociaux), with mostly consultative functions. A lot could be added, and has been written, about this reform (Lesemann 1981; Renaud 1977; Renaud 1984; Government of Quebec 1988). In a nutshell, then, Quebec adopted in the early 1970s a strong social-democratic approach that integrated all health and welfare services into a state-controlled, well-coordinated system.

This system was created during a period when the provincial state was flourishing and the welfare-state approach to the delivery of services was at its peak. Today, in a political economy much less favorable to governmental intervention, and with the health and welfare expenditures of the Quebec government amounting to $8,971.8 mil-lion (Canadian dollars) for the 1987-88 budgetary year (29.58 percent of its total expenditures), (Government of Quebec 1988: 334), there is a strong temptation to reor-ganize the system on different ideological and financial bases, given the provincial Lib-eral government that got elected in 1985 and reelected in 1989 on a neoconservative political platform. To investigate the status of the social consensus on these matters, as well as to propose alternative ways to organize the system, a major governmental com-mission of inquiry, the Rochon commission, worked for three years and delivered its report to the Quebec government in December 1987 (Government of Quebec 1988). In reaction to this report, the Quebec government published in April 1989 a policy paper

(Government of Quebec 1989) describing the reforms it was ready to introduce in the system after about 20 years of relative stability, reforms that in early 1990 were introduced for debate in the legislative process. We will now look at how community participation has occurred and is likely to evolve in this system.

Community Participation in Quebec's Health System

Participation in the Castonguay-Nepveu Report

The reforms of the 1970s were undertaken after the recommendations of another major provincial commission of inquiry: the Castonguay-Nepveu commission. This commission worked from 1966 to 1970 and suggested, in the spirit of the late 1960s in North America, a very strong input of the population in the general reorientation of the system and in its daily management (Brassard 1987). This suggestion was considerably altered during the heavy political debates that occurred in reaction to the Castonguay-Nepveu recommendations. These debates occurred at a time when Quebec society was in a major political crisis (the October 1970 FLQ crisis and its aftermath, when Quebec was occupied by the Canadian army and civil liberties were suspended for one year); the debates led, among other events, to the unionization and the first strike of physicians. In the laws that were passed from 1970 to 1972 to organize the reform, the participatory mechanisms suggested by the commission of inquiry were not implemented; rather, a decision was made to limit public participation to the formal context of the boards of directors of the five types of agencies described earlier. In each agency, a certain number of seats were thus, by law, allotted to the public (Brassard 1987).

Although this involvement of the population was not as strong as hoped for by the commission of inquiry, it was a totally new situation in Quebec and is still unheard of in many other countries, where, even if the government pays the majority or the totality of the health care bill out of public monies, the population is not formally represented on the decision-making bodies. The actual capacity of Quebec citizens, since 1970, to influence the system through these board seats will be reviewed below. The case of CLSCs will be presented in detail because of its numerous peculiarities.

Community Participation in Non-CLSC Agencies

In the major piece of legislation that reformed the system in 1971, the number of seats on the boards of directors given to the population in agencies other than CLSCs was as follows: in hospitals, four of 14; in nursing homes, four of 13; in social work agencies, four of 17; in rehabilitation centers, four of 14. In each case, the general director of the agency was an "ex officio" additional member of the board, with no voting rights (Brassard 1987: 7–10). In all these agencies, the four seats reserved for citizens were divided into two categories: two seats were devoted to delegates elected by the general assembly of the people using the services of the agency or facility, and two were given to people chosen by the government to represent "socioeconomic groups" of the area where the agency was located.

After almost 20 years of experience, the overall assessment of citizens' capacity to influence the orientations of these agencies is clear: "The role of users and representatives of socio-economic groups consists more in managing the agencies than in defending the community's interests" (Brassard 1987: 5; free translation). A few technical changes in the law in 1978 and 1982 even reduced the number of citizen representatives on these boards. Hence analysts (such as Eakin 1984a; 1984b) who studied hospital boards of English-speaking hospitals in Quebec, for instance are unanimous in their opinion that the presence of citizens on the boards has not succeeded in empowering the community in such a way as to significantly influence the system. The population in general was not interested in participating because, in a minority position, its delegates were confronted by highly technical and complex issues and by a technoprofessional culture to which they did not belong. Running the health system was thus left in the hands of professionals and administrators, the population delegates being perceived as "creating time losses, impeding the speed and efficacy of the decision-making process as well as generating sterile conflicts between various groups in the agency or the facility" (Brassard 1987: 12; free translation).

This does not mean that the formal presence of citizens on boards has never been effective. Citizens sometimes made the difference when, for instance, delicate decisions had to be taken in hospitals on topics such as whether or not to allow abortions to be performed (O'Neill 1986). Brassard (1987: 22) also points out that in hospitals and nursing homes, the users on the board were sometimes able to promote different types of professional practices, to see that certain types of services were maintained despite budget cuts, to make sure that certain employees were fired, etc. More importantly perhaps, the presence of citizens created a kind of "symbolic cut" with the past, introducing slowly but surely into the public mind the fact that everyone could have a say in the operation of the system, and not just the elites as before the reform (Brassard 1987: 21).

Nevertheless, the power bases that allow the population to significantly influence the agencies have mainly been created outside these organizations, through the creation of health-related consumer groups, through political pressure on representatives in parliament, or through the use of the media (Brassard 1987). The capacity to take over the board seats devoted to citizens, in order to conduct battles from both within and without the agencies, was surely more an asset than if these seats had not existed. But, overall, participation in these agencies has been a failure, and the incredible growth of services outside the system (for instance, in alternative medicine) is, for Brassard (1987), eloquent proof that citizens were not able to shape the system to meet their needs.

What is the situation of community participation in the subregional network of community health agencies, the DSCs? For several reasons, this network has been almost sealed off from any public influence. First, being part of another organization (usually a hospital), the DSC does not have its own board of directors, where its services could be formally challenged; the hospital board thus acts as a buffer between the community and the DSC. Second, DSCs' territories are huge, and the concept of serving (and being accountable to) local communities is thus lost in the size of their operations. Finally, the role ambiguities within which the DSCs have lived most of their short lives, the strong medicalization of their community interventions, and the neoconservative political climate have created a sort of "straight-jacket" in which, but for a very few exceptions, these agencies have been forced to play the technocratic game more than the participatory game (O'Neill 1986: 299–327).

Community Participation in Local Community Service Centres

What Are CLSCs?

As conceived by the reformists of the early 1970s, the CLSCs were supposed to be the entry point for all health and social work services throughout the province. In addition, each CLSC was to have a "community organization" service, to be staffed mainly by social workers with a community-work type of expertise, in order to stimulate and help the local communities where the organization was based to tackle various social issues – the ideology of the reform taking for granted that health and social problems were two sides of the same coin. The original idea was thus to integrate in state-subsidized but locally run bodies serving a catchment area of about 20,000 people: (a) all the medical general practitioners in private practice, (b) all the personnel (mostly social workers) already active in various public or private social service agencies, and (c) all the personnel in governmental public health agencies (mostly nurses).

The CLSCs were expected to be very responsive to the needs of the communities they served and were given broad mandates. Their personnel were to work as a multi-disciplinary integrated team, offering all preventive, curative, and readaptive nonspecialized health and social services, referring to the appropriate health or social facilities those people that needed more specialized care. A network of about 210 CLSCs was thus mapped out in the early 1970s to cover the whole province, and the original plan was to complete this network within about five years, i.e., by 1976 or 1977.

The development of the CLSCs, however, did not go quite as smoothly as the reformists had hoped. Most physicians in private practice refused to be integrated in a state-subsidized organization and developed instead, at an extremely fast pace, their own network of private group practice clinics, totally altering the solo mode of practice still dominant before the reform. The community organization component was infiltrated very early by political activists of various kinds who "raised hell" and focused a lot of negative public attention on several CLSCs. Social workers, not wanting to be assimilated into medical personnel, fought and got their own series of agencies: the Social Services Centers (CSS). And a good part of the preventive services were temporarily given by the other public health agencies (the DSCs), for more than a decade in certain cases, because the creation of new CLSCs took a much longer period than foreseen at the outset.

To make a very turbulent and fascinating story short, the network of CLSCs was finally completed in 1989, but with about 160 rather than 210 organizations, many of them thus having a catchment area significantly larger than was originally planned. Most social work services have finally been integrated therein, as well as most public health preventive services. The community organization dimension of the CLSCs has been downplayed and mostly oriented toward outreach to hard-to-find clienteles in order to bring them to increasingly curative health and social services. This has led many to contend that the community orientation of these organizations has almost vanished. However, the survival of the CLSC network, often threatened during the 1970s and the 1980s, now seems beyond question. In most cases these agencies, whose services vary significantly, are appreciated and used by the population. Despite a new, rather curative orientation that these organizations have been strongly encouraged to take since 1987, following the advice of a governmental task force that studied them very closely (Brunet et al. 1987), CLSCs still have a lot of local autonomy and remain the major focal point for the interactions between the public system and communities in Quebec.

It is thus in CLSCs that the issue of community participation and community control is the most interesting to observe and has been most studied (Divay and Godbout 1979; Godbout and Martin 1974; Godbout 1981; Godbout 1983; Godbout 1987; Lesemann 1978a; Lesemann 1978b). Citizens were, by law, very strongly represented on CLSC boards (Brassard 1987; Godbout 1981): at the outset, they had a *majority* of seven of 12 voting seats (five users' delegates and two delegates of the community's "socioeconomic groups," nominated by the government); from 1982 on, this majority was taken away; the citizens still having seven of 14 voting seats (four users, two delegates of socioeconomic groups nominated by the government, one delegate of voluntary organizations active in the area, nominated by the CRSSS). In theory at least, there was thus a much bigger chance for the community to influence the CLSCs than any other type of agency in the system.

Community Participation in the Implementation of CLSCs

As Godbout (1981), who has studied this question closely, clearly indicates, public involvement in the implementation of CLSCs was very significant. The official process to start a CLSC in a neighborhood or a rural area required that a group of citizens made contact with the ministry and showed interest. This group was then given some seed money, was formally recognized as the provisional board of directors of the future CLSC, and with the technical support of a professional provided by the ministry, had to study the needs of the population, to propose a plan to implement the CLSC as well as to request the legal creation of the agency. The constituency of this group of citizens was supposed to be the general assembly of citizens in the area; in practice, at least in the cases studied by Godbout (1981), between 50 and 150 people (from catchment areas usually of about 20,000 people) showed up in meetings, elected the provisional board, approved the plan of implementation, etc.

Although most of these implementation processes did not generate widespread participation, they nevertheless allowed the citizens to really have control over the definition of the project (Godbout 1981). However as we shall see presently, once the CLSC was formalized and the official board of directors created, the nature of participation was transformed and the real power of citizens dwindled significantly.

Community Participation After a CLSC was Implemented

Godbout (1981) notes that, after the implementation phase, power decreased when the real operations began, despite the majority of citizens on the board. The general director and the staff were in a position to build up, consciously or not, their own power base along technocratic and professional lines and to effectively take over the orientation of the organization.

However, the empirical analyses conducted by Godbout show that, compared with the other types of agencies in the system, the boards of CLSCs remained a significant place for the population to influence the health services. Over the years, the real issue became how citizens on the board could influence the practices of professionals in these organizations. In several places there were conflicts, sometimes severe to the point of threatening the very survival of the agency, when citizens and professionals had different views on priorities. As pointed out by Godbout (1981), citizens were more often interested in the extension of curative services than in the type of preventive approaches that the progressive professionals frequently attracted by CLSCs wanted to adopt. In other instances, citizens on the board were able to influence the CLSC to begin to offer services that professionals were not always willing to provide, such as abortions for instance. By their presence on the committees that hired or fired the staff, among other mechanisms, citizens in CLSCs were thus often able to exercise an important influence on the evolution of the organization, in spite of the very strong powers of the professionals.

Despite the important limitations citizens had to face, Godbout (1981) shows that in CLSCs, community participation was not just the token participation it had been in the other types of agencies. In several cases, the power of citizens was able to match the power of the CLSCs' bureaucrats and professionals mainly (according to Godbout) because of the formal and autonomous source of power derived by citizens from the significant number of seats on the board guaranteed to them by governmental law. The community empowerment possibilities in CSLCs are thus limited but present, as confirmed by the more recent work of Belanger and coworkers (1987), who thoroughly scrutinized the links between these agencies and their communities around three issues: home care for the aged, occupational health and safety, and community organization.

CLSCs versus "People's Health Clinics"

At a more macrosocial level of analysis, however, the creation of CLSCs was interpreted by some critical analysts (Lesemann, 1981; Godbout and Martin 1974; Lesemann 1979) as a subtle way for the government to tame and integrate into the mainstream of society a special brand of grassroots organizations which, in urban settings (especially in the poor neighborhoods of Montreal and Quebec City), had begun at the end of the 1960s to self-organize various kinds of services, notably in the realm of health. Formal participation on the board of CLSCs is seen by these analysts as a way to curtail situations in which communities had created organizations over which they had total control, and as a more or less deliberate strategy by professionals and technocrats who had gained control over the state health apparatus through the reform to tame this threat to their newly acquired power (Lesemann 1978a; Lesemann 1978b; Lesemann 1979).

These grassroots organizations, called "groupes populaires," were prompted by two major social groups – unions and community organizers of various kinds – in the context of a socialist political radicalization that occurred in urban Quebec during the second half of the 1970s. The dynamics of these groups has been carefully studied (Godbout and Collin 1977; Hamel and Leonard 1981; McGraw 1978; Collin and Godbout 1987). At the end of the 1960s, before the reform of the health system, there were about ten such grassroots organizations across the province whose efforts were mainly devoted to health care. They called themselves "people's health clinics" (cliniques populaires).

At the outset, citizens generally had total control over these clinics, professional power was minimal, and everyone providing any kind of service was paid the same salary. As was the case for almost all urban "groupes populaires," the creation of such clinics was not prompted by citizens themselves, but by what McGraw (1978) called, after Gramsci, "organic intellectuals:" politically sensitive people from better-off neighborhoods that were willing to try out new forms of social relationships. A historical case study covering the period 1968-1988 describes the people's health clinic that resisted the longest (18 years) the temptation to be integrated into a CLSC (Bolvin 1988). This study shows that the phenomenon of professional dominance over citizen control (described earlier for CLSCs) was present there as well, but in a different manner and in a much less harsh form.

The history of the St-Jacques clinic has led an analyst who followed these events closely to what is in my opinion a realistic conclusion about the phenomenon of the clinics' integration into CLSCs. Belanger (1988) contends that even if it is true that CLSCs absorbed and transformed these people's health clinics, the latter would probably not have survived on their own and could hardly have been extended to the whole of Quebec's territory, especially to rural areas lacking the militancy present in urban poor neighborhoods. He suggests that, all in all, it was probably better for Quebec to have a widespread network of CLSCs where participation is possible, even if far from perfect, than to dream about hypothetical people's clinics where the power of citizens would have been greater but which would have probably not survived over the years.

The Future of Community Participation: Current Debates

Participation in the Report of the Rochon Commission of Inquiry

In its sophisticated analysis of the Quebec health system about 20 years after the reform of the early 1970s, the final report of the Rochon commission of inquiry points to eight major problems (Government of Quebec 1988: 407–425). One of them pertains precisely to the mechanisms of community participation, which are perceived as paralyzed ("un mecanisme democratique sclerose") (Government of Quebec 1988: 424). The commission thus accepted the analyses of Godbout and others saying that overall, public participation in the system had not worked.

Very intriguing though are the recommendations that were made in relation to this conclusion. The political context in which the commission worked consisted of the election of a liberal provincial government using a neoconservative electoral platform, forming a cabinet mainly staffed with people from the business community and quickly beginning to dismantle the welfare state by privatizing several state-run enterprises. It might have been expected, in such an environment that the commission would not bother any more about citizen participation in a strong, publicly subsidized health system and would propose, as certain ministers of the liberal cabinet had already suggested, modalities to privatize this system as well.

However, this was not at all the case. Basing its recommendations upon a very comprehensive consultation process, the commission perceived that the overwhelming consensus in Quebec was to maintain a strong, governmentally funded health and welfare system. The Rochon commission hence suggested six orientations to fine-tune the existing situation and did not propose a radically new vision. The second of these orientations pertains to mechanisms ensuring a better citizen input than had occurred over the previous 20 years. The key principle underlying these mechanisms is stated as follows: "In a system oriented toward achieving results, evaluation cannot be reduced to a tool for technocratic management. The administrative evaluation should be dependent upon a political evaluation, made at the national, regional and local levels" (Government of Quebec 1988: 479; free translation).

Among the several mechanisms suggested by the commission to implement this principle, the most important was to decentralize the management of the gigantic governmental resources devoted to health and social services to regional authorities, whose boards would be elected and directly accountable to the general population (Government of Quebec 1988: 479). It was also proposed that nobody working for an agency or a facility of the system should be allowed to run for office on these boards. Moreover, in all the agencies and the facilities of the region, the boards would be composed of a majority of citizens. The commission thus suggests that the management of the system be put in the hands of elected citizens, rather than of users and experts; this is already the case for the public education system in Quebec. By doing so the Rochon commission, at the end of the 1980s, was consciously or not going back to the ideology of the Castonguay-Napveu report of the end of the 1960s.

Participation in the April 1989 Policy Paper

Needless to say, the report of the Rochon commission generated a lot of debates when it was published in early 1988. Although it suggested the maintenance of the status quo for the general structure of the system, it nevertheless proposed important adjustments to pull the power out of the hands of professionals, bureaucrats, and administrators (none of them being very pleased about that) in order to make them accountable to the general public through electoral mechanisms. Given the fact that the commission's report was just a set of recommendations, however well documented, it could have been ignored by the liberal government in office, which had already ignored the report of another commission of inquiry that had worked for years on a reform of the labor code. Moreover, given that the president of the Rochon commission was strongly associated with the reform of the early 1970s (as were other members of the commission) of which he had been one of the main organizers, the report could also have been dismissed by the government as a biased interpretation of the current reality. No one knew exactly what the governmental reaction to the commission's recommendations would finally be.

It was thus a big surprise when, about a year after the end of the commission's inquiry, the minister of health and social services put out in April 1989 a policy paper on the reform of the health system (Government of Quebec 1989) using a vast majority of the commission's recommendations. As far as participation is concerned, the policy paper (called *Orientations*) goes beyond what was suggested by the Rochon commission. It suggests among other things that the individual boards of all governmental health and welfare agencies (hospitals, CLSCs, nursing homes, etc.) on a specific territory should be merged into one single board *totally composed of elected citizens* (thus excluding professionals and other employees of these agencies' boards), which would also participate in allocating the governmental money given to community organizations on this territory.

Even given some alterations in the political give-and-take that is taking place over the bill, which was put before the parliament in early 1990 to discuss *Orientations'* proposals, it seems that the lessons drawn by Godbout and others from the failure of participatory mechanisms from 1970 to 1990 have reached the ears of the government, and that it is ready to act on their basis by structurally guaranteeing an autonomous power base to citizens.

Conclusion: What Was Learnt in Quebec About Community Participation and Community Empowerment?

The following summarizes the Quebec experience and draws some practical implications for people who, in agreement with the concept of health promotion put forward by WHO, are currently interested in community participation and community empowerment ventures.

First, the case of Quebec is a clear demonstration that community participation and community empowerment are two different things indeed. In formal structures at least, the inescapable conclusion drawn by Godbout (1981) from his extensive empirical work on the subject is that, consciously or not, citizen participation usually ends up as consolidating the power of professionals or bureaucrats and not as a way to empower the community. According to Godbout, the only way for the population to acquire influence is to have a strong source of autonomous power (such as a majority on a board, for instance).

A second element that can be of practical use according to Brassard (1987), is to keep in mind the four major factors found by Godbout and Leduc (Bolvin 1988) to be associated with undertakings in which the citizen members on the boards of various agencies succeeded in influencing the organization, i.e., when participation really meant empowerment. The first factor is *adequate information* on the system in general and on the actual operation of the agency; finding mechanisms to double-check whether the information presented to the board by the general director was the only valid interpretation often proved necessary for citizens to propose sound alternatives. The second is to have a *strong mandate from the users or the community;* a user, talking only in his or her name, has much less impact than if he or she is widely known to have a constituency that can be mobilized if need be to create political pressure on certain issues. The third is the need to have a *strong personality,* so that the citizen can avoid being bullied by the jargon of administrators and professionals, can argue as long as needed to have the issues clarified, and can create conflictual situations when needed to achieve his or her ends. Finally, the existence of *mechanisms* (formal or informal) for the citizen board members to *access easily their constituencies* has generally been a major help in their capacity to exercise influence.

A third important lesson from the analysis of the Quebec experience is an invitation not to be naive about community participation. As a rule, the community as a whole does not participate, only certain subgroups or individuals do, whose representativeness can always be questioned. Moreover, especially in less privileged areas, participation usually does not occur spontaneously; it is generally triggered and nurtured by what Gramsci called "organic intellectuals," who can behave in a way to really empower people, as is the case when Freirean approaches are used (Freire 1968), or to enlist the population more or less consciously in activities that will just be a little more alienating. From the viewpoint of even the best-intentioned professional or organization, community participation usually ends up as being cumbersome and time-consuming; moreover, it can become extremely stressful when, for instance, citizens are powerful enough to force on the professionals or the organizations values that are not shared by the latter (for instance, imposing more curative care when professionals want to do preventive work; or imposing the obligation to perform abortions on organizations not agreeing to do so).

Citizen involvement is proposed by WHO as a key ingredient to succeed in health promotion (Kickbusch 1986; World Health Organization 1986; Kickbusch 1988). Ultimately, however, as seen in the discussion of the Quebec case, community participation and community empowerment are indeed directly concerned with power. And power is, by definition, the capacity of various individuals or groups (be they physicians, sociologists, managers, welfare mothers, self-help groups, or whatever) to force others in the way they think appropriate. In this respect, the power games at stake in the Quebec experience are interesting to watch. As Renaud (1977) and Lesemann (1981) have convincingly shown, the reform of the early 1970s was a successful effort of a new type of elite (the young French-speaking technocrats who took over the state apparatus as a power base) to gain power against anglophone economic elites as well as against old types of francophones elites (religious groups and liberal professions), in a society that had decided to "rationalize" and "modernize" its economy and its institutions. In this process, the idea of a "community"-based health system was not at all meant to empower communities, but was used by these new power-seekers as a symbolic ideological tool to get control over the health and social services system (Renaud 1978; Lesemann 1978b).

What is currently happening, 20 years later, is thus fascinating. In a period where the new francophone elites are now moving out of the state apparatus to invade the private sector, where the welfare state is being disorganized, and where the neoconservative ideology is becoming a dominant discourse, a business-oriented government proposes to give at long last real power to citizens over a health system it refuses to dismantle at the profit of private interests! What is thus needed, to grasp the possibilities and the limits of community participation and community empowerment in health promotion endeavors, is a framework to understand the dynamics of power relationships in postindustrial societies. In social sciences, several frameworks do exist for this purpose, but two are especially helpful and are briefly mentioned here as possible fruitful starting points to begin reconceptualizing these possibilities and limits.

The first one is Touraine's theory on social movements, in which society is seen as a set of subgroups competing for the definition of cultural dominance. Touraine (1978) suggests a precise way to analyze and interact with these movements that could be used to make sense of what is currently occurring in Quebec. It could, among other things, help to understand whether emerging movements in the health arena, such as the rebirth of midwifery (O'Neill 1988; Saillant and O'Neill 1987) or the growth of alternative medicine (Government of Quebec 1988; Rousseau et al. 1987), are the only real avenues to empower the population or are just a different way through which new dependencies and dominations are created. Touraine also helps us to understand how the movements that one day challenge the dominant order end up, if they succeed, as the dominant order themselves. The second framework is the feminist approach to power. It shows that the current form of power, with all the hardships and violence that it creates, is not "natural" or without alternatives, as Marilyn French (1986) suggests in her book *Beyond Power*. She argues convincingly that we should go beyond the patriarchal form of "power over" and move toward the feminist form of "power to," which would force us to completely rethink the ways to deal with participation and empowerment issues.

There is most likely a place for community participation and community empowerment ventures in health promotion work. And, if undertaken properly, they may make life much more palatable both for the population and for the professionals involved in these ventures. But, as has been shown by the Quebec experience, the road there is not straightforward or easy. Knowing this might make the journey more pleasant and more fruitful for those willing to undertake it.

Acknowledgements

The author thanks Dr. Ilona Kickbusch (WHO-EURO, Copenhagen), Dr. J. Warren Salmon, and two anonymous reviewers for comments and suggestions on earlier drafts of this article.

References

Belanger, JP. 1988. *L'histoire de la clinique des citoyens de St-Jacques: c'est aussi un peu celle des premiers CLSC a Montreal.* Unpublished paper. Federation des CLSC du Quebec, Montreal.

Belanger, PR, et al. 1987. *Flexibilite du travail et demande sociale dans les CLSC.* Universite du Quebec a Montreal, Departement de sociologic, Montreal.

Bolvin, R. 1988. *Histoire de Ia clinique des citoyens de St-Jacques (1968-1988): des comites de citoyens au CLSC du Plateau Mont-Royal.* Montreal: VLB Editeur.

Brassard, L. 1987. *La participation.* Commission d'enquete sur les services de sante et les Services sociaux (serie "Dossiers thematiques"), Quebec.

Brunet, J, et al. 1987. *Rapport du comite de reflexion et d'analyse sur les services dispenses par les CLSC.* Quebec: Ministere de la sante et des services sociaux du Quebec.

Collin, JP, and J Godbout. 1987. *Des experiences reussies de relation avec le milieu.* Montreal: Institut national de recherche scientifique/Urbanisation.

Divay, J, and J Godbout 1979. *La decentralisation en pratique, quelques experiences montrealaises 1970-77.* Institut national de recherche scientifique/Urbanisation, Montreal.

Eakin, J. 1984a. Survival of the fittest? The Democratization of Hospital Administration in Quebec. *International Journal of Health Services* 14: 397–412.

Eakin, J. 1984b. Hospital Power Structure and the Democratization of Hospital Administration in Quebec. *Social Science and Medicine* 18: 221–228.

Freire, P. 1968. *Pedagogy of the Oppressed.* New York: Seaburg Press.

French, M. 1986. *Beyond Power: On Women, Men and Morals.* London: Abacus.

Godbout, J. 1987. *La democratie des usagers.* Montreal: Boreal.

Godbout, J. 1983. *La participation contre la democratie.* Montreal: Editions St-Martin.

Godbout, J. 1981. Is Consumer Control Possible in Health Care Services? The Quebec Case. *International Journal of Health Services* 11: 151–167.

Godbout, J, and JP Collin. 1977. *Les organismes populaires en milieu urbain: contre-pouvoir ou nouvelles pratiques professionnelles?* Montreal: Institut national de recherche scientifique/ Urbanisation.

Godbout, J, and M Leduc. 1987. *Une vision de l'exterieur du reseau des Affaires sociales.* Montreal: Institut national de recherche scientifique/Urbanisation.

Godbout, J, and NV Martin. 1974. *Participation et innovation: l'implantation des Centres locaux de services communautaires et les organismes communautaires autonomes.* Montreal: Ecole Nationale d'Administration publique and Institut national de recherche scientifique/ Urbanisation.

Government of Quebec. 1989. *Orientations.* Quebec: Ministere de la sante et des services sociaux du Quebec.

Government of Quebec. 1988. *Rapport de la Commission d'enquete sur les services de sante et les services sociaux.* Quebec: Les publications du Quebec.

Hamel, P, and JF Leonard. 1981. *Les organismes populaires, l'Etat et la democratie.* Montreal: Nouvelle Optique.

Kickbusch, I. 1988. The Concept of Health Promotion. *Innovation* 1(2/3): 135–140.

Kickbusch, I. 1986. Health Promotion, a Global Perspective. *Canadian Journal of Public Health* 77: 321–327.

Lesemann, F. 1981. *Du pain et des services. La reforme de la sante et des services sociaux au Quebec.* Montreal: Editions St-Martin.

Lesemann, F. 1978a. De la communaute locale a la communaute multinationale: l'etat; des monopoles et ses politiques communautaires dans la gestion de la sante et des services sociaux. *International Review of Community Development* 39/40: 49–98.

Lesemann, F. 1978b. Decentralisation et services communautaires. *Service Social* 27(1): 24–45.

Lesemann, F. 1979. La prise en charge communautaire de la sante au Quebec. *Revue Internationale d'Action Communautaire* 49(1): 5–15.

McGraw, D. 1978. *Le developpement des groupes populaires a Montreal (1963-1973).* Montreal: Editions St-Martin.

O'Neill, M. 1988. Le combat des sages-femmes quebecoises. *L'Enfant* 4: 16–20.

O'Neill, M. 1986. *Innovative Practices in Governmentally Funded Community Health Agencies: The Case of Quebec's D.S.C.'s.* Quebec: Centre de Recherche sur les services communautaires de l'Universite Laval (Edition Speciale Series).

Renaud, M. 1984. The Adventures of a Narcissistic State: Quebec's Govemmental Interventions in Health. In V DeKervasdoue et al. eds. *The End of an Illusion.* Berkeley: University of California Press.

Renaud, M. 1978. Quebec New Middle Class in Search of Social Hegemony: Causes and Political Consequences. *International Review of Community Development* 39/40: 1–36.

Renaud, M. 1977. Reforme ou illusion? Une analyse des interventions de L'Etat quebecois dans le domaine de la sante. *Sociologie Societes* 9(1): 127–159.

Rousseau, N, et al. 1987. A propos de l'insertion des therapies douces dans les CLSC. *Sante et societe* 9(4): 11–16.

Saillant, F, and M O'Neill, eds. 1987. *Accoucher autrement: reperes historiques, sociaux et culturels sur la grossesse et l'accouchement an Quebec.* Montreal: Editions St-Martin.

Simard, J-J. 1979. *La longue marche des technocrates.* Montreal: Editions St-Martin.

Touraine, A. 1978. *La voix et le regard.* Paris: Seuil.

World Health Organization. 1986. Health and Welfare Canada, and Canadian Public Health Association. Ottawa Charter for Health Promotion. *Health Promotion* 1(4): iii–v.

World Health Organization. 1984. *Health Promotion. A Discussion Document on the Concept and Principles.* Copenhagen: WHO Regional Office for Europe. (Doc. No. ICP/HSR 602 (m01).)

Part VII
Society, Health and Health Care

Introduction

Although the costs, organization, and usefulness of health care systems are central issues in national or provincial government policies, methods or ways of viewing health care systems within their national and international context are still in their infancy. The common-sense view of health care systems as being explainable simply as reflections of the health needs of populations has to be rejected (however, its rejection as an overall explanation does not mean that "health needs" have no impact whatsoever). One alternative, that health care systems are what they are because of provider, largely medical, control the medical dominance thesis we noted regarding providers also contains some elements of truth but by itself is incomplete.

While views "internal" to health care such as those suggested above approach the issue "from below," using some form of pluralist interest group perspective, others tend to see health care as reflecting broader "welfare system" dynamics and demanding similar types of explanation. That is, medicine, or other health care actors, do not simply "pull themselves up by their own boot-straps." Many of these latter theories touch upon the crucial role of the state which, by its presence (or considered absence) shapes health and health care. Present views of the state, and of welfare system dynamics generally, vary along a continuum from "society oriented" perspectives such as those focusing on changes in the dynamics of capitalism and on class structure, those more oriented to the effects of institutions, particularly state-oriented theories in which the state is viewed as the originator of actions rather than as a reflection of class structure; and finally, to those theories at the level of interest-group analysis. Various theorists emphasize one or the other of these – viewing them as either-or perspectives. Others feel that each theory is better at analyzing a particular level of social interaction. The latter analysts might claim that, given the problems in integrating these approaches, each should be used for purposes for which it seems best suited. Ironically, one of the recent advocates of the latter approach is Alford who in his earlier work (Alford 1975) seemed to have the beginnings of a solution to the "levels" problem by analyzing major interest groups (corporate rationalizers, professional monopolists and community health advocates) as "embedded" within a particular social structure which favoured some rather than others of these.

Health care systems have historically appeared as one aspect of, though perhaps a very specific and, along with education, unique, part of welfare systems in general. The gamut of explanations for the nature of, and changes in, health care systems partially reflect theories of the welfare state. While some emphasize similarities among advanced capitalist countries in which a major explanation for welfare measures generally or health care in particular is simply increased national wealth, others, such as Esping-Andersen (1990), emphasize the differences. The most prominent and promising candidate for examining types of welfare systems

Typologies are an advance on those analyses of welfare states which simply used the degree of government expenditures on welfare items or some such measures to differentiate one system from another. The latter fail to differentiate types of expenditure – for example, fiscal expenditures to promote employment versus fiscal expenditures to pay the unemployed given a market-produced unemployment, as well as neglecting to take into account socio-historical variations in the production and nature of such systems.

The welfare state literature includes various "society-oriented" to "state-centric" explanations. However, within welfare systems, explanation of the variation from market-oriented to social-democratic almost always includes some version of class struggle or class coalitional perspective (that is, that welfare states arose in "stronger" or "weaker" forms as a result of conflict among classes or coalitions of classes). Class coalitions most often focus on the solidarity of the working class with farmers or with the petty bourgeoisie. The class argument is that the stronger, more organized, and more unified the working class and its partners and the weaker the bourgeoisie, the stronger the version of the welfare state. There are, however, alternatives to this view.[1] But health care, and education, do seem differentiated from other aspects of the welfare state such as social welfare measures and unemployment insurance, that is, anything touching on labour market dynamics. The latter are much more contentious and class contested than are the former. Certainly health and education are more universal in touching all segments of the population, as well as having powerful providers and clients supportive of continuing funding. Particular aspects of education and health seem a "necessary" part of producing and reproducing advanced capitalist economies, although the extent and form of this provision is important.

Canadians like to congratulate themselves on having a well-developed welfare state, but such congratulations become hollow when it is realized that Canada is only high on certain measures as compared with a 'worst case' scenario of the United States. Regarding health care, in which universal government health insurance seems almost to define the Canadian identity, Canada spends less per capita than does the United States, but more than most EC nations. Despite huge expenditures the United States case indicates that high costs and a market oriented system do not mean effective health care. In fact, much of the difference in per capita costs between Canada and the United States can be attributed to the enormous administrative overhead in the U.S. system with its complex array of insurance companies and funding agencies.

Welfare systems, of course, arose in a particular era and were once thought an immutable part of capitalism. Advanced capitalist countries had the best of all possible worlds through the productivity of a market system and the, often state-sponsored, safeguards of health and welfare systems for those harmed by the market system. Capitalism could be both productive and humane. The characteristic of advanced capitalism was the Keynesian welfare state (of various hues and types). How times have changed! Now, the globalization of capital, recession, and the rise of the New Right has altered the balance of class power. Business is supreme and has managed to make its own interests appear those of nations as a whole (the definition of ideological hegemony). With its increased mobility, and with the decline of alternative societal visions, corporations now can play off one government or region against another. National states have a decreased "relative autonomy." Globalization is now used to pressure states into accepting a market agenda, as well as to paralyze opposition by portraying such globalization as either inevitable or necessary. Globalization is thus an ideological construct, as well as containing varying degrees of real constraints on national governments.

Health care systems, however, while under attack for consuming state expenditures and for being ineffective and inefficient, are not necessarily under the same threat as are social welfare or measures to support the unemployed. While the latter are viewed as negatively influencing both corporate bottom lines and as influencing the power of labour *vis-a-vis* capital, education and health appear as necessary, if inefficient. And, although the ideology of business, large and small, is petty bourgeoisie and emphasizes market solutions to all difficulties, including recommodifying or privatizing health care, complete privatization is not necessarily in the interests of big capital – since government sponsored health insurance shifts the costs from corporate payrolls to the public in general. There are conflicts amongst class fractions, for example, between big and small business, private and public sector workers, and between general ideologies and specific interests. But, everywhere, states have an ally in big business in its attempts to make health care more efficient and less costly, although with varying degrees of market emphasis.

The somewhat overlapping concerns of governments and big business in rationalizing health care, in the United States said to be a corporate-government coalition, means, almost inevitably, that control by medicine over health care is under attack. Medicine now lacks its once solid congruence of interests and ideology with dominant classes. At the same time, there are pressures within all capitalist societies towards the commodification of everything, from drugs to health care services. These contradictions are embodied in the conflicting welter of proposals for "reform" of health care which range from "corporate rationalization," that is, leaner, more efficient health care, through an increased emphasis on competition or managed competition within health care systems, to calls for increased privatization. All of these pressures are taking place in an atmosphere in which health providers, and medicine in particular, have lost their unchallenged claim to expertise regarding "health system" matters. The latter are now the purview of health economists, health planners, and epidemiologists. Perhaps just as important the impact of health care on health status is being questioned as "health promotion" and "population health" experts focus on the social determinants of health.

We are thus faced with the question, after medical dominance, what? And, after health care what? As noted, many observers now argue that broader social factors are more determinant of health than are health care systems per se. In Chapter 30 Evans and Stoddard, for example, note that money poured into care may be being diverted from more productive (for health) usages. The congruence of such arguments with those who wish to reduce state expenditures in general surely is more than coincidental.

While a shrinking health care system may just off-load various tasks to unpaid female labour in the domestic sphere, there seems little argument against a better managed, more efficient, and more effective health care system. What seems clear from the latest evidence, however, is that "well-being" has to be viewed in a broad perspective and that such matters as a full-employment policy may do more than health care, or even than unemployment insurance, to ensure healthier Canadians.

In this Part

In "Limits to Health Insurance," Swartz first argues that hospital insurance and, later, insurance for physicians services historically arose either as a political preventive measure against socialism, or, in Canada, as a direct response to the threat of a rising working class or working class parties. However, the promise of medicare is based on the assumptions that medicare would improve access to health care for the poor and on the notion that health care leads to improved health status. Swartz contends that, whereas medicare led to an improved access for the poor relative to the well-off, this access still does not produce access according to need, since the needs of the poor are much greater than those of the rich. Second, Swartz argues that much of medical care is not of proven efficacy, that health and illness are primarily determined by social factors and that health care thus focuses on cure rather than prevention or care. Finally, Swartz shows how there has been an increasing tendency to restrict medicare and cut costs. The more individualizing and victim-blaming advocates of health promotion, for example, provide a partial ideological justification for cutting health care costs. Reducing costs has hurt health care workers and the system, but the system remains skewed towards cure rather than prevention or care.

In 1994 the Canadian Institute for Advanced Research produced a book, *Why are Some People Healthy and Others Not?* A much cited article by Evans and Stoddart, "Producing Health, Consuming Health Care," provided the framework for the volume. Evans and Stoddart's message is that we have, collectively, invested large sums of money in health care, yet the relationship between health care systems and the health status of populations is at best problematic – health care systems do not necessarily produce health. The authors thus feel that health care systems are either vastly over-rated as producers of health, or are part of the health problem rather than the solution. The CIAR approach is not as unproblematic as it might first appear. There have already been a number of critiques of the CIAR approach (see, for example, Coburn et al. 1996 & 1997). And, in another chapter in this part, Burke and Stevenson are somewhat cynical about whether monies cut from health care will actually be spent on more broad based social determinants of health.

The next chapter, by Olsen, places health care in a somewhat problematic relationship with the welfare system generally. While health care might be automatically identified with the welfare system and its fate, Olsen introduces caveats to such an identification. Olsen notes that the United States is usually characterized as a "liberal" society, emphasizing the free market, Sweden as more social democratic and preventive, and Canada somewhere in between. Olsen, however contends that this wholesale categorization does not conform to reality, as nations vary in the degree to which specific programs within the "welfare state mix" approximate the liberal or social democratic models. In fact, perhaps of most importance is not the total amount spent on welfare measures, but on what type of welfare measures is money spent – are these "preventive" (such as, in the labour market area the maintenance of full-employment) or more "reactive," i.e., the paying of unemployment insurance. Olsen notes that Canada is fairly liberal (i.e., private market oriented) regarding family policy but more social democratic regarding health care policy. Still, even in the latter case Canada shows a mixture of styles, being organizationally liberal; social democratic regarding health insurance coverage; and midway between these regarding the orientation (cure versus prevention) of the health care system. The point here is that health care and other forms of welfare may differ within the same country and that they have to be tied to an overall evaluation of welfare policies and cannot viewed in isolation.

In a comprehensive yet tightly argued chapter Burke and Stevenson tackle both the current state of health care and present health care issues. They argue that most health care issues are at present focused on costs. They point to various cost-containment strategies from user charges, through "public sector competition," to the new "health promotion." While these offer promise of restructuring health care in the name of effectiveness and efficiency, Burke and Stevenson caution that they are the product of contradictory impulses and have contradictory political implications. Although it is difficult to argue with such plans in the abstract, Burke and Stevenson show how such measures may produce creeping privatization and a therapeutic nihilism which aids those who want to cut rather than enhance or improve government services in general. They argue that the real issue is not costs but that of "protecting and extending the principles of medicare and the conditions enhancing health."

Finally, Coburn and Eakin examine the state of the sociology of health in Canada. The areas covered include the social determinants of health, health and illness behaviour, and the health care system. Apart from describing accomplishments, the authors note that a good deal of what is done in the sociology of health is descriptive rather than explanatory. They also point to a split between the more empirical and the more theoretical aspects of the discipline. A major practical issue is that there does not yet exist a community of scholars. There is a lack of communication amongst sociologists of health in Canada, although this may be more of a problem outside of Quebec, and amongst men rather than women researchers. A major challenge facing sociologists is linking descriptions and explanations of health and health care phenomena with the broader Canadian social structure and developing closer linkages amongst Canadian sociologists in the area just at a time when international linkages are expanding.

Note

1   While some form of class analysis is included in almost all views of the origins and functioning of welfare states, a variety of authors stress other factors. These factors range from the influence of war and depression to the contradictions faced by the state, the influence of the international sphere on national states, to welfare systems as simple reflections of increasing GNP and the like. The class perspective emphasized here is thus selective and necessarily highly over-simplified.

References

Alford, R. 1975. *Health Care Politics*. Chicago: University of Chicago Press.

Coburn, D, B Poland, and members of the Critical Social Science and Health Group. Comment on R Evans, M Barer and T Marmor eds. *Why are Some People Health and Others Not?* New York: Aldine de Gruyter, 1994. Forthcoming in the journal *Health and Canadian Society.*, 1997. For a shorter version see *Canadian Journal of Public Health* 1996; 87(5): 308–311.

Esping-Andersen, G. 1990. *The Three Worlds of Welfare Capitalism*. Princeton, NJ: Princeton University Press.

Evans, RG, ML Barer and TR Marmor. 1994. *Why are Some People Healthy and Others Not?* New York: Aldine de Gruyter.

29

The Limits of Health Insurance*

Donald Swartz

Health insurance is one of the core elements of the welfare state in Canada, accounting for almost 30 percent of provincial expenditures (Hall 1980). This essay is concerned with examining the limits of social reform through an analysis of the Canadian health insurance system established by the 1957 Hospital Insurance and Diagnostic Service Act and the Medicare Act of 1968. Enormously popular among Canadians generally as well as social reform advocates, the declared objective of these two acts was to promote the health of Canadians by making comprehensive health care available to all on the basis of need rather than the ability to pay.

Two issues have dominated recent discussions of the existing system of health insurance. One is its cost, with free enterprise ideologues in particular arguing that widespread abuse by patients has rendered the system unaffordable (Grubel 1982). The other is the related concern of the erosion of accessibility due to the appearance in several provinces of user fees and extra-billing by physicians. This concern prompted the short-lived 1979/80 Clark Federal Conservative government to ask Justice Emmett Hall to undertake a Health Services Review, and the subsequent Liberal government to pass the Canada Health Act in 1984 to buttress the original legislation.

While I will examine these concerns in some depth, they are not, in my view, the only problems, or even the most important ones to address. The recent controversy is exceedingly narrow in focus, and superficial in its analysis, confined as it is to recent developments in the operation/administration of the original programmes. Virtually without exception it is taken for granted, that health insurance as originally conceived and implemented was fundamentally sound. More specifically, two crucial assumptions have been integral to this controversy:

a. that health insurance results in ready access to health care for those needing it;
b. that the health care provided is effective in promoting health.

These two assumptions, of course, are the very foundation upon which health insurance as rational social policy rests. They are, in my view, dubious, and it is by understanding why, that we can begin to grasp the real limitations of health insurance. Consequently, I will attempt to develop a critique of the validity of these assumptions. This critique will form the basis for an analysis of the recent concerns regarding access to health care. To introduce this analysis, I will first discuss briefly the history of health insurance in Canada.

* Reprinted from 'The limits of health insurance'. D. Swartz. In *The Benevolent State* (eds.)
A. Moscovitch and J. Albert. Garamond Press, Toronto, 1987. Reprinted with permission from the publisher.

Health Insurance: Its Origins and Meaning

The architects of the modern welfare state tried to reform neither the worker nor the economic system in which he (sic) made his living. Rather they required him by law to provide for himself and his family so that he could better withstand the vagaries of capitalism. (Gilbert 1966)

Health insurance, both in its origins, and belated arrival in Canada was an outgrowth of working class struggles against the ravages of capitalist development. For workers, people who are dependent for their living on the sale of their ability to labour, disease and injury, no less than a shortage of buyers for labour generally, posed a threat to their survival. It was a threat that workers could not and did not ignore. One response was to create benevolent funds upon which its contributors could draw under specified conditions, such as sickness. The inadequacies of these undertakings, which were typically localized responses to acute problems – whether initiated by workers or their employers – tended to add credence to another response advocated by workers: the abolition of wage labour and its replacement with a socialist system.

It was with at least one eye clearly focused upon preserving capitalism in the face of a growing working-class socialist movement that health insurance, indeed the whole set of reforms – unemployment insurance, pensions, etc. – comprising the welfare state were conceived. As Kaiser Wilhelm I, the "grandfather" of the welfare state observed:

The cure for social ills must not be sought exclusively in the repression of social democratic excesses, but simultaneously in the positive advancement of the welfare of the working-class. (Health Insurance: Report ... 1943)

A similar logic was at work in Canada, even if it wasn't so bluntly expressed. It was in 1919, in the wake of the state's repressive response to the upsurge in working-class militancy symbolized by the Winnipeg General Strike that the Liberal Party, led by Mackenzie King, first promised a national health insurance programme.

King's rationale for such a programme is instructive:

Social insurance, which in reality is health insurance in one form or another, is a means employed in most industrial countries to bring about a wider measure of social justice, without, on the one hand disturbing the institution of private property and its advantage to the Community, or on the other, imperilling the thrift and industry of individuals. (King 1973: 222)

It follows that if some measure of social justice was to be established without disturbing the institution of private property and without altering capitalist relations of production and the exploitation of labour that these entail, then it was in the conditions of consumption that reform was to be sought. Within the framework of social insurance then, the issue became not the social conditions giving rise to disease but workers' inability to purchase health services once they were stricken by disease – one of the "vagaries of capitalism." The point to note here is not merely that health insurance was as much about insuring capitalism against socialism as it was about improving workers' health, but that health insurance need not, (and in Canada did not), even imply "nationalizing" the production and distribution of health services.

The long path of health insurance from a 1919 Liberal promise to the final establishment of a nationwide health insurance system in 1971 can be only briefly reviewed here (see Swartz 1977 for more details). The Liberal Party's promise notwithstanding, the first concrete step towards health insurance was not taken until 1948, and then only in Saskatchewan. "Ideas," as Leo Panitch has cogently put it, "if they are socially disembodied in the sense of not correlating with the nature and balance of class forces in a society, can themselves have little impact" (Panitch 1977). The working-class was not only relatively small in 1919, but in the following years the balance of class forces tilted sharply in capital's favour as well. It was not until the unprecedented tide of sustained working-class mobilization and politicization of the late 1930s and 1940s that health insurance returned to the national political agenda.

Despite its accomplishments, this surge of self-activity by Canadian working people failed to bring about a national health insurance scheme. Only in Saskatchewan, where the CCF won the 1944 election, were reforms implemented. Yet even these were limited as the Party abandoned its promise of a socialized health system (conceived as including salaried physicians) for a universal hospital insurance scheme (1948) and medical insurance for pensioners in 1950 (administered by a doctor-controlled commission).

In the 1950s, with the reformist unions and the CCF now the chief exponents, pressure for a national health insurance plan continued to grow; not least because in several provinces, notably Ontario, hospitals were incurring substantial deficits. Finally, in 1957, a rather reluctant Liberal government moved to introduce the Hospital Insurance and Diagnostic Services Act, in a futile bid to stave off electoral defeat. In essence, the legislation simply committed the federal government to sharing the cost with any province (health being a provincial responsibility under the BNA Act) of a public prepaid insurance plan covering the costs of acute hospital care for all residents.

With hospital insurance in place, attention then focused on medical insurance; in 1961 Saskatchewan's CCF government again took the first step. In the hope of preventing similar legislation elsewhere, the Canadian Medical Association convinced the Diefenbaker government to establish a Royal Commission on Health Services (known as the Hall Commission after its head Emmett Hall). Before the Commission's report was finished, Diefenbaker had been swept from office by the Pearson led Liberals, who were now quite committed to public medical insurance. Whether coincidence or not, the Hall Commission's report, when it finally appeared, firmly declared itself in favour of such legislation. The ensuing Medicare Act (Bill C227), introduced in July 1966, closely followed Hall's recommendations and the earlier hospital insurance legislation. Again the federal government offered to share the cost of any provincial medical insurance plan meeting federal criteria; namely that the plan be universal, cover all physicians services, be financially administered on a public, nonprofit basis and portable from province to province. In 1972, when Ontario joined, a national health insurance scheme covering hospital and medical care was finally in place.

What was in place, however, was anything but socialized medicine. The 1958 federal legislation merely socialized the cost of hospital care, not its provision. Undoubtedly, Liberal Health Minister Paul Martin had the CCF's precedent setting legislation clearly in mind when he explained the limits of the federal legislation: "In Canada, I do not think anyone seriously proposed that the title to our (sic) hospitals should be transferred from religious or private bodies to the state."[1] The Medicare Act based on the precedent established by the Saskatchewan CCF in 1961 was no different. The CCF's medical care plan did not entail a public medical system modelled along the lines of public education with locally elected boards overseeing salaried physicians as once envisioned. Rather it was based upon the existing model of medicine with individual self-employed physicians selling their services for a fee, while collectively enjoying a legal monopoly over the provision of medical care. Still, it did at least call for a significant public presence in the administration of the insurance scheme, including the set-ting of fees. Nonetheless, when Saskatchewan doctors undertook their infamous strike of 1961 over this latter issue, the CCF was prepared to compromise to achieve a settle-ment. The resultant system of health insurance became the model for all the provincial plans which followed the passage of Medicare, with the exception of Quebec. No moves were made to subject either the medical supply or the drug corporations so inti-mately involved in shaping hospitals and physicians health care practices to public con-trol.

Health insurance, then, was concerned only with personal health care – medical ser-vices to individuals as prescribed by physicians. It did *not* undertake to socialize the production and delivery of these services. Rather it merely socialized the costs of pro-viding them, under conditions, moreover, in which even indirect public control was minimal. In sum, what was in place was precisely what Dr. Norman Bethune had con-temptuously characterized 30 years earlier as a "bastard form of socialism produced by belated humanitarianism out of necessity" (Allan and Gordon 1971: 97).

This is not to deny that the realization of health insurance was a significant achieve-ment by working people with real benefits for them. Socializing the costs of health care at least weakened the link between individual consumption levels and ability to pay. Working people no longer had to live in fear of medical bills or experience the humilia-tion of seeking services for which they could not pay. Consequently, their access to health care was improved. Nor should the relative efficiency of public insurance be ignored. By eliminating profits, advertising, etc., inherent in private insurance, public insurance reduced administrative costs from an average of 27% to 5% of revenue, thus providing more medical services for a given level of expenditure (Swartz 1977: 329).

But, what health insurance failed to change, profoundly circumscribed its efficacy not only in regard to health but also in regard to the narrower objective of equalizing access to health care. In elaborating this argument, I will consider first the effect of health insurance on access to medical care and the relationship between medical care and health, and then explore the contradictions inherent in these reforms.

Access To Health Care

As our concern here is to understand as well as to describe the limited impact of health insurance on access to medical care, it is important to remind ourselves that health insurance itself only addresses the decision of individuals to seek care, and only elimi-nates the direct cost – the bill – from active consideration. Nothing else has changed. And it is with what has not changed that we must begin.

Medicine must be seen as part of the social structure. It is the product of any given social environment. Every social structure has an economic base, and in Canada this economic base is called capitalism, avowedly founded on individualism, competition and private profit ... Medicine is a typical, loosely organized, basically individualistic industry in this "catch as catch can" capitalist system operating as a monopoly on a private profit basis. (Allan and Gordon 1971: 93)

I will develop the broad ramifications of this quotation from Norman Bethune later. Here I want to concentrate only on certain aspects of it.

To begin with, the vast majority of doctors, as noted, are essentially self-employed business people, who live by selling medical services on a fee-for-service basis. They hold to the dominant values of Canadian society and its acquisitive ethos, probably more so than most in light of their middle class backgrounds, sex (male) and self-employed status. These factors – together with the fact, given the extreme inequality of wealth in Canadian society, that urban areas with a wealthy clientele provide the potential for a higher income – have profoundly shaped physicians' social availability. If medical insurance made it possible to earn a substantial income from treating other people in other places, it was hardly necessary to do so. As Roos et al. put it, in explaining why differences in the regional concentration of physicians were unchanged by health insurance: "while universal coverage gives the underdoctored areas more money to spend on health services, it provides the same benefit to overdoctored areas" (Roos et al. 1976).

The basic issue, of course, is not regional inequalities but class inequalities in medical care utilization. Health insurance ostensibly addressed under-utilization by lower income groups whose needs were not being met (consequently health costs ought to have risen). In fact, if consumption of medical services was based upon need we might expect that utilization rates would vary inversely with income. For there is no doubt that the incidence of morbidity and mortality is much greater among working-class people than the professional/managerial class and the employing class, given the relatively greater health risks associated with working-class life (Siemiatycki 1974). These risks also include the stress from job insecurity, financial worries and absence of control over one's work circumstances; popular mythology notwithstanding, the so-called "diseases of affluence" are much more common among working-class people than executives.

What is the record of health insurance in this regard? As already suggested, health insurance has resulted in increased access to medical care by lower income people. Professor Beck's (Beck 1973a, also see Manga 1978) analyses of the impact of medical insurance in Saskatchewan confirms this general point but the consumption of medical services by upper income groups is still much greater than by lower income groups. The former, moreover, seem to have shifted their consumption pattern, away from general practitioners and towards specialists, so much so that income class differences in the use of specialists seem to have widened.

These data are not surprising. In part they reflect the historic concentration of medical services in affluent communities. They also reflect the fact that out-of-pocket costs are not the only financial barrier to visiting the doctor. Since doctors' offices are overwhelmingly run on a 9 - 5 basis, working people must forego income from having to leave work; in addition the costs of transportation and child care also play a role. Further, differential utilization rates may be explained by differential knowledge of disease symptoms, and the formal value of different physicians' treatments. Finally, as Beck cautiously suggests, it appears that since seeing a specialist involves being referred by a general practitioner, such referrals seem to be based in part upon the social class of the patient.

Thus, at its best, health insurance did not substantially alter class-based inequalities in the use of medical care, and certainly did not lead to a consumption pattern which corresponds to the incidence of disease across income classes. I say "at its best" to indicate reference to the time when direct financial barriers to access were minimal. They were never wholly eliminated, particularly in provinces like Ontario where coverage was not automatic but required payment of a premium. In the last few years, direct financial barriers have made a comeback, in the form of user-charges levied by provinces, and extra-billing/opting out charges levied by physicians which will be addressed.

The Value of Medical Care

> Are you able to heal?
>
> When we come to you
> Our rags are torn off us
> And you listen all over our naked body
> As to the cause of our illness
> One glance at our rags would
> Tell you more. It is the same cause that wears out
> Our bodies and our clothes.
> The pain in our shoulder comes
> You say, from the damp, and this is also the
> reason for the stain on the wall of our flat
> So tell us:
> Where does the damp come from?

Bertolt Brecht, "A Worker's Speech to a Doctor"

If the image of workers clothed in rags in Brecht's poignant poem is somewhat dated, his searing criticism of the practice of medicine surely is not. Modern medicine is the product of a lengthy process of development, a development which was neither smooth nor continuous. What we understand as modern scientific medicine emerged to challenge existing theories about the same time as industrial capitalism arose. Now the dominant approach, its theory, no less than the organization of the medical industry, has been profoundly influenced by the society within which it developed.

Scientific medicine is rooted in the notion of the "specific etiology." That is, it views disease as an isolatable "thing" which attacks individuals so as to physically impair the normal functioning of the body (hence the term physician). The underlying theoretical assumption, patently derived from the system of factory-based production, and the machine age it gave rise to was, as Dr. Thomas McKeown has cogently expressed it, that:

A living organism could be regarded as a machine which might be taken apart and reassembled if its structure and function were fully understood. In medicine the same concept led further to the belief that an understanding of disease processes and of the body's response to them would make it possible to intervene therapeutically mainly by physical (surgical), chemical, or electrical methods. (McKeown 1971: 29)

One implication of this conception of the medical task is a dehumanized approach to treatment. Scientific medicine entails not just a tendency to segment people; it also entails establishing an authority relationship in which the patient is treated as a passive and ignorant object to be repaired, the means of which is the doctor's choice and the ensuing record the doctor's property. Its worth adding here that good patients are those who readily acquiesce to their "own objectification" while those (women in particular) who insist on control over their bodies are labelled "difficult." The parallels between the good patient and the good worker here are obvious, suggesting more than science is at work. A second implication is that progress, as with capitalist development generally, is seen to lie with the development of technology; ever more powerful means for intervention in the human body.

The triumph of scientific medicine over contending approaches signified that health primarily would be sought through efforts to cure individuals of disease, rather than by creating the socio-economic (and physical) conditions which could prevent disease and promote health. What has been its record? Here we must consider the impact of scientific medicine *per se* as well as the specifics of the medical system within which it is practiced.

The broad acceptance of the theory of scientific medicine was very much based upon the association of early scientific discoveries with declining mortality rates for infectious diseases – for which scientific medicine was credited. To a large extent this association, however, was spurious. In the last decade there have been several studies, primarily by British epidemiologists, of the decline in death rates due to infectious diseases (diptheria, scarlet fever) between 1850 and 1950 (Renaud 1975). These studies show that the decline in mortality rates was well under way before the discovery of the antibiotics used to treat them, and the trend of the decline was scarcely altered by that discovery. The major reasons for the decline were advances in sanitation and increased resistance to infection owing to improvements in nutrition; in short, prevention was more important than intervention. When one turns to chronic disease, one again finds that socioeconomic factors are much more important in explaining reductions in mortality and morbidity. Indeed, Dr. McKeown argues that the scientific medicine paradigm is simply inappropriate to the nature of most contemporary illness (McKeown 1979).[2]

The point of these considerations is not to suggest that antibiotics are useless, or that we would be worse off without physicians; indeed, even better off, as Ivan Illich (1975) would have us believe. It is rather that, following McKeown it is necessary to distinguish care from cure, or managing disease from advancing health (McKeown 1979, Ch. 10). Modern medicine can provide care (reassurance and comfort, ease from suffering) and indeed save limb and life particularly through treatment of acute emergency, given technical competence and proper service organization. Unfortunately, however, the specific features of the Canadian medical system are such as to overproduce costly curative services frequently at the expense of less costly services with more value to the patient.

This is due, above all, to the structure of the Canadian medical system which at every level is characterized by the competitive pursuit of private profit. In this regard, the organization of physicians has already been considered. Since they operate as individuals selling health care as a commodity on a fee-for-service basis, their economic interests lie with the provision of more, relatively costly curative services – and with the broadest purvue of their trade (Armstrong 1986). It's not surprising that virtually every study of medical practice shows that substantial proportions of physicians services – from drug prescriptions to major surgical procedures – were without medical justification, in the process exposing patients to the risks associated with powerful surgical and chemical interventions (see Swartz 1977 and Naylor 1981). It also appears that few medical procedures are supported by adequate evidence of their efficacy (Cochrane 1979, Naylor 1988 and Waitskin 1979).

Having said this, it is extremely important to stress that physicians themselves are but a part of the problem, and indeed are often unwitting victims of forces beyond their own control. They are not the only ones whose economic interests lie with the development of more costly medical services. The suppliers of medical equipment and drugs must also be considered. These profit-seeking corporations benefit directly from the development of high-powered capital-intensive medical care and the discovery of cures for new diseases which they promote by aggressive marketing as well as direct and sponsored research. Extensive time-consuming testing of medical procedures involving new products, let alone circumspect claims from the results obtained, are hardly in their interests. The individual physician – given the paradigm of modern medicine with its technological bias, given the prestige and income associated with being at the forefront of medical practice, and given patients who have heard about particular new drugs or procedures and threaten to go elsewhere for them – typically is in no position to judge or resist.

The same factors which foster the overproduction of curative services limit the quality of care that is provided. Here, only a few points can briefly be noted. The sale of medical care on a fee-for-service basis transforms care into a cost of doing business, both in physicians offices and in hospitals, exacerbating the de-humanizing tendency inherent in scientific medicine. Physicians have a real economic incentive to transform their office into medical assembly lines, and to acquiesce to (if not actively to promote) limits on the amount of patient contact time allowed nursing and other support staff in order to free hospital resources for hardware, and the personnel to operate it. The result is care which is less thorough, less reassuring, less prompt and more dangerous due to the greater fatigue and frustration levels of hospital staff than is desirable.

The fragmentation inherent in a system characterized by individualism and competition defies proper service delivery. On the one hand, the numerous cracks in the system repeatedly undermine the continuity of care. On the other, such organization ensures, however rational the behaviour of its constituent elements, the rationality of the whole will suffer. Emergency services are a case in point. It has long been clear that effective treatment of acute emergencies (accidents, heart attacks) entails the *prompt receipt* of basic medical attention by the victim. Consequently, the key to prompt delivery of emergency care lies with the development of a well-organized, accessible and skilled ambulance service. This is hardly what exists in most of Canada. The focus instead has been on the development of sophisticated emergency departments in hospitals, choc o'bloc with "state of the art" technology of dubious value. Ambulance services to get people to the hospital have been almost an afterthought, so much so that not infrequently, these are contracted out to small businessmen. These services are typically fragmented rather than operationally integrated. The accessibility of existing services, moreover, is compromised by the absence of a simple emergency call system (i.e., a 999 telephone number) in many major Canadian cities. Finally, for several reasons, not least the legal monopoly over medical practice enjoyed by physicians, ambulance attendants have been provided with limited training and equipment.

From Health Insurance to the Canada Health Act

Health Insurance, then, promised much more than it could deliver. Moreover, the design of provincial health insurance programmes was such that the benefits, however limited, could not be cheap. In 1956, prior to the enactment of hospital insurance, personal health care expenses accounted for 3.4 percent of GNP. By 1972, when medical insurance was in place across the country the figure was 6.4 percent, rising further to roughly 8 percent of GNP in the 1980s.[3] Several factors underlay this increase in health care expenditures, including the efforts of hospital workers to raise their wages above the poverty line, but the most important was physician behaviour.

Health insurance was little more than a blank cheque made out to physicians: the state guaranteed to foot the bill for any physician provided services (at rates formally set by physicians themselves) and for any associated hospital costs. Major increases in medical fee schedules in the 1960s (to win physicians' support for health insurance) led directly to major increases in physician incomes. In addition, physician incomes were further inflated not by an increase in numbers of patients but by a reorganization of their practices which "generated more income from a given number of initial patient contacts" (Evans 1975). This shift to more intensive medical practice entailing more tests, surgery, etc. increased the demand for hospital facilities, causing the whole health system to expand.

The growth in health care costs came as no surprise. In 1956, the Federal Director of Health Insurance Studies had warned that "if we have no control over the doctor under a pre-paid hospitalization plan, we have no control over unnecessary use of hospital beds." [4] However, in responding to rising costs, it was not physicians' control over hospital and medical services which the state challenged, but the limited benefits workers obtained from health insurance. As events would have it, this challenge was not long in coming.

The pursuit of social justice through welfare state reforms in capitalist societies has always been conditioned upon successful capital accumulation to provide a margin for the implied redistribution. Health Insurance, however, arrived just as advanced capitalist countries like Canada were passing from the postwar boom into a sustained period of economic crisis and stagnation, reminding (sometimes forgetful) governments that their primary concern is with the health of capital. Confronted by intense international competition, capital is restructuring/rationalizing its operations on a national and global scale, a central objective being to increase the productivity and/or decrease the cost of labour. In this context, the welfare state has posed a serious obstacle to capital's interests. As a source of employment, the welfare state kept the reserve army of labour, so useful in exerting downward pressure on wages, lower than it otherwise would have been. No less significantly welfare state programmes constituted a social wage, limiting the dependence of workers on their employer and the willingness of workers to acquiesce to capital's demands.

The counterattack on health insurance really began with the publication of *A New Perspective on the Health of Canadians* by the federal government, in 1974. Echoing with the criticisms of the limits of modern medicine and the need to address the socioeconomic causes of disease raised by the women's movement and leftwing critics of the welfare state, the document had a radical veneer to it. This, however, was deceptive, for at its heart was a fundamentally conservative message: "patient, heal thyself." The focus of the document (subsequently reinforced by federal programmes like *Participaction*) was on the importance of "lifestyle" – on the link between the incidence of disease and individual decisions to adopt "behaviour and living habits which adversely affect health" (Lalonde 1974). In seeking to establish that the sick were to a significant degree victims of their own malfeasance, the document tried to mobilize support for limiting public expenditures on health services, and intentionally or otherwise, opened the door to the introduction of user fees.

A number of substantive measures accompanied this ideological initiative. New restrictions were placed on the ability of foreign physicians to enter Canada. More importantly, the federal government undertook to stem the flow of federal funds into the health care system. In 1977, the open-ended shared cost programmes which allowed federal involvement in areas of provincial jurisdiction like health care, were replaced by the Established Programmes Financing and Fiscal Arrangements Act (EPF), which imposed ceilings on federal contributions to the financing of medicare and hospitalization.

Whatever the actual short run impact of EPF[5] on the level of federal expenditures, it provided a welcome justification for provincial governments, already engaged in a struggle to enhance their attractiveness to capital, to intensify their own efforts to reduce health expenditures. A number of provinces, notably British Columbia, Alberta and Nova Scotia imposed direct charges on some or all users of health services, in the name of discouraging abuse and/or providing an incentive for people to adopt a healthier lifestyle. Provinces exercised their "power of the purse" over hospitals to force reductions in the number of hospital beds per capita (Hall 1980). Hospitals were also urged, sometimes backed by budgetary incentives, to reduce staffing levels through contracting of work and adopting approaches to the organization of work based in "Scientific Management" (Armstrong 1986). Pay levels for the remaining staff were subject to strict control. Formal wage controls, indeed, were in place under the 1975-78 federal Anti-Inflation Programme (AIP). Restraint continued informally until 1982, when most provinces again imposed formal controls in the wake of federal legislation (C-124) suppressing collective bargaining rights for all workers under federal jurisdiction (Panitch and Swartz 1985).

The fee schedules according to which physicians were reimbursed for their services did not escape restraint either. Physicians claimed that being independent suppliers of services to the health system, their fees – like drug equipment prices – were their own business and not subject to negotiation with governments. Nonetheless, there have been regular provincial negotiations since medicare came into existence. Physicians' fees were subject to the 1975-78 AIP limits. Afterwards, provinces continued to insist on restraint, not least of all because of the difficulty of doing otherwise, in view of the hard line being taken against hospital workers. Given physicians' determination to assert their freedom to set their own fees, governments began to lower the percentage of the official fee schedule (originally 90 percent) that physicians received from public insurance. It was in this context that physicians began to resort to extra or balance billing, charging patients the difference between the fee schedule and what they actually received from the provincial plan, to obtain incomes commensurate with their own exalted sense of self-worth, while provincial governments (who more often than not shared the physicians' view) turned a blind eye.

Rationalizations of direct charges to patients as necessary to deter abuse of the system, or as appropriate, given the contribution of individual lifestyle decisions to disease rates, are ingenious to say the least, involving a resort to the crudest sort of "blame the victim" ideology. Yet how can people distinguish health from disease when physicians (together with the drug industry) have made virtually every physical and emotional sensation a symptom of something while keeping virtually all medical knowledge as their own exclusive preserve? As for individual culpability in the incidence of disease far more weight must be given to socio-economic conditions over which individuals have no control: working conditions, ecological conditions, family structures and income levels. "Exercise more" is rather pointless advice for a single parent, a manual worker or indeed, most urban wage and salary earners for whom work and getting there alone consume some ten hours daily.

The re-emergence of direct charges to patients has eroded significantly the benefit workers achieved from health insurance. The most thorough study of the effect of user fees was based on examination of the impact of a government imposed user fee initiated in the late 1960s by the Saskatchewan Liberals under Ross Thatcher. Overall, health services utilization fell 7 percent, virtually all of which was due to a utilization rate decline of 18 percent among the lowest income groups (Beck 1973b). Studies of extra-billing by physicians reveal similar effects. The patients of physicians who have opted-out of medicare are found to have incomes some 20 percent higher than those of non opted-out physicians. Furthermore, opted-out physicians report significantly greater proportions of patients who have delayed seeking treatment than their opted-in counterparts (Wolfson and Tuohy 1980).

Clearly, this exercise in cutting back the welfare state led to the stabilization of health care costs and at a level far below that in the U.S., much to the dismay of right-wing ideologues for whom the profligacy of government relative to the private sector is an article of faith. That the quality of care, as defined by McKeown, has suffered cannot be seriously disputed, with chronic and aged patients, in particular, frequently experiencing appalling levels of neglect. At the same time, by the late 1970s, direct financial charges to patients once again had become a common experience. With the gains achieved by health insurance so visably threatened, the labour movement could not but respond.

In 1979, the CLC initiated the formation of a broad coalition to counter this threat. As framed by the CLC, the coalition's response was unfortunately highly defensive in nature, essentially calling for the restoration of the status quo ante. Any improvements sought were limited in nature; the funding of more chronic beds, home care services and community health centres, was secondary to the central objective of "saving medicare." There was virtually no attempt by the left, inside or outside of the CLC's coalition, to advance a serious critique of the health care system which workers were being asked to finance. Those few voices trying to do so – the nursing associations which raised the need for putting physicians on salary stand out – were marginalized. Whatever the reasons for this reticence on the part of most of those socialists and feminists who had been developing such a critique over the past decade, it certainly suited the CLC who viewed the coalition primarily as a means of generating electoral support for the NDP.

The popular hostility to any weakening of health insurance so readily tapped by the CLC and the NDP undoubtedly helped prompt the newly elected Conservative government, in 1979, to once again ask Emmett Hall to undertake an inquiry, giving him a broad mandate to review health care policy generally. Hall, who was certainly not about to pick up where the CLC and NDP had left off, declined the opportunity, choosing instead essentially to confine his attention to the erosion of the principles underlying the original legislation. Condemning extra-billing as "a head tax on the sick" his principle recommendation was to call for it to be prohibited.

Despite having his report ready within a year, the Conservatives were not around to deal with this report of Hall's either, and it fell to the born-again Trudeau Liberal government to respond. They were in no hurry as the economic pressures which led them to undermine the very reforms they had authored, were, if anything, more intense. But finally, in a last ditch effort to stave off looming electoral defeat and reminiscent of the party's sudden embrace of hospital insurance in 1956, the Canada Health Act (1984) was introduced. This act attempts to eliminate user fees and extra billing by taxing the provinces in an amount roughly equal to the costs born by individuals in purchasing the services covered under the 1958 and 1966 legislation.

Any assessment of the Canada Health Act at this point could be premature, but it does appear that it will largely eliminate the various user fees which appeared since public health insurance was enacted. This is not to be confused with the restoration of the status quo ante. There can be no doubt that the health services now dispensed are less prompt and less humane than a decade ago, or that the working conditions, if not the wages, of hospital workers have sharply deteriorated. As well, all the other short-comings of the status quo remain. The structure of power within the health care sector remains intact at the expense of effective care. Private profit will still govern the production of medical services and the incidence of disease will not change as long as prevention remains subordinate to cure.

The limits of health insurance cannot be overcome by banning extra-billing, user-charges, or even insurance premiums. Naively or otherwise, many proponents of health insurance, and of the welfare state, believed that meaningful lasting reforms could be realized in the sphere of consumption while leaving capitalist relations of production intact: that what working people lost in the sphere of production (and in the case of women, in the sphere of reproduction – control over what is produced, how, and when); control of themselves – could be recaptured in the sphere of consumption. Shedding this illusion can at least help us to see what remains to be done.

Notes

1   Memo to the Deputy Minister of Health, 21 February 1952. P. Martin Papers, vol. 28.
2   Lest anyone attribute the centering of Canadian health care policy on such a limited model to ignorance, it is important to note that the observations of McKeown and others are neither novel or recent. During World War II, when the Liberal government believed it might be necessary to carry out its long-standing promise of health insurance to gain working class acquiescence to the continued rule of capital, the Federal Health Department was asked to develop a plan. In addition to an insurance fund to cover medical costs, the proposal developed called for an extensive public health programme. Testifying before a parliamentary committee in 1943 regarding this plan, Dr. Heagerty observed with respect to Britain that while their health insurance plan of 1911 had been a political success, it had done nothing to improve the health of British workers, something which rested on yet to be enacted public education and preventive measures.
3   The figures for 1956 and 1972 are from Swartz (1977) Table 2, page 331. For the 1980s, see The Globe and Mail, 17 September, 1986 (one of an excellent series of articles comparing the U.S. and Canadian health care systems, by Anne Silversides, September 15-17, 1986). See also Angus (1987).
4   Memo to the Deputy Minister of Health, 21 February 1952. *P. Martin Papers*, Public Archives of Canada, vol. 28.
5   For a discussion of this impact, see G. Weller and P. Manga (1983).

References

Allan, T, and S Gordon. 1971. *The Scalpel, The Sword: The Story of Dr. Norman Bethune.* Toronto: McClelland and Stewart.

Angus, D. 1987. Health Care Costs: A Review of Past Experience and Potential Impact of the Aging Phenomenon. In D Coburn et al. eds. *Health and Canadian Society: Sociological Perspectives,* 2nd ed., 57-72. Toronto: Fitzhenry and Whiteside.

Armstrong, P. 1986. Female Complaints: Women, Health and the State, unpublished manuscript. Vanier College, Montreal.

Beck, R. 1973a. Economic Class and Access to Physician Services Under Public Medical Care. *International Journal of Health Services* 3: 341–355.

Beck, R. 1973b. The Effects of Co-payment on the Poor. *Journal of Human Resources* 9: 129–142.

Cochrane, A. 1979. *Effectiveness and Efficiency: Random Reflections on Health Services.* London: Nuffield Provincial Hospitals Trust.

Evans, R. 1975. Beyond the Medical Market place. In S. Andrepoulos ed. *National Health Insurance: Can We Learn from Canada?.* Toronto: John Wiley.

Gilbert, B. 1966. *The Evolution of National Insurance in Great Britain: The Origins of the Welfare State.* London: Joseph.

Grubel, H. 1982. The Costs of Social Insurance. In G Larmer ed. *Probing Leviathan.* Vancouver: Fraser Institute.

Hall, EM. 1980. *Canada's National-Provincial Health Program for the 1980s.* Ottawa: Canada, Special Commission on Health Services.

Health Insurance: Report of the Advisory Committee on Health Insurance. 1943. Canada, Parliament, House of Commons, Special Committee on Social Security (Also known as the *Heagerty Report).*

King, WLM. 1973. *Industry and Humanity.* Toronto: University of Toronto Press.

Lalonde, M. 1974. *A New Perspective on the Health of Canadians: A Working Document.* Ottawa: Canada, Department of National Health and Welfare.

Manga, P. 1978. The Income Distribution Effects of Medical Insurance in Ontario. Toronto: Ontario Economic Council, Occasional Paper 6.

McKeown, T. 1971. A Historical Appraisal of the Medical Task. In G McLachlin and T McKeown eds. *Medical History and Medical Care.* London: Oxford University Press for Nuffield Provincial Hospitals Trust.

McKeown, T. 1979. *The Role of Medicine.* London: Oxford University Press for the Nuffield Provincial Hospitals Trust.

Naylor, CD. 1981. Medical Aggression. *The Canadian Forum* (April): 5-9.

Panitch, L. 1977. The Role and Nature of the Canadian State. In L Panitch ed. *The Canadian State: Polictical Economy and Political Power,* 311-344. Toronto: University of Toronto Press.

Panitch, L, and D Swartz. 1985. *From Consent to Coercion: The Assault on Trade Union Freedoms.* Toronto: Garamond.

Renaud, M. 1975. On the Structural Constraints to State Intervention in Health. *International Journal of Health Services,* 5(4): 559–72.

Roos, N, et al. 1976. The Impact of the Physician Surplus on the Distribution of Physicians Across Canada. *Canadian Public Policy 2.*

Siemiatycki, J. 1974. The Distribution of Disease. *Canadian Dimension* (June) 15-25.

Swartz, D. 1977. The Politics of Reform: Conflict and Accommodation in Canadian Health Policy. In L Panitch ed. *The Canadian State: Political Economy and Political Power.* Toronto: University of Toronto Press.

Waitzkin, H. 1979. A Marxist Interpretation of the Growth and Development of Coronary Care Technology. *American Journal of Public Health* 69: 1260–1268.

Weller, G, and P. Manga. 1983. The Development of Health Policy in Canada. In M Atkinson and M Chandler ed. *The Politics of Canadian Public Policy,* 223-246. Toronto: University of Toronto Press.

Wolfson, A, and C Tuohy. 1980. *Opting Out of Medicare.* Toronto: Ontario Economic Council.

30

Producing Health, Consuming Health Care*

Robert G. Evans and Gregory L. Stoddart

Introduction

People care about their health, for good reasons; and they try in a number of ways to maintain or improve it. Individually and in groups at various levels – families, associations, work groups, communities and nations – they engage in a wide range of activities which they believe will contribute to their health. People also attempt to avoid activities or circumstances which they see as potentially harmful. Implicit in such behaviour are theories, or more accurately loosely associated and often inconsistent collections of causal hypotheses, as to the determinants of health.

In particular, but only as a sub-set of these health-oriented activities, modern societies devote a very large proportion of their economic resources to the production and distribution of 'health care,' a particular collection of commodities which are perceived as bearing a special relationship to health. The 'health care industry' which assembles these resources and converts them into various health-related goods and services is one of the largest clusters of economic activity in all modern states (Schieber and Poullier 1989; OECD Secretariat 1989). Such massive efforts reflect a widespread belief that the availability and use of health care is central to the health of both individuals and populations.

This concentration of economic effort has meant that public or collective health policy has been predominantly health *care* policy. The provision of care not only absorbs the lion's share of the physical and intellectual resources which are specifically identified as health-related, it also occupies the centre of the stage when the rest of the community considers what to do about its health.

Health care, in turn, is overwhelmingly *reactive* in nature, responding to perceived departures from health, and identifying those departures in terms of clinical concepts and categories – diseases, professionally defined. The definition of health implicit in (most of) the behaviour of the health care system, the collection of people and institutions involved in the provision of care, is a negative concept, the absence of disease or injury. The system is in consequence often labelled, usually by its critics but not unjustly, as a "sickness care system."[1]

* Reprinted from *Social Science and Medicine,* Vol. 31, Robert G. Evans and Gregory Stoddard, 'Producing health, consuming health care,' pp. 1347–1363, 1990, with permission from Elsevier Science Ltd., Oxford, England.

Yet this definition of health was specifically rejected by the World Health Organization (WHO) more than 40 years ago. Its classic statement, "Health is a state of complete physical, mental, and social well-being, and not merely the absence of disease or injury" expressed a general perception that there is much more to health than simply a collection of negatives – a state of *not* suffering from any designated undesirable condition.

Such a comprehensive concept of health, however, risks becoming the proper objective for, and is certainly affected by, *all* human activity. There is no room for a separately identifiable realm of specifically health-oriented activity. The WHO definition is thus difficult to use as the basis for health policy, because implicitly it includes all policy as health policy. It has accordingly been honoured in repetition, but rarely in application.

Moreover, the WHO statement appears to offer only polar alternatives for the definition of health. Common usage, however, suggests a continuum of meanings. At one end of that continuum is well-being in the broadest sense, the all-encompassing definition of the WHO, almost a platonic ideal of "The Good." At the other end is the simple absence of negative biological circumstances – disease, disability or death.[2]

But the biological circumstances identified and classified by the health care disciplines as diseases are then experienced by individuals and their families or social groups as illnesses – distressing symptoms. The correspondence between medical disease and personal illness is by no means exact. Thus the patient's concept of health as absence of illness need not match the clinician's absence of disease. Further, the functional capacity of the individual will be influenced but not wholly determined by the perception of illness, and that capacity too will be an aspect, but not the totality, of well-being.

There are no sharply drawn boundaries between the various concepts of health in such a continuum; but that does not prevent us from recognizing their differences. Different concepts are neither right nor wrong, they simply have different purposes and fields of application. Whatever the level of *definition* of health being employed, however, it is important to distinguish this from the question of the *determinants* of (that definition of) health (Marmor 1989).

Here too there exists a broad range of candidates, from particular targeted health care services, through genetic endowments of individuals, environmental sanitation, adequacy and quality of nutrition and shelter, stress and the supportiveness of the social environment, to self-esteem and sense of personal adequacy or control. It appears, on the basis of both long-established wisdom and considerable more recent research, that the factors which affect health at all levels of definition include but go well beyond health care *per se* (Dutton 1986; Levine and Lilienfeld 1987; Marmot 1986; McKeown 1979; McKinlay et al. 1989; Townshend and Davidson 1982).

Attempts to advance our understanding of this broad range of determinants through research have, like the health care system itself, tended to focus their attention on the narrower concept of health – absence of disease or injury. This concept has the significant advantage that it can be represented through quantifiable and measurable phenomena – death or survival, the incidence or prevalence of particular morbid conditions. The influence of a wide range of determinants, in and beyond the health care system, has in fact been observed in these most basic – negative – measures.

Precision is gained at a cost. Narrow definitions leave out less specific dimensions of health which many people would judge to be important to their evaluation of their own circumstances, or those of their associates. On the other hand, it seems at least plausible that the broad range of determinants of health whose effects are reflected in the 'mere absence of disease or injury,' or simple survival, are also relevant to more comprehensive definitions of health.

The current resurgence of interest in the determinants of health, as well as in its broader conceptualization, represents a return to a very old historical tradition, as old as medicine itself. The dialogue between Asclepios, the god of medicine, and Hygieia, the goddess of health – the external intervention and the well-lived life – goes back to the beginning. Only in the twentieth century did the triumph of 'scientific' modes of inquiry in medicine (as in most walks of life) result in the eclipse of Hygieia. Knowledge has increasingly become defined in terms of that (and only that) which emerges from the application of reductionist methods of investigation, applied to the fullest extent possible in a 'Newtonian' frame of reference (Reiser 1978).

The health care system has then become the conventional vehicle for the translation of such knowledge into the improvement of health – more, and more powerful, interventions, guided by better and better science. Nor have its achievements been negligible in enhanced ability to prevent some diseases, cure others and alleviate the symptoms or slow the progress of many more. Thus by mid-century the providers of health care had gained an extraordinary institutional and even more an intellectual dominance, defining both what counted as health, and how it was to be pursued. The WHO was a voice in the wilderness.

But the intellectual currents have now begun to flow in the other direction. There has been a continuing unease about the exclusive authority of classically 'scientific,' positivist methods, both to define the knowable and to determine how it may come to be known (McCloskey 1989; Dreyfus and Dreyfus 1988), an unease which has drawn new strength from developments in sub-atomic physics and more recently in artificial intelligence and mathematics.[3] In addition, the application of those methods themselves to the exploration of the determinants of health is generating increasing evidence in the most restricted scientific sense of the powerful role of contributing factors outside the health care system (House et al. 1988; Dantzer and Kelley 1989; Bunker et al. 1989; Renaud 1987; Sapolsky 1990).

Simultaneously, the more rigorous evaluation of the health care system itself has demonstrated that its practices are much more loosely connected with scientific or any other form of knowledge, than the official rhetoric would suggest (Banta et al. 1981; Eisenberg 1986; Feeny et al. 1986; Lomas 1990). And finally, the very success of that system in occupying the centre of the intellectual and policy stage, and in drawing in resources, has been built upon an extraordinarily heightened set of social expectations as to its potential contributions. Some degree of disappointment and disillusion is an inevitable consequence, with corresponding concern about the justification for the scale of effort involved – the rhetoric of 'cost explosions.'

There is thus a growing gap between our understanding of the determinants of health, and the primary focus of health policy on the provision of health care. This increasing disjunction may be partly a consequence of the persistence, in the policy arena, of incomplete and obsolete models, or intellectual frames of reference, for conceptualizing the determinants of health. How a problem is framed will determine which kinds of evidence are given weight, and which are disregarded. Perfectly valid data – hard observations bearing directly on important questions – simply drop out of consideration, as if they did not exist, when the implicit model of entities and inter-relationships in people's minds provides no set of categories in which to put them.

There is, for example, considerable evidence linking mortality to the (non)availability of social support mechanisms, evidence of a strength which House et al. (1988) describes as now equivalent to that in the mid-1950s on the effects of tobacco smoking. Retirement, or the death of a spouse, are documented as important risk factors. Similarly some correlate or combination of social class, level of income or education, and position in a social hierarchy is clearly associated with mortality (Dutton 1986; Marmot 1986). None of this is denied, yet no account is taken of such relationships in the formulation of health (care) policy.

Such policy is, by contrast, acutely sensitive to even the possibility that some new drug, piece of equipment, or diagnostic or therapeutic manoeuvre may contribute to health. That someone's health may perhaps be at risk for lack of such intervention, is *prima facie* grounds for close policy attention, and at least a strong argument for provision. Meanwhile the egregious fact that people are suffering, and in some cases dying, as a consequence of processes not directly connected to health care, elicits neither rebuttal nor response.

The explanation cannot be that there is superior evidence for the effectiveness, still less the cost-effectiveness, of health care interventions. It is notorious that new interventions are introduced, and particularly disseminated, in the absence of such evidence (Banta et al. 1981; Eisenberg 1986; Feeny et al. 1986). If (some) clinicians find it plausible that a manoeuvre might be beneficial in particular circumstances, it is likely to be used. The growing concern for 'technological assessment' or careful evaluation *before* dissemination, is a response to this well-established pattern. But those who might wish to restrain application, fearing lack of effect or even harm, find themselves bearing the burden of rigorous proof. If the evidence is incomplete or ambiguous, the bias is toward intervention.

This heavy concentration of attention and effort on a sub-set of health-related activities, and *de facto* dismissal of others, may be a product of the conceptual framework within which we think about the determinants of health. A simple mechanical model captures the causal relationships from sickness, to care, to cure. The machine (us) is damaged or breaks, and the broken part is repaired (or perhaps replaced). Although this mental picture may be a gross oversimplification of reality, it is easy to hold in mind.

By contrast, it is not at all obvious how one should even think about the causal connections between 'stress' or 'low self-esteem,' and illness or death – much less what would be appropriate policy responses. The whole subject has a somewhat mysterious air, with overtones of the occult, in contrast to the (apparently) transparent and scientific process of health care.[4] There being no set of intellectual categories in which to assemble such data, they are ignored.

In this paper, therefore, we propose a somewhat more complex framework, which we believe is sufficiently comprehensive and flexible to represent a wider range of relationships among the determinants of health. The test of such a framework is its ability to provide meaningful categories in which to insert the various sorts of evidence which are now emerging as to the diverse determinants of health, as well as to permit a definition of health broad enough to encompass the dimensions which people – providers of care, policy makers and particularly ordinary individuals – feel to be important.

Our purpose is *not* to try to present a comprehensive, or even a sketchy, survey of the current evidence on the determinants of health. Even a taxonomy for that evidence, a suggested classification and enumeration of the main heads, would now be a major research task. Rather, we are trying to construct an analytic framework within which such evidence can be fitted, and which will highlight the ways in which different types of factors and forces can interact to bear on different conceptualizations of health. Our model or precedent is the federal government's White Paper, *A New Perspective on the Health of Canadians* (Department of National Health and Welfare 1974), which likewise presented very little of the actual evidence on the determinants of health, but offered a very powerful and compelling framework for assembling it.

We will also follow the *White Paper* in offering no more than the most cursory indication of what the implications of such evidence might be for health policy, public or private. Policy implications will arise from the actual evidence on the determinants of health, not from the framework *per se.* If the framework is useful it should facilitate the presentation of evidence in such a way as to make its implications more apparent. But there is of course much more to policy than evidence; 'the art of the possible' includes most importantly one's perceptions of who the key actors are and what their objectives might be. We will be addressing these issues in subsequent work, but not here.

Finally, we must emphasize that the entities which form the components of our framework are themselves categories, with a rich internal structure. Each box and label could be expanded to show its complex contents. One must therefore be very careful about, and usually avoid, treating such categories as if they could be adequately represented by some single homogeneous variable, much less subjected to mathematical or statistical manipulations like a variable. Single variables may capture some aspect of a particular category, but they are not the same as that category. Moreover, in specific contexts it may be the *interactions* between factors from different categories of determinants that are critical to the health of individuals and populations.

Disease and Health Care: A (Too) Simple Foundation

We build up our framework component by component, progressively adding complexity both in response to the demonstrable inadequacies of the preceding stage, and in rough correspondence to (our interpretation of) the historical evolution of the conceptual basis of health policy over the last half century. The first and simplest stage defines health as absence of disease or injury and takes as central the relation between health and health care. The former is represented in terms of the categories and capacities of the latter. The relationship can be represented in a simple feedback model, as presented in Figure 1, exactly analogous to a heating system governed by a thermostat.

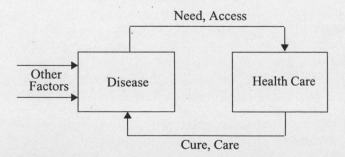

Figure 1

In this framework, people 'get sick' or 'get hurt' for a variety of unspecified reasons represented by the unlabelled arrows entering on the left hand side. They may then respond by presenting themselves to the health care system, where the resulting diseases and injuries are defined and interpreted as giving rise to 'needs' for particular forms of health care. This interpretive role is critical, because the definition of 'need' depends on the state of medical technology. Conditions for which (it is believed that) nothing can be done may be regrettable, and very distressing, but do not represent 'needs' for care. The patient feels the distress, but the health care system defines the need.

Potential 'needs' for health care are, however, prefiltered before they reach the care system, an important process which is reflected explicitly neither in Figure 1 nor in most of health policy.[5] Whether or not people respond to adverse circumstances by contacting the health care system, seeking 'patient' status, will depend on their perceptions of their own coping capacities, and their informal support systems, relative to their expectations of the formal system. These expectations and reactions are thus included among the "other factors" that determine the environment to which the health care system responds.

The health care system then combines the functions of thermostat and furnace, interpreting its environment, defining the appropriate response and responding. The level of response is determined by the "access" to care which a particular society has provided for its members. This access depends both on the combination of human and physical resources available – doctors, nurses, hospitals, diagnostic equipment, drugs, etc. – and also on the administrative and financial systems in place which determine whether particular individuals will receive the services of these resources, and under what conditions.[6]

The top arrow in Figure 1 thus reflects the positive response of the health care system to disease – the provision of care. But the form and scale of the response is influenced, through a sort of 'two-key' system, both by the professional definition of needs – what should be done to or for people in particular circumstances, suffering particular departures from health – and by the whole collection of institutions which in any particular society mobilize the resources to meet the needs, and ensure access to care.

Those organizing and financing institutions have very different structures from one society to another, but their tasks are essentially similar, as are the problems and conflicts they face. The actual technologies, and the institutional and professional roles, in health care also show a remarkable similarity across modern societies, suggesting that those societies share a common intellectual framework for thinking about the relationship between health and health care.

The feedback loop is completed by the lower arrow, reflecting the presumption that the provision of care reduces the level of disease, thereby improving health. The strength of this negative relationship represents the effectiveness of care. These effects include: the restoration and maintenance of health (providing 'cures'); preventing further deterioration; relieving symptoms, particularly pain; offering assistance in coping with the inevitable; and providing reassurance through authoritative interpretation.

The important role of health care in providing comfort to the afflicted fits somewhat ambiguously in this framework, since services which can clearly be identified as making people feel good, but having no present or future influence on their health status however defined, can readily be seen to include a very wide range of activities, most of which are not usually included as health care (Evans 1984).

The provision of services which *are* generally recognized as health care should obviously take place in a context that preserves a decent consideration for the comfort of those served. There is no excuse for the gratuitous infliction of discomfort, and patients should not be made any more miserable than they have to be. But for those services which represent *only* comfort, it is important to ask both: Why should they be professionalized, by assigning 'official' providers of health care a privileged right to serve? and Why should the clients of the health care system be awarded privileged access to such services? There are many people, not by any sensible definition ill, who might nevertheless have their lives considerably brightened by comforting services at collective expense.[7]

In this conceptual framework, the level of health of a population is the negative or inverse of the burden of disease. This burden of disease in Figure 1 is analogous to the temperature of the air in a house in a model of a heating system. The health care system diagnoses that disease and responds with treatment; the thermostat detects a fall in air temperature and turns on the furnace. The result is a reduction in disease/increase in room temperature. The external factors – pathogens, accidents – which 'cause' disease are analogous to the temperature outside the house; a very cold night is equivalent to an epidemic. But the consequences of such external events are moderated by the response of the heating/health care systems.[8]

The thermostat can, of course, be set at different target temperatures, and the control system of the furnace can be more or less sophisticated depending on the extent and duration of permissible departures from the target temperature. Similarly access to care can be provided at different levels, to meet different degrees of 'need' and with tighter or looser tolerances for over- or under-servicing.

The systems do differ, insofar as the house temperature can be increased more or less indefinitely by putting more fuel through the furnace (or adding more furnaces). In principle the expansion of the health care system is bounded by the burden of remediable disease. When each individual has received all the health care which might conceivably be of benefit, then all needs have been met, and 'health' in the narrow sense of absence of (remediable) disease or injury has been attained. Health is bounded from above; air temperature is not. The occupants of the house do not of course want an ever-increasing temperature, whether or not it is possible. Too much is as bad as too little. Yet no obvious meaning attaches to the words 'too healthy.' More is always better, a closer approximation to the ideal of perfect, or at least best attainable, health.[9]

The differences are more apparent than real, however, since in practice the professionally defined needs for care are themselves adjusted according to the capacity of the health care system, and the pressures on it. The objective of health, René Dubos' mirage (1959), ever recedes as more resources are devoted to health care. As old forms of disease or injury threaten to disappear, new ones are defined. There are always 'unmet needs.'[10]

Furthermore, obvious meanings *do* attach to the words 'too much health care,' on at least three levels. First, too much care may result in harm to health in the narrow sense – iatrogenic disease – because potent interventions are always potentially harmful. But even if care contributes to health in the narrow sense – keeping the patient alive, for example – it may still be 'too much.' Painful interventions which prolong not life but dying are generally recognized as harmful to those who are forced to undergo them. More generally, the side effects of 'successful' therapy may in some cases be, for the patient, worse than the disease.

Second, even if the care *is* beneficial in terms of both health and well-being of the recipient, it may still represent 'too much' if the benefits are very small relative to the costs, the other opportunities foregone by the patient or others. If health is an important, but not the only, goal in life, it follows that there can be 'too much' even of effective health care (Woodward and Stoddart 1990).

And finally, an important component of health is the individual's *perception* of his or her own state. An exaggerated sense of fragility is not health but hypochondria. Too much emphasis on the number of things than can go wrong, even presented under the banner of 'health promotion,' can lead to excessive anxiety and a sense of dependence on health care – from annual check-up to continuous monitoring. This is very advantageous economically for the 'health care industry,'[10] and *perhaps* may contribute in some degree to a reduction in disease, but does not correspond to any more general concept of health (Illich 1975; Haynes et al. 1979; Toronto Working Group on Cholesterol Policy 1989).

Unlike a heating system, however, health care systems do not settle down to a stable equilibrium of temperature maintenance and fuel use. The combination of the 'ethical' claim that all needs must be met, and the empirical regularity that, as one need is met, another is discovered, apparently *ad infinitum*, leads to a progressive pressure for expansion in the health care systems of all developed societies. It is as if no temperature level were ever high enough, more and more fuel must always be added to the furnace(s).[11]

Concerns About Cost, Effectiveness and the Marginal Contribution of Health Care

The result is shown in Figure 2, in which the top arrow, access to health care, has been dramatically expanded to reflect a "health care cost crisis."[12] A comparison of international experience demonstrates that the perception of such a crisis is virtually universal, at least in Western Europe and North America. It is interesting to note, however, that the countries which perceive such a crisis actually spend widely differing amounts on health care, either absolutely or as a proportion of their national incomes (Schieber and Poullier 1989; OECD Secretariat 1989).

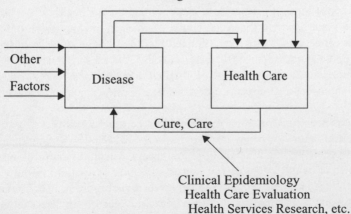

Figure 2

Nevertheless, whether they spend a little or a lot, in all such countries there is an expressed tension between ever-increasing needs, and increasingly restrained resources. Even in the United States, one finds providers of care claiming that they face more and more serious restrictions on the resources available to them (Reinhardt 1987), despite the egregious observation that the resources devoted to health care in that country are greater, and growing faster, than anywhere else in the world.

We interpret this observation as implying that perceptions of 'crises' in health care finance arise from conflicts over the level of expenditure on health care (and thus by definition also over the levels of incomes earned from its provision). Such conflicts develop whenever paying agencies attempt to limit the rate of increase of resources flowing to the health care system. They are independent of the actual level of provision of health care to a population, or of its expense, let alone of the level of health, however defined, of that population. They also appear to develop independently of the particular form taken by the payment system in a country.

Nor, as the American example shows, does it matter whether the attempts to limit cost escalation are successful. Perceptions of crisis emerge from the attempt, not the result. Accordingly one should not expect to find any connection between the health of a population, and allegations of 'crisis' in the funding of its health care – or at least not among the countries of Western Europe and North America.

On the lower arrow, and intimately connected with the perceptions of 'cost crisis,' we find increasing concern for the effectiveness with which health care services respond to needs. The development and rapid expansion of clinical epidemiology, for example, reflects a concern that the scientific basis underlying much of health care is weak to non-existent. More generally, the growing field of health services research has accumulated extensive evidence inconsistent with the assumption that the provision of health care is connected in any systematic or scientifically grounded way with patient 'needs' or demonstrable outcomes (Banta et al. 1981; Eisenberg 1986; Feeny et al. 1986; Lomas 1990; Ham 1988; Andersen and Mooney 1990). Accordingly, the greatly increased flow of resources into health care is perceived as not having a commensurate, or in some cases any, impact on health status. Nor is there any demonstrable connection between international variations in health status, and variations in health spending (Culyer 1988).

If there were a commensurate impact, then presumably efforts to control costs would be less intense (and perhaps more focussed on relative incomes). As Culyer (1989) emphasizes, " ... cost containment in itself is not a sensible objective." The rapid increase in spending on computers has not generated calls for cost caps. A care system which could 'cure' upper respiratory infections, colds and flu, for example, would have an enormous positive impact on both economic productivity and human happiness, and would be well worth considerable extra expense. So would a 'cure' for arthritis. Offered such benefits, we suspect that few societies would begrudge the extra resources needed to produce them; indeed these resources would to a considerable extent pay for themselves in higher productivity.[13]

The combination of virtually universal concern over cost escalation, among payers for care, with steadily increasing evidence from the international research community that a significant proportion of health care activity is ineffective, inefficient, inexplicable, or simply unevaluated, constitutes an implicit judgement that the 'expanding needs' to which expanding health care systems respond are either not of high enough priority to justify the expense, or simply not being met at all.

It is not that no 'needs' remain, that the populations of modern societies have reached a state of optimum health – that is obviously not the case. Nor is it claimed that medicine has had no effect on health – that too is clearly false. The concern is rather that the remaining shortfalls, the continuing burden of illness, disability, distress, and premature death, are less and less sensitive to further extensions in health care – we are reaching the limits of medicine. At the same time the evidence is growing in both quantity and quality that this burden may be quite sensitive to interventions and structural changes outside the health care system.

These concerns and this evidence are by no means new – they go back at least two decades. Yet most of the public and political debate over health policy continues to be carried on in the rhetoric of 'unmet needs' for health care. There is a curious disjunction in both the popular and the professional 'conventional wisdom,' in that widespread concerns about the effectiveness of the health care system, and acceptance of the significance of factors outside that system, co-exist quite comfortably with continuing worries about shortages and 'underfunding.'

The current 'shortage of nurses' in Canada and indeed in much of the industrialized world, provides a good example. Nursing 'shortages' have been cause for periodic concern in Canada for more than a quarter century. Yet throughout that period, there has been virtually uniform agreement among informed observers that utilization of inpatient beds in Canada is substantially higher than 'needed,' and efforts have been ongoing to reduce such use. Taking both positions together, this suggests that there is a 'shortage' of nurses to provide 'unnecessary' care!

The significant point is not the validity or otherwise of either perception, but the fact that they do not confront one another. In terms of the thermostatic model, public discussion still consists almost entirely of claims by providers (with considerable public support) that the room temperature is not high enough, or is in danger of falling, or that a severe cold spell is on the way ... but in any case it is imperative that we install more and bigger furnaces immediately, and buy more fuel. Meanwhile payers – in Canada provincial governments – wring their hands over the size of the fuel bill and seek, with very little external support, ways of making the existing heating system more efficient.

A more efficient heating system is indeed a laudable objective, although it is understandable that the providers of health care, as the owners of the fuel supply companies, may give it a lower priority than do those who are responsible for paying the bills. But there is a much more fundamental question. The people who live in the building are primarily concerned about the level and stability of the room temperature, not the heating system per se. They become drawn into an exclusive focus on the heating system, if they perceive that this is the only way to control the room temperature. But as was (re)learned in North America after the oil shock of 1974, this is not so.

Similarly the health care system is not, for the general population, an end in itself. It is a means to an end, maintenance and improvement of health (Evans 1984). And while few have followed Illich (1975) in arguing that the health care system has no positive – and indeed net negative – effects on the health of those it serves, nevertheless as noted above, the evidence for the importance of health-enhancing factors outside the health care system is growing rapidly in both quantity and quality.

But the intellectual framework reflected in Figures 1 and 2 pushes these other, and perhaps more powerful, determinants of health off the stage and into the amorphous cluster of arrows entering from the left hand side of the diagram. By implication they are unpredictable, or at least uncontrollable, so there is no point in spending a great deal of intellectual energy or policy attention on identifying or trying to influence them.

For most of the twentieth century, rapid advances in the scientific, organizational and financial bases of health care have encouraged, and been encouraged by, this dismissal. We have given almost all our attention to the heating contractor and the fuel salesman, and have had no time or interest to consider how the house is insulated.

By the early 1970s, however, all developed nations had in place extensive and expensive systems of health care, underpinned by collective funding mechanisms, which provided access for all (or in the United States, most) of their citizens. Yet the resulting health gains seemed more modest than some had anticipated, while the 'unmet needs,' or at least the pressures for system expansion, refused to diminish.

Simple trend projections indicated that, within a relatively short span of decades, the health care systems of modern societies would take over their entire economies. As public concerns shifted from expansion to evaluation and control, the alternative tradition began to reassert itself. In such an environment, a growing interest in alternative, perhaps more effective, hopefully less expensive, ways of promoting health was a natural response.

The resurgence of interest in ways of enhancing the health of populations, other than by further expansion of health care systems, was thus rooted both in the observation of the stubborn persistence of ill-health, and in the concern over growing costs. The latter development has been particularly important in recruiting new constituencies' for the broader view of the determinants of health. Financial bureaucrats, both public and private, have become (often rather suspect) allies of more traditional advocates (Evans 1982; McKinlay 1979).

The Health Field Concept: A New Perspective

The broader view was given particularly compact and articulate expression in the famous Canadian *White Paper* referred to above which came out, presumably by complete coincidence, in the same year as the first 'energy crisis.' Its 'Four Field' framework for categorizing the determinants of health was broad enough to express a number of the concerns of those trying to shift the focus of health policy from an exclusive concern with health care. In Figure 3 this framework is superimposed upon the earlier 'thermostat/furnace' model of health care and health.

The *New Perspective* proposed that the determinants of health status could be categorized under the headings of Lifestyles, Environment, Human Biology and Health Care Organization. As can be seen in Figure 3, the first three of these categories provided specific identification for some of the 'other and unspecified' factors entering on the left hand side of Figures 1 and 2. By labelling and categorizing these factors, the *White Paper* drew attention to them and suggested the possibility that their control might contribute more to the improvement of human health than further expansions in the health care system. At the very least, the health field framework emphasized the centrality of the objective of health, and the fact that health care was only one among several forms of public policy which might lead towards this objective.

The *White Paper* was received very positively; no one seriously challenged its basic message that who we are, how we live and where we live are powerful influences on our health status. But the appropriate policy response was less clear, because the document could be read in several different ways. At one end of the ideological spectrum, it was seen as a call for a much more interventionist set of social policies, going well beyond the public provision of health care *per se* in the effort to improve the health of the Canadian population and relieve the burden of morbidity and mortality.

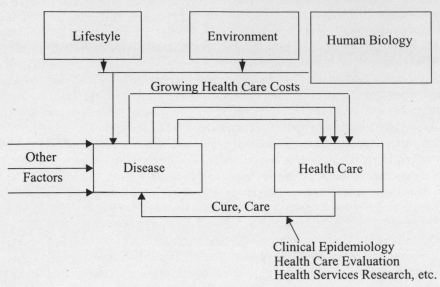

Figure 3

At the other end, however, the assumption that lifestyles and to a lesser extent living environments are chosen by the persons concerned could be combined with the *White Paper* framework to argue that people are largely responsible for their own health status – have in fact chosen it. If so, then the justification for collective intervention, even in the provision of health care, becomes less clear.[14] This appears to have been far from the intention of the authors of the paper, but the framework in Figure 3 lends itself to 'victim-blaming' as well as to arguments for more comprehensive social reform (Evans 1982).

Whatever the original intent, however, the White Paper led into a period of detailed analysis of *individual risk* factors, i.e., both individual hazards and individual persons, as contributors to 'disease' in the traditional sense.[15] The potential significance of processes operating on health at the level of groups and populations was obscured, if not lost (Buck 1988). Smoking, for example, was viewed as an individual act predisposing to specific diseases. Specific atmospheric pollution contributes to lung disease. Genetic defects result in well-defined genetic diseases. The central thermostatic relationship is preserved, with health as absence of disease, and health care as response to disease in order to provide 'cures' or relieve symptoms, individual by individual.

To illustrate the distinction, one can formulate health policy to address cancer across a spectrum from the individual to the collective. One can increase facilities for the treatment of cancer patients, a wholly individualized, reactive response. One can increase research on cancer treatment, an activity with a 'collective' focus only insofar as the specific recipients of new treatments may not be known in advance. One can launch anti-smoking campaigns, trying to induce certain individuals whose *characteristics* are known – they smoke – to change their behaviour voluntarily. These campaigns may in turn be wholly individualized – paying or otherwise encouraging physicians to provide counselling, for example – or advertising campaigns aimed at the general population. Or one can try to limit involuntary exposures by regulating the presence of carcinogens in the environment, establishing mandatory smoke-free zones (hospitals, restaurants, aircraft, workplaces ...) or regulating industrial processes.

The focus on individual risk factors and specific diseases has tended to lead, not away from but back to the health care system itself. Interventions, particularly those addressing personal lifestyles, are offered in the form of 'provider counselling' for smoking cessation, seat-belt use or dietary modification (American Council of Life Insurance and Health Insurance Association of America (1988); Lewis 1988). These in turn are subsumed under a more general and rapidly growing set of interventions attempting to modify risk factors through transactions between clinicians and individual patients.

The 'product line' of the health care system is thus extended to deal with a more broadly defined set of 'diseases' – unhealthy behaviours. The boundary becomes blurred between, e.g., heart disease as manifest in symptoms, or in elevated serum cholesterol measurements, or in excessive consumption of fats. All are 'diseases' and represent a 'need' for health care intervention. Through this process of disease redefinition, the conventional health care system has been able to justify extending outreach and screening programmes, and placing increased numbers of people on continuing regimens of drug therapy and regular monitoring.

The emphasis on individual risk factors and particular diseases has thus served to maintain and protect existing institutions and ways of thinking about health. The 'broader determinants of health' were matters for the attention of individuals, perhaps in consultation with their personal physicians, supported by poster campaigns from the local public health unit. The behaviour of large and powerful organizations, or the effects of economic and social policies, public and private, were not brought under scrutiny. This interpretation of the *White Paper* thus not only fitted in with the increasingly conservative zeitgeist of the late 1970s and early 1980s, but protected and even enhanced the economic position of providers of care, while restricting sharply the range of determinants, and associated policies, considered. Established economic interests were not threatened – with the limited exception of the tobacco industry.

This tendency was reinforced by attempts to estimate the relative contribution of the four different fields or sets of factors to ill-health. As Gunning-Schepers and Hagen (1987) have pointed out, a simple partitioning of sources of mortality, morbidity or care utilization into four discrete 'boxes' is fundamentally misguided. Nevertheless, 'expert opinion' suggested that, of the three fields external to the health care system, 'Lifestyles' had the largest and most unambiguously measurable effect on health. 'Lifestyles' – diet, exercise, substance use – were also the factors most readily portrayed as under the control of the individual. They thus lent themselves to the politically innocuous, inexpensive, highly visible and relatively ineffective intervention of health education campaigns – carried on through the public health arm of the health care system.

Smoking cessation provides a partial counter-example, which illustrates the difficulty of breaking out of the disease-health care intellectual framework. Tobacco is not only toxic, but addictive, and addiction most commonly commences in childhood. Consequently the presumption that users rationally and voluntarily 'choose' smoking as a 'lifestyle' is particularly inappropriate. Furthermore, the observation that smoking behaviour is very sharply graded by socioeconomic class undercuts the argument that it represents an individual choice, and indicates instead a powerful form of social conditioning.[16]

Partly for these reasons, Canadian health policy has gone beyond educational campaigns to spread information about the ill effects of smoking and includes limitations on the advertising and marketing of tobacco products. The political resistance to these limitations has been much more intense, suggesting prima facie that the marketers of such products fear that they might be effective. But the broader question, of the social determinants of tobacco use, is still left open.[17]

The intellectual framework of the *White Paper*, at least as it has been applied and as represented in Figure 3, has thus supplemented the thermostatic model of health as absence of disease, and health care as response, but has failed to move beyond the core relationship. Since as noted above, 'disease' is defined through the interpretation of individual experience by the providers of health care, it is perhaps not surprising that the Health Care Organization field tended to take over large parts of the other three, when they were presented as determinants of disease.

Extending the Framework: Health and its Biological and Behavioural Determinants

Yet in the years since the publication of the *White Paper*, a great deal of evidence has accumulated, from many different sources, which is difficult or impossible to represent within this framework. The very broad set of relationships encompassed under the label of 'stress,' for example, and factors protective against 'stress' (Dantzer and Kelley 1989; Sapolsky 1990), have directed attention to the importance of social relationships, or their absence, as correlates of disease and mortality. Feelings of self-esteem and self-worth, or hierarchical position and control, or conversely powerlessness, similarly appear to have health implications quite independent of the conventional risk factors (Dutton 1986; Marmot 1986; House et al. 1988; Sapolsky 1990).

These sorts of factors suggest explanations for the universal finding, across all nations, that mortality and (when measurable) morbidity follow a gradient across socioeconomic classes. Lower income and/or lower social status are associated with poorer health.[18]

This relationship is not, however, an indication of deprivation at the lower end of the scale, although it is frequently misinterpreted in that way. In the first place, the socioeconomic gradient in health status has been relatively stable over time (Townshend and Davidson 1982), although average income levels have risen markedly in all developed societies. The proportion of persons who are deprived of the necessities of life in a biological sense has clearly declined. But even more important, the relationship is a *gradient*, not a step function. Top people appear to be healthier than those on the second rung, even though the latter are above the population averages for income, status or whatever the critical factors are (Marmot 1986).

It follows that the variously interpreted determinants of health which lie outside the health care system are not just a problem of some poor, deprived minority whose situation can be deplored and ignored by the rest of us. *De te fabula narratur,* we are all (or most of us) affected. And that in turn implies that the effects of such factors may be quantitatively very significant for the overall health status of modern populations. The issues involved are not trivial, second-, or third-order effects.

Moreover, the fact that gradients in mortality and morbidity across socioeconomic classes appear to be relatively stable over long periods of time, even though the principal causes of death have changed considerably, implies that the underlying factors influence susceptibility to a whole range of diseases. They are general rather than specific risk factors. Whatever is going round, people in lower social positions tend to get more of it, and to die earlier – even after adjustment for the effects of specific individual or environmental hazards (Marmot 1984).

This suggests that an understanding of the relationship between social position, or 'stress,' and health, will require investigation at a more general level than the aetiology of specific diseases. It also raises the possiblity that disease-specific policy responses – through health care or otherwise – may not reach deeply enough to have much effect. Even if one 'disease' is' 'cured,' another will take its place.

An attempt to provide a further extension to our intellectual framework, to encompass these new forms of evidence, is laid out in Figure 4.

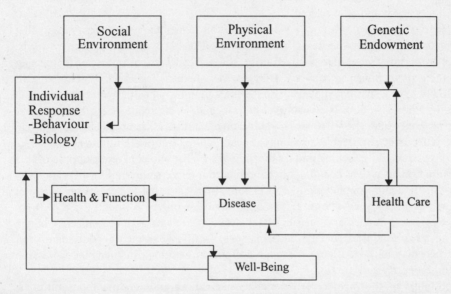

Figure 4

In Figure 4, two major structural changes are introduced. First, a distinction is drawn between disease, as recognized and responded to by the health care system, and health and function as experienced by the individual person. Such a distinction permits us to consider, within this framework, the common observation that illness experienced by individuals (and their families or other relevant social groups) does not necessarily correspond to disease as understood by the providers of care. Persons with 'the same' disease, from the point of view of the health care system – similar biological parameters, prognoses and implications for treatment – may experience very different levels of symptoms and distress, and very different effects on their ability to function in their various social roles. Arthritis, and musculo-skeletal problems more generally, are leading examples of conditions for which the patient's sense of 'illness' bears no very close relationship to the clinician's interpretation of 'disease.'

This is not to say that one perspective is 'right' and the other 'wrong'; the two modes of interpretation simply have different purposes. The clinician's concept of disease is intended to guide the appropriate application of available medical knowledge and technology, so is formulated in terms of that knowledge and technology. The patient, on the other hand, is ultimately concerned with the impact of the illness on his/her own life. The clinician's disease may be an important part of that impact but is by no means the only relevant factor.

Moreover, from the point of view of the individual's well-being and social performance – including economic productivity – it is the individual's sense of health and functional capacity which is determinative – as shown in Figure 4. The 'diseases' diagnosed and treated by the health care system are important only insofar as they affect that sense of health and capacity – which of course they do. But health, even as interpreted by the individual, is not the only thing in life which matters. Figure 4 introduces the category of 'well-being,' the sense of life satisfaction of the individual, which is or should be (we postulate) the ultimate objective of health policy. The ultimate test of such policy is whether or not it adds to the well-being of the population served.

Going back to the original WHO definition of health, we are relabelling that broad definition as well-being. Our concept of health is defined, in narrow terms but from the patient's perspective, as the absence of *illness* or injury, of distressing symptoms or impaired capacity. Disease, as a medical construct or concept, will usually have a significant bearing on illness, and thus on health, but is not the same thing. Illness, in turn, is a very important (negative) influence on well-being – but not the only one. The WHO broad definition of 'health' is, as noted above, so broad as to become the objective, not only of health policy, but of all human activity.

Hypertension screening and treatment gives a clear and concrete example of this distinction, as well as bringing out the limitations of the static framework expressed in all the accompanying figures. It is sometimes said that hypertension does not hurt you, it only kills you. Target organ damage proceeds silently and without symptoms; a sudden and possibly fatal stroke announces both the presence of the long-term condition, and its consequences. Until that point the individual concerned may have no illness, although a clinician who took his/her blood pressure might identify a disease.

Studies of the impact of hypertension screening and treatment programmes, however, have made it clear that the fact of *diagnosis*, 'labelling,' makes the patient ill, in ways which are unambiguous and objectively measureable (Haynes et al. 1979). Treatment exacerbates the illness, through drug side effects, although those who comply with treatment may suffer less severe labelling effects. Screening and treatment of hypertension thus spread illness among the beneficiaries and reduce their functional capacity, in a real and literal sense, even as their disease is alleviated.

Of course such screening is not carried out from clinical malice! The long-term consequences of hypertension as a disease may be expressed in very definite forms of illness, including death. The immediate consequences of discovery and treatment of disease may be increased illness; the longer term consequences are reduction in illness, and very severe illness at that, for some of those under care. There is substantial evidence that screening and treatment of moderate to severe hypertension have very significantly reduced both morbidity and mortality from stroke; this is widely regarded as one of the leading 'success stories' in clinical prevention (Hypertension Detection and Follow-up Program Cooperative Group 1979). But regardless of their relative strength, the static framework of Figure 4 does not reflect this pattern of off-setting movements in different time periods.

Indeed there is an implicit time structure to all of the figures. 'Cures' are rarely instantaneous, so health care has its negative effect on disease only with a time lag of variable length. The lifestyle and environmental factors displayed in Figures 3 and 4 have long-term and cumulative effects on health/disease. But the extra problem in Figure 4 arises because the relationship being displayed may reverse itself over time. Health care can have a negative effect on health in the short term, and a positive one in the longer term.[19]

The possibility of 'long-term gain' may, but does not necessarily, justify the 'short-term pain,' and analysts and evaluators of preventive programmes are acutely aware of the necessity of weighing the health benefits and health costs against each other. Over-zealous intervention can do significant harm to the health of those treated, even if at some later date it can be shown to have 'saved lives,' or more accurately postponed some deaths.

The debate over cholesterol screening, and the contradictory recommendations arising from 'experts' in different jurisdictions is a current case in point (Toronto Working Group on Cholesterol Policy 1989; Moore 1989; Anderson et al. 1989). At issue are not merely differing interpretations of the epidemiological evidence, or different weightings of 'lives and dollars' – programme resource costs versus mortality outcomes. The prospect of converting a quarter of the adult population of North America into 'patients' with chronic illness requiring continuous drug therapy gives at least some clinicians (and others!) pause.

The framework of Figure 4 enables, indeed encourages, one to consider this distinction. Large-scale cholesterol screening and drug therapy, in this framework, would represent an epidemic of new illness, with negative impacts on health and function from both labelling effects and drug side effects. As the hypertension studies remind us, these negative effects are real and concrete, measurable in people's lives. Against this, there would be a reduction in disease, as measured first in serum cholesterol, and subsequently in heart disease. The latter would then contribute positively to health, but the conflicting health effects of disease reduction, i.e., deterioration in health now, improvement later, must be weighed against each other in assessing their net impact on well-being.

In addition to distinguishing explicitly 'disease' from 'illness,' Figure 4 extends the categorization of the determinants of health provided in the *White Paper* framework. This permits us to incorporate within the framework the diverse and rapidly-growing body of research literature on the determinants of health which does not fit at all comfortably within the *White Paper* categories.

The key addition is the concept of the individual 'host response,' which includes but goes beyond the usual epidemiological sense of the term. The range of circumstances to which the organism/individual may respond is also wider than is usually encompassed within epidemiology (Cassel 1976). This 'host response' now includes some factors or processes which were previously assembled under the labels of 'Lifestyle' and 'Human Biology.'

The implications of this change can be seen when one considers (yet again) smoking behaviour. In the *White Paper* framework, tobacco use is labelled as a 'Lifestyle,' from which one can draw the implication that its use is an 'individual choice.' That in turn leads not only to victim-blaming, but also to an emphasis on informational and educational strategies for control, which are notoriously ineffective. The powerful ethical overtones of 'choice,' with its connections to 'freedom' and 'individual self-expression,' introduce not only political but also intellectual confusions into the process of control of an addictive and toxic substance.

Yet it is widely observed that tobacco use is powerfully socially conditioned. Income, status and prestige rankings in modern societies have become strongly negatively correlated with smoking, such that differential smoking behaviour is now a significant factor in the social gradient in mortality. This was not always so; prior to the widespread dissemination of information about its health effects, smoking was positively correlated with status. It seems clear that, far from being simply an 'individual' choice, smoking is an activity engaged in – or not – by groups of people in particular circumstances. Understanding why some people smoke, and others do not, and *a fortiori* developing successful strategies to discourage this self-destructive behaviour, requires that one explore these group processes, and their conditioning circumstances. To treat smoking as 'individual choice' is simply to throw away the information contained in the clustering of behaviour.

This is not to reduce the individual to an automaton, or deny any role for individual choice. Nor is smoking the only activity which is socially conditioned – far from it. But the well-defined clustering of smoking and non-smoking behaviour within the population suggests that such behaviour is also a form of 'host' (the smoker) response to a social environment which does or does not promote smoking. Heavy tobacco advertising promotes, for example, while legislated smoke-free environments discourage, quite separately from the 'individual choice.'

The psychological dynamics of status and class may have even more powerful, if subtler, effects. The sense of personal efficacy associated with higher social position encourages beliefs both in one's ability to break addictions, and in the positive consequences of doing so. Beliefs in the effectiveness (or lack of it) of one's own actions are both learned, and reinforced by one's social position.

The distinction between social environment and host response also permits us to incorporate conceptually factors which influence health in much less direct and obvious ways than smoking. It has been observed that the death of a spouse places an individual at increased risk of illness, or even death. This may be due to a reduction in the competence of the immune system, although the causal pathways are by no means wholly clear. Evidence is accumulating rapidly, however, that the nervous and immune systems communicate with each other, each synthesizing hormones that are 'read' by the other, so that the social environment can, in principle, influence biological responses through its input to the nervous system. Data from animal experiments have shown the power of these effects (Dantzer and Kelley 1989).

Biological responses by the organism to its social environment are not restricted to the immune system. Forms of stress which one feels powerless to control – associated with hierarchical position, for example – may be correlated with differences in the plasma levels of reactive proteins such as fibrinogen (Markowe et al. 1985), or with the efficiency of the hormonal responses to stress (Sapolsky 1990). The adequacy or inadequacy of nutrition in early infancy may 'programme' the processing of dietary fats in ways which have consequences much later in life (Barker et al. 1989; Birch 1972). The range of possible biological pathways is only beginning to emerge, and is at present still quite contentious, but it seems clear that the sharp separation between 'Human Biology' and 'other things' is crumbling.

Accordingly we have in Figure 4 unbundled that field, and restricted it to the genetic endowment. This endowment then interacts with the influences of the social and physical environments, to determine both the biological and the behavioural responses of the individual (Baird and Scriver 1990). Some of these responses will be predominantly unconscious – few of us are aware of how our immune systems are performing (unless they are overwhelmed), much less can deliberately affect them. Other responses will be behavioural – smoking, for example, or buckling seatbelts. Both forms of response, or rather the continuum of such responses, will influence the ability of the individual to deal with external challenges, either to resist illness or to maintain function in spite of it. They will also affect the burden of disease, separately from illness, insofar as the decision to seek care, compliance with therapy, and response to therapy (or to self-care) are also part of the host response.

An example of the significance of changes in such host responses may be given by the decline in tuberculosis in the United Kingdom over the last century. This dramatic change in mortality patterns occurred prior to the development of any effective responses from either public health measures or medical therapy (McKeown 1979); Sagan (1987) notes that the decline was apparently *not* due to a reduced rate of exposure to the bacillus, as the majority of the population continued to test positive for the TB antibody as late as 1940. The resistance of the population simply increased. McKeown offers improved nutrition as an explanation, but the issue still seems to be open (McKeown 1979; Sagan 1987).[20] The point for our purposes is that the *biological* response of the organism is malleable.

Indeed, progress in genetics is also extending the older picture of a fixed genetic endowment, in which well-defined genetic diseases follow from single-gene defects. It now appears that particular combinations of genes may lead to predispositions, or resistances, to a wide variety of diseases, not themselves normally thought of as "genetic." Whether these predispositions actually become expressed as disease, will depend *inter alia* on various environmental factors, physical and social (Baird and Scriver 1990).

The insertion of the host response between environmental factors, and both the expression of disease and the level of health and function, provides a set of categories sufficiently flexible to encompass the growing but rather complex evidence on the connections between social environment and illness. Unemployment, for example, may lead to illness (quite apart from its correlation with economic deprivation) if the unemployed individual becomes socially isolated and stigmatized. On the other hand, if support networks are in place to maintain social contacts, and if self-esteem is not undermined, then the health consequences may be minimal.

The correlation of longevity with hierarchical status may be an example of reverse casualty – the physically fitter rise to the top. But it is also possible that the self-esteem and sense of coping ability induced by success and the respect of others results in a "host response" of enhanced immune function or other physiological strengthening. The biological vulnerability or resilience of the individual, in response to external shocks, is dependent on the social and physical environment in interaction with the genetic endowment. While as noted the biological pathways for this process are only beginning to be traced out, the observed correlations continue to accumulate. Figure 4 provides a conceptual framework within which to express such a pattern of relationships.

In this extended framework, the relationship between the health care system and the health of the population becomes even more complex. The sense of self-esteem, coping ability, powerfulness, may conceivably be either reinforced or undermined by health care interventions. Labelling effects may create a greater sense of vulnerability in the labelled, which itself influences physiological function. Such a process was an important part of Ivan Illich's message. Yet the initiation of preventive behaviour, or of therapy, may also result in positive 'placebo' effects, perhaps reflecting an increased sense of coping or control, independently of any 'objective' assessment of the effectiveness of such changes.

The possibility that medical interventions may have unintended effects is inevitable. Our framework includes both placebo and iatrogenic effects in the causal arrow from care to disease. But there is also a potential effect, of ambiguous sign, from care to host response.

At yet another level, the protective sense of self-esteem or coping ability seems to be a collective as well as an individual possession. Being a 'winner,' being on a 'winning team,' or simply being associated with a winning team – a resident of a town whose team has won a championship – all seem to provide considerable satisfaction, and may have more objectively measurable influences on health.

A Further Extension: Economic Trade-Offs and Well-Being

But there is still another feedback loop to be considered. Health care, and health policy generally, have economic costs which also affect well-being. Once we extend the framework, as in Figure 4, to reflect the fact that the ultimate objective of health-related activity is not the reduction of disease, as defined by the health care system, or even the promotion of human health and function, but the enhancement of human well-being, then we face a further set of trade-offs which are introduced in Figure 5.

Health care is not 'free'; as noted above the provision of such services is now the largest single industry or cluster of economic activities in all modern societies. This represents a major commitment of resources – human time, energy, and skills, raw materials and capital services – which are therefore unavailable for other forms of production. To the extent that health care makes a positive contribution to health, it thereby contributes to human happiness both directly and through the economic benefits of enhanced human function and productivity.

The latter effect is frequently referred to as an "investment in health"; spending on health care may even pay for itself through increased capacity of the population to work and produce wealth. The increasing concentration of health care on those outside the labour force, the very elderly or chronically ill, has however severely weakened this form of linkage. For most health care now provided, the benefits must be found in the value of the resulting improvements in health, not in some further productivity gains.

Whatever the form of the pay-off to health care, the resources used in its provision are inevitably a net drain on the wealth of the community. The well-being and economic progress of the larger society are thus affected *negatively* by the extension of the health care system *per se*. The fallacious argument frequently put forward by the economically naive, that health care, or any other industry, yields economic benefits through the creation of jobs, rests on a confusion between the job itself – a resource-using activity or cost – and the product of the job, the output. It is in fact an extension into the general economic realm of a common confusion in health care, between the process of care and its outcome.[21]

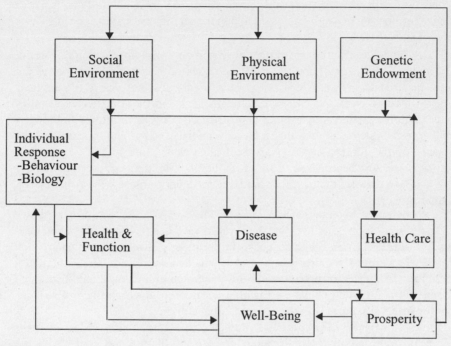

Figure 5

Yet 'job-creation' is very easy; one can always hire people to dig holes in the ground and fill them in again. (Keynes suggested burying bottles filled with banknotes, thereby creating opportunities for profitable self-employment.) The creation of wealth, however, depends upon the creation of jobs whose *product* is valued by the recipient. This understanding is implicit in references to 'real jobs,' as distinct from make-work, or employment purely for the sake of keeping people busy – and remunerated. In a complex modern economy, large numbers of people can be kept busy, apparently gainfully employed, and yet adding little or nothing to the wealth of the population as a whole. [22]

This distinction between the cost of an activity, its net absorption of productive resources, and the benefits which flow from it in the form of valued goods and services, is not unique to health care. It applies to any economic activity, as reflected in the generality of the techniques of cost-benefit analysis. The situation of health care is different, however, for a variety of complex and interrelated reasons which are implicit in the chain of effects from health care, to disease reduction, to improved health and function, to well-being.

As a commodity, health care has characteristics which make it intrinsically different from 'normal' commodities traded through private markets, and this is reflected in the peculiar and complex collection of institutional arrangements which surround its provision. As a consequence both of these intrinsic peculiarities, and of the institutional responses to them, the mechanisms which for most commodities maintain some linkage between the resource costs of a commodity and its value to users are lacking.

These problems are discussed in detail in the literature on the economics of health care (Evans 1984: Ch.1–5). For our purposes, however, the important point is that over-expansion of the health *care* system can in principle have negative effects not only on the well-being of the population, but even on its *health*. These dual effects are shown in Figure 5.

The possible negative impact of over-provision on well-being is straightforward. As emphasized, the provision of health care uses up economic resources which could be used for other valued purposes. Canadians spend nearly 9% of their national income on health care – 1 dollar in 12 – and these resources are thus unavailable for producing consumer goods like clothing or furniture, or building rapid transit systems, or improving the educational system, etc. (expanding the capacity of the Toronto airport!). In the United States, nearly 12% of national income is spent on health care; in Japan, about 6%. The Japanese correspondingly have a larger share of their income available for other purposes, the Americans a smaller proportion.

Less obviously, but implicit in Figure 5, the expansion of health care draws resources away from other uses which may also have health effects. In public budgets, for example, rising health care costs for the elderly draw funds which are then unavailable for increased pensions; rising deficits may even lead to pension reductions. Increased taxes or private health insurance premiums lower the disposable income of the working population. Environmental clean-up programmes also compete for scarce resources with the provision of health care.

Once we recognize the importance and potential controllability of factors other than health care in both the limitation of disease and the promotion of health, we simultaneously open for explicit consideration the possibility that the direct positive effects of health care on health may be outweighed by its negative effects through its competition for resources with other health-enhancing activities. A society which spends so much on health care that it cannot or will not spend adequately on other health-enhancing activities may actually be *reducing* the health of its population through increased health spending.

Two points of clarification may be helpful here, along with one of qualification.

First, we are *not* referring to iatrogenesis, the direct negative effects of health care on health. Powerful interventions have powerful side effects; the growing reach of medical technology often brings with it increased potential for harm.[23] Clinical judgement includes the balancing of probabilities for benefit and harm; the best care will sometimes work out badly. Moreover, all human systems involve some degree of error – inappropriate and incompetent care, or simply bad luck. Expansion of the health care system thus carries with it a greater potential for harm as well as good, as a direct result of care, but that is not the point here.

Second, the potential effects we are postulating are the economist's *marginal* effects. The global impact of health care, on either health or resource availability, is not addressed. Perhaps Ivan Illich is right, and the health care system as a whole has a net negative impact on the health of the population it serves. But we do not know that, and we do not know how one could come to know it.

The point we are making is a much more limited one, and one which within the framework of Figure 5 may be self-evident. The health of individuals and populations is affected by their health care, but also by other factors as well. Expansion of the health care system uses up resources which would otherwise be available to address those other factors. (Whether they would be so used or not, is another matter.) It follows that an expansion of the health care system may have negative effects on health. A *health* policy, as opposed to policies for *health care*, would have to take account of this balance.

The qualification, however, arises from the fact that when we speak of the health of a population, we are aggregating across all the individuals in it. Different policies benefit different individuals. A decision to reallocate resources from health care to other health-enhancing or productivity-enhancing activities might indeed result in a population which was in aggregate both healthier and wealthier, but particular individuals in it will be worse off. Most clearly, of course, these will include persons who either make or intended to make their living from the provision of health care. But in addition, health care services respond to the circumstances of identified individuals, in the present. A more limited commitment of resources to health care might leave such persons worse off, even though in future there might be fewer people in their position.

Such trade-offs, between the interests of those who are now ill, and those who may become so, may be inevitable. In any case it is important to note their possibility, because they are hidden from view in the aggregate framework. But conversely, it should also be noted that there is no obvious ethical, much less prudential, basis for resolving this trade-off in favour of more health care. We need to be clear as to whether we have, as a community, undertaken a collective obligation of concern, and support, for each other's *health*, or only for those aspects of health which can be enhanced through *health* care. If the latter, we may find that we are as a society both poorer, and less healthy, than we could otherwise be, and we may want to re-think the details of our (self-imposed) ethical obligation.

In this context, as in so many others, the Japanese experience is startling, and may provide an illustration of the feed-back loop from prosperity to health included in Figure 5. The extraordinary economic performance of Japanese society is not a new observation; the phenomenon goes back 40 years, and indeed a similar period of extraordinary modernization and growth began after the Meiji restoration in 1868. What is new, is that within the last decade Japan has begun to shift from the very successful copying of innovations elsewhere in the world, to being increasingly on the leading edge of both economic growth and technological change.

Over the same period there has been a remarkable growth in Japanese life expectancy, which in the 1980s has caught up with and then surpassed that of the rest of the developed world (Marmot and Smith 1989). Like the Japanese economy and per capita wealth, average life expectancy is continuing to rise on a significantly faster trend than in other industrialized countries. This experience is now setting new standards for the possible in human populations.

On the other hand, the Japanese health care system absorbs one of the lowest shares of national income in the industrialized world, and has been described by a recent American observer as 'an anachronism' in the context of modern Japanese society (Iglehart 1988). And the popular external image is that life in Japan is very crowded, highly stressful and quite polluted. How then does one explain the extraordinary trends in life expectancy?

One causal pattern suggested in Figure 5 would lead from outstanding economic performance, to rapid growth in personal incomes and in the scope and variety of life, to the greatly enhanced sense of individual and collective self-esteem and hope for the future. A number of observers, concerned not with comparative health status but with international economic competitiveness, have noted the extraordinary

Japanese sense of self-confidence and pride arising from their rapid progress toward world economic leadership. Individually and as a nation the Japanese are seeing themselves as harder-working, brighter, richer and just plain better than the rest of the world; could this attitude be yielding health benefits as well?

Conversely the centrally planned economies of Eastern Europe and the Soviet Union have on most measures of economic success performed dismally for many years, to the extent that their rulers as well as their populations have been willing to undertake a massive and indeed revolutionary political restructuring. Corresponding to this extended period of economic decline, measures of life expectancy in those nations have been stagnant or even falling, in marked contrast to the universal improvements in Western Europe (Hertzman 1990).

Uncontrolled environmental pollution and unhealthy lifestyles are commonly cited explanations, but the observation is at least consistent with the hypothesis of a relationship between collective self-esteem and health – a relationship which could be expressed in part through unhealthy lifestyles.

The factors underlying the shift in world economic leadership are no doubt complex and diverse. One of several recurring explanatory themes, however, is the Japanese advantage in access to low-cost long term capital, which is channelled into both research and development, and plant and equipment investment embodying the latest technology. This low-cost capital is generated by the very high savings rates of the Japanese people. The United States, by contrast, reports a savings rate close to zero, and now relies heavily on savings borrowed from the rest of the world – particularly Japan.

To maintain a high savings rate, one must limit the growth of other claims on social resources – such as health care.[24] The difference between Japanese and United States rates of spending on health care amounts to over 5% of national income, and could account for a significant proportion of the large difference between Japanese and American aggregate savings rates. (The difference in military spending accounts for another large share.)

Very speculatively, then, one can suggest that by limiting the growth of their health care sector, the Japanese have freed up resources which were devoted to capital investment both physical and intellectual. The consequent rapid growth in prosperity, particularly relative to their leading competitors, has greatly enhanced (already well developed) national and individual self-esteem, which has in turn contributed to a remarkable improvement in health.

It must be emphasized that this is a rough sketch of a possible argument, not a well developed case, much less a 'proof.' There are other candidate explanations for Japanese longevity – diet, for example, or the peculiar characteristics of Japanese society which may be protective against the ill effects of stress. (On the other hand, there are different forms of stress, and the stress of success is much less threatening to health than the stress of frustration and failure.)

Equally problematic, there is good evidence that environmental effects on morbidity and mortality may operate with very long lags, so that present Japanese life expectancies may reflect factors at work over the past 50 years. And in any case, what has been observed is that the Japanese live a long time, whether they are relatively healthy in any more comprehensive sense is another matter. On the other hand, the Japanese gains in life expectancy are occurring across the age spectrum, with both the world's lowest infant mortality, and extended lives among the elderly, consistent both with some contemporaneous effects, and with more general increases in health.

Whatever the explanation, it is clear that something very significant is happening (or has happened) in Japan – something reflected in trends in life expectancy which are remarkable relative to any other world experience. These observations are at least consistent with the rough sketch above. A good deal of closer investigation would seem warranted.

It is not our intent in this paper to lay 'The Decline of the West' at the feet of the health care system of the United States, or even those of North America and Western Europe combined. Rather our point is to show that the framework laid out in Figure 5 is capable of permitting such a relationship to be raised for consideration. Its network of linkages between health, health care, the production of wealth and the well-being of the population is sufficiently developed to encompass the question, without overwhelming and paralyzing one in the 'dependence of everything upon everything.'

Frameworks in Principle and in Practice

As noted above, the test of such a framework will be the extent to which others find it useful as a set of categories for assembling data and approximating complex causal patterns. The understanding of the determinants of population health, and the discussion and formulation of health policy, have been seriously impeded by the perpetuation of the incomplete, obsolete and misleading framework of Figure 1. There is a bigger picture, but clearer understanding, and particularly a more sensible and constructive public discussion, of it requires the development of a more adequate intellectual framework. The progression to Figure 5 is offered as a possible step along the way.

In this paper we have suggested several important features of such a framework. It should accommodate distinctions among disease, as defined and treated by the health care system, health and function, as perceived and experienced by individuals, and well-being, a still broader concept to which health is an important, but not the only, contributor. It should build on the Lalonde health field framework to permit and encourage a more subtle and more complex consideration of both behavioural and biological responses to social and physical environments. Finally, it should recognize and foster explicit identification of the economic trade-offs involved in the allocation of scarce resources to health care instead of other activities of value to individuals and societies, activities which may themselves contribute to health and well-being.

To date, health care policy has in most societies dominated health policy, because of its greater immediacy and apparently more secure scientific base. One may concede in principle the picture in Figure 5, then convert all the lines of causality into 'disease' and 'health and function' into thin dotted ones, except for a fat black one from 'health care.' That is the picture implicit in the current emphasis in health policy, despite the increasing concern among health researchers as to the reliability and primacy of the connection from health care to health.

One lesson from international experience in the post-Lalonde era is that appropriate conceptualization of the determinants of health is a necessary, but not a sufficient, condition for serious reform of health policy. Intellectual frameworks, including the one offered here, are only a beginning. Simply put, to be useful, they must be used.

Notes

1   The rhetoric of 'prevention' has penetrated the health care system to a significant degree; reactive responses to identified departures from health may be labelled secondary or tertiary prevention insofar as they prevent further deterioration of an adverse condition. But even when components of the health care system move from a reactive to a promotive strategy – screening for cholesterol, for example, or hypertension – the interventions still consist of identifying departures from clinically determined norms for particular biological measurements, and initiating therapeutic interventions. Elevated blood pressure or serum cholesterol measurements become themselves identified as "diseases," to be "cured."

2   The representation of mental illness is always troublesome – where is the borderline between clinical depression, and the 'normal' human portion of unhappiness? The difficulty of definition persists, however, across the whole continuum; the WHO definition of health does not imply perpetual bliss.

3   This does not represent a rejection of rational modes of enquiry; the universe is still seen as, on some levels, a comprehensible and orderly place. But there appear to be fundamental limits on its comprehensibility – not just on our ability to comprehend it – and the relevant concepts of order may also be less complete than was once hoped. Whether or not Nietzsche turns out to be right about the death of God (Hawking 1988), Laplace's Demon appears definitely defunct (Dreyfus and Dreyfus 1988; Gleick 1987; Holton 1988). (But has he met his maker?)

4   The actual interventions themselves may be very far from transparent; 'medical miracles' are an everyday occurrence, and the processes are presented as beyond the capacity or ken of ordinary mortals. But the application of a high degree of science and skill is still within the conceptually simple framework of a mechanical model – fixing the damaged part.

5   To the extent that overt policy does recognize this process, it tends to respond with marketing activities encouraging people to seek care. A surprising proportion of so-called 'health promotion' includes various forms of 'see your doctor' messages, and might more accurately be called 'disease promotion.' Measures to encourage 'informal' coping should *inter alia* include recommendations not to contact the health care system in particular circumstances; the latter are virtually unheard of.

6   The experience of the United States is a clear demonstration of the distinction between the resource and administrative/financial dimensions of access. The United States devotes a much larger share of its national resources to producing health care than does any other nation, and spends much more per capita (Schieber and Poullier 1989; OECD Secretariat 1989). Yet the peculiarities of its financing system result in severely restricted (or no) access for a substantial minority of its citizens. On the other hand, nominally universal 'access' to a system with grossly inadequate resources would be equally misleading.

7   Providers of care, particularly nurses, often emphasize their 'caring' functions. The point here is not at all that caring is without importance or value, but rather that it is by no means the exclusive preserve of providers of health care. Furthermore, the 'social contract' by which members of a particular community undertake collective (financial) responsibility for each other's health narrowly defined, does not necessarily extend to responsibility for their happiness. 'Caring' independently of any contemplated 'curing,' or at least prevention of deterioration, represents an extension of the 'product line' – and sales revenue – of the health care system. If collective buyers of these services, public or private, have never in fact agreed to this extension, its ethical basis is rather shaky.

8   Best attainable health begs the question of by which means health may be attained. A hypothetical situation in which the members of a population had each received all the health care

which might benefit them, might nevertheless be one in which the population fell well short of attainable health because other measures outside the health care system were neglected.

9 A classic example has been provided by the response of pediatrics to the collapse of the baby boom in the mid-1960s. The 'New Paediatrics' – social and emotional problems of adolescents – was discovered just in time to prevent underemployment. At the other end of the paediatric age range, progress in neonatology will ensure a growing supply of very low birthweight babies surviving into childhood, with a complex array of medical problems requiring intervention. We do not suggest that these system responses are the result of conscious and deliberate self-seeking by providers; such is almost certainly not the case. But the outcome is what it is.

10 The quotes are needed because the health care system, and the people in it, are not simply an 'industry' in the sense of a set of activities and actors motivated solely by economic considerations. But to the extent that they are – and it is undeniable that economic considerations do matter, even if they are not the exclusive motivations – then this observation holds.

11 If building environmental standards were set by fuel supply companies, would we have similar problems with the regulation of thermostats?

12 The rhetoric of 'cost crises' rarely if ever recognizes an extremely important distinction between expenditures or outlays, and the economist's concept of resource or opportunity costs. Expenditures on health care may rise (fall) either because more (fewer) resources of human time, effort, and skills, capital equipment and raw materials, are being used in its production, or because the owners of such resources are receiving larger (smaller) payments for them – higher (lower) salaries, fees, or prices. The arrow from health care to disease represents a response in the form of actual goods and services provided – real resources. But much of the public debate over 'underfunding' and 'cost crises' is really about the relative incomes of providers of care, not about the amount and type of care provided. For obvious political reasons, income claims are frequently presented as if they were assertions about levels of care (Evans 1984; Reinhardt 1987).

13 There might still, however, be quite justifiable interest in the patterns of prices and incomes generated by such care. A competitive marketplace can generate intense pressures which automatically control prices and incomes, as the computer example has demonstrated. Health care, however, is nowhere provided through such a marker (not even in the United States), and has not been for at least a hundred years. There are excellent reasons for this (e.g., Evans 1984; Culyer 1982), and the situation is not in fact going to change in the foreseeable future. It follows that other mechanisms, with associated controversy, will remain necessary to address issues of income distribution.

14 Not nonexistent. There is no basis in ethical theory or institutional practice for the proposition which creeps into so much of normative economics, that individual choice is the ultimate and even the only ground of obligation (Etzioni 1988).

15 We do not mean to imply that the authors of the White Paper had the relatively limited view which we present below, still less that all of their subsequent interpreters have been so intellectually constrained. But it is our perception that the principal impact of the White Paper framework on debates about, and the development of, health policy, has been limited in the way we describe.

16 None of which is news to tobacco marketers.

17 One should note, however, that the very limited experience in the early 1970s with anti-smoking advertising on television appeared to be sufficiently successful that tobacco companies were willing voluntarily to abandon this medium in order to get the 'opposition' off the air.

18 Wilkins et al. (1989) and Wolfson et al. (1990) provide recent Canadian data.

19   One might point out that this is true of much therapy. Surgery, for example, typically has a very powerful negative effect on health and function in the immediate intervention and recovery phase, while (when successful) yielding later improvements. In the hypertension case, however, healthy individuals are introduced to prolonged low-level illness, in order to receive large but uncertain benefits in the farther future. Such a difference of degree becomes one of kind.

    For people with short time horizons, painful or disabling interventions with longer term payoffs may not be justified. Elderly people, in particular, will quite rationally discount future benefits more heavily. The finding that elderly cancer patients are more likely to choose radiation treatment over surgery, even if the latter has a greater five-year survival rate (McNeil et al. 1978) illustrates the point. The enthusiasm among dentists to provide 'optimum' oral health to residents of nursing homes, raises similar concerns. Would you want to spend a day in a dentist's chair if you expected to die tomorrow? Next week? Next month? ...

20   'Improved' nutrition is ambiguous. For impoverished and deprived populations better is simply more, and more nutritious. But for a high proportion of modern populations better is probably less, and particularly less fats. It is not clear when in the historical record 'better' shifted from more to less, for the majority of industrialized populations, such that (from a health perspective) nutrition may have begun to deteriorate.

21   The operation was a success, but the patient died.

22   The common identification between private sector jobs as by definition 'real', and public sector ones as 'unreal' is however simply ideological nonsense – 'real' and 'unreal' exist in both sectors, wherever activity is being carried on with no output, or none of any value. It includes, but is not restricted to, the caricature of the lazy or obstructionist bureaucrat.

    A strong argument can be made, for example, that most of the jobs in the private health insurance sector in the United States – complex, demanding and highly paid – are not 'real jobs,' because they actually yield nothing of value and in all other health care funding systems are dispensed with. That is, of course, another story, but one which emphasizes the invalidity of an equation between 'unreal jobs' and 'lazy public servants.' One can work quite hard and conscientiously, both individually and as a group, and yet be completely useless or even get in the way. Parallels with public bureaucracies in centrally planned economies are not inapt.

23   Often, but not always. Improvements in the techniques of diagnostic imaging, for example, have reduced the degree of risk and distress associated with earlier forms of diagnostic imaging; and the substitution of lithotripsy for kidney surgery has yielded similar benefits. On the other hand, less risky or uncomfortable procedures tend to be offered to many more patients.

24   It would, of course, be quite possible for a nation to maintain both high savings rates, and high spending on health care – or the military – simply by cutting back on consumption. But there is strong resistance at both bargaining table and ballot box to a reduction in current consumption through higher taxes or lower wages. Citizens do not want to accept a reduction in present living standards to pay for more health care.

    A neo-classical economist might argue that the living standard is not reduced; what is given up in smaller houses, poorer roads or fewer electronic gadgets is gained in more cardiac bypass grafts, laboratory tests, MRI procedures and months in nursing homes. But the average individual is, quite rightly, unconvinced. Health care, like military spending, is not valued for its own sake. What, after all, are the direct satisfactions from a tonsillectomy, or a tank? Each is simply a regrettable use of resources, a service for which in a better world one would have no need. Hence the tendency for health spending increases to be drawn from savings, whether through government budget deficits or reduced corporate retained earnings.

Acknowledgments

We wish to thank colleagues in the CIAR Population Health Program, the Health Polinomics Research Workshop at McMaster University, and the Health Policy Research Unit at the University of British Columbia for stimulating comments on earlier versions of this paper. We take responsibility for remaining errors or omissions.

References

American Council of Life Insurance and Health Insurance Association of America. 1988. *INSURE Project – Lifecycle Study, Press Kit*, 25 April.

Andersen, TF, and G Mooney eds. 1990. *The Challenge of Medical Practice Variations*. London: MacMillan.

Anderson, GM, S Brinkworth, and T Ng. 1989. *Cholesterol Screening: Evaluating Alternative Strategies*. Health Policy Research Unit 89: 10D, University of British Columbia, Vancouver, August.

Baird, PA and CR Scriver. 1990. *Genetics and the Public Health*. Internal Document No. 10A, Program in Population Health, Canadian Institute for Advanced Research, Toronto, January.

Banta, HD, C Behney, and JS Willems. 1981. *Toward Rational Technology in Medicine: Considerations for Health Policy*. New York: Springer.

Barker DJP, PD Winter, C Osmond, et al. 1989. Weight in Infancy and Death from Ischaemic Heart Disease. *Lancet* (9 Sept): 577–580.

Birch, HG. 1972. Malnutrition, Learning and Intelligence. *American Journal of Public Health* 62: 773–784.

Buck, C. 1988. Beyond Lalonde: Creating Health. *Canadian Journal of Public Health* 76 (Suppl. 1): 19–24.

Bunker JP, DS Gomby and BH Kehrer. 1989. *Pathways to Health: The Role of Social Factors*. Menlo Park, CA: Henry J. Kaiser Family Foundation.

Cassel, J. 1976. The Contribution of the Social Environment to Host Resistance. *American Journal of Epidemiology* 104: 107–123.

Culyer, AJ. 1989. Cost Containment in Europe. *Health Care Financing Review* (Suppl.): 21–32.

Culyer, AJ. 1988. *Health Expenditures in Canada: Myth and Reality, Past and Future*. Toronto: Canadian Tax Foundation.

Culyer, AJ. 1982. The NHS and the Market: Images and Realities. In A Maynard and G McLachlan eds. *The Public-Private Mix for Health: The Relevance and Effects of Change*, 23–55. London: Nuffield Provincial Hospitals Trust.

Dantzer, R, and KW Kelley. 1989. Stress and Immunity: An Integrated View of Relationships Between the Brain and the Immune System. *Life Sciences* 44: 1995–2008.

Department of National Health and Welfare. 1974. *A New Perspective on the Health of Canadians* (Lalonde Report). Ottawa.

Dreyfus, HL, and SE Dreyfus. 1988. Making a Mind Versus Modelling a Brain: Artificial Intelligence Back at a Branchpoint. *Daedalus* 117: 1543.

Dubos, R. 1959. *Mirage of Health*. New York: Harper and Row.

Dutton, DB. 1986. Social Class and Health. In LH Aitken and D Mechanic ed. *Applications of Social Science to Clinical Medicine and Health Policy,* 31–62. New Brunswick NJ: Rutgers University Press.

Eisenberg, JM. 1986. *Doctors' Decisions and the Cost of Medical Care.* Ann Arbor, MI: Health Administration Press.

Etzioni, A. 1988. *The Moral Dimension: Toward a New Economics.* New York: The Free Press.

Evans, RG. 1984. *Strained Mercy: The Economics of Canadian Health Care.* Toronto: Butterworths.

Evans, RG. 1982. A Retrospective on the "New Perspective". *Journal of Health Politics, Policy and Law* 7: 325–344.

Feeny, D, G Guyatt, and P Tugwell. 1986. *Health Care Technology: Effectiveness, Efficiency and Public Policy.* Montreal: Institute for Research on Public Policy.

Gleick, J. 1987. *Chaos: Making a New Science.* New York: Viking.

Gunning-Schepers, LJ, and JH Hagen. 1987. Avoidable Burden of Illness: How Much Can Prevention Contribute to Health? *Social Science and Medicine* 24: 945–951.

Ham, C ed. 1988. *Health Care Variations: Assessing the Evidence.* London: The King's Fund Institute.

Hawking, S. 1988. *A Brief History of Time.* Toronto: Bantam Books.

Haynes, RB, DL Sackett, DW Taylor, ES Gibson, and AL Johnson. 1979. Increased Absenteeism from Work after Detection and Labelling of Hypertensive Patients. *New England Journal of Medicine* 229: 741–744.

Hertzman, C. 1990. *Poland: Health and Environment in the Context of Socioeconomic Decline.* Health Policy Research Unit 90: 2D. University of British Columbia, Vancouver, January.

Holton, G. 1988. The Roots of Complementarity. *Daedalus* 117: 151–197.

House, J, KR Landis, and D Umberson. 1988. Social Relationships and Health. *Science* 241: 540–545.

Hypertension Detection and Follow-up Program Cooperative Group. 1979. Five-Year Findings of the Hypertension Detection and Follow-up Program, I: Reduction in Mortality of Persons with High Blood Pressure, Including Mild Hypertension. *Journal of the American Medical Association* 242: 2562–2571.

Iglehart, JK. 1988. Japan's Health Care System – Part Two, Health Policy Report. *New England Journal of Medicine* 319: 1166–1172.

Illich, I. 1975. *Medical Nemesis: The Expropriation of Health.* Toronto: McClelland and Stewart.

Levine, S, and A Lilienfeld. 1987. *Epidemiology and Health Policy.* London: Tavistock Press.

Lewis, CE. 1988. Disease Prevention and Health Promotion Practices of Primary Care Physicians in the United States. *American Journal of Preventive Medicine.* 4(Suppl): 9–16.

Lomas, J. 1990. Promoting Clinical Policy Change: Using the Art to Promote the Science in Medicine. In TF Andersen and G Mooney eds. *The Challenge of Medical Practice Variations,* 174–191. Toronto: MacMillan.

Marlowe, HJJ, MG Marmot, MJ Shipley et al. 1985. Fibrinogen – A Possible Link Between Social Class and Coronary Heart Disease. *British Medical Journal* 291: 1312–1314.

Marmor, TR. 1989. *Healthy Public Policy: What Does That Mean, Who is Responsible For it, and How Would One Pursue it?* Program in Population Health, Internal Document No. 6A, Canadian Institute for Advanced Research, Toronto, August.

Marmot, MG and GD Smith. 1989. Why are the Japanese Living Longer? *British Medical Journal* 299: 1547–1551.

Marmot, MG. 1986. Social Inequalities in Mortality: the Social Environment. In RG Wilkinson ed. *Class and Health: Research and Longitudinal Data,* 21–33. London: Tavistock Press.

Marmot, MG. 1984. Inequalities in Death – Specific Explanations of a General Pattern. *Lancet 1* (8384): 1003–1006.

McCloskey, DN. 1989. Why I Am No Longer a Positivist. *Review of Social Economy* 47: 225–238.

McKeown, T. 1979. *The Role of Medicine: Dream, Mirage or Nemesis?* 2nd ed. Oxford: Blackwell.

McKinlay, JB, SM McKinlay, and R Beaglehole. 1989. A Review of the Evidence Concerning the Impact of Medical Measures on Recent Mortality and Morbidity in the United States. *International Journal of Health Services* 19: 181–208.

McKinlay, JB. 1979. Epidemiological and Political Determinants of Social Policies Regarding the Public Health. *Social Science and Medicine* 13A: 541–558.

McNeil, BJ, R Weichselbaum, and SG Pauker. 1978. Fallacy of the Five-Year Survival in Lung Cancer. *New England Journal of Medicine* 299: 1397–1401.

Moore, TJ. 1989. *Heart Failure: A Critical Inquiry into American Medicine and the Revolution in Heart Care, Part II: Prevention.* New York: Random House.

OECD Secretariat. 1989. Health Care Expenditure and Other Data: An International Compendium From the Organization for Economic Cooperation and Development. *Health Care Financing Review.*

Reinhardt, UE. 1987. Resource Allocation in Health Care: The Allocation of Lifestyles to Providers. *Milbank Quarterly* 65: 153–176.

Reiser, SJ. 1978. *Medicine and the Reign of Technology.* New York: Cambridge University Press.

Renaud, M. 1987. De l'Epidemiologie Sociale a la Sociologie de la Prevention: 15 ans de Recherche sur l'Etiologie Sociale de la Maladie. *Revue D Epidemiologie et de Sante Publique* 35: 3–19.

Sagan, LA. 1987. *The Health of Nations.* New York: Basic Books.

Sapolsky, RM. 1990. Stress in the Wild. *Scientific American* 262: 116–123.

Schieber, GJ, and JP Poullier. 1989. Overview of International Comparisons of Health Care Expenditures. *Health Care Financing Review.*

Toronto Working Group on Cholesterol Policy. 1989. *Detection and Management of Asymptomatic Hypercholesterolemia.* Prepared for the Task Force on the Use and Provision of Medical Services, Ontario Ministry of Health and Ontario Medical Association, Toronto.

Townshend, P, and N Davidson eds. 1982. *Inequalities in Health: The Black Report.* London: Penguin.

Wilkins, R, OB Adams, and A Brancker. 1989. *Mortality by Income in Urban Canada, 1971 and 1986: Diminishing Absolute Differences, Persistance of Relative Inequality.* Joint Study, Health and Welfare Canada and Statistics Canada. Ottawa.

Wolfson, MC, G Rowe, JF Gentleman, and M Tomiak. 1990. *Earnings and Death – Effects Over a Quarter Century.* Program in Population Health, Internal Document No. 5B. Canadian Institute for Advanced Research, Toronto, February.

Woodward, CA, and GL Stoddart. 1990. Is the Canadian Health Care System Suffering from Abuse? A commentary. *Canadian Family Doctor* 36: 283–289.

31

Locating the Canadian Welfare State: Family Policy and Health Care in Canada, Sweden, and the United States[*]

Gregg M. Olsen

It is commonplace to note that the American and Swedish welfare states exemplify antipodal forms of public provision. While the latter is identified by "cradle-to-grave" coverage, the former is widely recognized for its fragmented and meagre support. Portrayals of the Canadian welfare state suggest that it may be somewhat more difficult to situate. Few students of comparative social policy would seriously contend that the Canadian welfare state approximates Sweden's in terms of generosity, comprehensiveness, or efficacy. John Myles and Dennis Forcese (1981: 24), for example, note "a clear division between the two North American countries on the one hand and Sweden on the other."[1] Others, however, such as Seymour Martin Lipset (1990: 136; 1986), have clearly distinguished Canada from the United States on the basis of its "communitarianism," by which Lipset means "the public mobilization of resources to fulfill group objectives." As well, most Canadians believe that their welfare system is, generally speaking, much more developed than the American counterpart.[2]

The conclusions reached regarding the nature of the welfare state in Canada have largely depended upon the particular types of social policy under scrutiny. While social security programs have received a great deal of attention, social services often have not been included in comparative studies of the Canadian welfare state. In the present paper, an attempt will be made to redress this deficiency and locate the Canadian welfare state by contrasting it with its American and Swedish counterparts in two broad social policy areas – family policy and health care – with a particular emphasis upon the latter. It will be demonstrated that an accurate characterization of the Canadian welfare state must be based upon an examination of both social security and social service programs. This comparative examination of Canadian social policies will be preceded by a critical review of the most commonly used approaches to classify or categorize modern welfare states.

* Reprinted from *Canadian Journal of Sociology*, Vol. 19, No. 1, Gregg M. Olsen, 'Locating the Canadian welfare state: Family policy and Health care in Canada, Sweden and the United States, pp 1-20, 1994, with permission from the publisher.

From Social Spending to "Welfare Worlds"

Comparative analyses of welfare states have, until fairly recently, evaluated and ranked them along a simple leader-laggard continuum based upon the size, scope, and precocity of national welfare efforts. Accordingly, a number of European nations, which had already emplanted several major social security (income maintenance/social transfer) programs by WWI or earlier and routinely spent a significant proportion of their GDP on such measures by the early 1980s, tended to cluster at one end. Situated at the other extreme was, of course, the American welfare state – its celebrated "exceptionality" signifying the absence, inadequacy, or belated and reluctant introduction of these programs and relatively low levels of social expenditure. Canada was also identified as a welfare laggard. In contrast with nations such as the Netherlands, Belgium, and Sweden which, as a percentage of their GDP, spent 27.8 percent, 23 percent, and 17.9 percent respectively on social security in 1983, expenditures in Canada and the United States were quite similar at only 12.9 percent and 11 percent of GDP respectively during the same year (Gordon 1990).

While useful, such categorizations on the basis of social security spending paid insufficient attention to the policy instruments used and their impact and were thus often misleading. The creation of a variety of proactive and preventive social services and policies allowed the Scandinavian nations, for example, to achieve their goals while spending considerably less on reactive and redistributive social transfer payments. It is widely known that Sweden has maintained low levels of unemployment largely through the creation of an elaborate array of active labour-market policies while other countries, such as Canada and the United States, have *responded* to rising unemployment levels, primarily through unemployment insurance programs (Olsen 1988). When such proactive measures are examined, it becomes evident that Sweden was the undisputed spending leader in 1983 (25.3 percent of GDP) while Canada (18.6 percent) and the United States (11.7 percent), the welfare "laggards," appeared more dissimilar than they had when only social security measures were considered (O'Connor 1989).

Gosta Esping-Andersen's (1990) threefold typology of "welfare worlds" represents a significant advance over these earlier leader-laggard models and has rapidly become the predominant approach in the field of social welfare research. In this approach, the welfare states of various nations are categorized as "social democratic," "liberal" or "conservative" on the basis of the general nature of their income security and employment policies.[3] Social democratic welfare regimes are characterized by benefits with particular features. First, they are provided mainly through the public sector and are relatively generous. Second, they provide universal coverage as a right of citizenship. Third, they tend to stress prevention, rather than simply responding to need. Social policies based on these interrelated traits serve to weaken workers' dependence upon the labour market and to foster support for the welfare state and social solidarity among the citizenry. Moreover, these policies – best typified in Sweden – tend to form a coherent package of compatible programs and policies.

Social policy in the liberal world virtually mirrors social democratic policy. Here, the private production and provision of benefits plays a leading role, supplemented by modest, means-tested public assistance programs.[4] Welfare provision in the private market may be obtained through direct payment for goods and services (for example, daycare), private insurance plans (for old-age, health, etc.), employment-based welfare (a wide variety of occupational or "fringe" benefits), or voluntary, charitable organizations. However, all of these forms imply a much greater dependence upon the employer and/or the market generally than that seen in the social democratic world. Coverage is not universally provided but is, rather, highly dependent upon place of employment, ability to purchase or, in the case of public provision, need, and is thus subject to means- or needs-testing. Finally, social welfare measures are largely reactive, not proactive or preventive, and often contradict one another. The United States provides the purest example of this type of welfare regime.

Despite its strengths, this reconceptualization of welfare states into ideal-types conceals significant differences between Canada and the United States. Although they are both viewed as belonging to the liberal "world," the Canadian and American welfare states are, in some ways, notably distinct. For example, while private employment-based welfare plays an important role in both countries, it is somewhat more prominent in the United States than in Canada.[5] In a recent study it was noted that employer contributions to three major "occupational" welfare programs (public and private health insurance, private pension plans, and legislated income maintenance plans) in 1984 were approximately 50 percent higher in the United States, where benefits are usually purchased privately, than in Canada, where a greater proportion of the cost is borne by the government (Du Broy 1986). Employee benefit costs as a percentage of gross payroll were almost 6 points higher in the United States than in Canada in 1989 (Courchene 1989).

In addition, the Canadian welfare state has greater scope than its American counterpart. It is commonly noted that welfare state development in the United States has been "episodic," the first "big bang" occurring in 1935 with the creation of the Social Security Act (SSA). This first step into the field of welfare reform was to be the biggest step taken and, apart from some important amendments to the SSA, little subsequent development took place until the next episode in the 1960s.[6] In contrast, the Canadian welfare state developed in a more steady and deliberate manner and introduced a number of important universal social programs which still do not exist in the United States.[7]

The welfare worlds approach has also led to two other important problems with regard to the placement of the Canadian welfare state because it categorizes nations primarily on the basis of the *general* trends and tendencies of *certain types* of policies and programs. First, the model obscures the fact that the various social policies and programs which exist in Canada may differ widely from one another. Some, for example, clearly belong to the liberal world while others are more properly classified as social democratic. This will be demonstrated through an examination of two different components of the Canadian welfare state – family policy (liberal) and the health care system (social democratic) – from a comparative perspective.

Second, the welfare worlds model fails to acknowledge that any one particular social welfare policy or program may exhibit concurrently some "liberal world" tendencies (private provision, selective benefit distribution or a reactive or curative orientation) and some "social democratic world" tendencies (public provision, universal distribution, or a preventive orientation). This oversight is partly due to the almost exclusive emphasis on "social security" by researchers in this school. While the model has been applied primarily to old age pensions (Deviney 1984; Palme 1990) and the major income security programs – sickness insurance, accident insurance ("compensation") and unemployment insurance (Kangas 1991; Korpi 1989) – other important areas such as education, housing, health care, and family policy/day care have not yet been included. By ignoring the central "social service" components of the welfare state, nations like Canada may be too readily misclassified. This problem will be demonstrated here through a detailed examination of the Canadian health care system from a comparative perspective.[8] It will be argued that, while Sweden and the United States constitute the definitive social democratic and liberal worlds, respectively, Canada can only be uneasily categorized into either of these two ideal types. The development of an alternative approach which builds upon the strengths of both the leader-laggard and welfare world models is therefore suggested.

Family Policy in the 1980s

Family policy is comprised of two major types of benefits. The more familiar of these is the family allowance which is an income transfer to families with children that may be provided by the state or by an employer.[9] The other major type of family support measure is the tax benefit, or what has been referred to as "fiscal welfare."[10] Since 1950, Sweden has relied exclusively upon income transfers while the United States has provided only tax reductions as the means of family support. Canada has implemented both types of family support measures. Nevertheless, upon closer scrutiny, it becomes clear that family policy in Canada shares many more similarities with the United States than with Sweden in this regard and fits easily into the liberal sphere.

Universal, publically provided family allowances were introduced in Canada in 1944 with the Family Allowances Act, three years before they were created in Sweden. However, by 1985 Sweden provided family allowances that were almost 13 percent of net family income. This was among the most generous of the allowances provided by the sixteen advanced capitalist countries with family allowance programs.[11] In contrast, Canada provided less than 4 percent of net family income – the lowest level of cash benefits provided by the same sixteen nations (Wennemo 1992). Because of its Family Allowance program, Canada appears to differ from the United States, where the absence of such a plan makes it almost unique among the advanced capitalist nations. However, the meagre amount of financial support provided by the Family Allowance program in Canada clearly qualifies it for membership in the liberal world.[12] Moreover, by 1985 Canada had begun to rely more upon a variety of tax allowances and tax deductions than cash benefits as a means of family support.[13]

In terms of the social services aspect of family policy – the provision of day care – Canada shares few similarities with Sweden and is virtually identical to the United States. The influx of woman, and especially mothers, into the workforce over the past two decades has intensified the need for day care in all three nations. This is particularly true in Sweden, where women comprised 50 percent of the workforce and 80 percent of all Swedish women worked outside the home by the mid-1980s.[14] The corresponding employment figures for female workers in Canada and the United States were 44 percent and 44.8 percent, respectively (Anderson 1991).

While Sweden has not yet achieved its goal of universal public day care provision, public sector day care was available in all of the large- and medium-sized cities (35 municipalities) for 75 percent of pre-school children whose parents were employed or studying by the late 1980s (Hwang and Broberg 1992). There also exist more market-oriented forms of day care such as organized child-minding schemes (in which municipalities pay childminders directly and are reimbursed by parents) and private care in the home, although these forms do not predominate. In addition to family allowances and public day care, Sweden provides its widely admired "parental insurance" scheme.[15]

Day care in Canada and the United States is woefully inadequate and is provided primarily in the private sphere. The most widespread form of day care provision in these countries involves care by relatives; private, informal, and unregulated day care centres; or employer-sponsored workplace centres (Goelman 1992; Lamb et al. 1992; Mayfield 1990). Both countries are characterized by a shortage of spaces in licensed or regulated day care facilities. These tendencies were confirmed in a recent Canadian task force report which examined day care provision in the advanced capitalist nations in the 1980s (Cook 1986).

In Canada and the United States, the state's role is linked to a variety of funding mechanisms which parents may use to help pay for day care costs on the market. Such mechanisms, like the Canada Assistance Plan or Title XX of the Social Security Act in the United States, are not available universally as a right, but are aimed only at low-income families and are thus means-tested. Moreover, the benefits they have provided are quite modest. In addition, neither country provides "parental insurance." However, Canada provided mothers with fifteen weeks of "maternity" leave benefits in the late 1980s at 60 percent of their earnings (up to a maximum) through the unemployment insurance program, while there have been no statutory requirements in the United States (Bronfenbrenner 1992; National Council of Welfare 1988).[16] These characteristics of Canadian family policy bear the hallmarks of the liberal world. The Canadian health care system, in striking contrast, is much more social democratic in orientation while remaining somewhat liberal according to some policy dimensions.

The Health Care System in the 1980s

Expenditures and Outcomes

It is common knowledge today that health care expenditure in the United States is astronomically high – the highest in the world in both absolute and relative terms. At 11.2 percent, *total* expenditure on health in the United States, as a proportion of GDP, was significantly higher than Canadian (8.6 percent), Swedish (9 percent), or average OECD (7.3 percent) spending levels by 1987.[17] However, as would be expected, public spending on health, as a proportion of GDP, was almost twice as high in social democratic Sweden (8.2 percent) as it was in liberal United States (4.6 percent). Public health spending in Canada, at 6.5 percent, fell approximately mid-way between these two extreme expenditure cases and was somewhat higher than the OECD average of 5.6 percent. As a proportion of total health spending, public health expenditures in Sweden, Canada, and the United States were 90.6 percent, 74.8 percent, and 41.4 percent respectively, the same year (OECD 1990; Schieber and Poullier 1989). Moreover, despite record high expenditures in the United States, "output" measures, while somewhat crude, suggest that the American health care system is among the least effective. As illustrated in Table 1, Canada has been more successful than the United States with respect to infant mortality rates, life expectancy at birth, and mortality rates from chronic conditions, but has not performed as well as Sweden.

The three nations under consideration here also differ markedly regarding their delivery of health care. The United States and Sweden represent two almost entirely dissimilar approaches to health care. While the former emphasizes plurality and provision in the private market, the latter is sometimes characterized as "socialized medicine." As will become apparent from the following overview, health care delivery in Canada shares some features with both, but has more in common with the Swedish health system, despite Canada's common designation as a member of the liberal world.

TABLE 1

Health care output in the United States, Canada, and Sweden, 1982

Health Care	Country		
	United States	Canada	Sweden
Infant mortality rates[a]	11.5	9.1	6.8
Life expectancy at birth (in years)	74.7	75.5	76.6
Mortality rates from chronic conditions[b]	842.4	761.8	757.5

a   Death of infants per 1,000 live births.
b   Age-standardized death rates per 100,000. These data must be interpreted cautiously
     since they apply to different periods (1982 for the United States, 1984 for Canada and Swe-
     den), may be subject to yearly fluctuations (e.g., epidemics), categories are highly aggre-
     gated, and death may result from multiple cases.

Source: OECD 1987

Organization: Public Sector/Private Sector

The delivery of health care in Sweden has much in common with Britain's more familiar National Health Service (NHS).[18] Like Britain, Sweden has allowed administrative
coordination and public planning to supplant the market to a great extent. Hospitals are
publicly owned and administered and, apart from some nursing homes, there exist few
private alternatives for in-patient care. Ninety-percent of hospital admissions, for
example, are public and over 90 percent of Sweden's physicians (and 50 percent of its
dentists) are salaried employees. While the pharmaceutical industry itself remains
largely privately owned, the Swedish government nationalized one company (Kabi) in
the late 1960s, and in 1971 organized the retail drug industry (pharmacies) into a single
corporation (Apoteksbolaget), two-thirds of which is owned by the state and one-third
by the pharmacists' association (Kurian 1990; OECD 1990). This has made it easier for
the government to control the price of drugs in Sweden.

Unlike the NHS, however, the Swedish health care system is surprisingly decentralized, a feature that has characterized it since its inception. As Odin Anderson (1972)
points out, health care has been "informally regionalized" since the 1800s when the
counties and municipalities took over responsibility for the financing and operation of
hospitals from the local parishes. Today, hospitals are still owned and administered sub-
nationally, rather than by the central government, and provide their services to all,
largely free of charge. The central government, however, does assume the financial
responsibility for their operation and Sweden's health system, like the NHS, relies
heavily on tax-financing.

Given its mix of private and public sector ownership, variety of organizational
forms, numerous sources of funding, and decidedly market orientation, the American
health care system could not be much more dissimilar from Sweden's. A network of
private hospitals, owned largely by non-profit corporations sponsored by private citizens and sectarian groups, and public hospitals, run jointly by various levels of government, are complemented by a throng of private health insurance providers and public
health agencies and clinics. Most physicians (and dentists) practice privately in their
own offices using their own equipment. The pharmaceutical industry (manufacturers

and retailers) also operates almost exclusively in the private sphere. The combination of uninformed consumers and multimillion-dollar advertising campaigns by drug companies contributes to the high medical costs seen in the United States.[19]

Sometimes described as socialized medicine by organizations and individuals with an interest in maintaining the status quo in the United States, the health economy in Canada actually closely resembles its American counterpart.[20] As in the United States, health care is provided largely in the private sector. While some government-owned and administered hospitals exist, the great majority of hospitals in Canada (90 percent) are private non-profit corporations, although their global operating budgets are provided largely by provincial governments. Ninety-five percent of all physicians maintain private practices and earn their income on a fee-for-service basis. As in the United States, doctors are paid by a third party – although in Canada, the third party is the government, rather than a plethora of private insurance companies (General Accounting Office 1991). Finally, as would be expected given the central role of foreign (especially American) branch plants in Canada, the pharmaceutical industry operates almost entirely in the private sector, under relatively little public control.[21] Therefore, with respect to the organization of its health economy, Canada, like the United States, is situated in the liberal world.

Coverage: Universal/Selective

Low cost health care is available for the entire population in Sweden through a compulsory health insurance plan which operates largely at the regional (county/municipal) level. In 1955, Sweden created its mandatory National Health Insurance plan by converting existing voluntary, state-subsidized sickness funds and employer-financed schemes into public funds, which became part of the existing social security insurance system in 1963 (Serner 1980). Regional councils, originally established in the 1860s to operate the hospitals, administer the existing twenty-six regional (twenty-three county and three municipal) funds today. Financed primarily by employer payroll fees and, to a lesser extent, the state, these funds largely subsidize the provision of out-patient medical services in Sweden. Patients pay only a standard nominal fee to the regional council for each visit to a public clinic regardless of the amount of treatment or number of tests provided, and are partially reimbursed for their travel costs. Compensation is also received for a portion of the costs of drugs and dental care (Olsson 1988). Despite decentralization in the Swedish system, regional hospitals and councils are monitored closely by the Ministry of Health and Social Affairs through the National Board of Health and Welfare to ensure uniformity in the quality of health care, if not in its delivery (Borgenhammar 1984).

The United States is commonly known as the only industrial country without a national health insurance system. This, of course, does not mean that a majority of Americans are not covered by insurance. In fact, 85 percent of the American population have some form of health insurance protection. However, 35 to 37 million Americans are without health insurance. Although it includes the unemployed, the majority of this uninsured group consists of the working poor and their families – that is, those who are not old enough or poor enough to qualify for existing public programs. Many millions more have only partial coverage. Fifty million Americans have such poor coverage that a serious illness would mean financial devastation (Bernard 1992).

Only about 20 percent of Americans are covered by one of the two major public programs created in 1965 or by the military and veterans' programs. Medicare, a federal health insurance program for the elderly and disabled, covers about 12 percent of the population while Medicaid, a state- and federally-funded program for the indigent, provides benefits to another seven percent. These programs illustrate the tendency toward decentralization and fragmentation in the United States and the conviction, held at least among policy-makers, that health care is not a right of citizenship, as it is in Sweden and elsewhere, but a benefit of group membership (KIass 1985). Also, they ensure that it is the state, not the employers, that takes on the high cost of caring for those segments of the population with the greatest need.

Most American citizens obtain health protection in the private sphere. By the early 1980s, private insurance handled 81 percent of private consumer hospital expenditures and approximately 62 percent of physicians' charges (Gordon 1990). Today, about 57 percent of Americans are covered through occupational health insurance programs purchased for them by their employers from "third parties" as part of their benefits package. Another eight percent of Americans purchase health insurance directly from the commercial insurance industry on an individual basis. Contrary to popular belief, it is thus collective rather than individual purchases which predominate in the United States. Today over 1,500 companies are involved in health insurance. However, the major private nonprofit agencies, Blue Cross (for hospital insurance) and Blue Shield (for medical expenses), and the approximately 300 companies which comprise the Health Insurance Association of America are the major providers.[22]

Employment-based health insurance programs first began to spread in the 1930s and multiplied rapidly during the 1940s. Wartime wage controls and favourable tax legislation encouraged employers to offer a variety of "fringe benefit" programs as an alternative to wage increases. This expansion was given further impetus when the American Federation of Labour, thwarted in its attempts to expand public welfare protection, concentrated its efforts on the attainment of workplace welfare (Stevens 1990). But, while they are widespread today, employers are under no legal obligation to provide health insurance. More importantly, private occupational welfare serves to increase a worker's dependence upon the employer and the market. Workers seeking to change jobs may risk losing their benefits. Those individuals who must purchase their own insurance are, of course, even more dependent upon the market. Even those who can afford insurance are sometimes hesitant to risk increasing their premiums by using it. Facing soaring medical costs, insurance companies have recently become much less willing to continue to cover or take on those in poor health.

The Canadian approach to health care delivery diverged sharply from the American over two decades ago. With the passage of the Medical Care Insurance Act in 1966, and Ontario's entry into the federal scheme in 1972, Canada established a national, compulsory, health insurance system which is, in its essentials, very similar to the Swedish plan. While privately provided, health care in Canada is publicly funded, with costs shared by the provincial and federal governments, and administered by the provincial and territorial governments rather than the federal.[23] The passage of the Canada Health Act in 1984 ensured that Canada's health care system remained affordable by outlawing the "extra-billing" of patients above and beyond insurance coverage.[24] Most important, Canada's health insurance system is both compulsory and comprehensive. It includes all Canadians as a right of citizenship and covers most types of medical care (with a few exceptions such as eyeglasses, outpatient medications for those under 65 years of age, and cosmetic surgery). On the basis of these aspects of its health care system, Canada, like Sweden, falls within the social democratic world.

Orientation: Intervention/Prevention

One of the most definitive characteristics of social democratic regime policies is the emphasis placed on preventive measures. With regard to health care, this involves a recognition that ill-health is closely tied to a variety of interrelated "environmental" conditions such as poverty, unemployment, homelessness, and poor education which must be addressed before individual intervention can be effective. Sweden's social and economic policies and its elaborate welfare state are part of a coherent program which has been remarkably successful in altering those conditions by virtually eliminating poverty and unemployment. Specific problems, such as drug abuse and childhood disorders, are targeted through a variety of public preventive educational programs provided for students and parents (Nikelly 1987). By allowing parents to care for their sick children, the public provision of "parental insurance" discourages the development of minor ailments into more serious illnesses.[25]

In addition to the benefits and preventive measures described above, Sweden's national health insurance plan provides compensation for income lost due to disability or illness. Indeed, when the national health insurance plan was introduced, "cash sickness benefits" were easily the most important and expensive component. Today, these earnings-related sickness insurance benefits cover over 90 percent of economically active Swedes between the ages of 15 and 64. Stay-at-home spouses and unmarried parents of children under 16 years of age are also eligible for a flat-rate cash benefit which can be "topped up" with voluntary insurance. A recent study demonstrated that, of those nations offering such coverage, Sweden was among the most generous in terms of replacement levels (90 percent of gross income up to a ceiling), length of compensation period (no maximum), length of waiting period before benefits can be collected (0 days) and other qualifying conditions (Kangas 1991).[26] In keeping with the public orientation of health care, the private provision of such sickness benefits plays only a very minor role in Sweden (Kangas and Palme 1991).

Health and other programs in the United States are highly fragmented and largely geared toward intervention. There is a much greater tendency to hold individuals, rather than their environments, responsible for their plight. Americans are, for the most part, expected to manage their own health care and seek treatment when they become ill. However, preventive programs, designed to reduce many companies' rapidly increasing health care expenditures, have recently begun to proliferate in the private sphere.[27] Two out of three firms in the United States employing over fifty workers now provide some type of "wellness" plan which may provide prenatal/nutritional courses, fitness centres, or rebates for those individuals who manage to stay well (Schwartz and Padgett 1989). Finally, given the absence of a national public sector income maintenance insurance program, most Americans must rely on their employers for sick leave, although a few states (California, Hawaii, New Jersey, New York, and Rhode Island) do offer compulsory temporary disability insurance (Gordon 1990).

By virtue of its health insurance program alone, health care in Canada is oriented somewhat more strongly toward prevention than is that in the United States. The existence of "free" universal care allows those Canadians most vulnerable to illness, such as the poor and the unemployed, to make precautionary visits to their physicians and to take other prophylactic measures. Indeed, the numbers of checkups and prenatal consultations carried out among low-income Canadians increased dramatically with the introduction of medicare. Although there is, strictly speaking, no sickness insurance in Canada, provisions for time-limited sickness benefits have been provided since 1971 through the Unemployment Insurance Act. Nevertheless, compared to its Swedish counterpart, the Canadian health care system, like its welfare state generally, is geared more toward cure than care. Canada clearly falls between Sweden and the United States on this measure of health care provision.

Conclusion

The Canadian welfare state has been viewed by some as "advanced" while others have depicted it as stunted. An attempt has been made here to reconcile such disparate judgements and locate Canada's welfare state. The conclusions reached regarding the nature of social policy in Canada have much to do with the particular model used and the types of policies and dimensions (e.g., expenditures) emphasized. The most popular of these, the welfare worlds approach, has focused primarily upon social security and suggests that Canada and the United States are much more similar than different. However, despite Canada's increasingly common designation as a liberal welfare regime, certain social service programs, such as the Canadian health care system, are not so easily categorized. While it closely resembles the liberal regime along one dimension (organization of the health economy), it is much closer to the social democratic regime in terms of the second (coverage), and falls somewhere between the two models on the third dimension (orientation). It is also positioned midway between Sweden and the United States in terms of expenditures and outcomes.

The comparative overview of health care systems here suggests that the welfare worlds approach has not adequately represented the various dimensions of particular social policies, ignoring social services in favour of examining income transfer programs. In order to adequately represent various national welfare states, the welfare worlds approach must include this central element. While the focus here has been on health care, studies comparing other social service elements of the welfare state, such as education and housing, must also be conducted if the model is to reflect adequately the nature of welfare states. In addition, it has been suggested here that studies of welfare programs can more accurately classify them if they more closely examine the various dimensions of particular social policies. It may be useful, therefore, to re-introduce into such analyses the concept of multiple continua. As demonstrated in the present paper, a particular policy may be classified as liberal on one dimension but as social democratic on another. A multidimensional conceptualization not only permits a more precise evaluation of social policies and welfare states but also makes it easier to track abrupt or incremental changes in the direction of particular social policies and the gradual restructuring of the welfare state currently under way in most capitalist nations, reflecting significant changes in the balance of power in each.[28]

It would be entirely premature to suggest that we are witnessing a gradual "convergence" of the three welfare states under consideration here toward a more "mixed" approach. However, significant developments are taking place that cannot be ignored. In Sweden, where a strong labour movement and decades of social democratic rule have served to entrench the welfare state, changes to the health system have been, so far, much less dramatic than those seen in other European nations or in North America during the recent period of retrenchment and welfare "crisis." Yet even Sweden has not been totally immune to change. A privatization campaign organized by powerful business interests in the 1980s bore fruit beginning with the creation of new private health insurance schemes by companies such as Skandia, and the takeover of a hospital in Stockholm (Sophiahemmet) by the Wallenberg Empire in 1987. With the election of the "bourgeois coalition" government in September 1991, employer demands for changes to the public sickness insurance plan are beginning to be realized as well.[29] Even more recently, a variety of market-oriented reforms have been introduced or proposed for health care delivery in Stockholm county through the so-called "Stockholm Model" (Diderichsen 1993). In the United States, as numerous companies cutback contributions to their private health care programs and increasingly stringent eligibility rules ensure that ever fewer Americans are covered by public insurance, many of the leaders of the large corporations (such as Bethlehem Steel, Chrysler, and General Motors) have expressed a strong desire for the creation of some type of public insurance system which would shift the financial burden from their shoulders onto the state. As the Clinton government cautiously engages in health care reform, the Canadian health care system has been beset by federal and provincial cutbacks and calls for user-fees are now the order of the day. The distinction between the Canadian and American welfare systems outlined here soon may be only academic if the current trends continue.

Notes

1   The gradual unstringing of the safety net since the mid-1980s through a series of cutbacks and "clawbacks" (family allowances and Old Age Security), the elimination of federal contributions to Unemployment Insurance and the eventual "replacement" of the Family Allowance program, has further "Americanized" the welfare state in Canada. For an overview of some of these developments see Gray (1990) and Mishra (1990).

2   According to a recent Environics poll, Canadians ranked health care "first out of 15 items that made Canada superior to the U.S." (quoted in Armstrong and Armstrong 1991: 3–4). Another survey indicated that, while 61 percent of Americans would prefer the Canadian health care system to their own, only 3 percent of Canadians would prefer the American health care system to their own (Blendon 1989; Blendon and Taylor 1989).

3   Given the nations under scrutiny here, the conservative social policy regime will not be examined. In this "corporatist" regime-type, the concern with market efficiency and commodification that characterizes liberal regimes is not salient. Occupational welfare and private insurance thus play a minimal role. Instead, welfare provision occurs largely through the state. However, benefits are provided in a manner that serves to maintain status differences within the population, rather than to redistribute wealth. Austria, France, Germany, and Italy would be considered conservative welfare regimes.

4   However, a high level of private welfare does not necessarily imply a low level of public welfare. For example, the growth of public welfare may trigger further development of occupational welfare, rather than replace or curtail it. Or, as is presently the case in many capitalist societies, public and private welfare may be pared back simultaneously as the state and private enterprises attempt to cut costs.

5   Occupational pensions, for example, covered approximately 37 percent of the total labour force in Canada in 1984 and almost 42 percent in the United States in 1985 (Deaton 1989).

6   The Social Security Act of 1935 established three main programs: (1) federally subsidized, state-administered public assistance programs for the elderly poor (replaced by Supplemental Security Income (SSI) in 1971), dependent children (Aid to Families with Dependent Children (AFDC) or "welfare"), and the blind; (2) federal unemployment insurance based on employer taxes set by the states; and (3) national, contributory old-age insurance (OAS or "social security"). Survivors' benefits for widows and children of the insured were added to

the latter in 1939 (OASI), as was Disability Insurance (OASDI) for severely disabled workers in 1956.

7   The Canadian welfare state "evolved" through the gradual establishment of major social programs – old age assistance (1927), industrial accident insurance (1930), unemployment insurance (1940), family allowances (1944), old age security (1951), hospitalization insurance (1961), sickness insurance (1971) and health insurance (1972) – as in Europe, if at a somewhat slower pace and later date. The United States, in contrast, has no public, universal family allowance, old age, pensions, or sickness and health insurance (Kudrle and Marmor 1984; Lemen 1977).

8   Following public pensions, public health care is the second most expensive element of the welfare state (OECD 1987; 1988). Although the health care information introduced here may not be new to those with an interest in social policy and health care, the purpose of the comparative presentation of the various traits of social welfare is to help characterize and situate the Canadian welfare state.

9   These were formerly called children's allowances because the amount of income they provided depended upon the number of children in the family (Gordon 1990).

10 In his widely cited work on the welfare state, Richard M. Titmuss (1963) distinguished between "social welfare," "occupational welfare," and "fiscal welfare." These labels are still quite useful as a means of distinguishing between types of welfare measures.

11 Only Austria and France paid out higher levels of cash benefits.

12 There is a parallel here with the pension system. Old age security in Canada is provided through a Swedish style three-tier system (universal public pensions, earnings-related pensions, occupational pensions) but public pension payments are grossly inadequate, as they are in the United States (Myles 1989).

13 As a result of their partial "de-indexation," the value of the Family Allowances provided in Canada was eroding through inflation and many families were losing most of their benefits in a "clawback" when they filed their annual income tax returns. As of January 1993, Canada's universal family allowance system ("baby bonus") was eliminated altogether and replaced by tax credits, a change that ended a long-standing universal program in Canada.

14 While women have a relatively high rate of labour force participation in Sweden, it should be noted that, during the late 1980s, approximately 43.5 percent of these women worked part-time. However, almost all of these female part-time workers worked "long" part-time hours (between 20 and 34 hours per week) (Persson 1990).

15 Introduced in 1973, it included the following entitlements by the latter part of the 1980s: (1) ten days leave of absence at 90 percent of pay for new fathers upon the birth of a child to allow them to care for their partners and newborns; (2) a total of twelve months parental leave (taken by either parent or shared) at 90 percent of salary and an additional three months at the national flat-rate pay level; and (3) two paid "contact days" per child per year off work to enable parents to spend time with their children to get acquainted with day care facilities and make contact with the staff. As discussed below, it also provides "sick leave" for parents when their children are sick (Hwang and Broberg 1992; Persson 1990). For a critique of the parental insurance program from a feminist perspective see Karin Widerberg (1991).

16 A new law implemented by the Clinton administration now provides women with twelve weeks of unpaid maternity leave. However, it does not cover women employed in small businesses (fewer than fifty employees).

17 Newhouse (1977) and others (OECD 1990) maintain that health care expenditure is positively associated with per capita income. This would appear contrary to arguments by Sombart (1976 [1906]) and Anderson (1978), among others, which suggest that high income

levels were partly responsible for the relative underdevelopment of the American welfare state.

18 Founded in 1948 by the Labour government, the National Health Service was created to provide free, quality medical treatment financed through taxation.

19 A recent examination of the pharmaceutical industry in the United States described it as the most profitable business in America. Moreover, Drake and Uhlman (1993: 4) note that "prescription drug prices rose three times faster than inflation in the last decade, and [that] the industry has circumvented every effort by the government to contain prices." The American government has, however, had some success in regulating the delivery of health care in the United States more directly since 1983 when it introduced diagnostic related groups (DRG). The DRG system provides the government with some control over physicians and hospitals by setting fixed prices for the treatment of certain categories of illnesses (see Ruggie 1992).

20 For many years, lobbying efforts by the American Medical Association and the pharmaceutical and insurance industries as well as numerous government officials were highly successful in short-circuiting any discussion of the Canadian health care system by equating it with "socialism" (Kudrle and Marmor 1984).

21 However, while Canada has not been as successful as Scandinavia or other European countries in keeping down the costs of drugs, wholesale prices in Canada are, on average, 30 percent lower than those in the United States largely as result of government efforts (Drake and Uhlman 1993). This may change with the introduction of a new bill (C-91) which dramatically and retroactively extends the patent period on prescription drugs to twenty years.

22 The existence of myriad insurance providers and the administrative costs implied by the attendant multitude of fee schedules and variations in eligibility, deductibles, and co-payments is one reason commonly cited for exorbitant health care expenditures in the United States. Woolhandler and Himmelstein (1991), for example, note that the proportion of health care costs consumed by administration in 1983 was 60 percent higher in the United States than in Canada. By 1987, administrative costs amounted to 19.3 to 24.1 percent of total health costs in the United States but only 8.4 to 11 percent in Canada. In addition to the rising health costs associated with expensive new technologies, high-income physicians, and the increasing numbers of aged that affected most industrial societies, other important factors which are more specific to the United States include the duplication of services and technology utilized by competing medical institutions, and the malpractice system (the number of suits filed each year and the consequent need for malpractice insurance) (Public Agenda Foundation 1992).

23 Critics of public sector health care systems maintain that they stifle innovation, are technologically less well-equipped, and result in longer waiting periods for treatment (OECD 1990). Supporters of such systems point out in response that waiting lists may exist for elective, cosmetic and diagnostic surgery, but not for life-saving procedures. Moreover, they maintain that public health care systems have adequate levels of technological support (Rublee 1989). See Diderichsen and Lindberg (1989) and Ingemar Stahl (1981) for a critical evaluation of health care delivery in Sweden.

24 Critics charge that this only encourages doctors, who are paid on a fee-for-service or "piecework" basis, to further increase the numbers of patients seen, tests administered, etc.

25 In the 1980s parental insurance in Sweden allowed either parent to take up to 60 days per year off work to care for their sick children and receive 90 percent of their pay. This was gradually increased to 90 days – up to 120 days per year if the child was unable to stay in the place where care was normally provided (Hwang and Broberg 1992; Persson 1990). However, these benefits recently have been reduced.

26 Critics of Sweden's cash sickness program charge that its overly generous provisions are primarily responsible for the internationally high levels of absenteeism there; at 23.4 sick days for the average worker, the absentee rate in 1989 was almost 3 times as high as it was in North America. However, supporters of the plan suggest that, unlike workers in North America, workers in Sweden are not economically constrained from staying home when they are sick. As a result, workers are less likely to develop more serious illnesses and are less of a financial burden on the welfare state.

27 In 1990 General Motors, for example, spent more on health care benefits ($3.2 billion) than it spent on steel.

28 Accounts of policymaking in capitalist society have become increasingly sophisticated, taking a variety of social and political factors into consideration. Approaches examining the balance of power between capital and labour have contributed significantly to our understanding of the origins and development of welfare states. On this approach see Esping-Andersen (1985), Korpi (1983), O'Connor (1989), and Stephens (1980). For constructive critiques of this model see Baldwin (1989), Kelman (1990), and Olsen (1990; 1991; 1992).

29 The new Prime Minister and Conservative Party leader of the new four-party right-wing coalition (Carl Bildt) introduced a one-day waiting period for cash sickness benefits and made employers responsible for compensation during the first fourteen days of a period of illness. Forcing employees to apply to their employer for benefits during this period, they maintain, will cut down on "abuse" of the benefit program and lower rates of absenteeism. In addition, cash sickness benefits have been reduced from 90 percent replacement level to 80 percent while fees for visits to the doctor and charges for prescriptions were increased.

Acknowledgements

The author would like to thank Bob Brym, Joan Durrant, Julia O'Connor and the anonymous reviewers from the Canadian Journal of Sociology for their helpful comments.

References

Andersen, O. 1972. *Health Care: Can There Be Equity? The United States, Sweden, and England.* New York: Wiley.

Anderson, D. 1991. *The Unfinished Revolution: The Status of Women in Twelve Countries.* Toronto: Doubleday Canada.

Anderson, M. 1978. *Welfare: The Political Economy of Welfare Reform in the U.S.* Stanford, Calif: Hoover Institute Press.

Armstrong, P, and H Armstrong. 1991. *Health Care as a Business: The Legacy of Free Trade.* Ottawa: Canadian Centre for Policy Alternatives.

Baldwin, P. 1989. The Scandinavian Origins of the Social Interpretation of the Welfare State. *Comparative Studies in Society and History* 31(1): 3–24.

Blendon, RJ. 1989. Three Systems: A Comparative Survey. *Health Management Quarterly* 11(2): 2–10.

Blendon, RJ, and H Taylor. 1989. Views on Health Care: Public Opinion in Three Nations. *Health Affairs* 8(1): 149–157.

Bernard, E. 1992. The Politics of Canada's Health Care System. *New Politics* 3(4): 101–108.

Borgenhammar, E. 1984. Sweden. In M Raffel ed. *Comparative Health Systems.* University Park: Pennsylvania State University Press.

Bronfenbrenner, U. 1992. Child Care in the Anglo-Saxon Mode. In ME Lamb, KJ Sternberg, C P Hwang, and AG Broberg eds. *Child Care in Context: Cross-Cultural Perspectives.* Hillsdale, NJ: Lawrence Erlbaum.

Cook, K. 1986. *Report of the Task Force on Child Care.* Ottawa: Ministry for the Status of Women.

Courchene, M. 1989. *The Current Industrial Relations Scene in Canada: Wages, Productivity and Labour Costs.* Kingston: Industrial Relations Centre, Queen's University.

Deaton, RL. 1989. *The Political Economy of Pensions: Power, Politics and Social Change in Britain, Canada and the United States.* Vancouver: University of British Columbia Press.

Deviney, S. 1984. The Political Economy of Public Pensions: A Cross-National Analysis. *Journal of Political and Military Sociology* 12(Fall): 295–310.

Diderichsen, F. 1993. Market Reforms in Swedish Health Care: A Threat or Salvation for the Universalistic Welfare State? *International Journal of Health Services* 23(1): 185–87.

Diderichsen, F, and G Lindberg. 1989. Better Health – But Not For All: The Swedish Public Health Report. *International Journal of Health Services* 19(2): 221–255.

Drake, D, and M Uhlman. 1993. *Making Medicine Making Money.* Kansas City: Andrews and McMeel.

DuBroy, R. 1986. *A Comparison of Compensation in Canada and the United States: Report 08-86.* Ottawa: Conference Board of Canada.

Esping-Andersen, G. 1985. *Politics Against Markets.* Princeton: Princeton University Press.

Esping-Andersen, G. 1990. *The Three Worlds of Welfare Capitalism.* Princeton: Princeton University Press.

General Accounting Office. 1991. *Canadian Health Insurance: Lessons for the United States.* Washington: General Accounting Office.

Goelman, H. 1992. Day Care in Canada. In ME Lamb et al. eds. *Child Care in Context: Cross-Cultural Perspectives.* Hillsdale, NJ: Lawrence Erlbaum.

Gordon, MS. 1990. *Social Security Policies in Industrial Countries: A Comparative Analysis.* Cambridge: Cambridge University Press.

Gray, G. 1990. Social Policy by Stealth. *Policy Options* (March): 17–29.

Hwang, CP, and AG Broberg. 1992. The Historical and Social Context of Child Care in Sweden. In ME Lamb, KJ Sternberg, CP Hwang, and AG Broberg eds. *Child Care in Context: Cross-Cultural Perspectives.* Hillsdale, NJ: Lawrence Erlbaum.

Kangas, O. 1991. *The Politics of Social Rights.* Stockholm: Swedish Institute for Social Research.

Kangas, O, and J Palme. 1991. Statism Eroded? Labour Market Benefits and Challenges to the Scandinavian Welfare States. In EJ Hansen, S Ringen, H Usitalo, and R Erikson eds. *Welfare Trends.* New York: Sharpe.

Kelman, H. 1990. Social Democracy and the Politics of Welfare Statism. *The Netherlands' Journal of Social Sciences* 26(1): 17–34.

Klass, GM. 1985. Explaining America and the Welfare State: An Alternative Theory. *British Journal of Political Science* 15: 427–450.

Korpi, W. 1983. *The Democratic Class Struggle.* London: Routledge and Kegan Paul.

Korpi, W. 1989. Power, Politics and State Autonomy in the Development of Social Citizenship: Social Rights During Sickness in 18 OECD Countries Since 1930. *American Sociological Review* 54(3): 309–328.

Kudrle, RT, and TR Marmor. 1984. The Development of Welfare States in North America. In P Flora and AJ Heidenheimer eds. *The Development of Welfare States in North America.* London: Transaction Books.

Kurian, GT. 1990. *Facts on File National Profiles: Scandinavia.* Oxford: Facts on File.

Lamb, ME, K Sternberg, CP Hwang, and AG Broberg. 1992. The Child Care in the United States: The Modern Era. In ME Lamb et al. eds. *Child Care in Context: Cross-Cultural Perspectives.* Hillsdale, NJ: Lawrence Erlbaum.

Lemen, C. 1977. Patterns of Policy Development: Social Security in the United States and Canada. *Public Policy* 25(2): 261–291.

Lipset, SM. 1986. Historical Traditions and National Characteristics: A Comparative Analysis of Canada and the United States. *Canadian Journal of Sociology* 11(2): 113–155.

Lipset, SM. 1990. *Continental Divide: The Values and Institutions of the United States and Canada.* New York: Routledge.

Mayfield, M. 1990. *Work-related Child Care in Canada.* Ottawa: Labour Canada.

Mishra, R. 1990. *The Welfare State in Capitalist Society: Policies of Retrenchment in Europe, North America and Australia.* Toronto: University of Toronto Press.

Myles, J. 1989. *Old Age in the Welfare State: The Political Economy of Public Pensions.* Lawrence: University of Kansas Press.

Myles J, and D Forcese. 1981. Voting and Class Politics in Canada and the United States. *Comparative Social Research* 4: 3–31.

National Council of Welfare. 1988. *Child Care: A Better Alternative.* Ottawa: Minister of Supply and Services.

Newhouse, JP. 1977. Medical Expenditure: A Cross-National Survey. *The Journal of Human Resources* 12(1): 115–125.

Nikelly, AG. 1987. Prevention in Sweden and Cuba: Implications for Policy Research. *Journal of Primary Prevention* 7(3): 117–131.

O'Connor, JS. 1989. Welfare Expenditure and Policy Orientation in Canada in Comparative Perspective. *Canadian Review of Sociology and Anthropology* 26(1): 127–150.

OECD. 1987. *Financing and Delivery of Health Care: A Comparative Analysis of OECD Countries.* Paris: OECD,

OECD. 1988. *Reforming Public Pensions.* Paris: OECD.

OECD. 1990. *Health Care Systems in Transition: The Search for Efficiency.* Paris: OECD.

Olsen, GM. ed. 1988. *Industrial Change and Labour Adjustment in Sweden and Canada.* Toronto: Garamond Press.

Olsen, GM. 1990. Swedish Social Democracy and Beyond: Internal Obstacles to Economic Democracy. In L Haiven, S McBride, and J Shields eds. *Regulating Labour: The State, Neo-Conservatism and Industrial Relations.* Toronto: Garamond.

Olsen, GM. 1991. Labour Mobilization and the Strength of Capital: The Rise and Stall of Economic Democracy in Sweden. *Studies in Political Economy* 34: 109–145.

Olsen, GM. 1992. *The Struggle for Economic Democracy in Sweden.* Aldershot: Avebury.

Olsen, GM, and RJ Brym. 1994. Between American Exceptionalism and Social Democracy: Public and Private Pensions in Canada. In M Shalev ed. *Occupational Welfare and the Welfare State in Comparative Perspective.* New York: Plenum Press.

Olsson, S. 1988. Social Welfare in Economically Advanced Countries: Social Services and Social Security in Sweden. In J Dixon and R Scheurell eds. *Social Welfare in Developed Market Countries.* London: Croom Helm.

Olsson, S. 1990. *Social Policy and the Welfare State in Sweden.* Lund: Arkiv.

Persson, I. 1990. The Third Dimension – Equal Status Between Men and Women. In I Persson ed. *Generating Equality in the Welfare State: The Swedish Experience.* Oslo: Norwegian University Press.

Public Agenda Foundation. 1992. *The Health Care Crisis: Containing Costs, Expanding Coverage.* New York: McGraw Hill.

Rublee, DA. 1989. Medical Technology in Canada, Germany and the United Stares. *Health Affairs* 8(3): 178–181.

Ruggie, M. 1992. The Paradox of Liberal Intervention: Health Policy and the American Welfare State. *American Journal of Sociology* 97(4): 919–44.

Schieber GJ, and JP Poullier. 1989. International Health Care Expenditure Trends: 1987. *Health Affairs* 8(3): 169–177.

Schwartz, J, and T Padgett. 1989. Wellness Plans: An Ounce of Prevention. *Newsweek,* January 30.

Serner, U. 1980. Swedish health legislation: Milestones in reorganization since 1945. In AJ Heidenheimer and N Elvander eds. *The Shaping of the Swedish Health System.* New York: St. Martin's Press.

Sombart, W. 1976. *Why is There no Socialism in the United States?* New York: ME Sharpe Inc.

Stahl, I. 1981. Can Equality and Efficiency be Combined? The Experience of the Planned Health Care System. In Ma Olsen ed. *A New Approach to the Economics of Health Care.* Washington: American Institute for Public Policy Research.

Stephens, JD. 1980. *The Transition From Capitalism to Socialism.* London: Macmillan.

Stevens, B. 1990. Labor Unions, Employee Benefits, and the Privatization of the American welfare state. *Journal of Policy History* 2(3): 233–260.

Titmuss, RM. 1963. *Essays on the Welfare State.* London: Allen and Unwin.

Widerberg, K. 1991. Reforms for Women – on Male Terms – the Example of the Swedish Legislation on Parental Leave. *International Journal of the Sociology of Law* 19: 27–44.

Wennemo, I. 1992. The Development of Family Policy: A Comparison of Family Benefits and Tax Reductions for Families in 18 OECD Countries. *Acta Sociologica* 35: 201–217.

Woolhandler, S, and DU Himmelstein. 1991. The Deteriorating Administrative Efficiency of the U.S. Health Care System. *New England Journal of Medicine* 324(18): 1253–1258.

32

Fiscal Crisis and Restructuring in Medicare: The Politics of Health in Canada*

M. Burke, and H. Michael Stevenson

Introduction

Health care in Canada is very much a political issue. As in all modern states, government in Canada is involved in such matters as the regulation of the health professions, the financing of hospitals and other medical research and educational facilities, the regulation of health and safety standards, and the legislation of workers' disability insurance. Most obviously, health care is political as a result of the complex federal-provincial arrangements for government insurance of hospital and medical services put in place between the late 1950s and the early 1970s. The development of this system of public health insurance politicized health care issues by increasing conflict between the state and the medical profession, and by helping to make the provision of universally accessible and high quality medical services a key public value and expectation.

The full-scale development of Canadian medicare had barely been completed before Canadian governments were faced with a fiscal crisis resulting from the global constraints on growth in capitalist countries that have persisted since the mid 1970s. Heavy public expenditures in the health sector pushed against the constraints of fiscal incapacities. The inevitable consequences for the increased politicization of health issues have been dramatized by physician strikes, government caps on health budgets, and a series of initiatives to restructure the provision of health services.

Although health policy and politics are for these reasons interesting topics for professional students of politics, they do not attract great attention from Canadian political scientists. An informal poll of departments of political science in Canada shows that there are only two in which a course on health issues is offered. Further, a review of the literature suggests that there is very little work on such issues done by political scientists using the theoretical perspectives of their discipline. Rather than systematically reviewing this sparse literature, this paper seeks to suggest ways in which the current fiscal crisis and restructuring in Canadian medicare can

* Reprinted from *Health and Canadian Society*, Vol. 1, No. 1, M. Burke and H. Michael Stevenson, 'Fiscal crises and restructuring in medicare: The politics of health in Canada,' pp. 51–80, 1993, with permission from the publisher.

be illuminated from the point of view of contemporary political theory, specifically the theory of the welfare state.

Capitalist welfare states developed over a long period from the late nineteenth century, but with particular intensity just before and after World War II (Cox 1987). Their development involved a qualitative change in the role of government in the economy and society, with greater government intervention in the economy, following Keynesian principles; a more articulated system of labour relations, with greater government regulation of unions and labour disputes; and a massive expansion of the role of government in the areas of health, education, and welfare.

The timing and scope of these changes varied substantially across countries, but some such change occurred in all advanced capitalist states. The variation reflected differences in economic development and in associated class relations and political organization; but the regularity reflected the need in all such societies to solve the problems of laissez-faire, entrepreneurial capitalist development, culminating in the Great Depression. The "solution" was found in a Fordist regime of accumulation based on the synchronization of mass production and mass consumption, stabilized by a mode of regulation in which government took on the range of social and economic functions just described.

These arrangements in the welfare state were part of the solution, but also part of future problems. They led to a significant blurring of the real and ideological distinctions between public and private, which had protected the private realm of exploitation from public attack. They entailed a progressive expansion of the delivery through bureaucratic institutions of noncommodified goods and services in support of the reproduction of social relations needed to sustain the expanded reproduction of commodities. The contradictions of the welfare state were concentrated in this conflict between commodification and decommodification, with the latter initially sustaining but eventually undermining the former (Offe 1984; Gough 1979). In turn, these contradictions of the Fordist-Keynesian arrangement led to moves towards a new regime of accumulation and mode of regulation, exemplified by the post-Fordist emphasis on flexible accumulation and the neo-conservative concern with deregulation, privatization, recommodification, and retrenchment (Harvey 1989; Jessop 1989; King 1989; Myles 1988).

This kind of general argument about the inherent incompatibilities of welfare state capitalism is a common theme in contemporary political analysis, whether expressed in the essentially Marxist language of the "fiscal crisis of the state," resulting from contradictions between accumulation and legitimation (O'Connor 1973; Habermas 1973), and the political problems of the state, resulting from crises of representation (Poulantzas 1978) or what post-Marxists call the problem of hegemony (Laclau and Mouffe 1985); or whether expressed in the terms of liberal political sociology, as the problem of "demand overload" (Crozier et al. 1975), the "social limits to growth" (Hirsch 1978), or the "cultural contradictions of capitalism" (Bell 1978).

The development and current crisis of the Canadian government health insurance system clearly illustrate the contradictions and conflicts of welfare states in capitalist societies. Essentially a public insurance system that guarantees payment for medical services provided by private medical practitioners, Canadian medicare is consumed by the cost containment imperatives of the fiscal crisis. And it is constantly embroiled in conflict arising out of contradictory discourses which characterize health care either as a commodity sold on a market, albeit a highly regulated market, or as a decommodified public good provided through political arrangements.

This paper presents an overview and critique of contemporary Canadian studies of controlling health costs and restructuring health services in the light of this general perspective on the nature of the welfare state. It argues that without this perspective, and its focus on embedding the politics of health care in the systemic contradictions and conflicts of the wider political economy, such studies suffer from serious limitations. Specifically, we suggest that scholarly discussions of health costs in Canada tend to localize, isolate and compartmentalize health and related social issues as a self-contained policy field and an unassailable component of public expenditure. They also fail to apprehend the contradictory policy implications of their proposals for restructuring Canadian health care. We suggest, for instance, that the new social and environmental paradigm of health, on which many of the restructuring schemes are based, may have social consequences that are not only unintended but in direct opposition to the stated goals and objectives of those who wish to move beyond the constraints of the medical model. The new paradigm is itself an object of political and ideological struggle, invoked, variously, by the state and bureaucratic interests whose primary concern is to limit or reverse cost escalation and by activists and advocates whose main objective is to improve individual well-being and overall quality of life. The new paradigm's comprehensive conception of health can, through the politics of healthism, lead to a denial of the relevance of health as an objective of public policy. And its discursive themes of disease prevention, health promotion, iatrogenesis, individual and community empowerment, social networks, and family and home care can as easily become ideological justifications for the privatization and deregulation of health services, with all that implies for the quality and equality of care, as they can become mobilizing frameworks for a progressive transformation and democratization of social policy.

More generally, this paper is an attempt to probe beneath the inconsistencies regarding health care that are expressed at the level of appearance, in political conflicts, popular attitudes, and public policy. Diagnosis of the primary cause of the crisis in health-care funding points to both the frivolous demand for services and the oversupply of practitioners. Proposals for change call for the reintroduction of market discipline and the protection or strengthening of state intervention. The federal government reduces its financial commitment to health care at the same time as it pledges to continue its "strong defense" of the five principles of the *Canada Health Act*. This paper shows that these inconsistencies are more than minor disagreements on the surface of the politics of health care. Rather, they are indicative of fundamental conflicts about the functioning of the current health-care system and the criteria to be used in evaluating proposals for change, and also reflect real contradictions in the political and ideological practices of the social forces active in the debate on health and health care in Canada.

Any attempt to review the study of health-care policy in Canada is immediately confronted with the problem of focus. The literature is too vast and too specialized and the issues too complex to consider in a relatively short paper. Focussing on the politics of cost containment and restructuring is, we believe, appropriate. The political and economic necessity of controlling costs attends all discussions of health-care policy in Canada, sometimes at the centre of concerns, sometimes at the periphery. Often, it is intertwined with intergovernmental tension about the disjunction between constitutional responsibility and fiscal (in)capacity. For instance, uncertainty about the cost of a national programme of medical care was a concern from the beginning, which led to a delay in the implementation of medicare, the introduction of a new tax to help pay for the system, and the deterioration of federal-provincial relations (Taylor 1987). Recent developments like the move to block funding in 1977, the conflict over extra-billing, and Ottawa's freeze on per capita transfer payments for health and higher education, have ensured that financial considerations remain closely tied to health policy proposals. Observers agree that cost is once again "the dominant issue in Canadian health care" (Stoddart 1985: 5) and that "the politics of medical care is the politics of cost control" (Van Loon 1978: 455). The terms of reference of national and provincial health-care task forces and commissions appointed since 1983-84 confirm the overwhelming predominance of the issues of costs and restructuring (Angus 1992).

This focus means that important issues like innovations in health administration and management or the details of provincial public policy can be considered only insofar as they bear directly upon the national debate about cost and restructuring. But, generally speaking, our focus is expansive rather than restrictive in that it calls for the integration of at least some of the issues related to the role of state intervention in the health sector, the scholarly and ideological reconstruction of the concept of health, changes in the dominance of the medical profession, the rise of other health professions and occupations, and the growth of alternative modes of health-care delivery.

The Canadian Health-Care System

There are many analyses and reviews of the origins and development of the Canadian health-care system (Crichton and Hsu 1990; Evans and Stoddart 1989; LeClair 1975; Naylor 1986; Soderstrom 1978; Taylor 1987). Our purpose in this section is not to provide another systematic historical account of the establishment of public health insurance, but rather to highlight those compromises and contradictions in the evolution of Canadian health policy that have contributed significantly to the contemporary debate about health expenditures.

Four historical developments had a profound impact on the nature of the current crisis in health-care funding (Coburn et al. 1983; Taylor 1981, 1987; Van Loon 1978; Weller and Manga 1983a). First, under the National Health Programme of 1948, the federal government actively encouraged hospital construction to address what was perceived to be a marked shortage of hospital beds. Second, a system of government-sponsored health insurance, based initially on shared-cost agreements between the federal and provincial governments, became the instrument of health-care policy. Third, the government supported hospital insurance a full decade before it moved into the field of medical care insurance. Fourth, the dominance of the medical profession and the hegemony of the medical model of health were established prior to the implementation of public programmes in hospital and medical care.

The effects of these developments can be seen in the kind of health-care system that took shape. The open-ended nature of intergovernmental shared-cost agreements coupled with the timing of public programmes in hospital construction and hospital insurance led to the creation of an institutionally-based pattern of practice heavily weighted in favour of acute care treatment. Medical dominance encouraged the consolidation of a system that was oriented to curative rather than preventive care. The dominant position of physicians within the health field was also one factor producing a medical-care system based on the "insurance approach" of the public payment of private medical practice. That is, the health-care system in Canada, like other welfare state measures, emerged from specific social struggles that were ended, or at least mitigated, by a political compromise that changed but did not transform the existing circumstance. Forming the alliance in support of some scheme of public medical care were organized labour, social democracy, and reformist liberalism. Opposing its introduction were the medical profession, the commercial insurance industry, and their allies in certain sectors of the federal and provincial states. The struggle was "settled" by the implementation of a publicly funded and administered medical care insurance programme that provided universal and comprehensive first-dollar coverage on uniform terms and conditions (Taylor 1987). The settlement seriously weakened the private health insurance industry. And it represented an outright rejection of the medical profession's attempt to limit state involvement to the subsidization of the health care premiums of the poor. But it also affirmed and entrenched the professional autonomy and power of physicians (Naylor 1986). The insurance approach was based on providing public funds to support the demand for health care and therefore avoided direct state intervention on the supply side of the medical market. Although public health insurance did fundamentally alter the mode of health-care financing, it did not affect "the supply and mix of institutions and personnel or their income, location, and habits" (Manga and Weller 1980: 255). Nor did it affect the fee for service method of remunerating physicians. Private decisions continued to determine the content and context of medical practice.

The 1977 change in health-care financing, from shared-cost to block funding, halted the open-ended nature of federal transfer payments, made the provincial governments major players in the area of health-care financing and increased their incentives to control costs, and led to an escalation of conflict both between governments and between the medical profession and government. Despite this profound shift in the public funding of health, the Canadian health-care system had yet to resolve the irrationalities of its historical development, which had entrenched the private organization of medical practice and a large and expensive hospital sector. Even in the face of increasingly aggressive third party (provincial government) intervention in the setting of fees, the private practice/fee for service system allowed physicians to behave in a manner consistent with a "target income" approach to the provision of medical services (Barer and Evans 1989: 84). For any given arrangement over fees, physicians could alter the quantity and mix of services they provided in order to hit, or come close to hitting, their income target. Such targeting points to a fundamental property of the market in health services in Canada (Evans 1975: 155–165). That market is characterized by what has been termed *supplier-induced demand* (Rachlis and Kushner 1989: 123) or "producer sovereignty" (Stoddart 1985: 18), a condition that allows the providers of health care to have a significant impact on the nature and extent of services "demanded," the rate of utilization of those services, and the overall level of health expenditure.

The health service market, then, imposed limitations on government efforts to slow down the rate of growth in health costs. And governments continued to be confronted with the problems of heavy costs in the hospital sector and an oversupply of expensive acute care beds (LeClair 1975; Taylor 1981; Van Loon 1978; Weller and Manga 1983a). In short, the broad outlines of health-care expenditure had not been altered from the pattern established much earlier: physicians and hospitals remained the two most expensive components of the health care system throughout the decade of the 1980s (Canada Health and Welfare 1991a; Barer and Evans 1989).

The level of conflict, confrontation, and confusion in the health-care sector since the 1970s is evidence of large shifts in the ideological, political, and social terrain. The medical profession was under strain from the increase in specialization and fragmentation within its ranks, the expanding role of the state, the new organizational power of the hospital administrator, and economic restructuring that was destroying the class base of the physician as independent entrepreneur (Blishen 1969, 1991; Coburn et al. 1983; Wahn 1987). Additionally, the new social and environmental paradigm of health challenged the validity of the medical model, which had provided ideological justification for medicine's claims to expertise and dominance and had served as the rationale for the construction of the curative and hospital-based system of health services.

Based on the work of authors like Ivan Illich (1976) and Thomas McKeown (1978, 1979), the alternative paradigm represents a frontal assault on the major assumptions and tenets of the medical world view. It follows Hygeia instead of Asclepius (Dubos 1959) in offering an expansive conception of positive health that goes well beyond the medical concern with freedom from disease and injury; a privileging of the lifestyle, social, and environmental as opposed to the medical and therapeutic determinants of health; and an emphasis on disease prevention and health promotion rather than diagnosis and cure. Its political implications are no less subtle for the new model suggests that the provision of additional health services in the conventional form of more doctors and more hospitals has, at best, diminishing marginal returns for health outcomes. From a less benign point of view, it asserts that such a narrow focus on the health-care system may be indirectly harmful to personal and community health, because it reduces the resources available to other sectors, like the environment or the economy, whose improvement would have health-enhancing effects (Evans and Stoddart 1990). At worst, it sees medical interventions and the whole curative system as contributing directly to ill health through clinical iatrogenesis and the disempowering effects of the hierarchical structure of organized medical care (Illich 1976).

The rise of new health professions and occupations and the articulation and incipient organization of alternative modes of health-care delivery also challenged the physician and hospital components of the health sector. In Canada, as in the United States, the health labour force was transformed in the postwar period. In addition to relatively steady growth in the primary health professions of medicine, dentistry, pharmacy, and optometry, the past few decades witnessed strong, sometimes spectacular, increases in the numbers in complementary occupations like nursing, physiotherapy, and laboratory, respiratory and radiation technology (Aries and Kennedy 1990; Lomas and Barer 1989). As these groups and others emerged and pursued a political strategy of professionalization, they placed increasing pressure on the structures maintaining medical dominance:

Across Canada, nurses, optometrists, pharmacists, chiropractors, and psychologists, among others, are all seeking a place or a renewed position in the medical sun. In order to enhance their own prestige, power, and rewards, many of these occupations seize on professionalization, which for them means wriggling out from under the restrictive domination of medicine. Medicine is thus faced with a whole series of occupations either defending or seeking to establish their autonomy and/or actively chipping away at medical territory. (Coburn et al. 1983: 420)

The number of hospital workers in administrative and support services also rose dramatically, as part of the general increase in state workers and in response to the specific division of labour within the hospital sector (Armstrong 1977; Torrance 1987). The 1970s saw large gains in union membership among these workers and within some professional and technical units. By the end of the decade some 80 per cent of registered nurses and non-office staff in the hospital sector were included in collective agreements (Rose 1984: 107). Hospital unions were an especially militant force in a newly assertive public sector as hospital employees demanded distributional changes in the structure of remuneration and the locus of power (Deverell 1982; Laxer 1976; Smith 1984).

The increasing interest in various forms of medical group practice funded by capitation payments or global budgets – Health Service Organizations (HSOs), Community Health Centres (CHCs), and Local Community Service Centres in Quebec (CLSCs) – posed real alternatives to the conventional delivery system based on inpatient hospital care and fee for service payment of the physician in solo practice (Canada Health and Welfare 1972; Hastings 1986; Pineault 1984; Vayda 1977). This interest in alternative forms has diverse social and political origins. It emerged from trade union struggles to provide adequate medical care in the period before medicare (Lomas 1985). It has social democratic roots in community efforts to maintain the delivery of health services during the Saskatchewan doctors' strike against public medical insurance in 1962 (Badgley and Wolfe 1967), and in Quebec's attempts to reform its health-care system (Renaud 1987). It is related to the rise of new social movements in the 1960s and 1970s, themselves the product of changes in the class structure effected by postwar capitalist restructuring. Activists in groups like the peace movement, the women's movement, and the environmental movement helped to articulate the new social paradigm's critique of the medical model of health, and saw alternative modes of health-care delivery as an institutional means of challenging the medical hierarchy, democratizing the health sector, and empowering local communities (Lomas 1985; Stevenson and Burke 1991). Finally, in the period of fiscal crisis, the forces of bureaucratic rationalization in Canada became interested in the cost-containment potential of alternative medical group practice partly because of the economic efficiencies associated with the development of Health Maintenance Organizations in the United States (Hastings and Vayda 1989).

Medical and hospital associations interpreted the emerging interest in alternative forms as a threat to their place of prominence in the traditional division of labour in the health sector. Organized medicine mounted campaigns to defend physicians' market strength, professional autonomy, and clinical authority (Vayda 1977; Hastings 1986). Hospitals were concerned about the shift in emphasis to community centres and the general drift towards regional planning (Hastings and Vayda 1989). Curative, hospital-based medicine was weakened but far from defeated by the various forces assailing it. Measures of its continuing strength include the suppression of health occupations, like that of the nurse practitioner, whose members could substitute for physicians in the provision of certain medical services (Lomas and Barer 1989), the continued subordination of nursing (Warburton and Carroll 1988; Wotherspoon 1988), the medicalization of chiropractic as part of the price of (restricted) legitimation (Coburn and Biggs 1987), and the limited growth in the numbers and coverage of non fee for service medical groups (Hastings and Vayda 1989).

These diverse issues in the development of the Canadian health-care system are directly relevant to the current debate about containing health expenditures. That debate cannot be resolved without confronting questions regarding the efficiency and effectiveness of institutional and private practice care relative to alternative modes of delivery, the political power of the medical profession and the hospital sector, the level of organization and political strategy of health reformists, and the respective roles and responsibilities of the federal and provincial governments.

The Crisis in Health Care and Cost Containment Strategies

At the most basic level, the crisis in health care is directly related to the high cost of health services. And health care is expensive. In 1990, national health expenditures in

Canada amounted to some $60.2 billion, or $2,266 per capita (Canada Health and Welfare 1991a: 1–2). Comparatively, Canada's rate of per capita spending on health in 1987 was above that of every OECD country save the United States (Schieber and Poullier 1989). In 1987, total health expenditures in Canada were 8.6 percent of Gross Domestic Product and public health expenditures were 6.5 percent. Both shares stand above the OECD averages of 7.3 percent and 5.6 percent, respectively, although health spending in Canada is not markedly different from the pattern in Austria, France, Germany, the Netherlands, Ireland, Iceland, and Luxembourg (OECD 1990). At the provincial level, health-care costs account for approximately one-third of government budgets.

However large these figures may be, they can mystify as well as clarify the debate about health costs and restructuring. The "medicare crisis" is only partly about the absolute or relative level of expenditure on health. Consider the inconsistencies. The proposition that health-care costs were spiralling out of control became a political issue only in the 1970s, at the very moment that those costs stabilized, after two decades of steady growth, at just over 7 per cent of Gross National Product (Barer et al. 1979: 5–6; Barer and Evans 1989: 60–64; Canada Health and Welfare 1991a: 2; French 1978). Since that initial politicization, concern over expenditure escalation has remained high, seemingly unaffected by the many studies showing that, compared to the United States, the Canadian system of public health insurance has been remarkably successful in controlling costs (Detsky et al. 1990; Evans 1986, 1987; Evans et al. 1989, 1990; Himmelstein and Woolhandler 1986; Iglehart 1986; Manga and Broyles 1986; Marmor and Mashaw 1990; Woolhandler and Himmelstein 1991).

Across the Canadian health literature as a whole, the health-care crisis is portrayed as a sometimes contradictory amalgamation of the four components of escalation, underfunding, inefficiency, and ineffectiveness. First, governments are concerned that the already weighty costs of health care are rising too rapidly. Second, providers, especially physicians, contend that the health sector is seriously underfunded. Third, health economists suggest that health funding is wasteful and inefficient because the nature of the medical marketplace in Canada – the mixed system of private practice and public payment of first-dollar insurance coverage – provides no structural incentives for controlling costs. Fourth, health analysts also suggest that allocating funds to the existing health-care system may not be the most effective way of enhancing health.

Not surprisingly, given this multi-dimensional conception, the literature suggests several reasons for the onset and persistence of the crisis in funding health care, many of which have been mentioned above: ongoing federal-provincial conflict over the heavy financial responsibility for the health-care sector (Tuohy 1989a), increased political activity of the medical profession in the light of deteriorating incomes and threats to professional autonomy (Barer et al. 1979; Taylor 1981), a corresponding escalation in the organization and activity of non-medical professions and occupations within health services (Deber and Vayda 1985), the realization by some stakeholder groups that increasing expenditures on the health-care system may be a relatively ineffective way of improving health status and well-being (Evans and Stoddart 1990; Stoddart 1985), and the hegemony of free market ideology that constructs government intervention in health (and other social sectors) as an unnecessary and malign imposition on market forces (Evans 1984, 1987; Weller and Manga 1983b). There is also a direct expenditure component to the pervasive concern with a cost crisis: a "health spending 'breakout'" in 1982 saw a significant increase, for the first time in a decade, in the ratio of health expenditures to GNP (Barer and Evans 1989: 63; Evans et al. 1990). Proposals for controlling costs and restructuring health services proliferated as health expenditures became a constant focus of public policy.

It is not possible to review all of the attempts at, and proposals for, resolving the crisis in health-care funding. This section will mention only briefly those options, like user charges and partial controls on the physician and hospital sectors, that have been analyzed and evaluated in detail elsewhere. It will concentrate instead on describing those increasingly popular strategies that make explicit calls for profound change and have not yet been subjected to systematic political evaluation. These strategies will be the object of the critical analysis of the final section of this paper.

Direct Charges to Patients

The medical profession, often in alliance with the state, is the most consistent advocate of direct charges to patients, which may take various forms including extra billing, user fees, coinsurance, and deductibles. For instance, the 1977 joint report of the Ontario Medical Association and the Ontario Government recommended both subscriber charges for hospital admission and "balance billing" for payment of physicians (Ontario 1977). The justification for such charges is two-fold. First, the increase in health costs is defined as a demand problem that can be addressed by making patients pay a portion of the cost, thereby increasing their "awareness of, and responsibility for, use of the health care system" (Ibid. 13), curbing abuse, and moderating frivolous utilization. In this case, patient charges are a means of reducing the overall level of health-care spending. Second, and in direct opposition to the first rationale, user charges are viewed as a way of increasing total health expenditures by the addition of private funds (Barer et al. 1979: 2–3). For organized medicine, increased levels of funding from private sources offer the dual advantage of maintaining professional incomes and protecting professional autonomy from government encroachment (Weller and Manga 1983b).

However forcefully direct user charges are supported by organized medicine and government, even in the wake of the Canada Health Act, the verdict of the literature is unambiguous: "the direct charge concept is indeed an idea whose time has gone" (Barer et al. 1979: x). Extra billing, user fees, and the like impede equality of access to medical care, deter utilization by the poor, redistribute the burden of paying for health care from taxpayers to the sick, violate the principles on which the Canadian medical care system was established, do not make a contribution to overall expenditure control, and serve the interests of not the public, but providers, private insurance companies, and provincial governments (Barer et al. 1979; Manga 1983; Soderstrom 1987; Stoddart and Labelle 1985; Taylor 1981).

Adjustments to the Physician and Hospital Sectors

Proposals for adjustments to the physician and hospital sectors are responding in part to the historical overdevelopment of these components of the health-care system. They also emphasize the impact of supply on utilization and total expenditure, especially in regard to physicians:

The most important determinant of total health cost is the number of physicians practicing in the system. The costs attributable to physicians are not only their remuneration but also a sum, greater in amount, reflecting expenditures elsewhere in the system which result from professional decisions. The physician decides admission to hospital, duration of stay, the use of diagnostic and therapeutic procedures, prescription of drugs, referral to specialists and the pattern of further examinations. (LeClair 1975: 79)

The federal government, by agreement with the provinces, has attempted to limit overall supply by placing restrictions on the immigration of foreign physicians. Provincial governments have tried to affect the supply of physicians by placing controls on enrollments to medical schools, reducing the number of residency posts, and limiting the availability of new "rights" to bill the public medical plan. Efforts to hold down health costs have also caused governments to take a hard stand in negotiations with the medical profession, resulting in small increases in fees and in fee freezes and rollbacks. Other policy options used by government include "negotiated" caps on utilization to control total expenditures on medical services, increased monitoring of individual physicians to identify "anomalous" billing practices and discourage overservicing, and restrictions on the public compensation paid to physicians whose billings exceed a certain monetary threshold (Barer et al. 1992; Deber and Vayda 1985; LeClair 1975; Lomas and Barer 1989; Stoddart 1985; Tuohy 1989b).

In the hospital sector, governments have also employed various methods to limit increases in health expenditures, by using the relatively blunt instruments of closing hospitals, cutting beds, rearranging the system of budget allocation, and implementing freezes or ceilings on hospitals' capital and operating budgets. Hospitals have moved to alter the balance of service away from inpatient and acute care towards outpatient and chronic or rehabilitation care, contract out support services to the private sector, develop profit making ancillary services in areas like parking and catering, and encourage corporate management techniques emphasizing cost efficiencies (Auer 1987; Campbell 1988; Deber and Vayda 1985; Evans 1975; Hastings and Vayda 1989; Torrance 1987; Wahn 1987).

Such cost control mechanisms do not exhaust the options available to government. Governments use other means and health analysts propose other ways to manage health expenditures. But many of the options discussed in this section, and others like them, represent an ad hoc and incremental approach to resolving the crisis in health care funding (Auer 1987; Evans 1984; Hastings and Vayda 1989; Tuohy 1989a). Some policies, like rearranging hospital services and restraining physician fee increases, are opportunistic responses to immediate problems and do not represent a major challenge to the design of health-care delivery. Other options, however, pose more serious questions for the nature of health care. The privatization creep embodied in the practices of contracting out and corporate management will in the long run fundamentally alter the principles on which the health-care system was established. This threat to health and health care is addressed more fully in the final section of the paper. The proposals to be considered next, on the other hand, seek to protect those principles by promoting an explicit restructuring and redesign of health-care organization and delivery.

Restructuring Health Care

The proposals for cost containment and structural transformation discussed here, based on the new paradigm of health and health promotion, alternative modes of health-care delivery, alternative schemes of physician remuneration, and publicly financed competition, can be considered as a package of interrelated sub-strategies rather than as independent strategies for change. They emphasize the need for "the efficient production of health services" and "the provision of effective services in quantities sufficient to meet the health care needs of the population" (Stoddart and Labelle 1985: 6). Advocates of this package of proposals suggest that the savings engendered by such a move towards more efficient and effective production be reallocated within health services, or allocated to related sectors in which an influx of resources would produce outcomes beneficial to health and well-being (Rachlis and Kushner 1989).

An earlier section of this paper set out the broad outlines of the new paradigm of health and its themes of health promotion and disease prevention. In regard to the issue of expenditure control, the health promotion/disease prevention strategy offers to contain costs by discouraging those individual lifestyles and social conditions that produce ill health and encouraging those that foster well-being. In the long run, considerable savings may be achieved as the result of a decline in both the need for health care and the demand for health services. As the Minister of National Health and Welfare explains:

I am convinced that the focus of our system has to shift away from a curative approach to a preventive approach. It does not mean we will not continue to do anything we can to respond to disease after it occurs or respond to accidents after they occur. We have to do that, but it is infinitely cheaper for us to stop a child from ever starting to smoke than it is to treat somebody who contracts cancer. It is infinitely cheaper for us to educate people on how to avoid contracting AIDS than it is for us to provide services to them once they become infected with the disease. It is infinitely cheaper for us to prevent drug abuse and alcoholism in Canada than it is to treat the problem once it has occurred. (Cited in Canada 1991a: 27)

The discourse of health promotion also calls for a marked organizational shift from conventional to alternative modes of health-care delivery based on alternative methods of physician remuneration. Much of this discussion concerns the cost efficiencies of Health Service Organizations, Community Health Centres, and similar modes of medical practice. These efficiencies arise in two ways (Evans 1984). First, compared to conventional forms of medical practice, alternative organizations make better use of auxiliary personnel, nurse practitioners for instance, as substitutes for the high-cost option of care by a physician (Denton et al. 1983; Spitzer 1978). Second, the capitation or salary method of physician payment used by HSOs and CHCs does not encourage overservicing by practitioners and results in lower rates of hospital utilization than are found under fee for service arrangements (Boan 1966; Hastings et al. 1973; Hastings and Vayda 1989; but see Barer 1981, and Abelson and Lomas 1990).

The proposal to establish a system of publicly financed competition relies on these alternative forms of delivery and remuneration. It suggests that the lack of structural linkage is a critical deficiency of the Canadian health-care system: "The absence of any direct linkage between the authority to make production and utilization decisions and the financial responsibility for paying the bills for those decisions has led to unnecessarily high cost "styles of practice" (Stoddart and Labelle 1985: 60). The root of the problem lies in the incentive structure facing the public and the practitioner:

On one side of the coin, there is no incentive for patients to select a low-cost-style (efficient) provider – although that choice would reduce aggregate costs–for there is no way individual patients can be appropriately rewarded for such a selection ... On the other side of the coin, there is little or no incentive for individual physicians to exercise their discretion to offer lower-cost (to the public purse) styles of medicine, for practitioners cannot benefit substantially from such decisions. (Stoddart and Seldon 1984: 127–128)

Publicly financed competition rejects the strategy of increased public regulation in favour of one that rearranges structural (economic) incentives by giving an enhanced role to market forces "within the umbrella of a publicly financed, publicly monitored health-care system" (Stoddart 1985: 28).

This proposal supports the establishment of a system of competition among the fee for service, capitation, and salary "'modalities' of service delivery" (Stoddart and Seldon 1984: 131). Under such a scheme patients would be financially penalized, by being charged higher insurance premiums for health care, for enrolling in the more costly (less efficient) modalities of health-care delivery. And providers would be given an incentive to produce efficiently because they would "be seeking their incomes in competition with each other" (Ibid: 129).

The Politics of Cost Containment

This section examines the contradictory implications of this last group of proposals for resolving the problem of expenditure control by restructuring the health-care system. It points out the major political limitations of these proposals, and integrates a critique of the Canadian literature on cost containment with a discussion of the threats of reprivatization and privatization creep. Specifically, it suggests that the limitations of localism, therapeutic nihilism, healthism, and health promotion may contribute to the political and ideological strength of the forces diluting Canadian health care.

As we noted in the introduction, the Canadian literature on controlling health expenditure has, with a few exceptions (Armstrong and Armstrong 1990; Manga and Weller 1980; Swartz 1977; Walters 1982; Weller and Manga 1983b), tended to examine the health-care system in isolation from the larger question of the welfare state and its relation to capital accumulation and political-ideological struggle. This analytical localism encourages two political errors. First, the Canadian debate tends to assume too easily, or conclude too readily, that any savings derived from the introduction of cost efficiencies in the health sector will be redirected to health or to other areas of social expenditure that have health-enhancing effects (Stoddart and Labelle 1985: 58, 65). Rachlis and Kushner, for instance, after demonstrating the magnitude of savings that could be generated, suggest:

Before going any further, we need to issue a word of caution. These 'savings' must not be used to pay down governments deficits, nor to reduce taxes, however appealing such options will be to provincial governments. They must be ploughed back into the system to make it better. The whole point of this exercise is to improve health status and quality of care, not to cut health spending. The good news is that we can fund these improvements within existing health budgets. (Rachlis and Kushner 1989: 312)

This "word of caution" fails to acknowledge sufficiently that the question of "ploughing back" savings into the system is one of the fundamental political issues in the rationalization of health care. Assuming that the ultimate destination of savings will be the health or social sector becomes increasingly suspect once it is realized, from the perspective of contemporary political theory, that the welfare state itself and all components of social expenditure, not just health, are experiencing crisis, retrenchment and recommodification (Banting 1987a, 1987b; O'Connor 1989). In a period of fiscal constraint, the renewed government emphasis on the objectives of flexible accumulation, productivity, and international competitiveness is purchased at the expense of cutbacks in the social wage.

The first error promotes and is compounded by the second, a Canadian manifestation of what Paul Starr more generally refers to as "the politics of therapeutic nihilism" (Starr 1981). Many strategies for restructuring are founded upon the new social and environmental paradigm of health, particularly on its critique of the medical model and its attack on the current direction and organization of health services. But these strategies may have contradictory political implications. The attack on health services can undercut arguments in favour of improving access to, or securing adequate funding for, those services, especially in periods of generalized welfare state retrenchment. Starr makes this point in relation to social services as a whole:

At a time of fiscal austerity, when public services to the poor are frequently in jeopardy, it becomes extremely difficult to resist cutbacks if one simultaneously concedes that schools and hospitals, welfare programs and mental health centers, legal services and employment bureaus don't make much difference in the long run, or are positively damaging to the interests of the poor. The more one questions the ultimate value of the social services, the less urgent, the less vital equal access to them appear; furthermore, the more difficult it becomes to argue persuasively that the government should spend more on domestic needs. (Ibid: 437–438)

The objective here is not to rescue the medical model or minimize the problems associated with a system of health care based on that model. Nor is it to stifle social criticism. Rather, it is to note that this kind of critique of social policy and social services yields inconsistent political implications and can be put to diverse and opposed political purposes.

The new paradigm's expansive conception of the determinants of health can also engender a kind of "politics of healthism" evident in Canadian proposals for restructuring health care. The new model asserts that, because health is determined not only by the organization of health services but also by such factors as individual lifestyles and social and environmental conditions, governments must take into account the health consequences of policies in various sectors. This new accounting may have effects on the distribution of public funds:

Expansion of the health care system uses up resources which would otherwise be available to address those other factors. (Whether they would be so used or not, is another matter.) It follows that an expansion of the health care system may have negative effects on health. A *health* policy, as opposed to policies for *health care,* would have to take account of this balance. (Evans and Stoddart 1990: 57)

There are political dangers inherent in making health a super value against which all or many public policies are to be assessed (Crawford 1980). If such healthism allows governments the discursive space to claim that almost every expenditure has a health-enhancing effect, then health loses its value as a meaningful criterion of evaluation. And the rhetorical claims of government may bear little relation to the results of careful and professional programme study. To researchers, finding the proper or "healthy" balance between various categories of expenditure is a matter of detailed analysis. To governments that are ideologically inclined or under pressure to decrease "unproductive" spending and promote competitiveness, it may be a matter of selecting a convenient rationale for cutting costs in areas of least social resistance.

This last point brings up the whole question of the state's contradictory appropriation of the discourse of the new paradigm in health. Nowhere is this more evident than in the federal government's articulation of the policy of health promotion at the very same time as it vacates the field of health. Ottawa's verbal support for a programme of health promotion is well established and spans the change of government in 1984. The Lalonde report constructed a "health field concept" that drew explicitly on the new interest in the lifestyle, social, and environmental causes of illness, and proposed a health promotion strategy to achieve national objectives in health improvement (Lalonde 1974). The Epp document set out a health promotion framework for meeting the pressing challenges in health and improving quality of life (Epp 1986). The report of the first international conference on health promotion, co-sponsored by Health and Welfare Canada, became a major statement of the meaning and aims of programmes in health promotion (Ottawa Charter 1987). And recently, in response to a standing committee report on funding health care, the federal government affirmed its commitment to the pursuit of policies in illness prevention and health promotion (Canada Health and Welfare 1991b).

This last document is an effective illustration of the extent to which the federal government has assumed the language of health promotion. It is replete with all of the appropriate (and appropriated) terms and phrases: "Prevention and health promotion ... enhance self-care services, the expansion of home care services and the more effective utilization of health care professionals such as nurses, dietitians and therapists" (p. 13); "'Healthy' public policies and multisectoral approaches to health are important in addressing the prerequisites for health" (p. 17); "The federal government recognizes the importance of all Canadians being informed and knowledgeable participants in matters affecting their health" (p. 21). These themes emphasized in the discourse of health promotion are easily captured by neoconservative forces articulating an ideology of decentralization, flexibility, the intrusive state, individual responsibility, and the sanctity of the family.

The contradictory nature of the federal interest in health promotion emerges when practice is counterposed to discourse. Despite the strength of its documentary support for health and health promotion, the federal government has been abandoning the field of health over the last 15 years. Between 1975 and 1990, the federal government's contribution to total health expenditure declined from 30.8 per cent to 27.7 per cent (Canada Health and Welfare 1991a: 6). The series of unilateral reductions that Ottawa made in Established Programmes Financing transfers to the provinces in the 1980s will lead to a shortfall of some $3.3 billion in health funding in 1991-92 (Thomson 1991: 24–25). The Ontario government estimates that "the federal share of health care and post secondary education spending in Ontario has been reduced from a high of 52 per cent in 1979-80 to about 31 per cent in 1992-93" (Laughren 1992: 13).

The federal effort in the more circumscribed fields of alternative health-care delivery and health promotion programme development is equally inconsistent. Ottawa's offer of financial support for the establishment of Community Health Centres collapsed with the failure of intergovernmental negotiations over cost-sharing. Neither in the shift to block funding in 1977 nor in the 1984 *Canada Health Act* did the federal government resurrect its offer of start-up and capital funding for innovative organizational alternatives like CHCs (Hastings and Vayda 1989). With respect to health promotion, federal interventions since the Lalonde report have encouraged a limiting and conservative emphasis on individual risk factors and lifestyles to the neglect of movement on structural conditions in the society, economy, and environment (Bolaria 1988; Buck 1985; Evans and Stoddart 1990).

In sum, the limitations inherent in these various proposals to restructure Canadian health care can produce contradictory and unintended political consequences. On the one hand, the proposals represent real attempts to improve the quality, equality, and efficiency of health care. And they point to concrete deficiencies in the health sector which have mobilized constituencies for social change and caused the state to respond with incipient reforms. On the other hand, the proposals suffer from the limiting effects of localism, therapeutic nihilism, healthism, and the discourse of health promotion. Localism can encourage a critically uninformed and compartmentalized view of the health sector. Therapeutic nihilism can create obstacles to the protection of social expenditures. Healthism can dissipate the pursuit of the objectives of health and well-being. The individualist core immanent in the very discourse of health promotion, and part of the legacy of writers like Illich and McKeown, can frustrate collective efforts at change. These weaknesses are compounded in the course of political and ideological struggle. When they are mediated and appropriated by a neoconservative state concerned with controlling costs and ideologically committed to expanding the scope of market forces in health, they become forceful arguments promoting reprivatization and recommodification, despite overwhelming scholarly evidence that change in this direction is not the solution to the crisis in health care.

These general concerns do not exhaust the range of political contradictions in restructuring strategies. The details of some specific proposals for change also pose problems. For instance, schemes like publicly financed competition, that dismiss the need for increased regulation and call for a change in the structure of economic incentives to foster efficiency, can also reinforce privatization creep by providing support for neoconservative images of "the sloppy public sector" and "the efficient private sphere" (Armstrong and Armstrong 1990: 1).

Such contradictions and inconsistencies, both general and specific, raise questions of political practices, social alliances, and meaningful change. In the health sector, conservative governments and the medical profession form one alliance of mutual interest, and hospital workers, health advocates and other progressive social forces form another. To the extent that privatizing health care, or parts of health care, injects private funds into the system, it allows the state to manage the rate of growth in social expenditure and physicians to maintain their incomes. For hospital workers, on the other hand, creeping privatization means layoffs, unemployment, underemployment, deteriorating working conditions, and an intensification of labour (Armstrong and Armstrong 1990). For them, and others who realize that the real crisis is not one of cost containment but of protecting and extending the principles of medicare and the conditions enhancing health (Bryce 1991; Manga 1983), privatization is not the answer. Neoconservative success in dismantling health care and other components of the welfare state can be checked by strengthening the social, ideological, and institutional resources of opposition forces (Jessop 1989; King 1989; Mishler and Campbell 1978; O'Connor 1989).

Overcoming the deficiencies in health care demands the same kind of political strategy. To realize the objectives of reducing class and gender inequalities in health (D'Arcy and Siddique 1987; Grant 1988; Manga 1987; Rodwin 1988; Trypuc 1988), improving the health of aboriginal peoples (Frideres 1988; Shah and Farkas 1985; Siggner 1986; Weller 1981; Young 1987), eliminating work-related injuries and deaths (Dickinson and Stobbe 1988), and breaking down the barriers to health care experi-

enced by the poor (Ambrosio et al. 1992) requires close attention to political implications and political practices. It also requires moving beyond a concentration on savings
to focus on the need for the additional allocation of public funds to health and related
social sectors.

References

Abelson, J, and J Lomas. 1990. Do Health Service Organizations and Community Health Centres
    have Higher Disease Prevention and Health Promotion Levels than Fee-For-Service
    Practices? *Canadian Medical Association Journal* 142 (15 March): 575–581.

Ambrosio, E, D Baker, C Crowe, and K Hardill. 1992. *The Street Health Report. A Study of the
    Health Status and Barriers to Health Care of Homeless Women and Men in the City of
    Toronto.* (May).

Angus, DE. 1992. A Great Canadian Prescription: Take Two Commissioned Studies and Call Me
    in the Morning. In RB Deber and GG Thompson eds. *Restructuring Canada's Health
    Services System: How Do We Get There From Here?,* 49–62. Proceedings of the Fourth
    Canadian Conference on Health Economics, August 27-29, 1990. Toronto: University of
    Toronto Press.

Aries, N, and L Kennedy. 1990. The Health Labor Force: The Effects of Change. In P Conrad and
    R Kern eds. *The Sociology of Health and Illness: Critical Perspectives,* 3rd ed., 195–206.
    New York: St. Martin's Press.

Armstrong, H. 1977. The Labour Force and State Workers in Canada. In L Panitch ed. *The
    Canadian State: Political Economy and Political Power,* 289–310. Toronto and Buffalo:
    University of Toronto Press.

Armstrong, P, and H Armstrong. 1990. 'Is This Any Way to Run a Business?' Health Care in the
    Era of Free Trade. Unpublished manuscript.

Auer, L. 1987. *Canadian Hospital Costs and Productivity.* A Study Prepared for the Economic
    Council of Canada. Ottawa: Minister of Supply and Services, Canada.

Badgley, RF, and S Wolfe. 1967. *Doctors' Strike: Medical Care and Conflict in Saskatchewan.*
    Toronto: Macmillan.

Banting, KG. 1987a. *The Welfare State and Canadian Federalism,* 2nd ed. Kingston and
    Montreal: McGill-Queen's University Press.

Banting, KG. 1987b. The Welfare State and Inequality in the 1980s. *Canadian Review of
    Sociology and Anthropology* 24 (August): 309–338.

Barer, ML. 1981. *Community Health Centres and Hospital Costs in Ontario.* Occasional Paper
    13. Toronto: Ontario Economic Council.

Barer, ML, RG Evans, and GL Stoddart. 1979. *Controlling Health Care Costs by Direct Charges
    to Patients: Snare or Delusion?.* Occasional Paper 10. Toronto: Ontario Economic Council.

Barer, ML, and RG Evans. 1989. Riding North on a South-Bound Horse? Expenditures, Prices,
    Utilization and Incomes in the Canadian Health Care System. In RG Evans and GL
    Stoddart eds. *Medicare at Maturity: Achievements, Lessons and Challenges,* 53–163.
    Calgary: Banff Centre for Continuing Education.

Barer, ML, RG Evans, and DS Haazen. 1992. The Effects of Medical Care Policy in B.C.: Utilization Trends in the 1980s. In Deber and Thompson eds. *Restructuring Canada's Health Services System: How Do We Get There From Here?*, 13–17. Proceedings of the Fourth Canadian Conference on Health Economics, August 27–29, 1990. Toronto: University of Toronto Press.

Bell, D. 1978. *The Cultural Contradictions of Capitalism.* New York: Basic Books.

Blishen, BR. 1969. *Doctors and Doctrines: The Ideology of Medical Care in Canada.* Toronto: University of Toronto Press.

Blishen, B. 1991. *Doctors in Canada: The Changing World of Medical Practice.* Toronto: University of Toronto Press, in association with Statistics Canada.

Boan, JA. 1966. *Group Practice.* Royal Commission on Health Services. Ottawa: Queen's Printer.

Bolaria, BS. 1988. The Politics and Ideology of Self-Care and Lifestyles. In BS Bolaria and HD Dickinson eds. *Sociology of Health Care in Canada,* 537–549. Toronto: Harcourt, Brace, Jovanovich.

Bryce, GK. 1991. Medicare on the Ropes. *Canadian Journal of Public Health* 82 (March/April): 75–76.

Buck, C. 1985. Beyond Lalonde-Creating Health. *Canadian Journal of Public Health* 76 (Suppl 1) (May/June): 19–24.

Campbell, M. 1988. Management as 'Ruling': A Class Phenomenon in Nursing. *Studies in Political Economy* 27 (Autumn): 29–51.

Canada Health and Welfare. 1972. Health and Welfare Canada. *The Community Health Centre in Canada.* Report of the Community Health Centre Project to the Conference of Health Ministers (Hastings Report). Ottawa: Information Canada.

Canada Health and Welfare. 1991a. House of Commons. Standing Committee of Health and Welfare, Social Affairs, Seniors and the Status of Women. *The Health Care System in Canada and Its Funding: No Easy Solutions. First Report to the House* (June).

Canada Health and Welfare. 1991b. *Building Partnerships. Government Response to the Standing Committee Report Entitled "The Health Care System in Canada and its Funding: No Easy Solutions".* Ottawa: Minister of Supply and Services Canada (November).

Coburn, D, GM Torrance, and JM Kaufert. 1983. Medical Dominance in Canada in Historical Perspective: The Rise and Fall of Medicine? *International Journal of Health Services* 13 (3): 407–432.

Coburn, D, and CL Biggs. 1987. Legitimation or Medicalization? The Case of Chiropractic in Canada. In D Coburn, C D'Arcy, GM Torrance, and P New eds. *Health and Canadian Society: Sociological Perspectives,* 2nd ed., 366–384. Markham: Fitzhenry and Whiteside.

Cox, RW. 1987. *Power and Production. Vol. 1, Production, Power, and World Order.* New York: Columbia University Press.

Crawford, R. 1980. Healthism and the Medicalization of Everyday Life. *International Journal of Health Services* 10 (3): 365–388.

Crichton, A, and D Hsu, with S Tsang. 1990. *Canada's Health Care System: Its Funding and Organization.* Ottawa: Canadian Hospital Association Press.

Crozier, M, SP Huntington, and J Watanuki. 1975. *The Crisis of Democracy.* New York: New York University Press.

D'Arcy, C, and CM Siddique. 1987. Health and Unemployment: Findings from a National Survey. In Coburn et al. eds. *Health and Canadian Society: Sociological Perspectives,* 239–261. Markham: Fitzhenry and Whiteside.

Deber, RB, and E Vayda. 1985. The Environment of Health Policy Implementation: The Ontario, Canada Example. In WW Holland, R Detels, and G Knox eds. *Oxford Textbook of Public Health. Vol. 3, Investigative Methods in Public Health,* 441–461. Oxford: Oxford University Press.

Denton, FT, A Gafni, BG Spencer, and GL Stoddart. 1983. Potential Savings from the Adoption of Nurse Practitioner Technology in the Canadian Health Care System. *Socio-Economic Planning Services* 17(4): 199–209.

Detsky, AS, K O'Rourke, CD Naylor, SR Stacey, and JM Kitchens. 1990. Containing Ontario's Hospital Costs under Universal Insurance in the 1980's: What Was the Record? *Canadian Medical Association Journal* 142(15 March): 565–572.

Deverell, J. 1982. The Ontario Hospital Dispute 1980–81. *Studies in Political Economy* 9(Fall): 179–190.

Dickinson, HD, and M Stobbe. 1988. Occupational Health and Safety in Canada. In Bolaria and Dickinson eds. *Sociology of Health Care in Canada,* 426–438. Toronto: Harcourt, Brace, Jovanovich.

Dubos, R. 1959. *Mirage of Health.* Garden City, NY: Anchor Books.

Epp, J. 1986. (Minister of National Health and Welfare). *Achieving Health for All: A Framework for Health Promotion.* Ottawa: Minister of Supply and Services Canada.

Evans, RG. 1975. Beyond the Medical Marketplace: Expenditure, Utilization and Pricing of Insured Health in Canada. In S Andreopoulos ed. *National Health Insurance: Can We Learn Canada?,* 129–179. New York: Wiley.

Evans, RG. 1984. *Strained Mercy: The Economics of Canadian Health Care.* Toronto: Butterworths.

Evans, RG. 1986. Finding the Levers, Finding the Courage: Lessons from Cost Containment in North America. *Journal of Health Politics, Policy and Law* 11(4): 585–615.

Evans, RG. 1987. Hang Together, or Hang Separately: The Viability of a Universal Health Care System in an Aging Society. *Canadian Public Policy* 13(2): 165–180.

Evans, RG., J Lomas, ML Barer, RJ Labelle, C Fooks, GL Stoddart, GM Andrews, D Feeny, A Gafni, GW Torrance, and WG Tholl. 1989. Controlling Health Expenditures – The Canadian Reality. *New England Journal of Medicine* 320(9): 571–577.

Evans, RG, and GL Stoddart. 1990. *Producing Health, Consuming Health Care.* CIAR Population Health Working Paper No. 6. Toronto: Canadian Institute for Advanced Research. (April).

Evans, RG., ML Barer, and C Hertzman. 1990. *The Twenty Year Experiment: Accounting for, Explaining, and Evaluating Health Care Cost Containment in Canada and the United States.* CIAR Population Health Working Paper No. 14. Toronto: Canadian Institute for Advanced Research. (September).

Evans, RG, and GL Stoddart, eds. 1989. *Medicare at Maturity: Achievements, Lessons and Challenges.* Calgary: Banff Centre for Continuing Education.

French, S. 1978. *The Cost Containment Literature: Index and Summary.* Prepared (as Appendix D) for the Select Committee on Health Care Financing and Costs. Ontario. (15 September).

Frideres, JS. 1988. Racism and Health: The Case of the Native People. In Bolaria and Dickinson ed. *Sociology of Health Care in Canada*, 135–147. Toronto: Harcourt, Brace, Jovanovich.

Gough, I. 1979. *The Political Economy of the Welfare State*. London: Macmillan.

Grant, KR. 1988. The Inverse Care Law in Canada: Differential Access under Universal Free Health Insurance. In Bolaria and Dickinson eds. *Sociology of Health Care in Canada,* 118–134. Toronto: Harcourt, Brace, Jovanovich.

Habermas, J. 1973. *Legitimation Crisis*. Translated by Thomas McCarthy. Boston: Beacon Press.

Harvey, D. 1989. The *Condition of Postmodernity*. Oxford: Basil Blackwell.

Hastings, JEF. 1986. Organized Ambulatory Care in Canada: Health Service Organizations and Community Health Centers. *Journal of Public Health Policy* 7(Summer): 239–247.

Hastings, JEF, FD Mott, A Barclay, and D Hewitt. 1973. Prepaid Group Practice in Sault Ste. Marie: Part I: Analysis of Utilixation Records. *Medical Care* 11(2):91–103.

Hastings, JEF, and E Vayda. 1989. Health Services Organization and Delivery: Promise and Reality. In Evans and Stoddart eds. *Medicare at Maturity,* 337–384. Calgary: Banff Centre for Continuing Education.

Himmelstein, DU, and S Woolhandler. 1986. Cost Without Benefit: Administrative Waste in U.S. Health Care. *New England Journal of Medicine* 314(7): 441–445.

Hirsch, F. 1978. *Social Limits to Growth*. Cambridge: Harvard University Press.

Iglehart, JK. 1986. Canada's Health Care System. Three-part article. *New England Journal of Medicine* 315(3): 202–208; 315(12): 778–784; 315(25): 1623–1628.

Illich, I. 1976. *Limits to Medicine–Medical Nemesis: The Expropriation of Health*. Toronto and London: McClelland and Stewart, in association with Marion Boyars.

Jessop, B. 1989. Conservative Regimes and the Transition to Post-Fordism: The Cases of Great Britain and West Germany. In M Gottdiener and N Komninos eds. *Capitalist Development and Crisis Theory: Accumulation, Regulation and Spatial Restructuring,* 261–299. New York: St. Martin's Press.

King, D. 1989. Economic Crisis and Welfare State Recommodification: A Comparative Analysis of the United States and Britain. In Gottdiener and Komninos eds. *Capitalist Development and Crisis Theory: Accumulation, Regulation and Spatial Restructuring,* 237–260. New York: St. Martin's Press.

Laclau, E, and C Mouffe. 1985. *Hegemony and Socialist Strategy.* London and New York: Verso.

Lalonde, M. 1974. (Minister of National Health and Welfare). *A New Perspective on the Health of Canadians: A Working Document*. Ottawa: Minister of Supply and Services Canada.

Laughren, F. 1992. (Treasurer of Ontario). *Ontario Fiscal Outlook: Meeting the Challenges*. Toronto: Queen's Printer for Ontario. (January).

Laxer, R. 1976. *Canada's Unions*. Toronto: James Lorimer and Company.

LeClair, M. 1975. The Canadian Health Care System. In S Andreopoulos ed. *National Health Insurance: Can We Learn from Canada?,* 11–93. New York: Wiley.

Lomas, J. 1985. *First and Foremost in Community Health Centres: The Centre in Sault Ste Marie and the CHC Alternative*. Toronto: University of Toronto Press.

Lomas, J, and ML Barer. 1989. And Who Shall Represent the Public Interest? The Legacy of Canadian Health Manpower Policy. In Evans and Stoddart eds. *Medicare at Maturity,* 221–286. Calgary: Banff Centre for Continuing Education.

McKeown, T. 1978. Determinants of Health. *Human Nature* (April): 6.1–6.5

McKeown, T. 1979. *The Role of Medicine: Dream, Mirage or Nemesis?*, 2nd ed. Princeton: Princeton University Press.

Manga, P. 1983. *The Political Economy of Extra-Billing.* Working Paper 83–68. Ottawa: Faculty of Administration, University of Ottawa.

Manga, P. 1987. Equality of Access and Inequalities in Health Status: Policy Implications of a Paradox. In Coburn et al. eds. *Health and Canadian Society,* 637–648. Markham: Fitzhenry and Whiteside.

Manga, P, and GR Weller. 1980. The Failure of the Equity Objective in Health: A Comparative Analysis of Canada, Britain, and the United States. *Comparative Social Research* 3: 229–267.

Manga, P, and R Broyles. 1986. Evaluating and Explaining U.S.-Canada Health Policy. In SS Nagel ed. *Research in Public Policy Analysis and Management,* Vol. 3, 213–242. London: JAI Press.

Marmor, TR, and JL Mashaw. 1990. *Canada's Health Insurance and Ours: The Real Lessons, the Big Choices.* CIAR Population Health Working Paper No. 10. Toronto: Canadian Institute for Advanced Research. (Fall).

Mishler, W, and DB Campbell. 1978. The Healthy State: Legislative Responsiveness to Public Health Care Needs in Canada, 1920-1970. *Comparative Politics* 10 (July): 479–497.

Myles, J. 1988. Decline or Impasse? The Current State of the Welfare State. *Studies in Political Economy* 26(Summer): 73–107.

Naylor, CD. 1986. *Private Practice, Public Payment: Canadian Medicine and the Politics of Health Insurance, 1911-1966.* Kingston and Montreal: McGill-Queen's University Press.

O'Connor, J. 1973. *The Fiscal Crisis of the State.* New York: St. Martin's Press.

O'Connor, JS. 1989. Welfare Expenditure and Policy Orientation in Canada in Comparative Perspective. *Canadian Review of Sociology and Anthropology* 26(February): 127–150.

Offe, C. 1984. *Contradictions of the Welfare State.* Edited and with an Introduction by J Keane. Cambridge: MIT Press.

Ontario. 1977. *Report of the Joint Advisory Committee of the Government of Ontario and the Ontario Medical Association on Methods to Control Health Care Costs.* (Taylor Report).

OECD (Organisation for Economic Cooperation and Development). 1990. *Health Care Systems in Transition: The Search for Efficiency.* Social Policy Studies No. 7. Paris: OECD.

Ottawa Charter for Health Promotion. 1987. *Health Promotion* 1(4): iii–v.

Pineault, R. 1984. The Place of Prevention in the Quebec Health Care System. *Canadian Journal of Public Health* 75(January/February): 92–97.

Poulantzas, N. 1978. *State, Power, Socialism.* Translated by P Camiller. London: NLB.

Rachlis, M, and C Kushner. 1989. *Second Opinion: What's Wrong with Canada's Health Care System and How to Fix it.* Toronto: Collins.

Renaud, M. 1987. Reform or Illusion? An Analysis of the Quebec State Intervention in Health. In Coburn et al. eds. *Health and Canadian Society,* 590–614. Markham: Fitzhenry and Whiteside.

Rodwin, VG. 1988. Inequalities in Private and Public Health Systems: The United States, France, Canada and Great Britain. In WA Van Horne ed. *Ethnicity and Health,* 12–35. Madison, WI: University of Wisconsin System, Institute on Race and Ethnicity.

Rose, JB. 1984. Growth Patterns of Public Sector Unions. In M Thompson and G Swimmer eds. *Conflict or Compromise: The Future of Public Sector Industrial Relations,* 83–119. Montreal: Institute for Research on Public Policy.

Schieber, GJ, and J-P Poullier. 1989. International Health Care Expenditure Trends: 1987. *Health Affairs* 8(Fall): 169–177.

Shah, CP, and C Spindell-Farkas. 1985. The Health of Indians in Canadian Cities: A Challenge to the Health Care System. *Canadian Medical Association Journal* 133(1 November): 859–863.

Siggner, AJ. 1986. The Socio-Demographic Conditions of Registered Indians. In JR Ponting ed. *Arduous Journey: Canadian Indians and Decolonization,* 57–83. Toronto: McClelland and Stewart.

Smith, DA. 1984. Strikes in the Canadian Public Sector. In Thompson and Swimmer eds. *Conflict or Compromise,* 197–228. Montreal: Institute for Research on Public Policy.

Soderstrom, L. 1978. The *Canadian Health System.* London: Croom Helm.

Soderstrom, L. 1987. *Privatization: Adopt or Adapt?.* Un rapport pour la Commission d'enquete sur les services de sante et les services sociaux. 36 Synthese critique. Quebec: Government of Quebec.

Spitzer, WO. 1978. Evidence that Justifies the Introduction of New Health Professionals. In P Slayton and M J Trebilcock eds. *The Professions and Public Policy,* 211–236. Toronto: University of Toronto Press.

Starr, P. 1981. The Politics of Therapeutic Nihilism. In Conrad and Kern eds. *The Sociology of Health and Illness,* 434–448. New York: St. Martin's Press.

Stevenson, HM, and M Burke. 1991. Bureaucratic Logic in New Social Movement Clothing: The Limits of Health Promotion Research. *Health Promotion International* 6(4): 281–289.

Stoddart, GL. 1985. Rationalizing the Health-Care System. In TJ Courchene, DW Conklin, and GCA Cook, eds. *Ottawa and the Provinces: The Distribution of Money and Power, Vol. 2,* 3–39. Toronto: Ontario Economic Council.

Stoddart, GL, and JR Seldon. 1984. Publicly Financed Competition in Canadian Health Care Delivery: A Viable Alternative to Increased Regulation? In JA Boan ed. *Proceedings of the Second Canadian Conference on Health Economics,* 121–143. Regina: University of Regina.

Stoddart, GL, and RJ Labelle. 1985. *Privatization in the Canadian Health Care System: Assertions, Evidence, Ideology and Options.* Ottawa: Health and Welfare Canada, (October).

Swartz, D. 1977. The Politics of Reform: Conflict and Accommodation in Canadian Health Policy. In Panitch ed. *The Canadian State,* 311–343. Toronto and Buffalo: University of Toronto Press.

Taylor, MG. 1981. The Canadian Health System in Transition. *Journal of Public Health Policy* 2(June): 177–187.

Taylor, MG. 1987. *Health Insurance and Canadian Public Policy: The Seven Decisions that Created the Canadian Health Insurance System and Their Outcomes.* 2nd ed. Kingston and Montreal: McGill-Queen's University Press.

Thomson, A. 1991. *Federal Support for Health Care: A Background Paper.* Prepared for the Health Action Lobby (HEAL). (June).

Torrance, GM. 1987. Hospitals As Health Factories. In Coburn et al. *Health and Canadian Society: Sociological Perspectives,* 479–500. Markham: Fitzhenry and Whiteside.

Trypuc, JM. 1988. Women's Health. In Bolaria and Dickinson eds. *Sociology of Health Care in Canada,* 154–166. Toronto: Harcourt, Brace, Janovich.

Tuohy, C. 1989a. Conflict and Accommodation in the Canadian Health Care System. In Evans and Stoddart eds. *Medicare at Maturity,* 393–434. Calgary: Banff Centre for Continuing Education.

Tuohy, C. 1989b. Federalism and Canadian Health Policy. In WM Chandler and CW Zollner eds. *Challenges to Federalism: Policy-Making in Canada and the Federal Republic of Germany,* 141–160. Kingston: Institute of Intergovernmental Relations, Queen's University.

Van Loon, RJ. 1978. From Shared Cost to Block Funding and Beyond: The Politics of Health Insurance in Canada. *Journal of Health Politics, Policy and Law* 2(Winter): 454–478.

Vayda, E. 1977. Prepaid Group Practice under Universal Health Insurance in Canada. *Medical Care* 15(5): 382–389.

Wahn, M. 1987. The Decline of Medical Dominance in Hospitals. In Coburn et al. eds. *Health and Canadian Society,* 422–440. Markham: Fitzhenry and Whiteside.

Walters, V. 1982. State, Capital, and Labour: The Introduction of Federal-Provincial Insurance for Physician Care in Canada. *Canadian Review of Sociology and Anthropology* 19(May): 157–172.

Warburton, R, and WK Carroll. 1988. Class and Gender in Nursing. In Bolaria and Dickinson eds. *Sociology of Health Care in Canada,* 364–374. Toronto: Harcourt, Brace, Jovanovich.

Weller, GR. 1981. The Delivery of Health Services in the Canadian North. *Journal of Canadian Studies* 16(Summer): 69–80.

Weller, GR, and P Manga. 1983a. The Development of Health Policy in Canada. In MM Atkinson and MA Chandler eds. *The Politics of Canadian Public Policy,* 223–246. Toronto: University of Toronto Press.

Weller, GR, and P Manga. 1983b. The Push for Reprivatization of Health Care Services in Canada, Britain, and the United States. *Journal of Health Politics, Policy and Law* 8(Fall): 495–518.

Woolhandler, S, and DU Himmelstein. 1991. The Deteriorating Administrative Efficiency of the U.S. Health Care System. *New England Journal of Medicine* 324(18): 1253–1258.

Wotherspoon, T. 1988. Training and Containing Nurses: The Development of Nursing Education in Canada. In Bolaria and Dickinson eds. *Sociology of Health Care in Canada,* 375–392. Toronto: Harcourt, Brace, Jovanovich.

Young, TK. 1987. The Health of Indians in Northwestern Ontario: A Historical Perspective. In Coburn et al. eds. *Health and Canadian Society,* 109–126. Markham: Fitzhenry and Whiteside.

33

The Sociology of Health in Canada[*]

David Coburn and Joan Eakin

Introduction

Health, illness and health care are of central concern to Canadians. On an individual level we are all faced with the uncertainty of health and the sometimes sudden and often seemingly arbitrary nature of disease and death. Collectively, Canadians display a profound attachment to their particular form of the financing of health care, national health insurance. Indeed, "medicare" seems the bedrock of our continuing efforts to define ourselves as different from the United States. The sociology of health should thus be a highly salient area within the social sciences, and health and health care seems fertile ground for the development of sociology. In this brief survey of the field in Canada we point to areas in which this is true and others where such potential has not yet been realized.

We base our review primarily on the journal literature and the major Canadian texts and readers in the field produced in the past decade (there have been few reviews since Badgley 1976, 1973, 1971).[1] Our definition of "the sociology of health" has been inclusive regarding what is considered sociology, and who might be called a sociologist.

We first examine the shape and direction of the recent literature on the sociology of health in Canada, providing illustrative examples[2] before pulling out common themes and drawing tentative conclusions about the field as a whole. While space considerations preclude contextualization here (we do allude to issues of context in the conclusions), it is important to note that the sociology of health in Canada reflects, and in turn influences, developments in the discipline, in health and health care, and in the Canadian political economy. In the last decade, the sociology of health has been influenced by profound changes in Canada and in what it means to be a Canadian. There have also been a greater institutionalization of sociology in universities at a time of budget cutbacks and transformations within sociology theory such as the rise of feminist theory and postmodernism.

Despite the varied nature of the sub-discipline and the disparate topics covered we note one theme which ties together very diverse levels of analyses and specific areas of study. This theme is a concern with equality and equity. Because health is a prerequisite for most other activities, health is a domain in which equality of opportunity, if not equality of condition, is a mark of a civilized society. Struggles over equity and equality, and sociologists' documentation of those struggles and of the

[*] This is a much revised version of an article that first appeared in *Health and Canadian Society*, 1993; 1.

forces underlying them, are, we believe, a central, if occasionally submerged, theme in the sociology of health in Canada.

There are two other specific characteristics of the field which deserve mention, its applied nature and the increasing institutionalization of sociology in Canadian universities. The discipline thus, increasingly, has two "poles," one applied, one more academic. We note some of the consequences of such a division in what follows.

We divide our discussion of the sociology of health in Canada into three areas: health status; health and illness behaviour; and the health care system. These are, it is true, administrative rather than sociological categories. We argue that the practical nature of this division reflects the ways in which sociologists in this country have approached the topic.

The Social Determinants of Health Status

Concern with the social etiology of health and illness has a long tradition in Canada, from the 19th Century public health movements, to Social Progressivism and the Social Gospel early in the 20th century, through the reform movements of the pre-World War II era, to health promotion and the "new public health" of the 1980's and 1990's. In the policy area there has been a definite trend from a view of the health care system as the "producer" of health to one in which social factors are seen to be the most important determinants of health status (Government of Canada 1987; Government of Ontario 1992; Evans and Stoddart 1990). In recent years the findings of large scale epidemiological surveys and the work of the Canadian Institute for Advanced Research (Evans et al. 1994 – but, see also Coburn, Poland et al. 1997) have provided a major impetus to and legitimation of notions of the social determinants of health. Health promotion research in Canada has also contributed to the recognition of the social determinants of health. The focus in this field has moved "up-stream" from individual determinants (e.g., lifestyle behaviour) to environmental conditions (e.g., poverty, see Pederson et al. 1994). The theoretical and policy impact of the shift to social structural determinants will be of considerable interest to sociologists interested in the ebb and flow of social determinants discourses on health.

Much research is devoted to documenting and accounting for the health status of Canadians. The long-term increase in longevity is generally of less interest than the persistent inequalities in health status and health care. The majority of recent articles correlate health status variables, defined in disease or illness/disability terms, with various social factors, particularly socio-economic status, gender, age, and ethnicity, the underlying thesis generally being that of documenting social inequalities in health status.

Socio-economic status (SES) is widely used as one factor amongst others, or as a control variable in relating socio-demographic factors to health. This concern with SES reflects a continuing emphasis on equity in health status and in access to health care (see Badgley and Wolfe 1992; D'Arcy 1988). While there are attempts to ask why SES should be related to health (for example, does lower income lead to poorer health or the reverse and why?), the underlying bases of health inequalities are infrequently addressed. This may be associated with a general lack of attention to the difference between SES and social class. "Class" refers to structural *relations* between classes, while 'SES' emphasizes *stratification* with no apparent "real social connection" between strata. Only occasionally are Wright's (1979, 1989) more relational definitions of class used. Most often SES is used without any explicit acknowledgement of the theoretical burden it carries.

Most research on the SES-health link also focuses on the influence of immediate individual social location on health rather than on the impact of broader dimensions of SES or class. The literature generally ignores the notion that advanced capitalist countries such as Canada display historical patterns of health status which are related to the fundamental operation of, and changes within, society. For example, the success or failure of health-related action (even when made by members of social movements or interest groups that are not class based) may be heavily influenced by the way the interests and ideology of these groups fit into the existing power structure (we later give an example of this in the case of medical dominance).

The literature on health status does, of course, address other aspects of inequality besides SES. Gender issues and women's health, for example, have become major foci of attention. Canada is at the forefront of developments in feminist theory and research and these developments are permeating the health field. Recently, for example, several federally funded Centres for Excellence in Women's Health have been established across the country. Many other women's health research units connected to hospitals and medical science centres have been founded. Social scientists are included in most of these initiatives. For example, women's health is prominent in the McMaster Research Centre for the Promotion of Women's Health, and in a national network of researchers interested in women's occupational health (e.g., Messing et al. 1995). In the women, work and health area, emphasis has been on the sexual division of labour and its implications for health, women's differential access to organizational power, the compounding effects of "double shifts," and the invisibility of women's occupational health problems. Indeed, the pervasiveness of women's health themes in this volume is testimony to the vigour with which such issues have been taken up by contemporary sociologists of health.

The health care system has also been viewed as a determinant of health. Manga (1987) has noted the paradox that improved access to health care brought about by health insurance has not reduced existing inequalities in health status (there are arguments about the degree to which inequalities in access remain cf. Badgley and Wolfe 1992). In a parallel way, a few studies, not all by sociologists, point to the political and social forces pushing for an expanded health care sector despite the fact that ever-larger health systems are not necessarily associated with improved health (Evans and Stoddart 1990). Few sociologists in Canada pursue the claims of Illich (1975) and others that health care is itself "iatrogenic," and that the ever-proliferating number of health care professionals "disable" people by rendering them less competent regarding health matters (Illich et al. 1977). The illness-creating impact of labelling, such as that associated with hypertension screening, has been noted, as have the negative impact of the ever-proliferating use of pharmaceuticals (Lexchin 1990).

It is significant that the purported irrelevance of health care to health status has not been well documented after the initial flurry of assertions flowing from the historical work of McKeown (1979) and others. Has criticism of the health care system led to throwing the baby out with the bathwater? Might the influence of social factors on health vary historically? Perhaps it suits government policy makers intent on reducing health care costs to point to the failures of care, just as it is in the interests of powerful lobbies within health care to push for more. Health care administrators, the public and health researchers seem to share a fundamental ambivalence about things medical –

displaying a continued interest in access to health care despite doubts about its relevance to health status.

More focused exploration of the social determinants of health is represented in the literature on stress. Significant Canadian contributions have been made in this area. Although the link between chronic stress and mental and physical well-being has long been observed, researchers in Canada have made important contributions to unravelling the specifics of this relationship. Turner, Wheaton, and colleagues, for example, have explored the relevance of social roles and past social experience to how stress is experienced (Turner et al. 1995). The notion of social support as a buffer mechanism between stress and health, or as a determinant of (positive) health, is incorporated almost ritualistically into many studies, but direct research on the topic does not seem extensive in Canada. The notion of stress is seldom related to its structural determinants or to more general socially rooted concepts such as alienation or anomie. There has also been little recognition of the concepts of stress and social support as links between individual or group physiological response and broader social structures, or of the "permeability" of the boundaries between the social and the biological.

The health status determinants research identified so far generally approaches health and illness as relatively "objective" phenomena that are embedded in nature (the "nature speaks" school of science). If health status is approached more as a social construction, however, the process of social definition itself becomes the "determinant." Reflecting wider debates on the social construction of scientific knowledge, some sociologists of health are exploring how illness constructs are formulated at the societal level (e.g., through medicalization), at the institutional level (e.g., through practitioner-patient interaction), and at the individual level (e.g., through labelling). From this perspective the determinants of disease lie in the processes through which they are produced as "diseases."

Social constructionist approaches to health status tend to be more prevalent in areas of 'weak' bio-medical explanation, such as where physical explanations are less readily available (e.g., chronic fatigue syndrome and mental health generally), where bio-mechanical explanations are proving inadequate (e.g., repetitive strain injury, lower back pain), and where previously existing phenomena are being medicalized, or recast in health terms (domestic violence, anorexia, menopause). As yet, there has been less consideration of the social construction of core bio-medical categories where "real" physical properties so far remain sacrosanct from sociological meddling (cf. more generally Bloor 1991). The arguments of social constructionism itself can be applied to explaining why some topics have been researched and not others. The Women's Movement has had an important impact on social constructionist perspectives on the determinants of health. Conversely, the formulation of First Nation health research issues has, until recently, reflected the political weakness of the Native community. The role of power in the definition of research is also invisibly entrenched in the basic functioning of society rather than in the specific actions of particular organizations. The relative lack of emphasis on the workplace as a determinant of health is obviously related to its location in a social structure governed by the needs and principles of private enterprise and capitalism. Paradoxically, given the patriarchal character of Canadian society, one could ask what "invisible" forces account for the absence of research specifically examining the substantially higher mortality rate of men as compared with women?

In sum, a good deal of the literature on health status in Canada has been devoted to correlating various socio-demographic factors with health status, reflecting a strong, if often implicit, focus on equity. Many of these studies, however, are essentially asociological in nature. Correlations are often found, but less often explained. "Social" variables are not seen as real social entities but are used simply as statistical categories. For example, the notion of "population," popular in the social epidemiological literature, refers to an aggregate of individuals and misses the sociological significance of groups, communities or classes (that is, defined in terms of patterns of interaction, or with reference to some theoretical framework). Social factors are often examined in isolation from one another, torn out of the structural context within which they are located. Social constructionist accounts of health status do embody a degree of contextualization. A key sociological point in this approach is that "determinants" of health cannot be understood apart from the issue of how health is defined (and by whom), and that these definitions embody explicit or implicit social theories of what constitutes a healthy person, a healthy life, or a healthy society.

Health and Illness Behaviour

A second category of literature attempts not so much to explain the etiology of health and illness as much as analyze the behaviour that arises in relation to these states. The notion of "health and illness behaviour" refers to the way in which people perceive, understand and respond to health and illness related states or events.

"Health behaviour" can be distinguished from "illness behaviour." The former refers to the way in which people regard and respond to wellness as opposed to illness (e.g., how they conceive of health, how they understand threats to health), and what they do to preserve and protect and enhance their wellbeing (e.g., the risks they do or do not take). The latter incorporates an even broader array of phenomena, ranging from the perception of signs and symptoms, to entry into and experience within the health care system, to the social processes of disability and death (and, after death - bodies receive differential treatment depending on prior social standing and other social characteristics).

Canadian scholarship on health and illness behaviour is built on the earliest sociological contributions to our understanding of illness behaviour, the distinction between *disease* (the "objective" state of physiological disorder), *illness* (the "subjective" experience or feeling of disorder), and *sickness* (the social state associated with being diseased or ill). More recently there is increasing recognition that disease categories are themselves social products. The notion of the "sick role," one of the most enduring sociologic concepts in the field, and other core concepts, such as deviance and labelling, continue to be drawn upon in contemporary Canadian research. Classic and contemporary conceptualizations of health and illness behaviour share a common appreciation of health and health care as mediators of social relations and as mechanisms of social control.

Pearlin distinguished "structure seekers" from "meaning seekers" in medical sociology (Pearlin 1992). The former "seek to reveal structure in social life and its consequences for health" (usually through quantitative survey research) while the latter "seek to reveal the meaning of social life and its bearing on health" (typically through qualitative methodology). The predominant approach in Canadian scholarship in the area of health and illness behaviour has been "structure-seeking." For example, research has attempted to examine how, in particular populations, certain health and illness behaviours (as opposed to health status outcomes, as in the previous discussion), are related statistically to discrete social structural variables. The behaviours explored have most frequently been the utilization of health care services, while the "social vari-

ables" such as gender, ethnicity, age, rural-urban location reflect the concern noted earlier with issues of equity. This research tends to be framed from the vantage point of the
health care system (e.g., why people use medical services, why they do not comply
with professional advice) rather than from sociological theory (e.g., the relationship
between labelling practices and social class).

Forms of help-seeking outside of the medical orbit (e.g., consultations with pharmacists, use of alternative healers, self-care) have been infrequently explored, although
there are indications of increasing interest, particularly in relation to AIDS and chronic
illness. Recent growth in public policy commitment to health promotion and community health in Canada has been accompanied by a research focus on behaviours pertaining to health as opposed to illness, i.e., risk behaviour, the use of preventive health
services, and lifestyle health practices. The behaviours considered, however, remain
quite narrowly defined. For example, participation in health planning or workplace
health activism are not conceptualized as "health behaviours."

The limited scope of the behaviours considered probably reflects the fact that the
conceptualization of health and illness behaviour has been so closely tied to applied
health system concerns. It may also arise from the absence of an explicit theoretical
framework to guide the choice of behaviours for investigation. It is often not clear how
the various behaviours studied relate to each other, or why some and not others were
selected for study. The social variables are typically conceived of as psychosocial
attributes of the individual (e.g., cultural beliefs) rather than as dimensions of social
structure (e.g., power discrepancies between service providers users). The choice of
variables seems guided by administrative concerns, by the empiricist assumptions of
survey methodology, and by a risk factor approach to understanding behaviour.

Although social epidemiological approaches to health and illness behaviour predominate, there is an apparently growing shift to "meaning-centred" research, where interest lies less in "population" patterns of behaviour as much as in the meanings and
experiences attached to such behaviour. In the last few years interest in qualitative
methods has risen substantially within the health care research field (among social scientists and clinical researchers such as family medicine, nursing and health promotion). Such methods have had appeal in part because of the ideological compatibility of
such methods with praxis (Eakin and Maclean 1992), and in part because of disillusionment with positivist science more generally.

The behavioural phenomena studied in "meaning-centred" research is conceptualized not from the perspective of the health system or external observers, but from the
perspective of those doing the behaving (e.g., experiences, perceptions, accounts). The
different purchase on understanding associated with meaning-centered research is evident in Yoshida's (1993) study of the experiences of Canadians with spinal cord injury.
Adaptation to disability emerges, not as a once-and-for-all expression of "successful
coping" (as it is most frequently understood from a normative, professional rehabilitation standpoint), but as a constant *process* of readjustment and alignment, particularly
through transformations in personal identities.

The relationship between structure-seeking and meaning-seeking research embodies
one of the central problematics of sociology: the relationship between agency (individual experience) and structure (broader social institutions, collective forces). A number
of Canadian sociologists are exploring these relationships. For example, Pirie (1988)
explores the process whereby women actually adopt certain social labels and definitions related to their health and to their bodies and calls for research that links personal
biographies with the broader social context in which they are located (cf. Smith 1987).

Anderson (1985) describes the social, economic and political forces structuring the experiences of immigrant women *vis a vis* use of the health system. Kaufert and Locker (1990) have examined the structural context of the subjective experience of post-polio syndrome. Lippman (1991) has elaborated the consequences for women's experience of the "geneticization" of prenatal care and the discourse of new reproductive technologies. These and other studies make important contributions to the attempt to relate experience and personal meaning to their institutional, societal and ideological contexts.

In sum, Canadian research in the area of health and illness behaviour has been heavily directed towards the description of behaviours associated with the utilization of health services, and with the epidemiological search for their general social determinants. However, there are signs of growing interest in health as opposed to illness behaviour, in meaning-centred qualitative research approaches, and in broadening the range of behaviours studied and the social phenomena to which they are related. Particularly exciting are efforts to connect personal experience with broader social structures and conditions.

The Health Care System

The literature related to the health care system includes the largest part of the sociology of health in Canada. Contributions in this area can be divided into those that address topics at the micro (interpersonal) level, the meso (organizational) level, and the macro (societal) level of analysis.

At the micro level, the interests of sociologists in the Canadian health care system have again centered on issues of concern to practitioners and policy-makers or on those which have derived from concepts and theories readily transferable from the general corpus of sociology. Yet there has been change. For example, in relation to one of the most popular micro topics, patient-practitioner relationships, the initial focus on patient compliance with doctors orders has been supplemented by a perspective which emphasizes the power differences and exploitation, and possible "cultural" incongruence embodied in it.

A fair amount of recent work suggests that medicalization (the power to define both what public "needs" are and how these needs are to be met), impinges on individual patient autonomy. It is also proposed that medicine either acts directly as a mode of social control (directing "deviance" into controllable channels) or, individualizes, hence mystifies, what are at base "social" problems. Not all researchers, however, have the same findings or come to the same conclusions. For example, Cooperstock and Lennard (1987) found that physicians' prescription of tranquillizers to women had the effect of helping them adapt to what, from an observers perspective, appeared to be excessively stressful roles. P. Kaufert and Gilbert (1986), on the other hand, found that individual physicians did not "medicalize the menopause" (although medicine writ large might have).

Research at the micro level of the health care system includes study of the behaviour and experience of health care providers i.e., the social psychology of health care giving. Topics include the attitudes of professionals on various moral issues, the management of uncertainty in practice, the impact of various factors (e.g., financial incentives) on clinical behaviour, burnout, inter-professional conflict, strain related to the social control functions of medicine, and the implicit theories built into particular modes of professional knowledge.

Concern with health care "work" has focused on professionals or semi-professionals. Lower level health workers have received little research attention. Yet, the study of professionals may be limited by the prevailing tendency *not* to see them as workers on a continuum with other workers. That is, the health professions have been privileged as "unique" occupations.

A notable development in the study of health care providers has been the extension of the definition of "care-givers" to include informal care-givers, especially families caring for chronically ill or disabled members. A growing sociological literature in this area addresses both the social psychological dimensions of care-giving and the social/ political dimensions of policy in the area of home care, particularly its implications for women. Extension of the concept of "care-giving" outside of the professional domain reformulates the family's relationship to illness in health system terms. What may formerly have been considered "coping" or "the impact of illness on the family" is now 'informal care-giving.' Although the intent of broadening the conceptualization of care-giving is to acknowledge and support such experience, one could also ask if, by converting what is "private" to that which is "public," it also increases public surveillance and control. Is the "discovery" of informal care-giving itself part of a process of medicalization?

At the meso level of analysis, the health care system has most often been viewed in terms of its administrative elements: occupations and professions, hospitals, and other provider organizations such as medical schools. The focus on formal health care and on the health occupations and professions and on the most powerful profession, medicine, is a product of practical concerns but also may be induced by the existence of sociology courses and journals in work and occupations and the professions which permit a carry-over of concepts and methods.

The prevailing theme has been medical dominance, the power of medicine to define health and health care issues in terms of its own interests. This dominance, is, however, now generally viewed as contingent on the power of the state and/or social elites or classes. Most recently, the rise of a curatively oriented medicine is seen as tied to a congruence of ideology and interests between medicine and the dominant class as well as to the use of science as a justificatory ideology. An individualistic, curative medicine was seen to personalize what were essentially "social" problems (e.g. due to the factory system, poverty, etc.).

In the health occupations and professions area generally there has been a movement from a straightforward functionalist approach centered on "professionalization" – one which accepts at face value professional claims of altruism, esoteric knowledge, and self-regulation – to one which overwhelmingly emphasizes the power of providers to create monopolies to serve their own interests. The image now is of a "system of professions" in which medicine is losing its long-held position at the apex of this system, or at least is being challenged by resurgent or newly formed "other" occupations (though the roots of medical decline lie elsewhere).

The literature on various aspects of medicine as an occupation ranges from the socialization of medical students to the relationships between medicine and other occupations, health institutions, and the state. More recently, attention has turned to "non-medicine" occupations such as nursing, chiropractic, naturopathy, occupational therapy, midwifery, and others. The current interest in nursing and midwifery arises from the influence of women sociologists, the increasing number of sociologists who are, or were, nurses, the feminist movement, and the prominence of feminist theory in sociology.

Studies of nursing are particularly prevalent and interesting both because the occupation is undergoing great change and because its composition is overwhelmingly female. Early studies of nursing outside of Canada focused on the subordination of nursing to medicine as a reflection of the general dominance of women by men. Recent Canadian work, however, analyzes nursing in terms of professionalization. Although nurses often claim to be "patient advocates," Storch and Stinson (1988) are among the few who ask whether the professionalization of nurses is actually good for patients. Other studies view nursing more from the perspective of the industrialization of health care generally i.e., nursing as work. Campbell (1988), for example, proposes that the occupation is being "proletarianized" i.e., routinized and fragmented (but not necessarily deskilled). Recent cutbacks in health care, and particularly in hospitals, emphasize the dispensability of nursing and the intensification of nursing work (Armstrong et al. 1993).

Patients are largely absent in most Canadian theories, explanations, or descriptions of occupations and professions, or of other aspects of the health care system. Sometimes "the public" or various groups within it are viewed as challenging professional power. Elsewhere, patients are referred to in terms of a cultural "incongruence" between patients and health care providers. The salience of problems arising from Canada's increasingly multicultural population and more evident material inequality would predict growing future research interest in the provider-patient interface and a questioning of the very notion of an undifferentiated "public." Recently, there has been a revival of interest in examining the nature and determinants of public participation in all aspects of health care, from the practitioner-patient relationship to community involvement in planning (democratization of health care) and even to involvement in health research (participative health care research).

While high status health care providers have received much attention, one of the health system's major institutions, the hospital, has received very little. Although, as Torrance (1987) notes, Canadian hospitals, in 1981, employed more workers than the automobile, iron and steel, and pulp and paper industries combined, they have not been studied by sociologists in the same way as have other work organizations. Research on hospitals appears more substantial if one includes studies of the utilization of hospital services, although the emphasis here is generally not on the hospital as an organization. Neither the internal structure and functioning of hospitals, or their place in the larger formal health care system have been subject to sociological study. Nor is there much, if anything, on the role of the new medical-teaching complexes.

Other aspects of the health care system have also not been subject to scrutiny, including, for example, the nature and implications of the fast-growing bio-medical research and development enterprise. The selective neglect of certain aspects of the health care system may reflect the cachet of "science" as an "extra-human" activity which cannot be examined sociologically. Or, perhaps it stems from the difficulty of securing grants from those whose conceptions of an "objective" science remains intact, or who do not view such topics as relevant.

A new vision of health, embodied in the notion of health promotion, is being brought into sociological focus in Canada. Stevenson and Burke's (1992) examination of health promotion as "bureaucratic logic in new social movement clothing" is an example of the debate developing around whether health promotion is a reformist social movement, or simply an excuse for the state to cut down on expenditures for health care services.

Health policy is a further dimension of the health care system. In this area most analysts have been political scientists or economists, although a few sociologists (see e.g., Armstrong and Armstrong 1994), have tackled public policy issues. But, the underlying explanations for these, surely a part of the province of sociology, are relatively untouched.

At the macro level of analysis the health care system is approached as a whole. In Canada, curiously, sociologists have been the least involved in this level of analysis. Perhaps this is an example of the problems arising from exclusively disciplinary perspectives on health care, i.e., the "political economy" of care tends to be neglected. Some of the basic explanations for health phenomena are not necessarily specific to the domain of health (cf. inequality in access to or treatment within educational or legal systems) and would benefit from a more general explanatory framework.

Although the reorganization of health care and costs have been much described, sociological perspectives on the topic are less common. There is material on the historical development of and explanation for, the implementation of health insurance. This work ranges from pluralist interest group descriptions (e.g., health insurance was brought in by a benevolent state against a recalcitrant medical profession) to class based explanations. Regarding the latter, there is a interesting division between Swartz (1977), who argues that health insurance came about largely because of working class pressures (over a long period of time) and Walters (1982), who proposes that there was little working class pressure and not much opposition (at least from big business, which benefitted from having health care costs socialized and from the production of what was hoped would be a "healthy workforce"). Still, until very recently, few sociologists have examined the relationships between the supposedly powerful health occupations and the state (Coburn 1993) or business, or have carried out international comparisons of the Canadian health care system (apart from comparing access to health care in Canada and the United States).

There are few analyses within the sociology of health of the place of health insurance or of health care generally within the rise (and fall?) of the liberal or neo-liberal version of the welfare state that Canada displays. There is discussion about how and why health insurance has (so far) escaped the fate of other welfare state reforms, themselves once, but no longer, viewed as a permanent part of a new improved and "humane" capitalism. Some explanations for the preservation of health insurance include – working class struggles, powerful consumer and provider interests and the interests of big business in avoiding direct health care costs. Health care events, as with change in other aspects of "the welfare state" can be linked to changes in Canada as a whole brought about by its absorption into the international capitalist system (NAFTA, GATT). Very broad social considerations such as the influence of the internationalization of capital on the relative autonomy of the state and the consequences of this for social welfare and health policy, demands more attention from sociologists.

In sum, Canadian contributions in the area of the health care system include much on the utilization of health services (but this is not linked to the nature and functioning of the system, beyond analyses of insurance) and a great deal on professional or semi-professional health care occupations. Less well-covered is the nature and experience of health care "work" and the various components of the health system, such as hospitals. The area with the least to show concerns the dynamics of the health care system as a whole, the very area in which sociologists might be thought to have much to contribute. There is a changing national, continental, and world system which moulds and constrains the health of Canadians and health care in Canada. The underlying structural factors determining, or shaping, health and health care should, one would think, be the particular province of sociology.

Summary and Conclusions

The sociology of health covers a wide territory – from examination of the social construction of definitions of health to the role of the international mobility of capital and its effects on the autonomy of the state and on health care systems. The sociology of health, along with the other social sciences, helps us escape from perspectives which view health and illness as explainable simply as direct responses to changing health care "needs." Health needs and health care are brought into view as human and social products and as such open to social analysis and change.

There have been general trends in sociology in Canada, such as a shift from interpretations relying on "culture" to those relying on power (Brym and Fox 1989; Carroll et al. 1992). Parallel developments are reflected in the sociology of health in Canada in the movement from a predominantly medically oriented perspective towards broader approaches. But the medical perspective has not been replaced, it has simply been supplemented by various alternatives emphasizing the social determinants of health and health care. Methodologically, sociology in the health field relies on the somewhat stereotypic application of concepts from sociology, such as SES, and relies heavily on expertise in survey methods. Yet the use of surveys now contends with other methods, qualitative, documentary, historical. Sociologists are increasingly unwilling to accept the notion that broad understanding of health and health care will eventually emerge from the accumulation of seemingly endless lists of social "variables," themselves descriptive of disembodied and desocialized individuals. An overly rigid positivism is being undermined. Much has been done, but the absences are notable.

We considered research in three general areas: the social determinants of health, health and illness behaviour, and the health care system. There are clusters of researchers focused specifically on equity in health status and health care, on the study of stress and social psychological phenomena generally, and on the health occupations and professions. There is much description and measurement, little explanation or theory. There are many studies on the periphery of the sociology of health of a social epidemiology type. But, both micro settings and macro structures in health and health care have been relatively neglected as have their interrelationships. The whole is seldom seen as more than the sum of its parts.

Most obviously, health care has for too long been equated with the formal health care system and "practitioners" with doctors, nurses and others in the "healing occupations." The problem is not so much that the sociology of health is applied as it is that perhaps too many of these applications take place within the common-sense perspectives of health care administrators. More important than the applied-theory dichotomy is their separation and the lack of an arena in which these views might engage in constructive interaction and debate.

Many of the characteristics of the sociology of health in Canada can be traced to an early (and continuing) American influence. This through journals and the flood of American professors into Canada in the 1960s, and to later reaction to this associated with a Canadianization movement. An American social-psychological and survey research emphasis, and the prestige of publication in American journals, has had a powerful steering effect on Canadian scholarship.

In addition, many sociologists of health were employed in medical schools or government agencies. There was pressure to accept the problems of health as defined by the dominant health profession, i.e., medicine. The later institutionalization of sociology in universities did lead to a greater development of the sociology *of* health. But, the general tenor was set by the field rather than by the discipline. And, universities themselves are now the centre of efforts to make them more "relevant" and applied.

An applied orientation is encouraged by the policies of key funding agencies. The NHRDP and provincial funding organizations are increasingly interested in those matters which will have immediate application. There are few sources of support for research that is at some remove from immediate use. Added to these forces are pressures to rationalize the health care system with social scientists, today more usually economists than others, used to address real or officially defined health care system "crises." In the United States, the tendency to rely on research funds to support university faculty has produced an even more applied orientation in that country than in Canada. As Mechanic (1993) notes, the result is a reluctance to be critical or to take a more structural approach. There are tendencies in Canadian universities to move in the same direction. Our major point is that sociologists have a unique contribution to make, but this uniqueness is often lost in catering to those whose visions would exclude a decidedly sociological approach from the outset. The prime example is the use of sociological "variables" as simple individual characteristics rather than as denoting social relationships.

A characteristic of the field, one hindering its own development and its usefulness to Canadians, is a lack of identity and community. There are few publication outlets in Canada. Canadian sociologists of health write for American or international journals, publish in a diverse array of substantive areas, and orient their publications accordingly. A Canadian sociologist's publications in the health field are read by relatively few colleagues and there is seldom opportunity for direct comment or debate. Even within the same city, or the same university, there is little communication between sociologists in the health field, or amongst the whole spectrum of social scientists in the area – there is perhaps much more of a "community of scholars" in Quebec than elsewhere.

Regarding communication there may be emerging a "gender-gap." Certainly, women, we suspect, comprise a much larger proportion of researchers in the health area than they do in sociology in general. Perhaps there is still some gender stereotyping about the area in the same sense that we noted earlier regarding the sociology of the family. But women health researchers also are increasingly plugged into more "networks" than are male researchers (cf. the Centres of Excellence in Women's Health). While there may be a, somewhat fading, "old boys" network in sociology, there is a thriving "new girls" network in research in the sociology of health and particularly in research on women's health. The latter provides a focus around which women can see common concerns. Our comment about a lack of community thus probably applies more to men than to women.

Despite the fragmentation and isolation, we believe there is something tying together the separate areas we have examined. Whether examining health status differences, differences in health behaviours by patients or providers, or analyzing health care or health care embedded in its social context, Canadian sociologists have emphasized health inequalities and inequities. Whether the level or topic has concerned SES, women, aboriginal or ethnic groups, health care providers, health care policy, or the role of health insurance, there is a theme of equal treatment or equal access in the face of unequal power resources or social structures. This theme is, no doubt, partly a reflection of the core orientation of sociology as a discipline. Yet, the emphasis on equality and equity also emanates from the subject matter itself. After all, if health and access to health care is fundamental to human experience, equality becomes a basic human right. Equality and equity do provide an underlying unity. There is something of a common cause. The relationship between health inequalities and more general, structural inequality might provide a future major focus in the sub-discipline.

Finally, Whyte has argued that sociologists in this country are failing to "constitute Canadian Society" in the sense of articulating knowledge of the whole, of "constructing" Canada in academia and in the public eye, as a valuable and unique entity for study. Sociologists of health have shown the same tendency. Canadian sociologists in the health field have made significant contributions in particular areas. Individuals or small clusters of researchers have done much with relatively few resources. To date, however, as a collective, they – we – have failed to constitute a vision of health and health care within a unique socio-historical context from which we, and others, might learn. The sociology of health in Canada could be substantially strengthened with greater attention to the contextualizing of research and an enhanced concern with the way individual parts fit within the context of Canadian society.

Notes

1 We searched Canadian, British and American health-related journals, and sociological journals, for contributions by Canadian sociologists. We also examined the contents and references of four texts/readers (Clarke 1990; Edginton 1989; Bolaria and Dickinson 1988; Coburn, D'Arcy, Torrance and New 1987). We searched computer data bases (with Canada as a search term), and sought referrals from a number of sociologists of health across the country.
2 We have purposely avoided citing examples for every area we touch upon (this would require a reference list longer than the text). While central areas of research are noted, particular authors are not, except where a specific example is discussed. Thus, our reference list is decidedly not a list of key references (or writers) in the field.

References

Anderson, JM. 1985. Perspectives on the Health of Immigrant Women: A Feminist Analysis. *Advances in Nursing Science* 8(1): 61–76.

Antonovsky, A. 1979. *Health, Stress, and Coping.* San Francisco: Jossey-Bass.

Armstrong, P, J Choiniere, and E Day. 1993. *Vital Signs: Nursing in Transition.* Toronto: Garamond Press.

Armstrong, P, and H Armstrong. 1994. *Take Care: Warning Signals for Canada's Health System.* Toronto: Garamond Press.

Badgley, RF, and S Wolfe. 1992. Equity and Health. In CD Naylor ed. *Medicine and the State.* Montreal: McGill-Queens University Press.

Badgley, RF. 1991. Social and Economic Disparities Under Canadian Health Care. *International Journal of Health Services* 21(4): 659–671.

Badgley, RF, and SW Bloom. 1973. Behavioural Sciences and Medical Education: The Case of Sociology. *Social Science and Medicine* 7: 927–941.

Badgley, RF. 1976. The Sociology of Health in Canada. *Social Science and Medicine* 10: 3.

Badgley, RF. 1971. The Sociology of Health: Some Questions. *Milbank Memorial Fund Quarterly* 49(2), Part 1.

Bloor, D. 1991. *Knowledge and Social Imagery.* 2nd ed. Chicago: The University of Chicago Press.

Bolaria, BS, and HD Dickinson. 1988. *Sociology of Health Care in Canada.* Toronto: Harcourt, Brace, Jovanovich.

Boudreau, F. 1991. Partnership as a New Strategy in Mental Health Policy: The Case of Quebec. *Journal of Health, Politics, Policy and Law* 16(2)

Brym, RJ, and BJ Fox. 1989. *From Culture to Power: The Sociology of English Canada.* Toronto: Oxford University Press.

Campbell, M. 1988. Management as 'Ruling': A Class Phenomenon in Nursing. *Studies in Political Economy.* 27(Autumn) 29–51.

Carroll, WK, L Christiansen-Ruffman, RF Currie, and D Harrison. 1992. *Fragile Truths: 25 Years of Sociology and Anthropology in Canada.* Ottawa: Carleton University Press.

Clarke, JN. 1990. *Health, Illness, and Medicine in Canada.* Toronto: McClelland and Stewart.

Coburn, D, B Poland, and members of the Critical Social Science and Health Group. 1997. Comment on: 'Why are Some People Healthy and Others Not?. Forthcoming in *Health and Canadian Society* 1997.

Coburn, D. 1993. State Authority, Medical Dominance, and Trends in the Regulation of the Health Professions. *Social Science and Medicine* 37(7): 841–850.

Cooperstock, R, and HL Lennard. 1987. Role Strains and Tranquilizer Use. In D Coburn et al. eds. *Health and Canadian Society,* 2nd ed. Toronto: Fitzhenry and Whiteside.

D'Arcy, C. 1988. *Reducing Inequalities in Health.* Health Promotion Directorate, NHRDP, HSSPB 88–16, Ottawa.

Eakin, J, and H McLean. 1992. A Critical Perspective on Research and Knowledge Development in Health Promotion. *Canadian Journal of Public Health* 83(Suppl 1): S72–S75

Eakin, J. 1992. Leaving it up to the Workers: Sociological Perspectives on the Management of Health and Safety in Small Workplaces. *International Journal of Health Services* 22(4): 689–704.

Edginton, B. 1989. *Health, Disease and Medicine in Canada: A Sociological Perspective.* Toronto: Butterworths.

Edwards, RK. 1986. *Ideology and Canadian Medicine, 1880–1920.* Master's thesis in Environmental Studies, York University.

Evans, RG, ML Barer, and TR Marmor. 1994. *Why are Some People Healthy and Others Not?* New York: Aldine de Gruyter.

Evans, RG, and GL Stoddart. 1990. Producing Health, Consuming Health Care. *Social Science and Medicine* 31(12): 1347–1363

Government of Canada. 1986. *Achieving Health For All: A Framework for Health Promotion,* Department of National Health and Welfare, November.

Government of Ontario. 1991. Premier's Council on Health Strategy, *Nurturing Health: A Framework on the Determinants of Health,* March.

Horobin, G. 1985. Medical Sociology in Britain: True Confessions of an Empiricist. *Sociology of Health and Illness* 7: 94–99.

Illich, I. 1975. *Medical Nemesis.* London: Marion Boyars.

Illich, I, IK Zola, J McKnight, J Caplan, and H Shaiken. 1977. *Disabling Professions.* London: Marion Boyars.

Kaufert, P, and P Gilbert. 1986. Women, Menopause and Medicalization. *Culture, Mental Health, and Psychiatry.* 10: 7–21.

Kaufert, J, and D Locker. 1990. Rehabilitation Ideology and Respiratory Support Technology. *Social Science and Medicine.* 30(8): 867–877.

Levine, S. 1987. The Changing Terrains in Medical Sociology: Emergent Concern with Quality of Life. *Journal of Health and Social Behavior* 28: 281–286.

Lexchin, J. 1990. Drug Makers and Drug Regulators: Too Close for Comfort. A Study of the Canadian Situation. *Social Science and Medicine* 31(11): 1257–1263.

Lippman, A. 1991. Prenatal Genetic Testing and Screening: Constructing Needs and Reinforcing Inequities. *American Journal of Law and Medicine* 17(1&2): 15–50

Lock, M, and D Gordon eds. 1988. *Biomedicine Examined.* Dordrecht: Kluwer Academic.

Manga, P. 1987. Equality of Access and Inequalities in Health Status: Policy Implications of a Paradox. In D Coburn et al. eds. *Health and Canadian Society,* 2nd ed. Toronto: Fitzhenry and Whiteside.

McKeown, T. 1979. *The Role of Medicine: Dream, Mirage or Nemesis.* New Haven, NJ: Princeton University Press.

Mechanic, D. 1993. Sociological Research in Health and the American Socio-Political Context: The Changing Fortunes of Medical Sociology. *Social Science and Medicine* 36(2): 95–102

Messing, K, B Neis, and L Dumais eds. 1995. *Invisible: Issues in Womens Occupational Health/ La Sante des Travailleuses.* Charolottetown: Gynergy Books.

Parsons, T. 1957. *The Social System,* New York: Free Press.

Pearlin, L. 1992. Structure and Meaning in Medical Sociology. *Journal of Health and Social Behavior* 33(1): 1-9.

Pederson, A, M O'Neill, and I Rootman. 1994. *Health Promotion in Canada.* Toronto: WB Saunders.

Pirie, M. 1988. Women and the Illness Role; Rethinking Feminist Theory. *Canadian Review of Sociology and Anthropology* 25(4): 628–644.

Renaud, M, S Dore, and D White. 1989. Sociology and Social Policy: From a Love-Hate Relationship With the State to Cynicism and Pragmatism. *Canadian Review of Sociology and Anthropology* 26(3): 426–456.

Shortt, SED. 1983. Physicians, Science, and Status: Issues in the Professionalization of Anglo-American Medicine in the Nineteenth Century. *Medical History* 27(1): 51–68.

Smith, D. 1987. *The Everyday World as Problematic: A Feminist Sociology.* Toronto: University of Toronto Press.

Stevenson, HM, and M Burke. 1992. Bureaucratic Logic in New Social Movement Clothing: The Limits of Health Promotion Research. *Canadian Journal of Public Health* 83(Suppl 1) (March–April): S47–S53.

Storch, JL, and SM Stinson. 1988. Concepts of Deprofessionalization with Application to Nursing. In R White ed. *Political Issues in Nursing,* 3. London: John Wiley.

Swartz, D. 1977. The Politics of Reform: Conflict and Accommodation in Canadian Health Policy. In L Panitch ed. *The Canadian State: Political Economy and Political Power.* Toronto: University of Toronto Press.

Torrance, GM. 1987. Hospitals as Health Factories. In D Coburn, C D'Arcy, GM Torrance, P New eds. *Health and Canadian Society,* 2nd ed. Toronto: Fitzhenry and Whiteside.

Turner, RJ, B Wheaton, and DA Lloyd. 1995. The Epidemiology of Social Stress. *American Sociological Review* 60: 104–125.

Turner, RJ, and WR Avison. 1989. Gender and Depression: Assessing Exposure and Vulnerability to Life Events in a Chronically Strained Population. *The Journal of Nervous and Mental Disease* 177(8): 443–455.

Walters, V. 1991. State Mediation of Conflicts Over Work Refusals: The Role of the Ontario Labour Relations Board. *International Journal of Health Services* 21(4): 717–729.

Walters, V. 1982. State, Capital and Labour: The Introduction of Federal-Provincial Insurance for Physicians Care in Canada. *Canadian Review of Sociology and Anthropology* 19(2): 157–172.

Wheaton, B. 1990. Life Transitions, Role Histories, and Mental Health. *American Sociological Review* 55(April): 209–223.

Wright, EO. 1979. *Class, Crisis and the State*. London: Verso.

Wright, EO et al. 1989. *The Debate on Classes*. London: Verso.

Yoshida, K. 1993. Reshaping of Self: A Pendular Reconstruction of Self and Identity Among Adults With Spinal Cord Injury. *Sociology of Health and Illness* 15(2): 217–245.

About the Authors

David Coburn, a sociologist by training, is a professor in the Department of Public Health Sciences, University of Toronto.

Carl D'Arcy, trained as a sociologist, is a professor in the Department of Psychiatry and Director of Applied Research at the University of Saskatchewan, Saskatoon.

George Torrance, a sociologist by training, is a consultant in social epidemiology and health services, Ottawa.

Joan M. Anderson is a professor in the School of Nursing at the University of British Columbia, Vancouver.

Douglas E. Angus is at the Faculty of Administration, University of Ottawa.

Jane Aronson is with the School of Social Work, McMaster University, Hamilton.

William R. Avison is a professor in the Department of Sociology and Director, Centre for Health and Well-Being, University of Western Ontario, London, Ontario.

Sharon Batt is an award-winning journalist and a breast cancer survivor. She is a founding member of the advocacy organization Breast Cancer Action Montreal.

Cecilia Benoit teaches in the Department of Sociology at the University of Victoria.

Connie Blue is Project Co-ordinator with the Cross-Cultural Health Studies Project at the University of British Columbia, Vancouver.

Françoise Boudreau is in the Department of Sociology, Glendon College, York University, Toronto.

Gregory P. Brown is a team leader in the Research and Evaluation Unit of the Ontario Ministry of the Solicitor General and Correction Services. He is an adjunct professor of sociology at the University of Waterloo.

M. Burke is with the Institute for Social Research, York University, Toronto.

Ruth Cooperstock, now deceased, was a research scientist with the Addiction Research Foundation, Toronto.

Raisa B. Deber is in the Department of Health Administration at the University of Toronto.

Karin Domnick is with the Department of Public Health Sciences, University of Toronto.

Joan Eakin teaches in the Department of Public Health Sciences, University of Toronto.

Robert G. Evans is a professor in the Department of Economics at the University of British Columbia, Vancouver; a National Health Scientist (Health Canada); and a member of the Centre for Health Services and Policy Research.

David Gagan is Provost and Vice-President, Academic, Simon Fraser University, Burnaby, British Columbia, and a professor in the Department of History.

Jay Goldstein is an associate professor in the Department of Sociology at the University of Manitoba.

Betty Havens is now with the Centre on Aging at the University of Manitoba, Winnipeg.

Roy W. Hornosty, now retired, was a professor in the Department of Sociology, McMaster University, Hamilton.

Patricia A. Kaufert teaches in the Department of Community Health, Health Sciences, Faculty of Medicine, University of Manitoba, Winnipeg.

Joseph M. Kaurfert is a medical anthropologist in the Department of Community Health, Health Sciences, Faculty of Medicine, University of Manitoba, Winnipeg.

Annie Lau is a research assistant with the Cross-Cultural Health Studies Project at the University of British Columbia, Vancouver.

Henry L. Lennard, at the time of article writing, was in the Department of Sociology, Yeschiva University, and at the Center for Policy Research, New York.

Joel Lexchin is a physician with an interest in policy issues. He practises at the Emergency Department at the Toronto Hospital, and is a member of the Family and Community Medicine Department at the University of Toronto.

Margaret Lock is an anthropologist in the Department of Social Studies of Medicine, McGill University, Montreal.

Graham S. Lowe is a professor in the Department of Sociology, University of Alberta, Edmonton.

Shamila L. Mhatre, is a research associate with CIET Canada and CIET International, an international non-governmental, non-profit organization dedicated to building the community voice into planning. She is also an assistant professor in the Department of Medicine, University of Ottawa.

Sam Migliore currently teaches in the Department of Sociology and Anthropology, University College of Cape Breton, North Sydney, Nova Scotia.

Linda J. Muzzin is at the Ontario Institute for Studies in Education, University of Toronto.

Herbert C. Northcott is a professor in the Department of Sociology, University of Alberta, Edmonton.

John D. O'Neil is a medical anthropologist in the Department of Community Health, Health Sciences, Faculty of Medicine, University of Manitoba, Winnipeg.

Michel O'Neill is in the School of Nursing at Laval University, Quebec.

Gregg M. Olsen is an associate professor in the Department of Sociology, University of Manitoba, Winnipeg.

Nigel S.B. Rawson is a professor in the Division of Community Health, Faculty of Medicine, Memorial University of Newfoundland, St. John's.

Naralou P. Roos is Director of the Manitoba Centre for Health Policy and Evaluation and a professor in the Department of Community Health Sciences at the University of Manitoba, Winnipeg.

Alexander Segall is a professor in the Department of Sociology and a research associate at the Health, Leisure and Human Performance Research Institute at the University of Manitoba, Winnipeg.

Gregory J. Sherman is with the Laboratory Centre for Disease Control, Health Canada, Ottawa.

H. Michael Stevenson is Vice-President, Academic Affairs, York University, Toronto, and a professor in the Department of Political Science.

Gregory L. Stoddart trained as an economist and is a professor in the Department of Clinical Epidemiology and Biostatistics, Faculty of Health Sciences at McMaster University, Hamilton. He is also a member of the Centre for Health Policy Analysis.

Donald Swartz is in Administrative Studies, Carleton University, Ottawa.

R. Jay Turner is currently a research professor in the Department of Sociology, University of Miami, Coral Gables, Florida.

Eugene Vayda is a professor in both the Departments of Health Administration and Medicine, at the University of Toronto.

Russell Wilkins is a senior analyst with the Health Statistics Division, Statistics Canada, Ottawa.

A. Paul Williams is in the Department of Health Administration, University of Toronto.

638

T. Kue Young is a physician and a professor in the Department of Community Health Sciences, Faculty of Medicine, University of Manitoba, Winnipeg.